# DIGITAL COMMUNICATIONS

# DIGITAL COMMUNICATIONS

**I. Korn**

University of New South Wales,
Sydney, Australia

**Van Nostrand Reinhold Electrical/Computer Science and Engineering Series**

VNR VAN NOSTRAND REINHOLD COMPANY

*New York*

Softcover reprint of the hardcover 1st edition 1985
Library of Congress Catalog Card Number: 84-27047
ISBN 978-1-4684-1463-9 ISBN 978-1-4684-1461-5 (eBook)
DOI 10.1007/978-1-4684-1461-5



Manufactured in the United States of America

Published by Van Nostrand Reinhold Company Inc.
135 West 50th Street
New York, New York 10020

Van Nostrand Reinhold Company Limited
Molly Millars Lane
Wokingham, Berkshire RG11 2PY, England

Van Nostrand Reinhold
480 Latrobe Street
Melbourne, Victoria 3000, Australia

Macmillan of Canada
Division of Gage Publishing Limited
164 Commander Boulevard
Agincourt, Ontario M1S 3C7, Canada

15 14 13 12 11 10 9 8 7 6 5 4 3 2 1

**Library of Congress Cataloging in Publication Data**
Korn, I. (Israel)
Digital communications.

(Van Nostrand Reinhold electrical/computer science and engineering series)
Includes bibliographies and index.
1. Digital communications. I. Title. II. Series.
TK5103.7.K67 1985 621.38 84-27047
ISBN 978-1-4684-1463-9

*To my wife Nurit*
*and*
*my father Pinhas*

He transmits His message over earth,
His word propagates fast. (Psalms 147, verse 15)

**Van Nostrand Reinhold**
**Electrical/Computer Science and Engineering Series**
**Sanjit Mitra—Series Editor**

**HANDBOOK OF ELECTRONIC DESIGN AND ANALYSIS PROCEDURES USING PROGRAMMABLE CALCULATORS,** by Bruce K. Murdock

**COMPILER DESIGN AND CONSTRUCTION,** by Arthur B. Pyster

**SINUSOIDAL ANALYSIS AND MODELING OF WEAKLY NONLINEAR CIRCUITS,** by Donald D. Weiner and John F. Spina

**APPLIED MULTIDIMENSIONAL SYSTEMS THEORY,** by N. K. Bose

**MICROWAVE SEMICONDUCTOR ENGINEERING,** by Joseph F. White

**INTRODUCTION TO QUARTZ CRYSTAL UNIT DESIGN,** by Virgil E. Bottom

**DIGITAL IMAGE PROCESSING,** by William B. Green

**SOFTWARE TESTING TECHNIQUES,** by Boris Beizer

**LIGHT TRANSMISSION OPTICS, Second edition,** by Dietrich Marcuse

**REAL-TIME COMPUTING,** edited by Duncan Mellichamp

**HARDWARE AND SOFTWARE CONCEPTS IN VLSI,** edited by Guy Rabbat

**MODELING AND IDENTIFICATION OF DYNAMIC SYSTEMS,** by N. K. Sinha and B. Kuszta

**COMPUTER METHODS FOR CIRCUIT ANALYSIS AND DESIGN,** by Jiri Vlach and Kishore Singhal

**HANDBOOK OF SOFTWARE ENGINNERING,** edited by C.R. Vick and C.V. Ramamoorthy

**SWITCHED CAPACITOR CIRCUITS,** by Phillip E. Allen and Edgar Sanchéz-Sinencio

**SOFTWARE SYSTEM TESTING AND QUALITY ASSURANCE,** by Boris Beizer

**MODERN DC-TO-DC SWITCHMODE POWER CONVERTER CIRCUITS,** by Rudolf P. Severns and Gordon E. Bloom

**DIGITAL COMMUNICATIONS,** by I. Korn

# PREFACE

This book contains material that should interest students of electrical engineering and computer science specializing in digital communications and also practicing electrical engineers who apply digital communications techniques to telecommunication systems, digital radio, digital satellites, fiber optics, and the physical layer of computer networks.

This book is an outgrowth of lecture notes prepared over a number of years at various universities. In the earlier years I benefited immensely from the excellent textbooks and monographs in preparing my notes.[1–5] With passing time I had to rely more and more on the current periodical literature, mainly the *IEEE Transactions* and the *Bell System Technical Journal.*

Although the book is intended mainly for those who have already had an introduction to communications, as usually taught in an undergraduate course, it can also be used without this background. For that purpose I concentrated most of the necessary mathematics in Chapter 1. If the mathematics is not an obstacle, the reader can start with Chapter 2.

I tried, as far as possible, to make each chapter independent of the other chapters, and for that reason many concepts and notations have been defined several times. To keep the book at a reasonable length, however, it was impossible, in most cases, not to rely on derivations and results of previous chapters.

In addition to the theory, each chapter contains examples of application of the theory to specific cases. Each chapter is accompanied by a set of problems, some of which are very simple and serve mainly as additional examples, and others that require reading of the references—in some cases the solution is not yet known. Each chapter is followed by a list of references, which, although not always complete, together with the references within the cited papers, is quite comprehensive.

It is impossible to cover the material of this book in one or even two semesters. I have taught different parts of it in different courses. I do not recommend any particular selection of the material. The lecturer in charge of a course in which the book will be used as a textbook will make his own decisions on the appropriate material.

In digital communications the problems of bandwidth, signal-to-noise ratio, error probability, interference, synchronization, and complexity are interrelated. The error probability is the most important performance criterion of a digital communications system. The bandwidth is a natural resource whose availability is reduced with the expansion of the number of communications systems. The efficiency of the system is measured by the bit rate (number of binary symbols per unit time) it is able to transmit at an acceptable error probability in a given bandwidth. Thus the aim of the communications engineer is to design a system that, for a given error probability and signal energy, requires the least bandwidth, has the highest bit rate, and is simple or, in other words, for a given bandwidth and signal-to-noise ratio has the lowest error probability and highest bit rate. In this book I treat explicitly only the first four topics. Other, excellent books are devoted to synchronisation.[6–8] The cost and complexity of a given system depend often on the current state of hardware; hence only relative merits can be presented. In many cases a theoretical solution to the problem is not yet available, and simulations are used to obtain relevant engineering data. In this book a great majority of the results follow a theoretical analysis based on sound mathematical models of the communications systems.

The book has the following outline:

Chapter 1 presents the mathematical preliminaries. It covers such topics as deterministic and random signals; Fourier, Laplace, and Hilbert transforms; filters; effect of filters on signals; and bandpass and baseband equivalent signals and filters.

In Chapter 2 I give a very general definition of the various methods of digital modulation. It is assumed that $M$-ary symbols are transmitted every $T$ seconds. Each symbol is represented by a signal that we call a *shaping function*, the totality of which forms a baseband signal that in turn modulates the amplitude, phase, or frequency (or a combination of these) of a high-frequency carrier signal. The modulated signal is called ASK (amplitude shift keying), PSK (phase shift keying), and FSK (frequency shift keying), depending on the parameter of the carrier signal, which is varied. Two-dimensional signals can be generated by using two orthogonal carriers. The result is QASK (quadrature ASK) (also called QAM (quadrature amplitude modulation)), which can be viewed as a signal in which both the phase and amplitude are modulated. The shaping functions may be different for the different symbols, or they may have a common form and differ only in amplitude or time location. Their duration may often exceed $T$. Only a few of the shaping functions are used in practice currently, and for many of them we do not even have a mathematical analysis of the resulting error probability.

A very important factor in the design of a communications system is the knowledge of the power spectral density (PSD) and bandwidth of the signals. Chapter 3 is dedicated to this problem. Here we find the PSD of the baseband signal and the modulated signals defined in Chapter 2.

In Chapter 4 we compute the error probability of a baseband communications system in the presence of noise and intersymbol interference (ISI). ISI is caused by inadequate filter design, imperfect channels, and inaccurate timing synchronization. In many communications systems the effect of ISI is more important than the effect of noise. Various bounds and approximations for the error probability are presented.

Chapter 5 is devoted to ASK systems. The systems may be double side band, single side band, or vestigial side band.

Chapter 6 deals with QASK and OQASK (offset QASK). It also discusses MSK (minimum shift keying), which is both a special case of OQASK and FSK. PSK with rectangular shaping function can also be considered as a special case of QASK (with a circular symbol constellation); hence in fact this chapter contains materials pertinent to the majority of digital communications systems. In addition to ISI, we compute here also the effect of QCI (quadrature channel interference), caused by imperfect phase synchronization and filters, and ACI (adjacent channel interference), caused by signals in neighboring channels.

In Chapter 7 we analyze PSK with nonrectangular shaping functions and DPSK (differential PSK), in which the symbols are presented as phase changes and the demodulation of which does not require a coherent receiver.

In Chapter 8 we study both wideband and narrowband FSK with coherent, noncoherent, and discriminator detectors, with or without narrowband filters prior to or after detection. Because of the continuity of the phase in FSK, we also compute the effect of extension of the observation interval from a single symbol to a sequence of such symbols.

In Chapter 9 we define partial response signals that are spectrally efficient and whose inherent structure can be used in monitoring the system performance.

In Chapter 10 we discuss the problem of optimization of a digital communications system under various criteria. For example, we optimize the receiver for a given transmitter or optimize both under certain constraints. The conclusion is that the optimal receiver is always composed of a matched filter and a transversal filter with an infinite number of taps.

In Chapter 11 we present an analysis of fixed and adaptive equalizers. We optimize the tap gains under various criteria and show the convergence of adaptive, automatic equalizers to their optimal settings. A section is devoted to nonlinear equalization.

In Chapter 12 we discuss line coding. Such codes are required when the channel in the system has spectral characteristics that would prevent efficient transmission of uncoded symbols or where synchronization may be affected.

## REFERENCES

1 W. R. Bennett and J. R. Davey, *Data Transmission*, McGraw-Hill Book Co., New York, N.Y., 1965.

2 J. M. Wozencraft and I.M. Jacobs, *Principles of Communication Engineering*, John Wiley & Sons, Inc., New York, 1965.

3 M. Schwartz, W. R. Bennett and S. Stein, *Communication Systems and Techniques*, McGraw-Hill Book Co., New York, N.Y., 1966.

4 A. J. Viterbi, *Principles of Coherent Communication*, McGraw-Hill Book Co., New York, N. Y., 1966.

5 R. W. Lucky, J. Salz, E. J. Weldon, *Principles of Data Communication*, McGraw-Hill Book Co., New York, N.Y., 1968.
6 J. J. Stiffler, *Theory of Synchronous Communication*, Prentice-Hall, Inc., Englewood Cliffs, N.J., 1971.
7 W. C. Lindsey, *Synchronisation Systems in Communication and Control*, Prentice-Hall, Inc., Englewood Cliffs, N.J., 1972.
8 W.C. Lindsey and M. K. Simon, *Telecommunication Systems Engineering*, Prentice-Hall, Inc., Englewood Cliffs, N.J., 1973.

# CONTENTS


**Preface** vii

**1. Signals, Filters, Random Variables and Random Processes 1**

1.1 Introduction 1
1.2 Deterministic signals and their transforms 2
1.2.1 Real and complex signals 2
1.2.2 Properties of signals 6
1.2.3 Expansion of signals into orthogonal series 8
1.2.4 Fourier transforms 11
1.2.5 Laplace transforms 16
1.3 Linear systems and filters 19
1.3.1 Impulse response and transfer function 19
1.3.2 Nondistorting filters 22
1.3.3 Band-limiting filters 22
1.3.4 Time-variant, linear filters 24
1.3.5 Hilbert transform 24
1.4 Equivalence of baseband and bandpass signals and filters 26
1.4.1 Baseband and bandpass signals 26
1.4.2 Baseband and bandpass filters 28
1.4.3 Bandpass filters in tandem 32
1.4.4 Response of bandpass filters to bandpass signal 32
1.4.5 Equivalence with respect to different carrier frequencies 33
1.4.6 Baseband equivalence of arbitrary function 35
1.5 Random variables 38
1.5.1 Sets 38
1.5.2 Events and probabilities 40
1.5.3 Random variable 43
1.5.4 Function of random variable 50
1.5.5 Averages 52
1.6 Two random variables 55
1.6.1 Definition and probabilities 55
1.6.2 Averages 60
1.6.3 Tansformations 62
1.6.4 Complex random variables 65
1.7 Random vectors 66
1.7.1 Definition and probabilities 66

1.7.2 Transformation and averages 69
1.8 Random process 74
1.8.1 Definitions 74
1.8.2 Correlation 76
1.8.3 Effect of linear systems on random processes 77
1.8.4 Complex random process 83
1.8.5 Equivalence of bandpass and baseband random noise 84
1.9 Summary 89
1.10 Problems 90
1.11 References 99

**2. Baseband and Modulated Signals 101**
2.1 Introduction 101
2.2 Common, full-response, shaping function 105
2.2.1 Baseband signal 107
2.2.2 Modulated signal 108
2.2.3 Linear shift keying 109
2.2.3.1 Amplitude shift keying—double side band 109
2.2.3.2 ASK—single side band 111
2.2.3.3 ASK—vestigial side band 112
2.2.3.4 Quadrature amplitude shift keying 113
2.2.3.5 Offset quadrature amplitude shift keying 117
2.2.4 Phase shift keying 121
2.2.4.1 Differential phase shift keying 124
2.2.5 Frequency shift keying 126
2.2.5.1 Continuous phase frequency shift keying 126
2.2.5.2 FSK with noncontinuous phase 130
2.2.5.3 Multi-*h* frequency shift keying 132
2.2.5.4 Minimum shift keying 133
2.2.5.5 Equivalence of binary MSK and quaternary OQASK 134
2.2.5.6 Binary MSK as a form of DPSK 138
2.2.5.7 Equivalence of *M*-ary MSK and a modified OQASK 138
2.3 Nonoverlapping shaping function 139
2.3.1 Baseband signal 139
2.3.2 Modulated signal 141
2.3.3 LSK 142
2.3.4 PSK and FSK 142
2.3.5 MSK 142
2.4 Overlapping shaping function 144
2.4.1 Baseband signal 144
2.4.2 Modulated signal 148
2.4.3 LSK 148
2.4.4 PSK and FSK 149
2.4.5 MSK 149

2.5 Conclusions 150
2.6 Problems 152
2.7 References 156

**3. Power Spectral Density (PSD) and Bandwidth 159**
3.1 Introduction 159
3.2 PSD and bandwidth of modulated signal 160
3.3 PSD of complex envelope 162
3.3.1 Independent symbols 168
3.4 PSD of baseband signal 168
3.4.1 Common shaping function 169
3.5 PSD of LSK 172
3.6 Optimisation of shaping function 175
3.7 PSD of PSK 177
3.7.1 Shaping function of duration $T$ 177
3.7.2 Common shaping function of duration $T$ 177
3.7.3 Shaping function of duration $2T$ 186
3.7.4 Shaping function of duration $KT$ 193
3.8 PSD of FSK 194
3.8.1 Shaping function of duration $T$ 194
3.8.2 Shaping function of duration $2T$ 209
3.8.3 Shaping function of duration $KT$ 217
3.9 The PSD of MSK 224
3.9.1 Binary MSK and common shaping function 224
3.9.2 Optimisation problem 227
3.9.3 General MSK 229
3.10 The PSD of QASK and OQASK with nonlinear bandpass filtering 233
3.10.1 Bandpass, memoryless nonlinearity 233
3.10.2 The PSD 238
3.10.3 PSD of hard-limited QASK 240
3.10.4 PSD of hard-limited OQASK 244
3.11 Filter bandwidth for digital radio 246
3.12 Summary 248
3.13 Problems 251
3.14 References 256

**4. ASK Baseband System 259**
4.1 Introduction 259
4.2 Optimal decision region and error probability 261
4.2.1 Maximum likelihood decision rule 261
4.2.2 Matched filters 269
4.2.3 Signal-to-noise ratio 272
4.3 Nyquist condition for no ISI 275

4.3.1 Intuitive approach 275
4.3.2 Analytic approach 276
4.3.3 Minimum bandwidth 279
4.3.4 Bandwidth not exceeding R 279
4.3.5 Raised cosine family 280
4.3.6 Spectral efficiency 281
4.3.7 Equalization 284
4.4 Effect of ISI 285
4.4.1 Properties of interference 286
4.4.2 Eye diagram 288
4.4.3 Computation of error probability 290
4.4.3.1 Worst-case bound 292
4.4.3.2 Bounds by finite number of terms 293
4.4.3.3 Taylor series expansion 295
4.4.3.4 Legendre series expansion 296
4.4.3.5 Quadrature formulas 298
4.4.3.6 Bounds to probabilty densities 300
4.4.3.7 Chernoff bound 300
4.4.3.8 Bounds and approximations of Jenq et al 302
4.4.4 Bounds in systems with dependent symbols 306
4.4.5 Applications of bounds to systems with Nyquist function response 306
4.5 System with NRZ, HS, and SP shaping functions 309
4.5.1 Derivation of system response, $g(t)$ 311
4.5.1.1 Causal filters 311
4.5.1.2 Filters with a finite number of distinct poles 312
4.5.1.3 Butterworth filters 315
4.5.2 Derivation of noise variance 320
4.5.2.1 Causal filter 321
4.5.2.2 Filters with a finite number of distinct poles 321
4.5.2.3 Butterworth filters 322
4.5.3 Error probability 324
4.6 Approximations of Nyquist functions 332
4.7 Summary 333
4.8 Problems 333
4.9 References 339

**5. ASK Bandpass System 343**
5.1 Introduction 343
5.2 Bandpass and Baseband ASK 343
5.3 Error probability 346
5.4 Error probability for ASK-DSB with nonsymmetric bandpass filter 349
5.5 Summary and conclusions 353

5.6 Problems 353
5.7 References 354

**6. QASK and OQASK 355**
6.1 Introduction 355
6.2 Condition of no interference 360
6.3 Systems with no interference 364
6.3.1 Rectangular constellation 366
6.3.2 Circular constellation 370
6.3.3 General constellation 375
6.4 Effect of interference in rectangular constellations (QASK, OQASK) 382
6.4.1 Effect of QCI and ISI 384
6.4.1.1 System with Nyquist function response 386
6.4.1.2 System with Butterworth filters 387
6.4.2 Effect of ACI and ISI 390
6.4.2.1 System with Nyquist function response 391
6.4.2.2 System with distinct poles filters 396
6.4.2.3 MSK system with nonnegative impulse response filters 403
6.5 Effect of interference in circular constellations (PSK) 408
6.5.1 Extension of the method of Jenq et al to circular constellation 413
6.5.2 System with Nyquist function response 418
6.6 Channel with flat and frequency selective fading 422
6.7 Summary 430
6.8 Problems 433
6.9 References 436

**7. PSK and DPSK 439**
7.1 Introduction 439
7.2 PSK 439
7.2.1 The pdf of phase and amplitude of a complex Gaussian random variable 447
7.2.2 Exact error probability 450
7.3 DPSK 452
7.3.1 Ideal DPSK 455
7.3.2 Bounds to error probability 461
7.4 Summary 466
7.5 Problems 466
7.6 References 468

**8. FSK 471**
8.1 Introduction 471
8.2 Coherent FSK 476

8.2.1 Orthogonal FSK 476
8.2.2 An upper bound to the error probability 480
8.2.3 Binary coherent FSK 481
8.3 Noncoherent FSK 483
8.3.1 No detector filters 484
8.3.2 With detector filter 487
8.4 FSK with discriminator detector 494
8.4.1 The PDF of instantaneous frequency 495
8.4.2 Binary FSK 498
8.4.3 Condition of no ISI 500
8.4.4 Effect of filter on FSK signal 503
8.5 FSK with discriminator and detector filter 505
8.5.1 Error probability for NRZ shaping functions 510
8.5.1.1 No intersymbol interference 511
8.5.1.2 With intersymbol interference 513
8.5.2 Error probability for split phase shaping function 518
8.6 Observation interval longer than $T$ 520
8.7 Summary 524
8.8 Problems 531
8.9 References 534

**9. Partial Response Signals 537**
9.1 Introduction 537
9.2 Definition of PRS 537
9.3 Elimination of ISI by decision feedback 541
9.4 Elimination of ISI by precoding 545
9.5 Error monitoring 550
9.6 Summary 552
9.7 Problems 552
9.8 References 555

**10. System Optimization 557**
10.1 Introduction 557
10.2 Formulation of optimization problem 557
10.3 Optimal receiver and transmitter 561
10.3.1 Optimal receiver 562
10.3.2 Optimal transmitter 564
10.4 Minimization of the mean square error 566
10.4.1 Optimization of receiver 567
10.4.2 Optimization of receiver and transmitter 569
10.5 Summary 575
10.6 Problems 576
10.7 References 578

**11. Equalization 581**
11.1 Introduction 581
11.2 Definition of the problem 582
11.3 Structure of equalizers 585
11.3.1 Forward (nonrecursive) equalizer 587
11.3.2 Feedback (recursive) equalizer 587
11.3.3 Composite forward and feedback equalizers 587
11.3.4 Decision feedback equalizer 587
11.3.5 Composite forward and decision feedback equalizer 588
11.4 Minimum mean square error 589
11.4.1 Formal solution 590
11.4.2 Iterative solution 592
11.4.3 Practical solution 597
11.4.4 Automatic and adaptive equalization 603
11.4.5 Fast adaptive algorithm 608
11.4.6 Equalization of passband system 610
11.5 Zero-forcing equalizer 610
11.6 Nonlinear equalization 617
11.6.1 Small ISI 623
11.6.2 Large signal-to-noise ratio 624
11.7 Summary 627
11.8 Problems 628
11.9 References 628

**12. Line Coding 633**
12.1 Introduction 633
12.2 Binary codes 635
12.3 Linear ternary codes 641
12.4 Alphabetic codes 644
12.5 Nonalphabetic codes 649
12.6 Summary 653
12.7 Problems 653
12.8 References 655

**Commonly Used Functions and Symbols 657**

**List of Abbreviations 659**

**Index 661**

# DIGITAL COMMUNICATIONS

# 1 SIGNALS, FILTERS, RANDOM VARIABLES, AND RANDOM PROCESSES

## 1.1 INTRODUCTION

In this chapter I outline briefly the mathematical tools that are needed for the analysis and design of digital communications systems that are discussed in the other chapters of the book. I start with a review of deterministic signals and their transforms (Fourier, Laplace, Hilbert) and Fourier series for periodic signals. Then I define a linear system and discuss the interaction of signals and linear time-invariant systems. I present in more detail the relation and equivalence between baseband and bandpass signals and between baseband and bandpass filters. In doing that we first rely on intuition, assuming narrowband signals and filters, and, for those inclined more to mathematics, we use the Hilbert transform technique to achieve the same result. We also cover briefly random variables (discrete and continuous) and random processes. The chapter presents in more detail the relation between the correlation, power spectral density, energy and power of random processes, and the effect of linear filters. It also discusses in some detail the relation and equivalence of baseband and bandpass random processes.

This chapter is not a treatise on the subject of signals, filters, random variables, and random processes. Entire books have been dedicated to these topics, a partial list of which appears at the end of this chapter. Here, I present only the essentials needed for the other sections of the book.

Readers with a workable knowledge of the topics of this chapter are advised to follow directly from this point to Chapter 2. I made the chapters of the book, as far as possible, independent of the first chapter, but there are many cases where I have to quote results of this chapter.

Although we need many mathematical tools, the discussion of mathematics here is not as precise as some would like. For example we are not concerned very much with $\varepsilon$ and $\delta$ convergence. We do not present the necessary and sufficient conditions for a signal to have a transform. We simply assume that the transform is unique, and if the function does not have a transform it is not in the scope of this book. We exchange freely the order of summation, integration, and statistical expectation without specifying the conditions under which this is permitted, again under the assumption that if this is not allowed it is not within the scope of the book.

The chapter has the following outline. In Section 1.2 we define a deterministic signal and its transforms. In Section 1.3 we define a linear filter and show the interaction of such filters and signals. In Section 1.4 we derive an equivalence between bandpass signals and filters and baseband signals and filters. In Section 1.5 we define random variables, in Section 1.6, a pair of random variables (complex random variables); and in 1.7, a random vector. Section 1.8 is dedicated to random processes, where we also derive an equivalence between baseband and bandpass random processes. A summary is given in Section 1.9. Section 1.10 gives problems, and finally Section 1.11 lists references.

## 1.2 DETERMINISTIC SIGNALS AND THEIR TRANSFORMS

### 1.2.1 Real and complex signals

A *real signal* $x(t)$ is a real function of time. Some important signals are presented in Fig. 1.1. They are:

a. Unit step function

$$x(t) = u(t) = \begin{cases} 1 & t \geq 0 \\ 1 & t < 0 \end{cases} \tag{1.2.1}$$

b. Rectangular pulse of duration $T$

$$x(t) = u_T(t) = u(t) - u(t - T) \tag{1.2.2}$$

c. Sign function

$$x(t) = \text{sign } t = u(t) - u(-t) \tag{1.2.3}$$

d. One-sided exponential

$$x(t) = A \exp(-at)u(t) \tag{1.2.4}$$

e. Sinusoid

$$x(t) = A \cos(2\pi ft + \phi) \tag{1.2.5}$$

where $A$ is the amplitude, $f$ is the frequency, and $\phi$ is the phase.

f. Impuse

$$x(t) = \delta(t) = \begin{cases} \infty & t = 0 \\ 0 & t \neq 0 \end{cases} \tag{1.2.6}$$

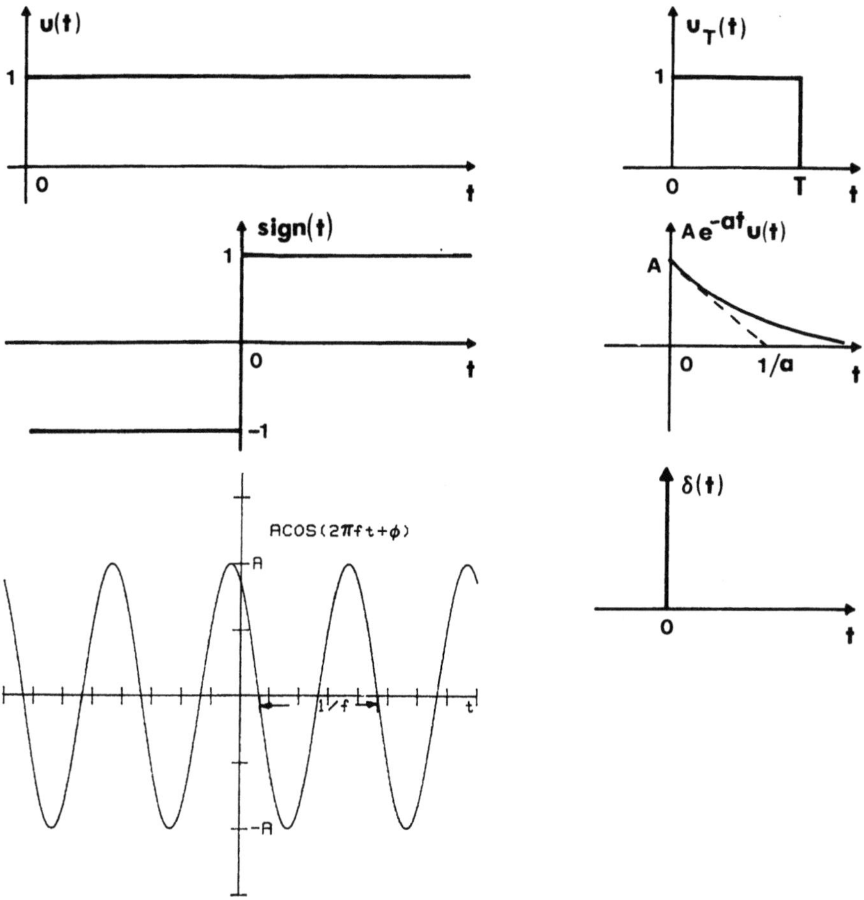


Fig. 1.1. Deterministic signals.

such that for all $\varepsilon > 0$

$$\int_{-\varepsilon}^{\varepsilon} \delta(t)\, dt = 1 \tag{1.2.7}$$

A *complex signal* $x(t)$ is the sum of two real signals $x_I(t)$, $x_Q(t)$

$$x(t) = x_I(t) + jx_Q(t) \tag{1.2.8}$$

where $j^2 = -1$. A complex signal can also be expressed by its amplitude and phase

$$x(t) = A_x(t) \exp (j\phi_x(t)) \tag{1.2.9}$$

The relations between the amplitude, $A_x(t)$, phase $\phi_x(t)$, inphase (or real) component $x_I(t)$, and quadrature (or imaginary) component $x_Q(t)$ are (see Fig. 1.2)

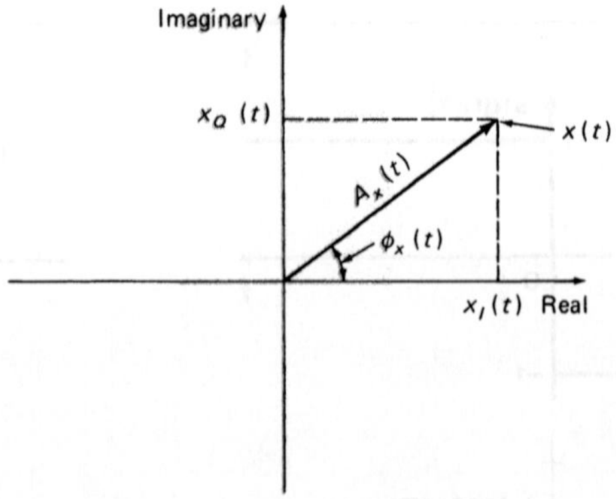


Fig. 1.2. Complex plane.

$$A_x(t) = |x(t)| = \{x_I^2(t) + x_Q^2(t)\}^{1/2} = (x(t)x^*(t))^{1/2} \tag{1.2.10}$$

$$\phi_x(t) = \tan^{-1}\{x_Q(t)/x_I(t)\} = \arg(x(t)) \tag{1.2.11}$$

$$x_I(t) = A_x(t)\cos\phi_x(t) \tag{1.2.12}$$

$$x_Q(t) = A_x(t)\sin\phi_x(t) \tag{1.2.13}$$

$$x_I(t) = \mathrm{Re}\{x(t)\} = 0.5\{x(t) + x^*(t)\} \tag{1.2.14}$$

$$x_Q(t) = \mathrm{Im}\{x(t)\} = 0.5\{x(t) - x^*(t)\}/j \tag{1.2.15}$$

where | | is the absolute value, arg( ) is the argument or phase, Re( ) is the real part, Im( ) is the imaginary part, and * denotes the complex conjugate.

For example, the function

$$\begin{aligned} x(t) &= A\exp\{\pm j(2\pi ft + \phi)\} \\ &= A\cos(2\pi ft + \phi) \pm jA\sin(2\pi ft + \phi) \end{aligned} \tag{1.2.16}$$

has as components two sinusoids in quadrature, because

$$\mp\sin(2\pi ft + \phi) = \cos(2\pi ft + \phi \pm \pi/2) \tag{1.2.17}$$

A signal is called *causal* if it is zero for $t < 0$, i.e.,

$$x(t) = x(t)u(t) \tag{1.2.18}$$

A signal has duration $T$ if it is nonzero in a time interval of duration $T$, i.e., for some $t_0$

$$x(t) = x(t)u_T(t - t_0) \tag{1.2.19}$$

A signal is *periodic* of fundamental period $T$ if $T$ is the smallest number such that

$$x(t) = x(t + T) \tag{1.2.20}$$

A periodic signal is shown in Fig. 1.3. Let

$$x_0(t) = x(t)u_T(t + 0.5\,T) \tag{1.2.21}$$

be the periodic signal confined to $|t| \leqq 0.5\,T$. The periodic signal can be written in the form

$$x(t) = \sum_n x_0(t - nT) \tag{1.2.22}$$

This is not the only way to define a periodic signal. Let

$$x_1(t) = x(t)u_T(t - t_0) \tag{1.2.23}$$

where $t_0$ is arbitrary; then again (1.2.22) is valid with $x_0(t)$ replaced by $x_1(t)$. In fact, there is even no need for the interval to be single. For example

$$x_2(t) = x(t)\{u_{0.5T}(t) + u_{0.5T}(t - 1.5\,T)\} \tag{1.2.24}$$

which is the periodic function confined to the two intervals $0 \leqq t < 0.5\,T$, and $1.5\,T \leqq t < 2\,T$ can also replace $x_0(t)$ in (1.2.22) in defining the periodic function. We can generalize: let $I_T$ be a set of intervals such that (a) if $t \in I_T \rightarrow t + kT \notin I_T$ for all nonzero integer $k$

(b)

$$\int_{t \in I_T} dt = T \tag{1.2.25}$$

and let $x_3(t)$ be $x(t)$ confined to this set, then again $x_3(t)$ can replace $x_0(t)$ in (1.2.22). Such a signal is shown in Fig. 1.3.

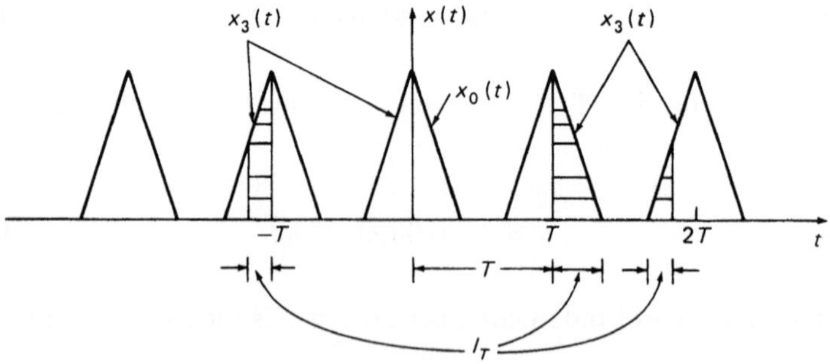


Fig. 1.3. Periodic signal.

### 1.2.2 Properties of signals

The *energy* of a complex signal is

$$E_x = \int_{-\infty}^{\infty} |x(t)|^2 \, dt = \int_{-\infty}^{\infty} \{x_I^2(t) + x_Q^2(t)\} \, dt = E_{xI} + E_{xQ} \quad (1.2.26)$$

The energy of a periodic signal is infinite (see Problem 1.2.1).

The *power* of a periodic signal is

$$P_x = \int_{t_0}^{t_0+T} |x(t)|^2 \, dt/T \quad (1.2.27)$$

The *convolution of two signals* $x(t)$ and $y(t)$ is

$$z(t) = x(t) * y(t) = \int_{-\infty}^{\infty} x(t - \tau)y(\tau)d\tau \quad (1.2.28)$$

The convolution is commutative (see Problem 1.2.2), i.e.

$$x(t) * y(t) = y(t) * x(t) \quad (1.2.29)$$

and if the signals are causal

$$z(t) = \int_{0}^{t} x(t - \tau)y(\tau) \, d\tau \quad (1.2.30)$$

Note that the outcome of the convolution of $\delta(t - t_0)$ (i.e., a shifted impulse function) and any function, continuous at point $t_0$, is

$$z(t) = \delta(t - t_0) * x(t) = \int_{-\infty}^{\infty} \delta(t - \tau - t_0)x(\tau)\,d\tau$$

$$x(t - t_0)\int_{-\infty}^{\infty} \delta(t - \tau - t_0)\,d\tau = x(t - t_0) \tag{1.2.31}$$

This is the so-called *sifting* property of the impulse function. Particularly for $t_0 = 0$

$$\delta(t) * x(t) = x(t) \tag{1.2.32}$$

The *cross-correlation* of two signals $x(t)$ and $y(t)$ is

$$R_{x,y}(\tau) = \int_{-\infty}^{\infty} x(t + \tau)y^*(t)\,dt \tag{1.2.33}$$

Note that (see Problem 1.2.3)

$$R_{x,y}(\tau) = R^*_{y,x}(-\tau) \tag{1.2.34}$$

The *autocorrelation* is a special case of cross-correlation with $y(t) = x(t)$. In this case

$$R_x(\tau) = R_{x,x}(\tau) = \int_{-\infty}^{\infty} x(t + \tau)x^*(t)\,dt \tag{1.2.35}$$

Note that

$$R_x(0) = E_x \tag{1.2.36}$$

A useful inequality to be used often is the *Schwartz inequality*

$$\left|\int_{-\infty}^{\infty} x(t)y(t)\,dt\right|^2 \leq E_xE_y \tag{1.2.37}$$

The proof is simple and short; hence we give it here

$$0 \leqq \int_{-\infty}^{\infty}\int_{-\infty}^{\infty} |x(t)y(\tau) - y(t)x(\tau)|^2 \, dt \, d\tau$$

$$= \int_{-\infty}^{\infty} |x(t)|^2 \, dt \int_{-\infty}^{\infty} |y(\tau)|^2 \, dt - \int_{-\infty}^{\infty}\int_{-\infty}^{\infty} x(t)y(\tau)y^*(t)x^*(\tau) \, dt \, d\tau$$

$$- \int_{-\infty}^{\infty}\int_{-\infty}^{\infty} x^*(t)y^*(\tau)y(t)x(\tau) \, dt \, d\tau + \int_{-\infty}^{\infty} |y(t)|^2 \, dt \int_{-\infty}^{\infty} |x(\tau)|^2 \, d\tau$$

$$= 2\left(E_x E_y - \left| \int_{-\infty}^{\infty} x(t)y(t) \, dt \right|^2\right)$$

Equality is achieved when

$$y(t) = cx^*(t) \tag{1.2.38}$$

which can be verified by substitution into (1.2.37). When we apply the inequality to (1.2.33), we obtain

$$R_{x,y}(\tau) \leqq (E_x E_y)^{1/2} \tag{1.2.39}$$

with equality only if

$$y(t) = cx(t + \tau) \tag{1.2.40}$$

When we apply Schwartz inequality to (1.2.35), we obtain

$$R_x(\tau) \leqq R_x(0) \tag{1.2.41}$$

because

$$x(t) = cx(t + \tau) \tag{1.2.42}$$

is possible only if $c = 1$, $\tau = 0$.

### 1.2.3 Expansion of signals into orthogonal series

Let $\{\phi_n(t)\}$ $-\infty < n < \infty$ or $n = 0, 1, \ldots,$ be a set of functions with the property of *orthogonality*, i.e.

$$\int_{-\infty}^{\infty} \phi_n(t)\phi_k^*(t)\,dt = C_k\delta_{n,k} = \begin{cases} C_k > 0 & n = k \\ 0 & n \neq k \end{cases} \tag{1.2.43}$$

The functions are called *orthonormal* if $C_k = 1$. We write $x(t)$ in the form of a series

$$x(t) = \sum_n x_n\phi_n(t) \tag{1.2.44}$$

and $x_k$ can be computed by multiplying both sides of (1.2.44) by $\phi_k^*(t)$, integrating, and applying (1.2.43). The result is

$$x_k = \int_{-\infty}^{\infty} x(t)\phi_k^*(t)\,dt/C_k \tag{1.2.45}$$

The energy in the function is

$$E_x = \int_{-\infty}^{\infty} |x(t)|^2\,dt = \sum_n\sum_k \int_{-\infty}^{\infty} x_n x_k^* \phi_n(t)\phi_k^*(t)\,dt$$

$$= \sum_n |x_n|^2\, C_n \tag{1.2.46}$$

Let $x_k(t)$ be the finite sum

$$x_K(t) = \sum_{n=-K}^{K} x_n\phi_n(t) \tag{1.2.47}$$

and let

$$\varepsilon_K(t) = x(t) - x_K(t) = \sum_{n=K+1}^{\infty} x_n\phi_n(t) \tag{1.2.48}$$

be the remainder, the energy of which is

$$E_{\varepsilon K} = \sum_{n=K+1}^{\infty} |x_n|^2\, C_n \tag{1.2.49}$$

In fact the function $x(t)$ can be expanded into this series if

$$\lim_{K\to 0} E_{\varepsilon K} = 0 \tag{1.2.50}$$

*Example* 1.2.1 *Legendre polynomials*
Let $\phi_n(t)$, $n = 0, 1, \ldots,$ be the set of real functions

$$\begin{aligned}\phi_0(t) &= 1, \qquad \phi_1(t) = t \\ \phi_n(t) &= \{(2n-1)t\phi_{n-1}(t) - (n-1)\phi_{n-2}(t)\}/n \qquad n \geqq 2\end{aligned} \tag{1.2.51}$$

defined for $|t| \leqq 1$. $\phi_n(t)$ is a polynomial in $t$ of order $n$. The energy in the polynomial is

$$C_n = \int_t \phi^2{}_n(t)\,dt = (n + 0.5)^{-1} \tag{1.2.52}$$

*Example* 1.2.2 Fourier series
Let

$$\phi_n(t) = \exp(j\,2\,\pi nt/T) \tag{1.2.53}$$

defined for $|t| \leqq 0.5\,T$. Here

$$\phi_{-n}(t) = \phi^*{}_n(t) \tag{1.2.54}$$

and

$$C_n = T \tag{1.2.55}$$

Hence any function $x(t)$, $|t| \leqq 0.5\,T$ can be expanded into

$$x(t) = \sum_n x_n \exp(j\,2\,\pi nt/T) \tag{1.2.56}$$

where

$$x_k = R\int_{-0.5T}^{0.5T} x(t)\exp(-j\,2\,\pi kt/T)\,dt \tag{1.2.57}$$

and

$$R = 1/T \tag{1.2.58}$$

$\{x_k\}$ are called Fourier coefficients. The energy is from (1.2.46) and 1.2.55)

$$E_x = T\sum_k |x_k|^2 \tag{1.2.59}$$

Because a periodic function is defined by its value at $|t| \leqq T/2$, (1.2.56) is an expansion of the periodic function for all $t$. The average power of this periodic function is

$$P_x = E_x/T = \sum_k |x_k|^2 \tag{1.2.60}$$

Note from (1.2.57) that if $x(t)$ is real and even then

$$x_k = R \int_{-0.5T}^{0.5T} x(t) \cos(2\pi kt/T)\, dt \tag{1.2.61}$$

and $x_k$ is real and even in $k$, i.e.

$$x_k = x_{-k} \tag{1.2.62}$$

while if $x(t)$ is real and odd

$$x_k = -jR \int_{-0.5T}^{0.5T} x(t) \sin(2\pi kt/T)\, dt \tag{1.2.63}$$

$x_k$ is imaginary and odd in $k$, i.e.

$$x_k = -x_{-k} \tag{1.2.64}$$

### 1.2.4 Fourier transforms

The Fourier transform (FT) of $x(t)$ is the function of frequency $X(f)$ (a lower-case letter replaced by a capital letter), defined by

$$X(f) = F\{x(t)\} = \int_{-\infty}^{\infty} x(t) \exp(-j2\pi ft)\, dt \tag{1.2.65}$$

and the inverse FT (IFT) is

$$x(t) = F^{-1}\{X(f)\} = \int_{-\infty}^{\infty} X(f) \exp(j2\pi ft)\, df \tag{1.2.66}$$

$x(t)$ and $X(f)$ form a FT pair, and we denote this fact by

$$x(t) \leftrightarrow X(f) \tag{1.2.67}$$

Note from (1.2.65) and (1.2.66) the duality property of FT and IFT, which is

$$x(t) = Y(t) \leftrightarrow X(f) = y(-f) \tag{1.2.68}$$

i.e., if we know the FT of a function we immediately know the IFT of the same function. In Table 1.1 we present some signals and their FT.

**Table 1.1 Signals and their Fourier transforms**

| $x(t)$ | $X(f)$ |
|---|---|
| $\delta(t)$ | 1 |
| 1 | $\delta(f)$ |
| $u_T(t + 0.5\,T)$ | $\dfrac{T \sin(\pi f T)}{\pi f T}$ |
| $\operatorname{sign} t$ | $(j\pi f)^{-1}$ |
| $\cos(2\,\pi f_c t)$ | $0.5\{\delta(f + f_c) + \delta(f - f_c)\}$ |
| $\sin(2\,\pi f_c t)$ | $-j\,0.5\{\delta(f + f_c) - \delta(f - f_c)\}$ |
| $\exp(j\,2\,\pi f_c t)$ | $\delta(f - f_c)$ |
| $\exp(-\pi t^2/\sigma^2)$ | $\sigma \exp(-\pi f^2 \sigma^2)$ |

The FT has various properties, some of which are listed in Table 1.2. The IFT has similar properties, which can be proved from the duality.

**Table 1.2 Properties of Fourier transforms**

| PROPERTY | $x(t)$ | $X(f)$ |
|---|---|---|
| Linearity | $\sum_i a_i y_i(t)$ | $\sum_i a_i Y_i(f)$ |
| Time shift | $y(t - t_0)$ | $Y(f) \exp(-j\,2\,\pi f t_0)$ |
| Frequency shift | $y(t) \exp(-j\,2\,\pi f_c t)$ | $Y(f + f_c)$ |
| Time scaling | $Y(at)$ | $Y(f/a)/\lvert a \rvert$ |
| Time derivative | $d^n y(t)/dt^n$ | $(j\,2\,\pi f)^n Y(f)$ |
| Frequency derivative | $(-j\,2\,\pi t)^n y(t)$ | $d^n Y(f)/df^n$ |
| Convolution | $y_1(t) * y_2(t)$ | $Y_1(f) Y_2(f)$ |
| Integral | $\int_{-\infty}^{t} y(\tau)d\tau$ | $0.5\,Y(0)\delta(f) + Y(f)/(j\,2\,\pi f)$ |
| Even | $x(t) = x(-t)$ | real |
| Odd | $x(t) = -x(-t)$ | imaginary |
| Real | real | $X^*(-f)$ |

Most of the Fourier transforms and their properties in Tables 1.1 and 1.2 are proved in the problems. We shall elaborate on some of them.

a. *Convolution*

$$z(t) = x(t) * y(t) \leftrightarrow X(f)Y(f) = Z(f) \tag{1.2.69}$$

It may be easier sometimes to computer the IFT

$$z(t) = \int_{-\infty}^{\infty} X(f)Y(f) \exp(j\,2\,\pi ft)\,df \tag{1.2.70}$$

rather then the convolution. This property simply states that an intergral in the time domain is equivalent to a product in the frequency domain. This property is one of the main reasons for using Fourier transforms.

b. *x(t) real*

$$X(f) = \int_{-\infty}^{\infty} x(t)\cos(2\,\pi ft)\,dt - j\int_{-\infty}^{\infty} x(t)\sin(2\pi ft)\,dt = X_e(f) - jX_0(f) \tag{1.2.71}$$

Note that $X_e(f)$ is even and real and $X_0(f)$ is odd and real; thus

$$X(-f) = X^*(f) \tag{1.2.72}$$

Note that if $x(t)$ is even, then $X_0(f) = 0$, and $X(f)$ is even and real, but if $x(t)$ is odd, then $X_e(f) = 0$ and $X(f)$ is odd and imaginary. If follows from (1.2.71) that $|X(f)|$ is even and arg $X(f)$ is odd. This is shown in Fig. 1.4, where the solid line represents $X_e(f)$ or $|X(f)|$, and the dashed line represents $X_0(f)$ or arg $X(f)$.

c. *x(t) complex*

It can be verified that (1.2.71) is not true, because the even part and the odd parts are not real. We shall need the FT of $x^*(t)$ and its relation to $X(f)$. Let, thus

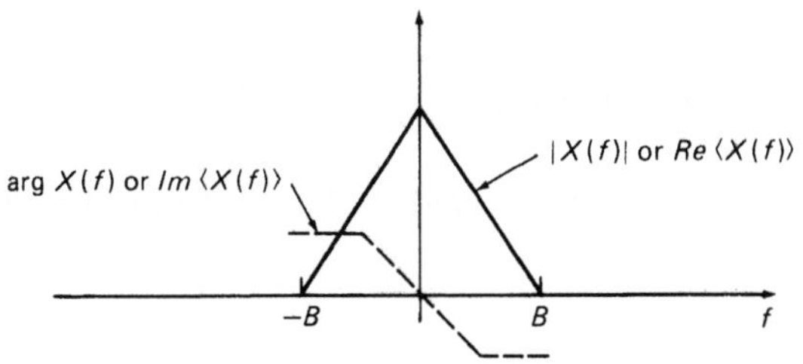


Fig. 1.4. Fourier transform of real signal.

$$y(t) = x^*(t) \tag{1.2.73}$$

$$Y(f) = \int_{-\infty}^{\infty} x^*(t) \exp(-j\,2\,\pi f t)\,dt$$

$$= \left(\int_{-\infty}^{\infty} x(t) \exp(j\,2\,\pi f t)\,dt\right)^* = X^*(-f) \tag{1.2.74}$$

Thus

$$x^*(t) \leftrightarrow X^*(-f) \tag{1.2.75}$$

d. <u>*Modulated signal*</u>

Let

$$y(t) = x(t) \cos(2\,\pi f_c t + \phi) \tag{1.2.76}$$

Because

$$\cos(2\,\pi f_c t + \phi) = 0.5\,\{\exp(j(2\,\pi f_c t + \phi)) + \exp(-j\,(2\pi f_c t + \phi))\} \tag{1.2.77}$$

$$y(t) = 0.5\,\{x(t) \exp(j(2\,\pi f_c t + \phi) + x(t) \exp(-j(2\,\pi f_c t + \phi))\} \tag{1.2.78}$$

When we use entry three of Table 1.2, the FT is

$$Y(f) = 0.5\,\{(f - f_c) \exp(j\phi) + X(f + f_c) \exp(-j\phi)\} \tag{1.2.79}$$

Similarly, it can be shown that since

$$\sin(2\,\pi f_c t + \phi) = -0.5\,j\{\exp(j(2\,\pi f_c t + \phi)) - \exp(-j(2\,\pi f_c t + \phi))\} \tag{1.2.80}$$

the FT of $x(t) \sin(2\,\pi f_c t + \phi)$ is

$$-0.5\,j\{X(f - f_c) \exp(j\phi) - X(f + f_c) \exp(-j\phi)\} \tag{1.2.81}$$

e. <u>*Periodic signal*</u>

Comparing (1.2.22) and (1.2.56), we obtain the equality

$$x(t) = \sum_k x_k \exp(j\,2\,\pi kRt) = \sum_n x_0(t - nT) \qquad (1.2.82)$$

We see from (1.2.65) and (1.2.57) that

$$x_k = RX_0(kR) \qquad (1.2.83)$$

where

$$R = 1/T \qquad (1.2.84)$$

is the fundamental frequency of the periodic signal

$$R\sum_k X_0(kR) \exp(j\,2\,\pi kRt) = \sum_n x_0(t - nT) \qquad (1.2.85)$$

Particularly, if

$$x_0(t) = \delta(t) \qquad (1.2.86)$$

which means that $x(t)$ is a sequence of delta functions separated in time by $T$, then

$$X_0(f) = 1 \qquad (1.2.87)$$

and we have the useful result

$$R\sum_k \exp(j\,2\,\pi kRt) = \sum_n \delta(t - nT) \qquad (1.2.88)$$

When we take the FT of (1.2.82), we obtain

$$X(f) = R\sum_k X_0(kR)\delta(f - kR) = X_0(f)\sum_n \exp(-j\,2\,\pi fnT) \quad (1.2.89)$$

The middle term is just

$$RX_0(f)\sum_k \delta(f - kR) \qquad (1.2.90)$$

Hence we have the equivalent expression to (1.2.88) in the frequency domain

$$R\sum_k \delta(f - kR) = \sum_n \exp(-j\,2\,\pi fnT) \qquad (1.2.91)$$

f. *Parseval's formula*

$$\int_{-\infty}^{\infty} x_1(t)x_2^*(t)\, dt = \int_{-\infty}^{\infty} X_1(f)X_2^*(f)\, df \tag{1.2.92}$$

*Proof*

This follows immediately from (1.2.69) and (1.2.70) with $t = 0$

$$z(0) = \int_{-\infty}^{\infty} x(\tau)y(-\tau)\, d\tau = \int_{-\infty}^{\infty} X(f)Y(f)\, df$$

Denoting

$$x_2^*(t) = y(-t)$$

we have

$$Y(f) = \int_{-\infty}^{\infty} x_2^*(-t) \exp(-j\, 2\, \pi f t)\, dt$$

$$= \int_{-\infty}^{\infty} x_2^*(t) \exp(j\, 2\, \pi f t)\, dt = \left( \int_{-\infty}^{\infty} x_2 \exp(-j\, 2\, \pi f t)\, dt \right)^* = X_2^*(f)$$

g. *Energy*

$$E_x = \int_{-\infty}^{\infty} |x(t)|^2\, dt = \int_{-\infty}^{\infty} |X(f)|^2\, df \tag{1.2.93}$$

This follows immediately from (1.2.92) by substitution

$$x_1(t) = x_2(t) = x(t)$$

Because both $|x(t)|^2$ and $|X(f)|^2$ are nonnegative and their integral is the energy, we can call $|x(t)|^2$ the *energy temporal density* and $|X(f)|^2$ the *energy spectral density*.

### 1.2.5 Laplace transforms

We assume that $x(t)$ is real and causal. The *Laplace transform* (LT) of such a function is defined by

$$X'(s) = \int_0^\infty x(t) \exp(-st)\, dt \tag{1.2.94}$$

where

$$s = \sigma + j\omega, \qquad \omega = 2\pi f \tag{1.2.95}$$

is a complex variable.

The LT is related to the FT in almost all cases by

$$X(f) = X'(j\,2\pi f) \tag{1.2.96}$$

The exception occurs when $X'(0) = \infty$.

The inverse LT (ILT) is

$$x(t) = (2\pi)^{-2} \int_{c-j\infty}^{c+j\infty} X'(s) \exp(st)\, ds \tag{1.2.97}$$

and $c$ is a real number that is greater than the real parts of all singular points, i.e., points for which $X'(s) = \infty$.

Many properties of LT are identical to those of FT. Some LT are given in Table 1.3, and the properties of LT are listed in Table 1.4.

*Example* 1.2.3 Linear differential equation

We have a differential equation with real coefficients and zero initial conditions, i.e.

$$\sum_{n=0}^{N} a_n \frac{d^n y(t)}{dt^n} = \sum_{m=0}^{M} b_m \frac{d^m x(t)}{dt^m} \tag{1.2.98}$$

with $a_N = b_M = 1$ and

$$\frac{d^n y(0)}{dt^n} = \frac{d^m x(0)}{dt^m} = 0$$

We take the LT of (1.2.98), and, using line 5 of Table 1.4, we obtain

$$\left(\sum_{n=0}^{N} a_n s^n\right) Y'(s) = \left(\sum_{m=0}^{M} b_m s^m\right) X'(s) \tag{1.2.99}$$

**Table 1.3 Signals and their Laplace transforms**

| $x(t)$ | $X'(s)$ |
|---|---|
| $\delta(t)$ | $1$ |
| $u(t)$ | $1/s$ |
| $\sin(\omega t)u(t)$ | $\omega(s^2+\omega^2)^{-1}$ |
| $\cos(\omega t)u(t)$ | $s(s^2+\omega^2)^{-1}$ |
| $\exp(-at)u(t)$ | $(s+a)^{-1}$ |

**Table 1.4 Properties of Laplace transforms**

| PROPERTY | $x(t)$ | $X'(s)$ |
|---|---|---|
| Linearity | $\sum_i a_i y_i(t)$ | $\sum_i a_i Y_i'(s)$ |
| Time shift | $y(t-t_0)$ | $Y'(s)\exp(-st_0)$ |
| Frequency shift | $y(t)\exp(-at)$ | $Y'(s+a)$ |
| Time scaling | $y(at)$ | $Y'(s/a)/a$ |
| Time derivative | $d^n y(t)/dt^n$ | $s^n Y'(s) - \sum_{k=1}^{n} s^{n-k}\frac{d^{k-1}y(0)}{dt^{k-1}}$ |
| Convolution | $y_1(t)*y_2(t)$ | $Y_1'(s)Y_2'(s)$ |
| Integral | $\int_{-\infty}^{t} y(\tau)\,d\tau$ | $Y'(s)/s + \int_{-\infty}^{0} y(\tau)\,d\tau/s$ |

The ratio is

$$H'(s) = Y'(s)/X'(s) = \frac{\sum_{m=0}^{M} b_m s^m}{\sum_{n=0}^{N} a_n s^n} = \frac{M(s)}{N(s)} \qquad (1.2.100)$$

The polynomials can be written as products of their roots

$$M(s) = \prod_{m=1}^{M}(s+z_m) \qquad (1.2.101)$$

$$N(s) = \prod_{n=1}^{N}(s+p_n) \qquad (1.2.102)$$

Thus

$$H'(s) = \prod_{m=1}^{M}(s+z_m) \Big/ \prod_{n=1}^{N}(s+p_n) \qquad (1.2.103)$$

The $\{-z_m\}$ are called the zeros of $H'(s)$, and the $\{-p_n\}$ are called the poles of $H'(s)$. The poles are singular points of $H'(s)$. Because $M(s)$ and $N(s)$ are polynomials with real coefficients the poles and zeros are either real or they appear in complex conjugate pairs. The zeros and poles may be distinct or multiple, i.e., $p_1$ are $p_2$ may be identical. If we assume that all poles are distinct, then we can rewrite (1.2.103) in the form

$$H'(s) = \sum_{n=1}^{N} \rho_n/(s + p_n) \tag{1.2.104}$$

where $\{\rho_n\}$, called *residua*, are obtained from (1.2.103) by

$$\rho_k = \lim_{s\to -p_k} H'(s)(s + p_k) = \frac{M(-p_k)}{\sum\limits_{\substack{n=1\\ n\neq k}}^{N} (p_n - p_k)} \tag{1.2.105}$$

If $p_n = p_k^*$, then (1.2.104) implies that $\rho_n = \rho_k^*$. From (1.2.103) and line 5 of Table 1.3, we obtain the ILT

$$h(t) = \sum_{n=1}^{N} \rho_n \exp(-p_n t)u(t) \tag{1.2.106}$$

which is a real function of time. This function has finite energy only if all $\{p_n\}$ have positive real parts, i.e., all poles $\{-p_n\}$ lie in the left-hand plane.

## 1.3 LINEAR SYSTEMS AND FILTERS

### 1.3.1 Impulse response and transfer function

We shall use the words *system* and *filters* interchangeably. A system or filter operates on a signal $x(t)$ to produce the signal $y(t)$

$$y(t) = L\{x(t)\} \tag{1.3.1}$$

A filter is called *linear* if

$$L\left\{\sum_i a_i x_i(t)\right\} = \sum_i a_i L\{x_i(t)\} \tag{1.3.2}$$

A filter is called *time-invariant* if for any $t_0$

$$L\{x(t - t_0)\} = y(t - t_0) \tag{1.3.3}$$

A filter is called *real* if the response $y(t)$ is real when the input $x(t)$ is real. A filter is called *causal* if the response is zero prior to the application of the input signal. If $x(t) = \delta(t)$, i.e., the input is an impulse, then the output, which is now the impulse response of the filter, will be denoted by $y(t) = h(t)$, i.e.

$$h(t) = L\{\delta(t)\} \tag{1.3.4}$$

Because the input $x(t)$ can be written (see 1.2.32))

$$x(t) = \int_{-\infty}^{\infty} x(\tau)\delta(t - \tau)\, d\tau = \lim_{\Delta\tau \to 0} \sum_i x(\tau_i)\delta(t - \tau_i)\Delta\tau \tag{1.3.5}$$

where $\tau_{i+1} = \tau_i + \Delta\tau$, we obtain from the linearity and time-invariant properties, that the response to $x(t)$ is

$$y(t) = \lim_{\Delta\tau \to 0} \sum_i x(\tau_i)h(t - \tau_i)\Delta\tau = \int_{-\infty}^{\infty} x(\tau)h(t - \tau)\, d\tau$$

$$= x(t) * h(t) \tag{1.3.6}$$

Taking the FT we obtain

$$Y(f) = X(f)H(f) \tag{1.3.7}$$

Equations (1.3.6) and 1.3.7) suggest that the impulse response of a filter can be treated as another signal. There is no mathematical difference between signals and filters. The FT of $h(t)$, $H(f)$ is called the *transfer function* of the filter. A filter is modeled in Fig. 1.5.

If the filter is real and the input is complex

$$x(t) = x_I(t) + jx_Q(t) \tag{1.3.8}$$

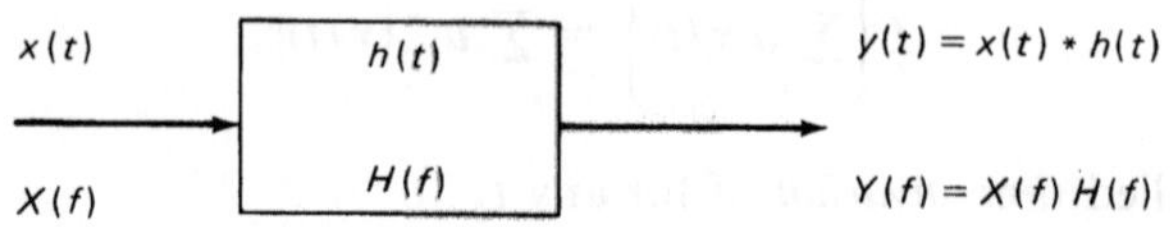


Fig. 1.5. Modeling of linear system.

the output will be complex

$$y(t) = y_I(t) + jy_Q(t) \tag{1.3.9}$$

with

$$Y_I(f) = X_I(f)H(f), \qquad Y_Q(f) = X_Q(f)H(f) \tag{1.3.10}$$

It is thus sufficient to compute

$$y(t) = \int_{-\infty}^{\infty} X(f)H(f) \exp(j\,2\,\pi f t)\, df \tag{1.3.11}$$

because

$$y_I(t) = \text{Re}\,\{y(t)\}, \qquad y_Q(t) = \text{Im}\,\{y(t)\} \tag{1.3.12}$$

*Example* 1.3.1 Response of linear filter to sinusoid
We want to computer the response of the real, linear, time-invariant filter to $A\cos(\omega t + \phi)$ or $A\sin(\omega t + \phi)$, $\omega = 2\,\pi f$. Instead we can compute the response to

$$x(t) = A\exp(j(\omega t + \phi)) = A\cos(\omega t + \phi) + jA\sin(\omega t + \phi) \tag{1.3.13}$$

and then use (1.3.12). The response to $x(t)$ is

$$\begin{aligned} y(t) &= \int_{-\infty}^{\infty} A\exp(j(\omega t - \omega\tau + \phi))h(\tau)\, d\tau \\ &= A\exp(j(\omega t + \phi)) \int_{-\infty}^{\infty} h(\tau)\exp(-j\omega\tau)\, d\tau \\ &= A\exp(j(\omega t + \phi))H(f) \end{aligned} \tag{1.3.14}$$

Thus the response to the cosine is

$$\text{Re}\,\{y(t)\} = A|H(f)|\cos(\omega t + \phi + \arg H(f)) \tag{1.3.15}$$

and the response to the sine is

$$\text{Im}\,\{y(t)\} = A|H(f)|\sin(\omega t + \phi + \arg H(f)) \tag{1.3.16}$$

We see from these formulas that the response of a real, linear, time-invariant system to a sinusoid of frequency $f$ is also a sinusoid of the same frequency, but a modified amplitude and phase.

### 1.3.2 Nondistorting filters

A filter normally distorts the input signal $x(t)$, because

$$\begin{aligned} y(t) &= x(t) * h(t) \neq x(t) \qquad \text{(temporal distortion)} \\ Y(f) &= X(f)H(f) \neq X(f) \qquad \text{(spectral distortion)} \end{aligned} \tag{1.3.17}$$

unless $h(t) = \delta(t)$ $(H(f) = 1)$.

In many cases we do not consider the output to be distorted if the output is a shifted in time and scaled in amplitude version of the input, i.e.

$$y(t) = Ax(t - t_0) \tag{1.3.18}$$

The transfer function of such a filter, which is found from FT of (1.3.18)

$$Y(f) = A \exp(-j\,2\,\pi f t_0)X(f) \tag{1.3.19}$$

$$H(f) = A \exp(-j\,2\,\pi f t_0) \tag{1.3.20}$$

Note that in such a filter

$$|H(f)| = A \tag{1.3.21}$$

i.e., the amplitude is a constant and

$$\arg H(f) = -(2\,\pi t_0)f \tag{1.3.22}$$

is a linear function of frequency. Particularly if $X(f)$ is nonzero for $f_L \leqq |f| \leqq f_H$, we do not care what the transfer function is for other frequencies, and (1.3.20)–(1.3.22) must be satisfied for these frequencies only.

### 1.3.3 Band-limiting filters

A filter is *band-limiting* if $H(f) = 0$ outside the frequency band $0 \leqq f_L \leqq |f| \leqq f_H$ with

$$f_H - f_L = B > 0 \tag{1.3.23}$$

the bandwidth of such filter. A band-limiting filter is called *ideal* if $H(f)$ satisfies (1.3.20) for all $f_L \leqq |f| \leqq f_H$. Such filters pass signals with no distortion, so long as the signals are confined to this frequency range. Outside this band, the output is zero even if the input signal contains nonzero components.

The band-limiting filter is called *lowpass* if $f_L = 0$ (hence $f_H = B$). If $f_L > 0$, the filter is called *bandpass*.

In practical filters the transition from passband to stopband is gradual rather then abrupt, i.e., (1.3.20) is satisfied only approximately in the passband, and $H(f)$ is not zero outside the passband. It is not difficult to show that band-limiting filters with finite $f_H$ are not causal.

*Example* 1.3.2 Butterworth filter
A Butterworth lowpass filter of order $N$ has a transfer function, the absolute value of which is

$$|H(f)| = (1 + (f/f_0)^{2N})^{-1/2} \tag{1.3.24}$$

Note that $|H(0)| = 1$, and $|H(f_0)| = 2^{-1/2}$. Thus

$$20 \log |H(f_0)/H(0)| = -10 \log 2 = -3 \text{ dB} \tag{1.3.25}$$

i.e., $f_0$ is the frequency at which the transfer function has a loss of 3 dB relative to its value at zero frequency. The filter passes approximately all input signals with frequencies up to $f_0$ and stops approximately all input signals with frequencies beyond this frequency. When $N \to \infty$, the Butterworth filter becomes an ideal lowpass filter. Note the gradual transition from passband to stopband for finite $N$ in Fig. 1.6.

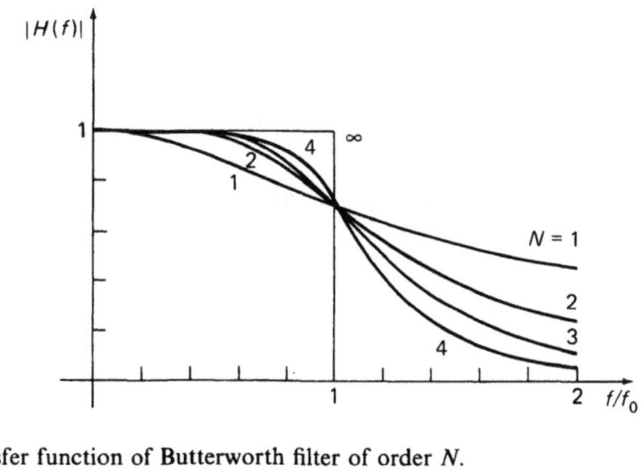


Fig. 1.6. Transfer function of Butterworth filter of order $N$.

### 1.3.4 Time-variant, linear filters

Let $h(t, \tau)$ be the response of the filter at time $t$ to an impulse applied at time $t - \tau$. The response of the filter to input $x(t)$ is, from (1.2.32) and (1.3.2)

$$y(t) = \lim_{\Delta\tau \to 0} \sum_i x(\tau_i)h(t, \tau_i)\Delta\tau = \int_{-\infty}^{\infty} x(\tau)h(t, \tau)\, d\tau \qquad (1.3.26)$$

In the future if we do not explicitly state it otherwise, the filters are linear and time-invariant.

### 1.3.5 Hilbert transform

The Hilbert transform (HT) is the result of operation with the filter

$$h(t) = (\pi t)^{-1} \leftrightarrow H(f) = -j \operatorname{sign} f \qquad (1.3.27)$$

on signal $x(t)$. We shall denote the HT by

$$X_h(f) = H\{x(t)\} = -j \operatorname{sign} f X(f) \qquad (1.3.28)$$

The physical interpretation of the HT is a change in phase by $-j = -90°$ for all signal components with positive frequencies.

*Example* 1.3.3 HT of sinusoid
Let

$$x(t) = A \cos(2\pi f_c t + \phi) \qquad (1.3.29)$$

Then

$$x_h(t) = A \cos(2\pi f_c t + \phi - \pi/2) = A \sin(2\pi f_c t + \phi)$$

Formally we can obtain this result from

$$X(f) = (1/2)A\{\delta(f - f_c) \exp(j\phi) + \delta(f + f_c) \exp(-j\phi)\}$$

$$\begin{aligned} X_h(f) &= (1/2)A\{-j\delta(f - f_c) \exp(j\phi) + j\delta(f + f_c) \exp(-j\phi)\} \\ &= (1/2)A\{\delta(f - f_c) \exp(j(\phi - \pi/2)) \\ &\quad + \delta(f + f_c) \exp(-j(\phi - \pi/2))\} \end{aligned}$$

$$x_h(t) = A \cos(2\pi f_c t + \phi - \pi/2)$$

*Example* 1.3.4 HT of bandpass signal
Let $x(t)$ be a real signal such that $X(f) = 0$ for $|f| \geqq B$, and let

$$y(t) = x(t) \cos (2 \pi f_c t + \phi) \tag{1.3.30}$$

with $f_c > B$, thus

$$Y(f) = X(f - f_c) \exp (j\phi) + X(f + f_c) \exp (-j\phi)$$

Note that $X(f - f_c)$ is confined to positive frequencies and $X(f + f_c)$ to negative frequencies; hence

$$\begin{aligned} Y_h(f) &= -jX(f - f_c) \exp (j\phi) + jX(f + f_c) \exp (-j\phi) \\ &= X(f - f_c) \exp (j(\phi - \pi/2)) + X(f + f_c) \exp (-j(\phi - \pi/2)) \end{aligned}$$

Therefore

$$y_h(t) = x(t) \cos (2 \pi f_c t + \phi - \pi/2) = x(t) \sin (2 \pi f_c t + \phi) \tag{1.3.31}$$

In Table 1.5 we present some HT pairs. In this table it was assumed that $Y(f) = 0$ for $|f| > f_c$.

**Table 1.5 Signals and their Hilbert transform**

| $x(t)$ | $x_h(t)$ |
|---|---|
| $\cos (2 \pi ft + \phi)$ | $\sin (2 \pi ft + \phi)$ |
| $\sin (2 \pi ft + \phi)$ | $-\cos (2 \pi ft + \phi)$ |
| $y(t) \cos (2 \pi f_c t + \phi)$ | $y(t) \sin (2 \pi f_c t + \phi)$ |
| $y(t) \sin (2 \pi f_c t + \phi)$ | $-y(t) \cos (2 \pi f_c t + \phi)$ |
| $\delta(t)$ | $(\pi t)^{-1}$ |
| $(1 + t^2)^{-1}$ | $t(1 + t^2)^{-1}$ |

A signal $x_a(t)$ is called *analytic* if its real and imaginary parts form a HT pair, i.e.

$$x_a(t) = x(t) + jx_h(t) \tag{1.3.32}$$

$$\begin{aligned} X_a(f) &= X(f) + jX_h(f) = X(f)\{1 + \text{sign} f\} \\ &= 2 X(f)u(f) \end{aligned} \tag{1.3.33}$$

Thus an analytic signal is obtained from the real signal $x(t)$ by removing its components with negative frequencies.

## 1.4 EQUIVALENCE OF BASEBAND AND BANDPASS SIGNALS AND FILTERS

### 1.4.1 Baseband and bandpass signals

A signal $x(t)$ is called baseband if $X(f) = 0$ for $|f| \geqq B$. Let $x_I(t)$, $x_Q(t)$ be real baseband signals, and let $\cos(2\pi f_c t + \phi)$, $\sin(2\pi f_c t + \phi)$ be two carriers in quadrature. A signal $x_M(t)$ is called bandpass around $f_c$ with bandwidth $2B$ if $x_M(f) = 0$ for $|f \pm f_c| > B$ and $f_c > B$. Such a signal can be generated by a process called *modulation*

$$\begin{aligned} x_M(t) &= x_I(t)\cos(\omega_c t + \phi) \pm x_Q(t)\sin(\omega_c t + \phi) \\ &= A_x(t)\cos(\omega_c t + \phi \mp \phi_x(t)) \end{aligned} \tag{1.4.1}$$

where the envelope and phase are

$$A_x(t) = (x^2_I(t) + x^2_Q(t))^{1/2} \tag{1.4.2}$$

$$\phi_x(t) = \tan^{-1}(x_Q(t)/x_I(t)) \tag{1.4.3}$$

and

$$\omega_c = 2\pi f_c \tag{1.4.4}$$

A bandpass signal and its envelope are shown in Fig. 1.7. If $f_c \gg B$, the bandpass signal is narrowband, and the envelope and phase are slowly varying functions of time compared with the carriers. The *complex envelope* is defined by

$$x(t) = A_x(t)\exp(j\phi_x(t)) = x_I(t) + jx_Q(t) \tag{1.4.5}$$

We obtain the envelope and phase from the complex envelope by

$$A_x(t) = |x(t)|, \qquad \phi_x(t) = \arg x(t) \tag{1.4.6}$$

The bandpass signal can be expressed as a function of the complex envelope by

$$\begin{aligned} x_M(t) &= \mathrm{Re}\,\{x(t)\exp(j(\omega_c t + \phi))\} \\ &= 0.5\,\{x(t)\exp(j(\omega_c t + \phi)) + x^*(t)\exp(-j(\omega_c t + \phi))\} \end{aligned} \tag{1.4.7}$$

Taking the Fourier transform, we obtain

$$X_M(f) = 0.5\,\{X(f - f_c)\exp(j\phi) + X^*(-f - f_c)\exp(-j\phi)\} \tag{1.4.8}$$

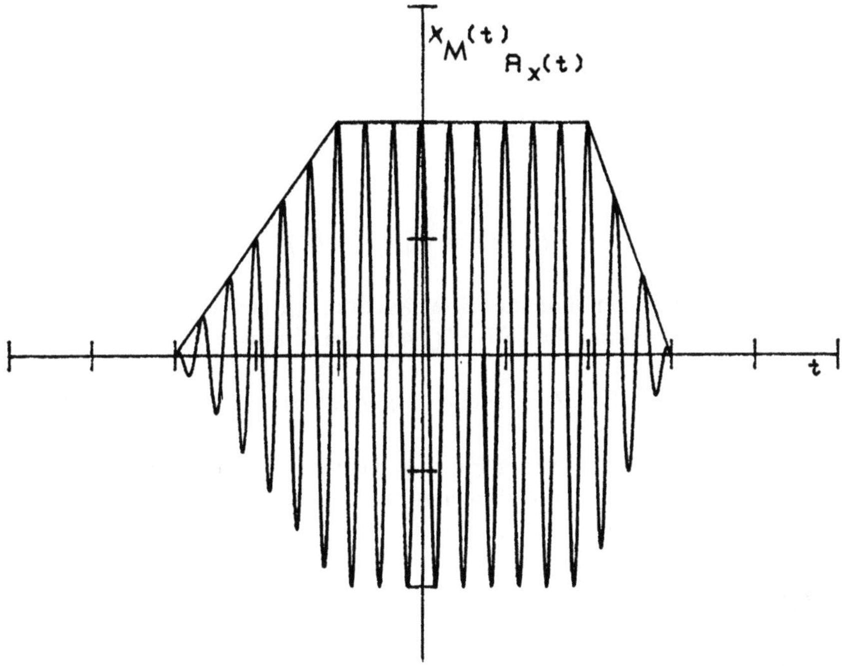


Fig. 1.7. Bandpass signal and envelope.

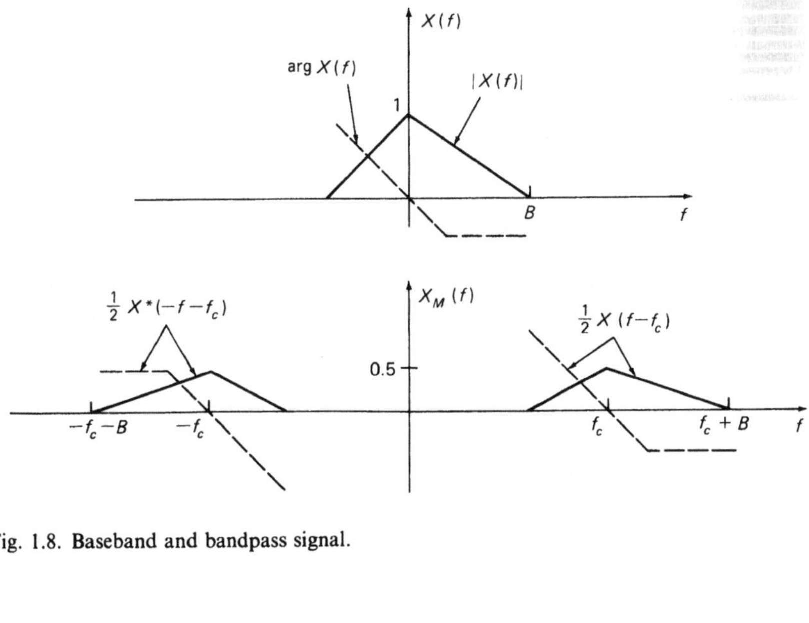


Fig. 1.8. Baseband and bandpass signal.

This is illustrated in Fig. 1.8 assuming $\phi = 0$. Note that the two terms in (1.4.8) do not overlap, and we can generate $X(f)$ from $x_M(f)$ by

$$X(f) = 2\, X_M(f + f_c)\, H_{\text{id}}(f) \exp(-j\phi) \tag{1.4.9}$$

where

$$H_{\text{id}}(f) = u_{2W}(f + W) \tag{1.4.10}$$

is the transfer function of an ideal lowpass filter with bandwidth $B < W < f_c$ and zero phase. Taking the IFT of (1.4.9), we obtain

$$x(t) = 2\, x_M(t) \exp(-j(\omega_c + \phi)) * h_{\text{id}}(t) \tag{1.4.11}$$

where $h_{\text{id}}(t)$ and $H_{\text{id}}(f)$ form a FT pair. Using (1.4.1) and (1.4.11), we can generated $x(t)$ and $x_M(t)$, and shown in Fig. 1.9. Because the bandpass signal and its complex enevelope are closely related when $f_c$ and $\phi$ are known, knowledge of one is equivalent to knowledge of the other, and we say that they are equivalent representation of the signals.

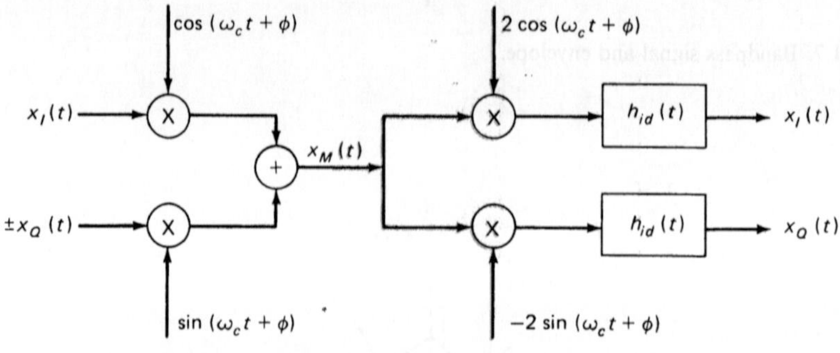


Fig. 1.9. Generation of bandpass signal and its complex envelope.

### 1.4.2 Baseband and bandpass filters

A filter is called baseband if $H(f) = 0$ for $|f| > B$. A filter is called bandpass if $H_M(f) = 0$ for $|f \pm f_c| > B$, $B < f_c$. A bandpass filter has a transfer function that can be written in the form

$$H_M(f) = H_M(f)H_{\text{id}}(f - f_c) + H_M(f)H_{\text{id}}(f + f_c) \tag{1.4.12}$$

We assume that the bandpass filter is real; hence

$$H_M^*(-f) = H_M(f) \tag{1.4.13}$$

and we can rewrite (1.4.12) in the form

$$H_M(f) = H_M(f)H_{id}(f - f_c) + H_M^*(-f)H_{id}^*(-f - f_c) \quad (1.4.14)$$

where we have also used the fact that $H_{id}(f)$ is even and real, i.e.

$$H_{id}(f) = H_{id}^*(-f) \quad (1.4.15)$$

Denoting

$$H(f) = H_M(f + f_c)H_{id}(f) \quad (1.4.16)$$

we obtain from (1.4.14)

$$H_M(f) = H(f - f_c) + H^*(-f - f_c) \quad (1.4.17)$$

$H(f)$ is a baseband filter equivalent to the bandpass filter, and they are related by (1.4.16) and (1.4.17). This is illustrated in Fig. 1.10. When we take the IFT of (1.4.16) and (1.4.17), we obtain

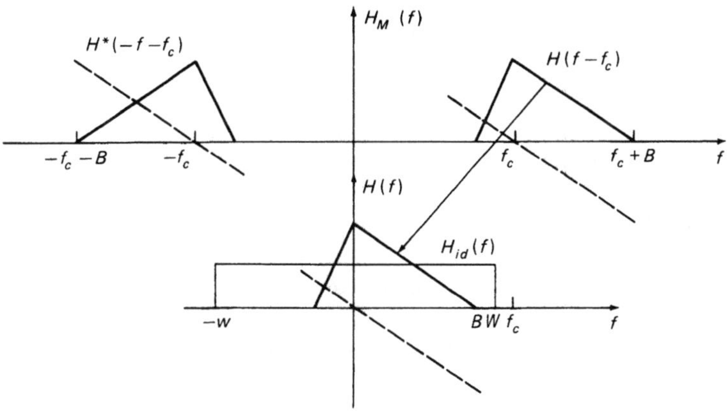


Fig. 1.10. Bandpass and equivalent baseband filters.

$$h(t) = h_M(t) \exp(-j\omega_c t) * h_{id}(t) = h_I(t) + jh_Q(t) \quad (1.4.18)$$

$$\begin{aligned} h_M(t) &= h(t) \exp(j\omega_c t) + h^*(t) \exp(-j\omega_c t) \\ &= 2 \operatorname{Re}\{h(t) \exp(j\omega_c t)\} \\ &= 2\, h_I(t) \cos(\omega_c t) - 2\, h_Q(t) \sin(\omega_c t) \end{aligned} \quad (1.4.19)$$

This is illustrated in Fig. 1.11. Because the input and output in Fig. 1.11 are the same bandpass function $h_M(t)$, that means that the scheme in Fig. 1.11 is

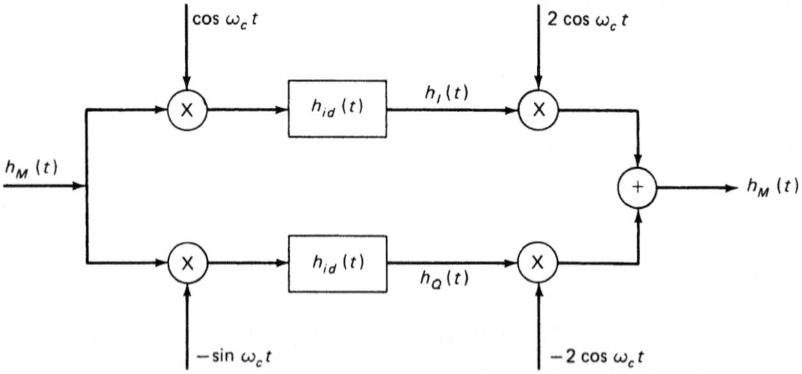


Fig. 1.11. Relation between impulse response of bandpass and equivalent baseband filter.

an ideal bandpass filter, the transfer function of which is 1 for $|f \pm f_c| < B$ and 0 otherwise. $h(t)$ is also the complex envelope of the bandpass function $h_M(t)$. If $H_M(f)$ is symmetric around $f_c$, i.e.

$$H_M(f_c + f) = H_M^*(f_c - f) \tag{1.4.20}$$

for $f_c \pm f > 0$, then it follows from (1.4.16) that

$$H(f) = H^*(-f) \tag{1.4.21}$$

i.e., the baseband equivalent filter is also symmetric, and $h(t)$ is a real function. In this special but very important case, (1.4.18) and (1.4.19) are simplified to

$$h(t) = h_I(t) \tag{1.4.22}$$

$$h_M(t) = 2\, h_I(t) \cos(\omega_c t) \tag{1.4.23}$$

*Example* 1.4.1 *Single side band filter*
A bandpass filter that eliminates the signal frequencies either below or above the carrier frequency $f_c$ is called a *single side band filter*. Such filters, which eliminate either the lower or upper sideband and their baseband equivalent filters, are shown in Fig. 1.12

*Example* 1.4.2 *Vestigial side band filter*
A bandpass filter that eliminates most of the signal frequencies below or above the carrier frequency in a symmetric way is called a *vestigial side band filter*, because a vestige of the signal at these frequencies is left. Such

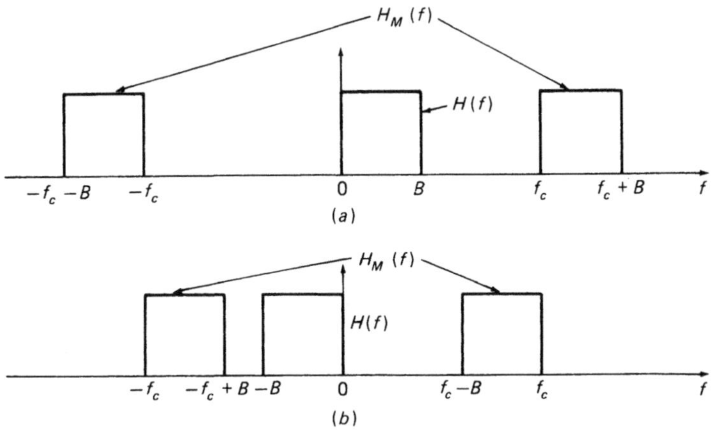


Fig. 1.12. Single side band filters and their baseband equivalent filters: (a) upper side band, (b) lower side band.

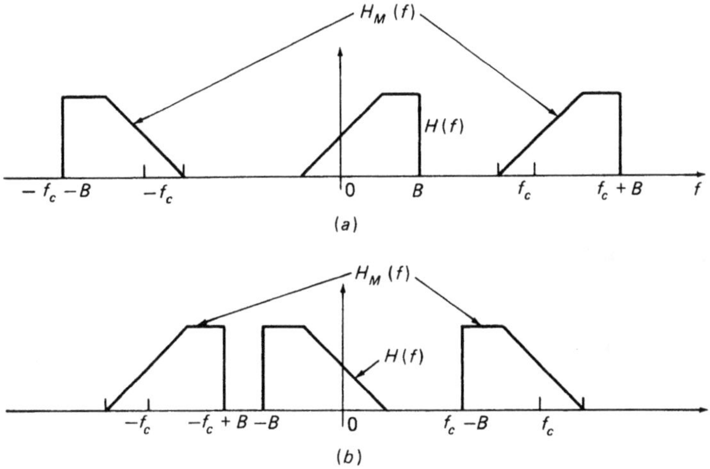


Fig. 1.13. Vestigial side band filters and their baseband equivalent filters: (a) upper side band, (b) lower side bands.

filters and their baseband equivalent filters are shown in Fig. 1.13. By symmetry we mean here the condition

$$H_M(f_c + f) + H_M(f_c - f) = 1$$

for all

$$|f_c \pm f| \leqq B$$

### 1.4.3 Bandpass filters in tandem

Let $H_{Mi}(f)$ $i = 1, \ldots, N$ be transfer functions of bandpass filters, and let $H_i(f)$ be their baseband equivalent filters. The transfer function of these filters in tandem is

$$H_M(f) = \prod_{i=1}^{N} H_{Mi}(f)$$
$$= \prod_{i=1}^{N} \{H_i(f - f_c) + H_i^*(-f - f_c)\} = H(f - f_c) + H^*(-f - f_c) \tag{1.4.24}$$

where

$$H(f) = \prod_{i=1}^{N} H_i(f) \tag{1.4.25}$$

The reason for equality in (1.4.24) is

$$H_i(f - f_c)H_k^*(-f - f_c) = 0 \qquad i, k = 1, \ldots, N \tag{1.4.26}$$

### 1.4.4 Response of bandpass filter to bandpass signal

Let $x_M(t)$ be the input to a bandpass filter, with impulse response $h_M(t)$, and let the output be $y_M(t)$. Thus, from (1.4.8) and (1.4.17)

$$Y_M(f) = X_M(f)H_M(f)$$
$$= 0.5\,\{Y(f - f_c)\exp(j\phi) + Y^*(-f - f_c)\exp(-j\phi)\} \tag{1.4.27}$$

where

$$Y(f) = X(f)H(f) \tag{1.4.28}$$

and in the time domain

$$y_M(t) = \mathrm{Re}\,\{y(t)\exp(j(\omega_c t + \phi))\} \tag{1.4.29}$$

This implies that in order to compute the response of a bandpass filter to a bandpass signal of known frequency and phase, it is sufficient to compute the baseband equivalent response $Y(f)$, which is obtained as a product of the complex envelopes of the signal and filter. This equivalency is shown in Fig. 1.14.

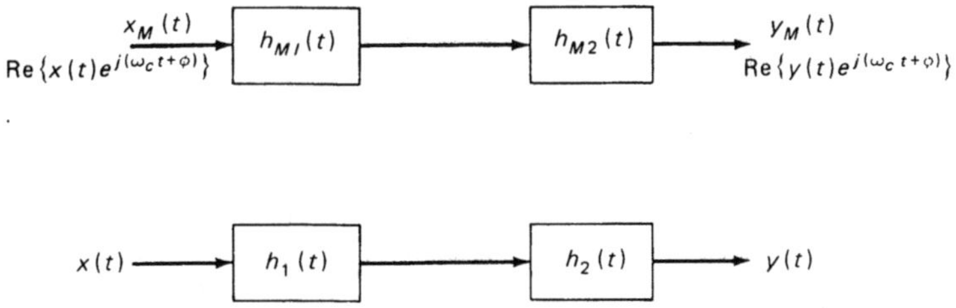


Fig. 1.14. Bandpass signals and filters and their baseband equivalents.

### 1.4.5 Equivalence with respect to different carrier frequencies

Let $y_M(t)$ be a bandpass signal with carrier frequency $f_T$ and phase $\phi_T$; thus similarly to (1.4.8) with $f_c$, $\phi$ replaced by $f_T$, $\phi_T$

$$Y_M(f) = 0.5\,\{Y(f - f_T)\exp(j\phi_T) + Y^*(-f - f_T)\exp(-j\phi_T)\} \quad (1.4.30)$$

The baseband equivalent signal with respect to carrier frequency $f_R$ and phase $\phi_R$ is from (1.4.9), with $f_c$, $\phi$ replaced by $f_R$, $\phi_R$

$$Y(f, \Delta f, \Delta\phi) = 2\,Y_M(f + f_R)H_{\text{id}}(f)\exp(-j\phi_R) \quad (1.4.31)$$

where

$$\Delta f = f_T - f_R \quad (1.4.32)$$

$$\Delta\phi = \phi_T - \phi_R \quad (1.4.33)$$

is the difference in the frequencies and phases. We substitute (1.4.30) into (1.4.31) and obtain

$$\begin{aligned} Y(f, \Delta f, \Delta\phi) = {} & Y(f - \Delta f)\exp(j\Delta\phi)H_{\text{id}}(f) \\ & + Y^*(-f - f_T - f_R)\exp(-j(\phi_T + \phi_R))H_{\text{id}}(f) \end{aligned} \quad (1.4.34)$$

which is illustrated in Fig. 1.15. We note from this figure that so long as

$$B + \Delta f \leqq W \leqq f_R \quad (1.4.35)$$

the second term in (1.4.34) is eliminated, and the result is

$$Y(f, \Delta f, \Delta\phi) = Y(f - \Delta f)\exp(j\Delta\phi)H_{\text{id}}(f) \quad (1.4.36)$$

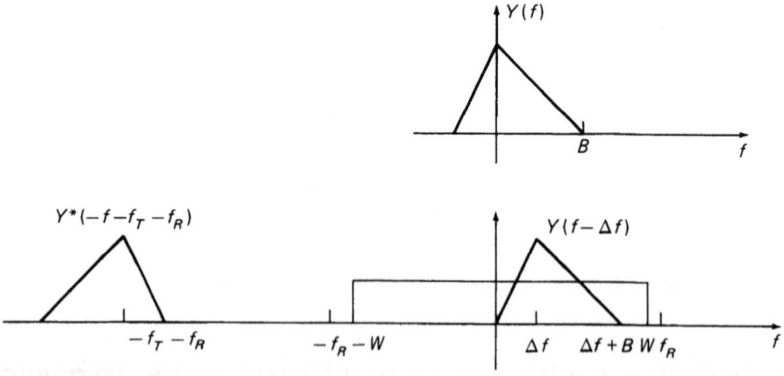


Fig. 1.15. Illustration of eq. (1.4.34).

Equation (1.4.36) gives the complex envelope of a signal with respect to $f_T$, $\phi_T$ in terms of the complex envelope with respect to $f_R$, $\phi_R$. The significance of this result will be explained shortly.

In a communications system $x_I(t)$, $x_Q(t)$ contain the information, and the carrier is only a means to transfer the information between two points at a distance. The information is transmitted using a carrier with frequency $f_T$ and phase $\phi_T$. At the receiver end of the system only $x_I(t)$ and $x_Q(t)$ are of interest. Therefore these two terms are extracted from the incoming signal $y_M(t)$, which is a distorted version of $x_M(t)$. The receiver side has no access to $f_T$, $\phi_T$; rather it has access to $f_R$, $\phi_R$, which ideally should be the same as $f_T$, $\phi_T$, but, because of errors, will drift around $f_T$, $\phi_T$. This system is shown in Fig. 1.16. Thus

$$\begin{aligned} z_I(t) = \{&2\, y_I(t) \cos(\omega_T t + \phi_T) \cos(\omega_R t + \phi_R) \\ &+ 2\, y_Q(t) \sin(\omega_T + \phi_T) \cos(\omega_R t + \phi_R)\} * h_{\mathrm{id}}(t) \end{aligned} \quad (1.4.37)$$

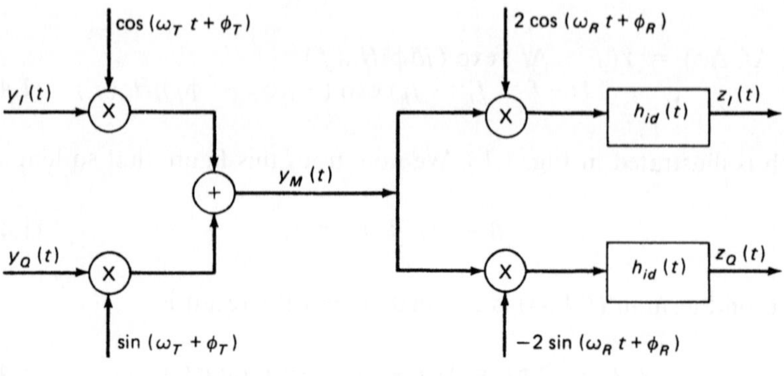


Fig. 1.16. System with different frequencies and phases at transmitter and receiver.

Using the sine and cosine relations

$$\cos\alpha\cos\beta = 0.5\{\cos(\alpha+\beta) + \cos(\alpha-\beta)\} \tag{1.4.38}$$

$$\sin\alpha\cos\beta = 0.5\{\sin(\alpha+\beta) + \sin(\alpha-\beta)\} \tag{1.4.39}$$

and noting that the ideal lowpass filter will not pass the

$$\alpha + \beta = (\omega_T + \omega_R)t + \phi_T + \phi_R$$

terms, we obtain

$$z_I(t) = \{y_I(t)\cos(2\pi\Delta f t + \Delta\phi) - y_Q(t)\sin(2\pi\Delta f t + \Delta\phi)\} * h_{\text{id}}(t) \tag{1.4.40}$$

Similarly

$$z_Q(t) = \{y_Q(t)\cos(2\pi\Delta f t + \Delta\phi) + y_I(t)\sin(2\pi\Delta f t + \Delta\phi)\} * h_{\text{id}}(t) \tag{1.4.41}$$

Now we return to (1.4.36) and take the IFT

$$y(t, \Delta f, \Delta\phi) = y(t)\exp(j(2\pi\Delta f t + \phi)) * h_{\text{id}}(t)$$
$$\{y_I(t) + jy_Q(t)\}\{\cos(2\pi\Delta f t + \phi) + j\sin(2\pi\Delta f t + \phi)\} * h_{\text{id}}(t) \tag{1.4.42}$$

Now it is a simple exercise to see that

$$y_I(t, \Delta f, \Delta\phi) = \text{Re}\{y(t, \Delta f, \Delta\phi)\} = z_I(t) \tag{1.4.43}$$

$$y_Q(t, \Delta f, \Delta\phi) = \text{Im}\{y(t, \Delta f, \Delta\phi)\} = z_Q(t) \tag{1.4.44}$$

We can thus replace the system of Fig. 1.16 by the equivalent baseband system of Fig. 1.17.

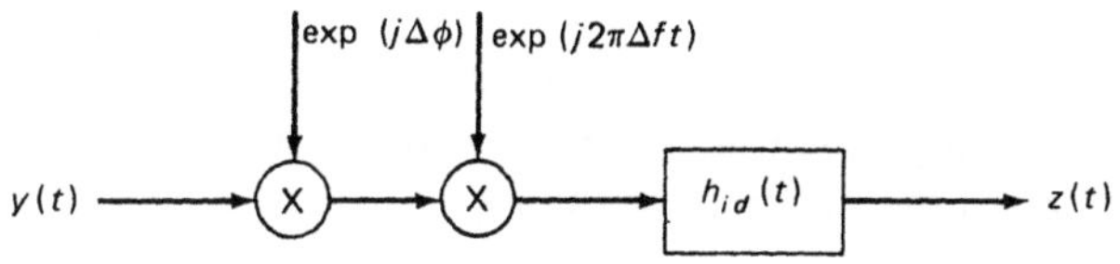


Fig. 1.17. Baseband equivalent system of Fig. 1.16.

### 1.4.6 Baseband equivalence of arbitrary function

Let $z_M(t)$ be a real function that represents both a signal $x_M(t)$ and an impulse response $h_M(t)$. The *FT*, $Z_M(f)$, can be separated into two nonoverlapping terms

$$Z_M(f) = Z_M(f)u(f) + Z_M(f)u(-f) \tag{1.4.45}$$

confined to positive and negative frequencies, respectively. Because $z_M(t)$ is real, we have

$$Z_M(f) = Z_M^*(-f) \tag{1.4.46}$$

and because $u(f)$ is real, we can also replace $u(-f)$ by $u^*(-f)$. Thus we can write (1.4.45)

$$Z_M(f) = Z_M(f)u(f) + Z_M^*(-f)u^*(-f) \tag{1.4.47}$$

Let $f_c > 0$ and $\phi$ be arbitrary and define

$$Z(f) = Z_M(f + f_c)u(f + f_c) \exp(-j\phi) \tag{1.4.48}$$

which is simply the term with the positive frequencies shifted to the left by $f_c$. We can now write (1.4.47)

$$Z_M(f) = Z(f - f_c) \exp(j\phi) + Z^*(-f - f_c) \exp(-j\phi) \tag{1.4.49}$$

which in the time domain is

$$\begin{aligned} z_M(t) &= z(t) \exp(j(\omega_c t + \phi)) + z^*(t) \exp(-j(\omega_c t + \phi)) \\ &= 2 \operatorname{Re}\{z(t) \exp(j(\omega_c t + \phi))\} = 2\, A_z(t) \cos(\omega_c t + \phi + \phi_z(t)) \end{aligned} \tag{1.4.50}$$

Similarly from (1.4.48)

$$z(t) = z_M(t) \exp(-j(\omega_c t + \phi)) * h_a(t) \tag{1.4.51}$$

where $h_a(t)$ is the IFT of $u(f + f_c)$.

When $z_M(t)$ is a bandpass function, we can replace $u(f)$ by $H_{id}(f - f_c)$ with $B < W < f_c$, as was done in Sections 1.4.1–1.4.5. We can still call $z(t)$ the complex envelope and $A_z(t)$ the envelope of the function $z_M(t)$; however they are not slowly varying functions of time compared with $\cos \omega_c t$, because the bandwidth of $Z(f)$ may be greater than $f_c$.

*Example* 1.4.3 Nonbandpass signal

Let $z_1(t)$ be a real baseband signal with bandwidth $B$. Let

$$z_M(t) = 2\, z_1(t) \cos(\omega_c t + \phi) \tag{1.4.52}$$

with $f_c < B$. The signal $z_M(t)$ is not a bandpass signal as defined in Section 1.4.1 because $f_c < B$, although $Z_M(f) = 0$ for $|f - f_c| > B$. This is

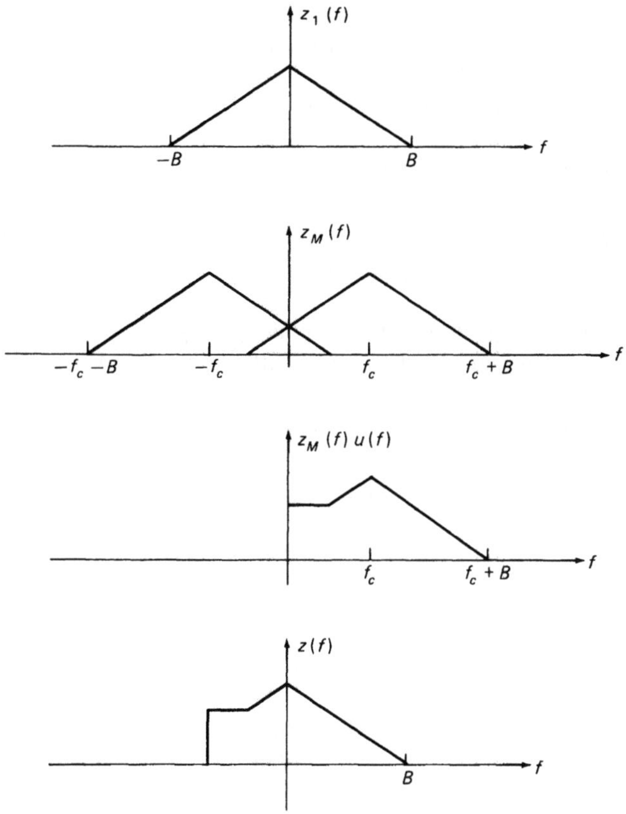


Fig. 1.18. Example of nonbandpass signal and its complex envelope.

illustrated in Fig. 1.18. The envelope of $z_M(t)$ is not $2\,|z_1(t)|$, but rather $|z(t)|$, the FT of which is shown in the figure. Note that $Z(f)$ and $Z_1(f)$ are not identical because $f_c < B$.

In fact $Z_M(f)u(f)$ is the analytic signal derived from $Z_M(f)$

$$2Z_M(f)u(f) = Z_M(f)\{1 + j(-j \, sign \, f)\} \tag{1.4.53}$$

and $Z(f)$ is the baseband equivalent of this analytic signal. All results of this section can be paraphrased in terms of the analytic signal, with the understanding that the complex envelope is the baseband equivalent of the analytic signal. The SSB and VSB filters can also be defined in these terms. In practice, however, we can assume that the signals and filters are bandpass ($f_c > B$) and even narrowband ($f_c \gg B$). The second assumption will imply that

$Z_M(f)$ is symmetric around $f_c$, and thus $z(t)$ is real. For example an upper side band SSB filter is obtained from an arbitrary signal $Z_M(f)$ by

$$Z_{\text{SSB}}(f) = Z_M(f)\{u(f - f_c) + u(-f - f_c)\} \tag{1.4.54}$$

which has a baseband equivalent

$$\begin{aligned} Z(f) &= Z_M(f + f_c)u(f) = 0.5\, Z_M(f + f_c)\{1 + j(-j \operatorname{sign} f)\} \\ &= Z_M(f + f_c)H_{\text{SB}}(f) \end{aligned} \tag{1.4.55}$$

A lower sideband is obtained by replacing $+j$ by $-j$.
Similarly, an upper side band VSB filter is obtained by

$$Z_{\text{VSB}}(f) = Z_M(f)\{H_{\text{VB}}(f - f_c) + H_{\text{VB}}(-f - f_c)\} \tag{1.4.56}$$

which has a baseband equivalent

$$Z(f) = Z_M(f + f_c)H_{\text{VB}}(f) \tag{1.4.57}$$

and

$$H_{\text{VB}}(f) = 1 + jH_{\text{VSB}}(f) \tag{1.4.58}$$

$$H_{\text{VSB}}(f) = \begin{cases} -j \operatorname{sign} f & |f| < f_v \\ -j\, H_{\text{od}}(f) & |f| > f_v \end{cases} \tag{1.4.59}$$

and $H_{\text{od}}(f)$ is an odd function of $f$, such that $H_{\text{od}}(f_v) = 1$, and $f_v$ is a fixed frequency.

## 1.5. RANDOM VARIABLES

### 1.5.1 Sets

Let $\Omega = \{\omega\}$ be a set of elements, called *sample space*. Subsets of $\Omega$ will be denoted by capital letters such as $A$, $B$. $\phi$ is the empty set, i.e., a set with no elements. From two sets we can form the union and intersection

$$B = A_1 \cup A_2 = A_2 \cup A_1 = \{\omega: \omega \in A_1 \text{ or } \omega \in A_2\} \tag{1.5.1}$$

$$C = A_1 \cap A_2 = A_2 \cap A_1 = \{\omega: \omega \in A_1 \text{ and } \omega \in A_2\} \tag{1.5.2}$$

The complementary of $A$ is

$$A^c = \{\omega: \omega \notin A\} \tag{1.5.3}$$

Note that $\Omega$ and $\phi$ are complementary sets. Sets $A_1$ and $A_2$ are disjoint if

$$A_1 \cap A_2 = \phi \tag{1.5.4}$$

Figure 1.19 is a diagram (called a Venn diagram) that shows $\Omega$, sets $A_1$, $A_2$, $A_3$, $A_4$, the union $C = A_3 \cup A_4$, and intersection $B = A_1 \cap A_2$. To simplify notation we shall denote

$$A_1 \cap A_2 = A_1 A_2 \tag{1.5.5}$$

and if the sets are disjoint

$$A_1 \cup A_2 = A_1 + A_2 \tag{1.5.6}$$

In Fig. 1.19, $A_7$ and $A_8$ are disjoint sets, and $D$ is their union. If the set $A$ contains all elements of set $B$, we shall denote

$$B \subset A \tag{1.5.7}$$

In Fig. 1.19 $A_6$ contains $A_5$, and $A_5$ is contained in $A_6$. The following properties can be easily proved (see problem 3.5.1)

$$\begin{aligned}
&\text{a. } A \cup A^c = A + A^c = \Omega \\
&\text{b. } A\phi = \phi \\
&\text{c. } A \cup \phi = A + \phi = A \\
&\text{d. } A\Omega = A \\
&\text{e. } A \cup \Omega = \Omega \\
&\text{f. } AB \subset A,\ AB \subset B \\
&\text{g. } A \cup B \supset A,\ A \cup B \supset B \\
&\text{h. } \phi \subset A \subset \Omega \\
&\text{i. } A \subset B \rightarrow AB = A
\end{aligned} \tag{1.5.8}$$

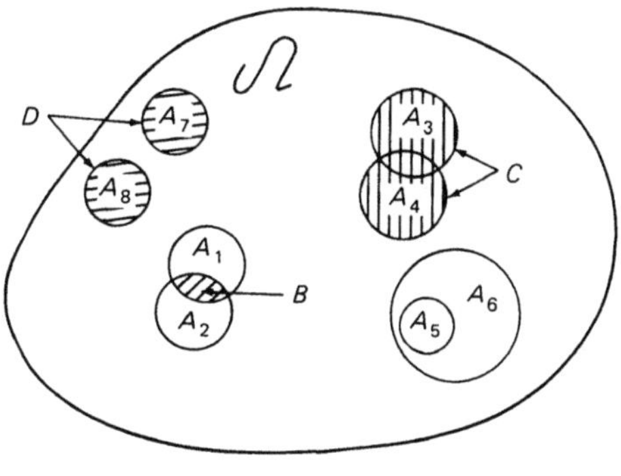


Fig. 1.19. Venn diagram of sets.

A partition of $\Omega$ is a collection of sets $A_1$, $i = 1, 2, \ldots$, such that

$$\sum_i A_1 = \Omega$$

*Example* 1.5.1

$$\begin{aligned}
&\Omega = \{1, 2, 3, 4, 5, 6\}\\
&A_1 = \{1, 2, 3\},\ A_2 = \{2, 3, 5\},\ A_3 = \{5\},\ A_4 = \{4, 5, 6\}\\
&A_1 \cup A_2 = \{1, 2, 3, 5\}\\
&A_1A_2 = \{2, 3\}\\
&A_1A_3 = 0,\ A_4 = A_1^c,\ A_4 \supset A_3,\ A_1 + A_4 = \Omega
\end{aligned}$$

*Example* 1.5.2

$$\begin{aligned}
&\Omega = \{0 \leqq \omega \leqq 5\}\\
&A_1 = \{0 \leqq \omega \leqq 2\} \qquad A_2 = \{1 \leqq \omega \leqq 3\}\\
&A_3 = \{4 \leqq \omega \leqq 5\} \qquad A_4 = \{2 \leqq \omega \leqq 5\}\\
&A_1 \cup A_2 = \{0 \leqq \omega < 3\}\\
&A_1A_2 = \{1 \leqq \omega < 2\}\\
&A_4 = A_1^c \qquad A_3 \subset A_4\\
&A_1 + A_4 = \Omega
\end{aligned}$$

### 1.5.2 Events and probabilities

Let $S$ be a collection of subsets of $\Omega$ including $\Omega$ and $\phi$ and such that if $A$, $B$ are in $S$ so are $AB$ and $A \cup B$. The elements of $S$ are called *events*. To each event, say $A$, we assign a nonnegative number between 0 and 1 called *probability*, $P(A)$, with the following properties

$$\begin{aligned}
&\text{a. } 0 \leqq P(A) \leqq 1\\
&\text{b. } P(\Omega) = 1\\
&\text{c. If } A, B \text{ are disjoint } P(A + B) = P(A) + P(B)
\end{aligned} \tag{1.5.9}$$

These properties imply

$$\begin{aligned}
&\text{a. } P(A^c) = 1 - P(A)\\
&\text{b. } P(\phi) = 0\\
&\text{c. } A \subset B \rightarrow P(A) \leqq P(B)\\
&\text{d. } P(A \cup B) = P(A) + P(B) - P(AB)\\
&\text{e. } P\left(\sum_1^N A_i\right) = \sum_1^N P(A_i)
\end{aligned} \tag{1.5.10}$$

We shall denote

$$P(AB) = P(A, B) \tag{1.5.11}$$

*Example* 1.5.3

$$\begin{aligned}
&\Omega = \{1, 2, 3, 4, 5, 6\} \\
&A = \{1, 2\} \qquad B = \{3, 4, 5, 6\} \\
&S = \{\Omega, \phi, A, B\} \\
&P(A) = 0.2 \qquad P(B) = 0.8
\end{aligned}$$

*Example* 1.5.4

$$\Omega = \{a \leqq \omega \leqq b\}, \qquad a \leqq a_1 \leqq b_1 \leqq b$$

Let $S$ be the collection of all subsets of $\Omega$, and let the probability of

$$A = \{a_1 \leqq \omega \leqq b_1\}, \qquad a \leqq a_1 \leqq b_1 \leqq b$$

be

$$P(A) = \frac{b_1 - a_1}{b - a}$$

In fact here we have

$$P(A) = \int_{\omega \in A} f(\omega)\, d\omega$$

where

$$f(\omega) = \begin{cases} (b - a)^{-1} & a \leqq \omega \leqq b \\ 0 & \text{otherwise} \end{cases}$$

In fact we can select any function $0 \leqq f(\omega)$, such that

$$\int_a^b f(\omega)\, d\omega = 1$$

The *conditional probability* of $A$ with respect to $B$ is defined as

$$P(A|B) = \frac{P(A, B)}{P(B)} \tag{1.5.12}$$

if $P(B) \neq 0$. Thus

$$P(A, B) = P(A|B)P(B) = P(B|A)P(A) \tag{1.5.13}$$

This equation is called *Bayes rule*. From (1.5.13)

$$P(A|B) = \frac{P(B|A)P(A)}{P(B)} \tag{1.5.14}$$

$A$ and $B$ are *statistically independent* if

$$P(A|B) = P(A) \rightarrow P(A, B) = P(A)P(B) \tag{1.5.15}$$

The implications of (1.5.12)–(1.5.15) are

a. $B \subset A \rightarrow P(A|B) = 1$ (1.5.16)

thus

$$P(A|A) = 1 \tag{1.5.17}$$

b. $P(A|B) = P(A) \rightarrow P(B|A) = P(B)$

c. Let $A_i$, $i = 1, \ldots, n$ be a partition of $A \supset B$; then

$$1 = P(A|B) = P\left(\sum_1^n A_i|B\right) = \sum_1^n P(A_i|B) \tag{1.5.18}$$

and the conditional probability has all properties of a probability.

d. Let $\sum_1^n B_i \supset B$; then

$$B = B\left(\sum_1^n B_i\right) = \sum_1^n BB_i \tag{1.5.19}$$

and

$$P(B) = P\left(\sum_1^n BB_i\right) = \sum_1^n P(B, B_i) = \sum_1^n P(B|B_i)P(B_i) \tag{1.5.20}$$

Thus from (1.5.14)

$$P(A|B) = \frac{P(B|A)P(A)}{\sum_1^n P(B|B_i)P(B_i)} \tag{1.5.21}$$

which is another form of the Bayes rule. Particularly with $A = B_i$

$$P(B_i|B) = \frac{P(B|B_i)P(B_i)}{\sum_{1}^{n} P(B|B_i)P(B_i)} \tag{1.5.22}$$

*Example* 1.5.5
Let $\Omega$ be the collection of points

$$\Omega = \{\omega_{i,j} = (a_i, R_j): i = 1, 2, \ldots, N, j = 1, 2, \ldots, M\}$$

and let $S$ be the collection of all subsets of $\Omega$ including $\Omega$ and $\phi$. The sets $A_i = \{a_i\}$ $i = 1, \ldots, N$ is a partition of $\Omega$, and also the sets $B_j = \{R_j\}, j = 1, \ldots, M$ is a partition of $\Omega$, as can be seen in Fig. 1.20 for $N = 2, M = 3$. We assign probabilities $P(a_i)$ and conditional probabilities $P(R_j|a_i)$. We can compute

| | $R_1$ | $R_2$ | $R_3$ |
|---|---|---|---|
| $a_1$ | $(a_1, R_1)$ | $(a_1, R_2)$ | $(a_1, R_3)$ |
| $a_2$ | $(a_2, R_1)$ | $(a_2, R_2)$ | $(a_2, R_3)$ |

Fig. 1.20. A two-dimensional sample space.

$$P(a_i|R_j) = \frac{P(a_i, R_j)}{P(R_j)} = \frac{P(R_j|a_i)P(a_i)}{\sum_{i=1}^{N} P(R_j|a_i)P(a_i)} \tag{1.5.23}$$

This example illustrates a digital communications system with input symbols $\{a_i\}$ and output decision intervals $\{R_j\}$. $P(a_i)$ is here the a priori probability of symbol $a_i$, and $P(a_i|R_j)$ is the a posteriori probability of $a_i$, i.e., after it is known that the output is in interval $R_j$.

### 1.5.3 Random variable

A mapping or function from $\Omega$ to the real line

$$x = x(\omega), \ -\infty < x < \infty \tag{1.5.24}$$

is called a *random variable* (rv). Usually we shall suppress for notational conveniences the dependence on $\omega$. The rv generates events in $S$, whose probabilities we can compute. For example $\{a_1 \leqq x \leqq a_2\}$ generates the event $A = \{\omega: a_1 \leqq x(\omega) \leqq a_2\}$; hence they have the same probability

$$P(a_1 \leqq x \leqq a_2) = P\{\omega: a_1 \leqq x(\omega) \leqq a_2\} \qquad (1.5.25)$$

where for notational convenience we adopted the convention

$$P(\{\text{event}\}) = P\{\text{event}\} = P(\text{event}) \qquad (1.5.26)$$

The probability of the events

$$\{\omega: -\infty < x(\omega) \leqq a\} = \{\omega: x(\omega) \leqq a\}$$

as a function of $a$ is called the ***probability distribution function*** (PDF) of $x$ and is denoted by

$$F_x(a) \,\Delta\, P(x \leqq a) = P\{\omega: x(\omega) \leqq a\} \qquad (1.5.27)$$

*Example* 1.5.6
Let

$$\Omega = \{\omega_1, \omega_2, \omega_3, \omega_4\}$$

and let the rv be as shown in Fig. 1.21, i.e.

$$x(\omega_1) = -3,\ x(\omega_2) = 4,\ x(\omega_3) = 0,\ x(\omega_4) = -3$$

with probabilities

$$P\{\omega_1\} = 1/2,\ P\{\omega_2\} = 1/4,\ P\{\omega_3\} = P\{\omega_4\} = 1/8$$

we obtain

$$\begin{aligned}
P(x < -3) &= P\{\omega: x(\omega) < -3\} = 0 \\
P(x \leqq -3) &= P(x < 0) = P\{\omega: x(\omega) < 0\} = P\{\omega_1 + \omega_4\} \\
&= P\{\omega_1\} + P\{\omega_4\} = 1/2 + 1/8 = 5/8 \\
P(x \leqq 0) &= P(x < 4) = P\{\omega: x(\omega) < 4\} = P\{\omega_1 + \omega_4 + \omega_3\} \\
&= P\{\omega_1\} + P\{\omega_4\} + P\{\omega_3\} = 6/8 = 3/4 \\
P(x \leqq 4) &= P(x < \infty) = P\{\omega: x(\omega) < \infty\} = P\{\omega_1 + \omega_4 + \omega_3 + \omega_2\} \\
&= P(\Omega) = 1
\end{aligned}$$

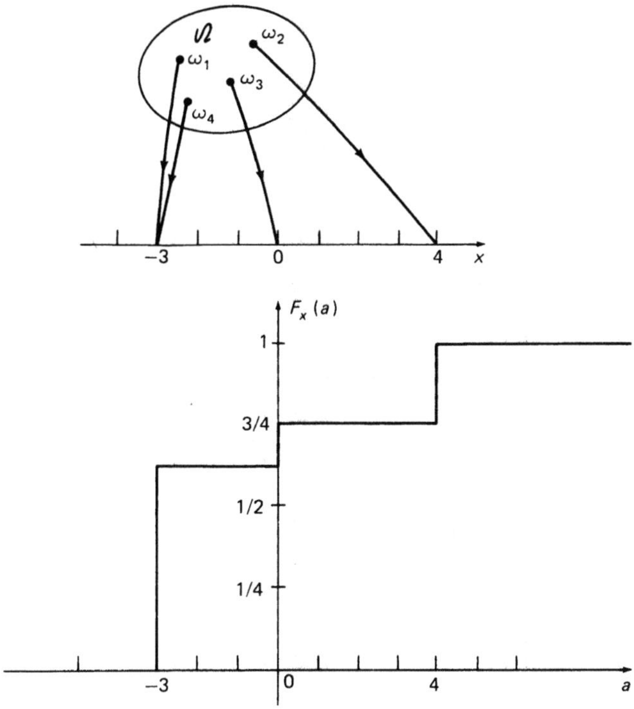


Fig. 1.21. Illustration of radom variable.

The following properties of PDF follow from the definition (1.5.27)

$$\begin{aligned}&\text{a. } 0 \leqq F_x(a) \leqq 1\\&\text{b. } F_x(-\infty) = 0\\&\text{c. } F_x(\infty) = 1\\&\text{d. } a_1 < a_2 \rightarrow F_x(a_1) \leqq F_x(a_2)\end{aligned} \tag{1.5.28}$$

The *complementary probability density function* (CPDF) is defined by

$$Q_x(a) = P(x > a) = 1 - F_x(a) \tag{1.5.29}$$

The *probability density function* (pdf) is defined as

$$p_x(a) = \frac{dF_x(a)}{da} \tag{1.5.30}$$

If $F_x(a)$ is continuous at point $a_1$, $p_x(a_1)$ is finite, and if $F_x(a)$ has a discontinuity of step $P_1$ at point $a_1$, $p_x(a)$ is an impulse at that point with

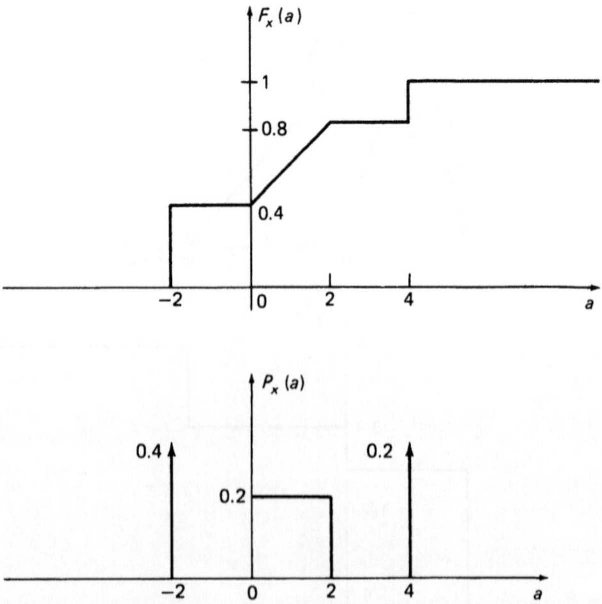


Fig. 1.22. Probability distribution function and probability density function.

value $P_1$, i.e.

$$p_x(a_1) = P_1\delta(a - a_1) \tag{1.5.31}$$

*Example* 1.5.7
Figure 1.22 shows a PDF and the corresponding pdf. In this example the pdf is

$$p_x(a) = 0.4\ \delta(a + 2) + 0.2\ \{u(a) - u(a - 2)\} + 0.2\ \delta(a - 4)$$

It follows from (1.5.27) and (1.5.30) that the pdf has the following properties

a. $p_x(a) \geqq 0$

b. $$F_x(a) = \int_{-\infty}^{a} p_x(a_1)\, da_1 \tag{1.5.32}$$

c. $$\int_{-\infty}^{\infty} p_x(a)\, da = 1$$

d. $P(a_1 \leqq x \leqq a_2) = \int_{a_1}^{a_2} p_x(a)\, da = F_x(a_2) - F_x(a_1)$

$x$ is a *symmetric* random variable if $p_x(a)$ is an even function. $x$ is a *discrete* rv (drv) if $p_x(a)$ is a sum of impulse functions

$$p_x(a) = \sum_{i=1}^{N} P_i\, \delta(a - a_i) \tag{1.5.33}$$

where $N$ may be infinite. For a discrete random variable

$$P(x = a_i) = \lim_{\Delta \to 0} P(a_i - \Delta < x < a_i + \Delta)$$

$$= \lim_{\Delta \to 0} \int_{a_i - \Delta}^{a_i + \Delta} p_x(a)\, da = P_i \lim_{\Delta \to 0} \int_{a_i - \Delta}^{a_i + \Delta} \delta(a - a_i)\, da = P_i \tag{1.5.34}$$

and from (1.5.32)

$$\sum_{i=1}^{N} P_i = 1 \tag{1.5.35}$$

For a drv it will be more convenient in some cases to deal with $\{a_i\}$ and $\{P_i\}$ rather then with $p_x(a)$. The set $\{P_i\}$ are the probabilities of $x$. A constant $x = a_1$ can be viewed as a drv with one value and $P(x = a_1) = 1$. $x$ is a *continuous* rv (crv) if $p_x(a)$ is finite for all $a$. For a crv

$$P(a = a_i) = \lim_{\Delta \to 0} P\{a_i - \Delta < x < a_i + \Delta\}$$

$$= \lim_{\Delta \to 0} \int_{a_i - \Delta}^{a_i + \Delta} p_x(a)\, da = \lim_{\Delta \to 0} p_x(a_i) 2\Delta = 0 \tag{1.5.36}$$

i.e., the probability of a single value is zero. If a rv is not discrete and not continuous, it is *mixed.* We say that $x$ and $y$ are identically distributed rvs if their pdf is identical.

Table 1.6 presents some useful probability density functions.

## Table 1.6 Probability density functions

| $p_x(a)$ | SKETCH | NAME |
|---|---|---|
| $(a_2 - a_1)^{-1}(u(a - a_1) - u(a - a_2))$ | 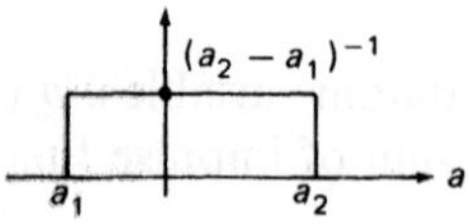  | uniform |
| $\lambda \exp(-\lambda a)u(a)$ | 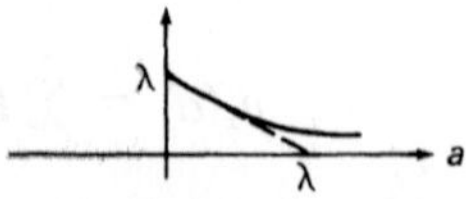  | exponential |
| $(a/\lambda^2) \exp(-0.5\, a^2/\lambda^2)u(a)$ | 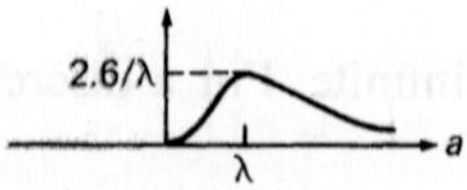  | Rayleigh |
| $(2\pi)^{-1/2} \exp(-a^2/2)$ | 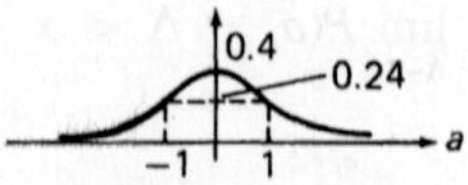  | Normal |
| $(2\pi\sigma^2)^{-1/2} \exp(-0.5(a - m)^2/\sigma^2)$ | 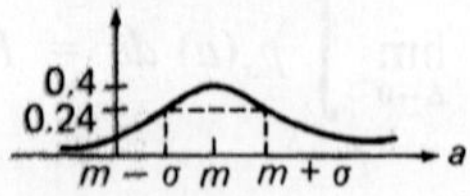  | Gaussian |
| $0.5\lambda \exp(-\lambda\lvert a\rvert)$ | 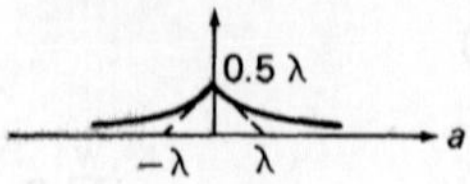  | Laplace |
| $\exp(-\lambda) \sum_{i=1}^{\infty} \lambda^i/i!\,\delta(a - i)$ | 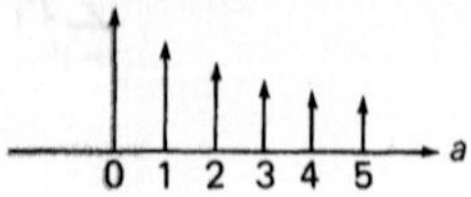  | Poisson |
| $N^{-1} \sum_{i=1}^{N} \delta(a - i)$ | 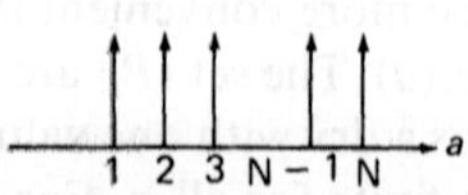  | uniform |
| $2^{-N} \sum_{i=1}^{N} \binom{N}{i} \delta(a - i)$ | 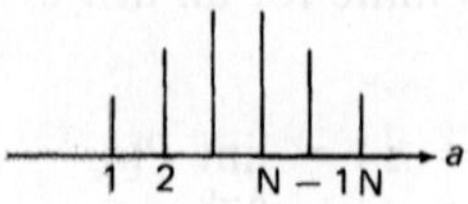  | binomial |
| $P\delta(a - a_1) + (1 - P)\delta(a - a_2)$ | 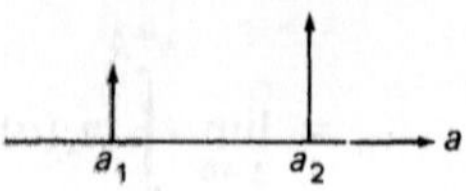  | binary |

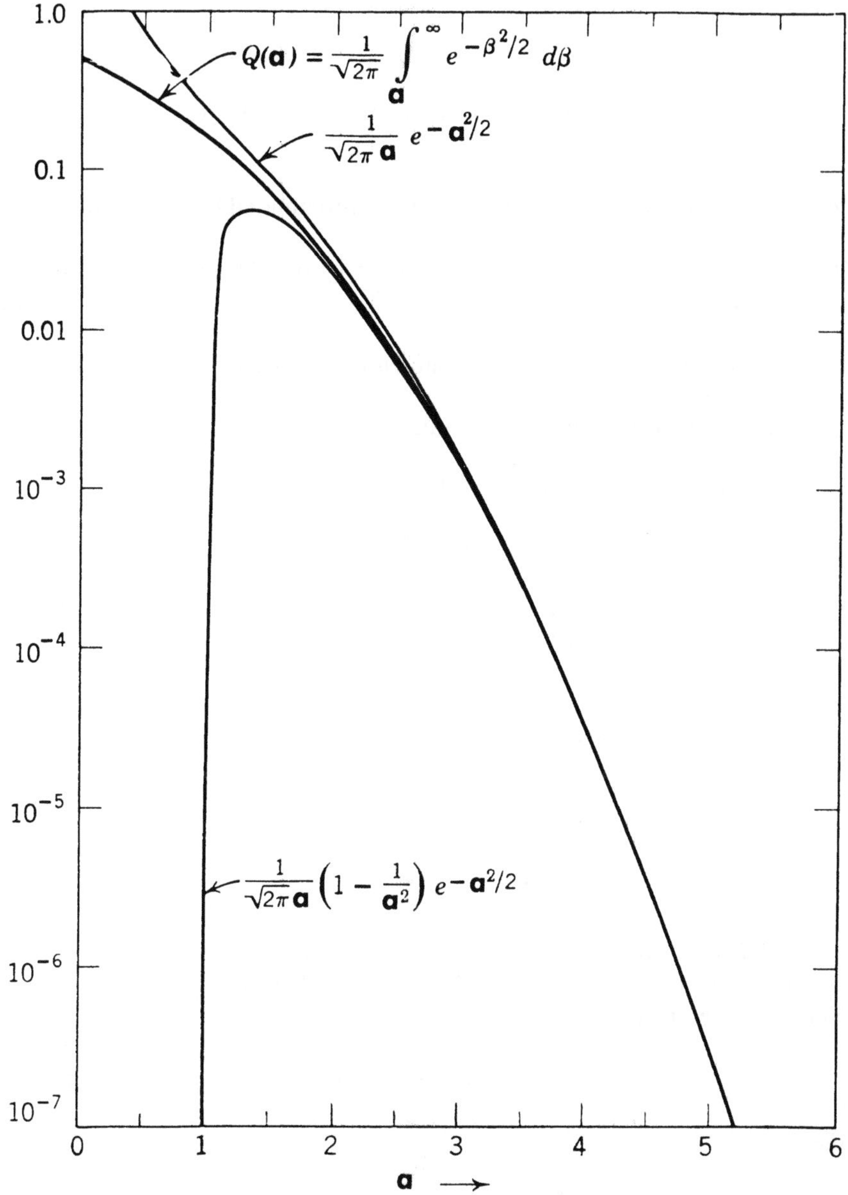


Fig. 1.23. Bounds to normal complementary probability distribution function.

The CPDF of the normal rv is

$$Q_x(a) = (2\,\pi)^{-1} \int_a^{\infty} \exp(-0.5\, a_1^2) da_1 = Q(a) \qquad (1.5.37)$$

$Q(a)$ is not a simple function, but it can be approximated by (see Problem 1.5)

$$\begin{aligned} Q_L(a) &= (1 - a^{-2})(2\,\pi a^2)^{-1/2} \exp(-0.5\, a^2) < Q(a) < (2\,\pi a^2)^{-1/2} \exp(-0.5\, a^2) \\ &= Q_U(a) \end{aligned} \qquad (1.5.38)$$

The bounds and the true value are shown in Fig. 1.23.

### 1.5.4 Function of random variable

Let $x$ be a rv with pdf $p_x(a)$, and let

$$y = f(x) \qquad (1.5.39)$$

Then $y$ is also a rv providing $\{y \leqq b\}$ are events and the pdf of $y$ is $p_y(b)$. To find $p_y(b)$, we first compute the PDF

$$F_y(b) = p(y \leqq b) = P\{x: f(x) \leqq b\} = \int_{X_b} p_x(a)\, da \qquad (1.5.40)$$

where

$$X_b = \{x: f(x) \leqq b\} \qquad (1.5.41)$$

and then take the derivative. If $f(x)$ is a continuous, increasing function of $x$, then $y = b$ corresponds to $a = f^{-1}(b) = g(b)$, where $x = g(y)$ is the inverse function. Therefore

$$X_b = \{x: x \leqq a\} \qquad (1.5.42)$$

and

$$p_y(b) = \frac{d}{db} \int_{-\infty}^{a} p_x(a_1)\, da_1 = p_x(a) \frac{da}{db} = \left. \frac{p_x(a)}{\dot{f}(a)} \right|_{a = g(b)} \qquad (1.5.43)$$

Similarly if $f(x)$ is a continuous but decreasing function of $x$, (1.5.43) is valid with $\dot{f}(a)$ replaced by its absolute value, because the pdf is nonnegative ($\dot{f}(x)$ is the derivative of $f(x)$).

*Example* 1.5.8 Gaussian rv
Let $x$ be a Gaussian rv, i.e.

$$p_x(a) = (2\,\pi\sigma_x^2)^{-1/2} \exp\left(-\frac{1}{2}\frac{(a - m_x)^2}{\sigma^2{}_x}\right)$$

and let

$$y = f(x) = \alpha x + \beta$$

Thus

$$x = g(y) = (y - \beta)/\alpha \rightarrow a = (b - \beta)/\alpha$$

Substitution into (1.5.43) leads to

$$p_y(b) = (2\,\pi\sigma_x^2\alpha^2)^{-1/2} \exp\left\{-\frac{1}{2}\frac{(b - \beta - \alpha m_x)^2}{(\sigma_x\alpha)^2}\right\}$$

$$= (2\,\pi\sigma_y^2)^{-1/2} \exp\left\{-\frac{1}{2}\frac{(b - m_y)^2}{\sigma_y^2}\right\} \tag{1.5.44}$$

with

$$m_y = \alpha m_x + \beta$$

$$\sigma_y^2 = (\alpha\sigma_x)^2$$

which shows that a linear function of a Gaussian rv is also a Gaussian rv.

If $x$ is a drv with values $a_i = 1, 2, \ldots N$ then $y = f(x)$ is also a drv. Let $a_i$, $i = 1, 2, \ldots, K \leqq N$ be the values of $x$ for which $y = f(a_i) = b_j$; then

$$P(y = b_j) = P\{x\colon f(x) = b_j\} = \sum_1^K P(a_i) \tag{1.5.45}$$

If $f(x)$ is in addition a 1 to 1 mapping, then for each value of $x = a_i$, there is one value of $y = f(a_i) = b_i$ and

$$P(y = b_i) = P(x = a_i) \tag{1.5.46}$$

$x$ may be a crv, and $y$ may be a drv. For example, if the interval $a_1 \leqq x \leqq a_2$ is mapped into a single point $y = b$, then

$$P(y = b) = \int_{a_1}^{a_2} p_x(a)\, da$$

*Example* 1.5.9 Discrete transformation
Let

$$y = b \text{ sign } x$$

then $y$ is a drv with two values $b_1 = -b$, $b_2 = b$ and

$$P(y = -b) = P(x \leq 0) = \int_{-\infty}^{0} p_x(a)\, da$$

$$P(y = b) = P(x > 0) = \int_{0}^{\infty} p_x(a)\, da$$

## 1.5.5 Averages

The *average* value (*mean* value, *expected value*) of the rv $y$ is

$$E(y) = \bar{y} = \int_{-\infty}^{\infty} b p_y(b)\, db \tag{1.5.47}$$

We would like to express the average value of $y = f(x)$ in terms of the pdf $p_x(a)$. The result is

$$\bar{y} = \int_{-\infty}^{\infty} f(a) p_x(a)\, da \tag{1.5.48}$$

which for a drv can be written as

$$\bar{y} = \sum_i f(a_i) P(x = a_i) \tag{1.5.49}$$

which we shall prove for decreasing or increasing functions only.

*Proof*
a. If $x$ is a drv and $b_i = f(a_i)$, then

$$\bar{y} = \sum_i b_i P(y = b_i) = \sum_i b_i P(x = a_i) = \sum_i f(a_i) P(a_i)$$

b. If $x$ is a crv, we partition the real line with intervals defined by $|x - a_i| \leqq \Delta/2$, $a_{i+1} = a_i + \Delta$ and $b_i = f(a_i)$. Thus

$$\bar{y} = \int_{-\infty}^{\infty} b p_y(b)\, db = \lim_{\Delta \to 0} \sum_i b_i P(y = b_i)$$

$$= \lim_{\Delta \to 0} \sum_i b_i P(|x - a_i| \leqq \Delta/2)$$

$$= \lim_{\Delta \to 0} \sum_i f(a_i) \int_{a_i - \Delta/2}^{a_i + \Delta/2} p_x(a)\, da = \int_{-\infty}^{\infty} f(a) p_x(a)\, da$$

The average value of a constant $x = a_1$ is $a_1$. The $k$ th moment of $x$ is defined as

$$E(x^k) = \int_{-\infty}^{\infty} a^k p_x(a)\, da \tag{1.5.50}$$

which for a drv is simplified to

$$E(x^k) = \sum_{i=1}^{N} a^k{}_i P(a_i) \tag{1.5.51}$$

The first moment is the same as the average value and is denoted by $m_x$. The second moment is also called the *mean square value*. The $k$th *central moment* is defined as

$$E(x - m_x)^k = \int_{-\infty}^{\infty} (a - m_x)^k p_x(a)\, da \tag{1.5.52}$$

The second central moment is called the *variance*

$$\sigma_x^2 = E(x - m_x)^2$$

and $\sigma_x$ is also called the *standard deviation* or *dispersion* of $x$.

If $x$ is a symmetric rv and $y = f(x)$ is an odd function of $x$, then $\bar{y} = 0$. The characteristic function of $x$ is the average value of exp $(jxv)$, i.e., is the IFT of the pdf (with $v = 2\pi f$)

$$C_x(v) = \overline{\exp(jxv)} = \int_{-\infty}^{\infty} p_x(a) \exp(jav)\, da \tag{1.5.53}$$

thus $p_x(a)$ and $C_x(v)$ are a FT pair. Note that

$$\frac{d^k C_x(v)}{du^k} = \int_{-\infty}^{\infty} (ja)^k \exp(jav) p_x(a)\, da \tag{1.5.54}$$

$$\frac{d^k C_x}{dv^k}(v = 0) = \overline{j^k x^k} \tag{1.5.55}$$

Thus

$$\overline{x^k} = j^{-k} \frac{d^k C_x}{dv^k}(0) \tag{1.5.56}$$

and we can obtain all moments from the derivative of the characteristic function.

*Example* 1.5.10 Average, variance, and characteristic function of Gaussian rv
Let $x$ be a Gaussian random variable with

$$p_x(a) = (2\pi b^2)^{-1/2} \exp(-0.5\, a^2 (a - c)^2/b^2)$$

The average value is

$$m_x = \int_{-\infty}^{\infty} a (2\pi b^2)^{-1/2} \exp(-0.5\,(a - c)^2/b^2)\, da$$

changing variables

$$z = (a - c)/b$$

$$m_x = \int_{-\infty}^{\infty} (2\pi)^{-1/2}(c + bz) \exp(-z^2/2)\, dz = c \int_{-\infty}^{\infty} (2\pi)^{-1/2} \exp(-z^2/2)\, dz$$

$$+\, b \int_{-\infty}^{\infty} z (2\pi)^{-1/2} \exp(-z^2/2)\, dz = c + 0 = c$$

This is the result, because the first integral is the total integral of a pdf (the normal pdf), which is 1, and the second integral is 0 because $z$ is odd, the pdf is even, and their product is an odd function of $z$.

The variance is

$$\sigma_x^2 = (2\,\pi b^2)^{-1/2} \int_{-\infty}^{\infty} (a - c)^2 \exp\,(-0.5\,(a - c)^2/b^2)\, da$$

$$= (2\,\pi)^{-1/2}\, b^2 \int_{-\infty}^{\infty} z^2 \exp\,(-z^2/2)\, dz$$

Because

$$\int_{-\infty}^{\infty} \exp\,(-\alpha z^2/2)\, dz = (2\,\pi/\alpha)^{1/2}$$

the first derivative with respect to $\alpha$ at $\alpha = 1$ is

$$-\int_{-\infty}^{\infty} z^2 \exp\,(-0.5\, z^2)/2\, dz = -0.5\,(2\,\pi)^{1/2}$$

hence

$$\sigma_x^2 = b^2$$

The characteristic function of a normal rv, $n$, is from Table 1.1

$$C_n(v) = \exp\,(-v^2/2)$$

Because $x$ is related to $n$ by

$$x = bn + c$$

we obtain

$$\begin{aligned} C_x(v) &= \overline{\exp\,\{jv(bn + c)\}} = \exp\,(jvc)\,\overline{\exp\,(jvbn)} \\ &= \exp\,(jvc)C_n(vb) = \exp\,(jvc)\exp\,(-v^2b^2/2) \end{aligned}$$

## 1.6 TWO RANDOM VARIABLES

### 1.6.1 Definition and probabilities

We can associate with $\Omega$ and $S$ two rvs, $x_1(\omega)$ and $x_2(\omega)$, which define events in $S$. For example, let for $i = 1, 2$

$$A_i = \{\omega\colon a_{i1} \leqq x_i(\omega) \leqq a_{i2}\} = \{x_i\colon a_{i1} \leqq x_i \leqq a_{i2}\} \qquad (1.6.1)$$

and let $A$ be the joint event

$$A = A_1 A_2 = \{\omega: a_{11} \leqq x_1 \leqq a_{12}, \quad a_{21} \leqq x_2 \leqq a_{22}\} \quad (1.6.2)$$

where the comma has here the same meaning as the logical and ($\cap$) statement. The probability of the event is well defined

$$P(A) = P(A_1 A_2) \quad (1.6.3)$$

The probability of the joint event

$$\{\omega: x_1 \leqq a_1, \quad x_2 \leqq a_2\} \quad (1.6.4)$$

as a function of $a_1$, $a_2$ is called the *joint PDF*

$$F_{x1,x2}(a_1, a_2) = P\{\omega: x_1 \leqq a_1, \quad x_2 \leqq a_2\} \quad (1.6.5)$$

and the order is not important, i.e.

$$F_{x1,x2}(a_1, a_2) = F_{x2,x1}(a_2, a_1) \quad (1.6.6)$$

The joint PDF has the following properties

a. $0 \leqq F_{x1,x2}(a_1, a_2) \leqq 1$
b. $F_{x1,x2}(\infty, \infty) = 1$
c. $F_{x1,x2}(a_1, a_2) = 0$ if either $a_1$ or $a_2$ or both are $-\infty$
d. Let $b_1 \geqq a_1$ and $b_2 \geqq a_2$, then

$$F_{x1,x2}(b_1, b_2) \geqq F_{x1,x2}(a_1, a_2) \quad (1.6.7)$$

e. $F_{x1,x2}(a_1, \infty) = F_{x1}(a_1)$, $F_{x1,x2}(\infty, a_2) = F_{x2}(a_2)$

Property (d) states that the joint PDF is a nondecreasing function of its arguments, and property (e) states that we can obtain the marginal PDF from the joint PDF by substitution of $\infty$ for the eliminated rv.

The *joint pdf* is defined as

$$p_{x1,x2}(a_1, a_2) = \frac{\partial^2 F_{x1,x2}(a_1, a_2)}{\partial a_1 \partial a_2} \quad (1.6.8)$$

hence

$$F_{x1,x2}(a_1, a_2) = \int_{-a}^{a_1}\int_{-a}^{a_2} p_{x1,x2}(b_1, b_2)\, db_1\, db_2 \quad (1.6.9)$$

The joint pdf has the following properties

a. $0 \leqq p_{x1,x2}(a_1, a_2)$

b. $$\int_{-\infty}^{\infty}\int_{-\infty}^{\infty} p_{x1,x2}(a_1, a_2)\, da_1\, da_2 = 1$$

c. $$p_1(a_1) = \int_{-\infty}^{\infty} p_{x1,x2}(a_1, a_2)\, da_2 \tag{1.6.10}$$

$$p_{x2}(a_2) = \int_{-\infty}^{\infty} p_{x1,x2}(a_1, a_2)\, da_1$$

*Example* 1.6.1 Jointly Gaussian rvs

$$p_{x1,x2}(a_1, a_2) = \{2\,\pi\sigma^2(1 + \rho^2)^{1/2}\}^{-1} \exp\left\{-\frac{1}{2}\frac{a_1^2 - 2\,\rho a_1 a_2 + a_2^2}{\sigma^2(1 - \rho^2)}\right\}$$

$$p_{xi}(a_i) = (2\,\pi\sigma^2)^{-1/2} \exp\,(-a_i^2/2\,\sigma^2) \qquad i = 1, 2$$

The rvs may be discrete, continuous, or mixed. If $x_1$ and $x_2$ are discrete (continuous), the joint pdf is also discrete (continuous).

*Example* 1.6.2 Discrete rvs
Let $x_1$ have $K_1$ values and $x_2$ have $K_2$ values.

$$p_{x1,x2}(a_1, a_2) = \sum_{i=1}^{K_1}\sum_{j=1}^{K_2} P_{ij}\delta(a_1 - a_{1i})\delta(a_2 - a_{2j})$$

The probabilities are

$$P(x_1 = a_{1i}, x_2 = a_{2j}) = P_{ij}$$

$$P(x_I = a_{1i}) = \sum_{j=1}^{K_2} P_{ij},\ P(x_2 = a_{2j}) = \sum_{i=1}^{K_1} P_{ij}$$

$$\sum_{i=1}^{K_1}\sum_{i=2}^{K_2} P_{ij} = 1$$

The PDF of $x_1$ conditioned on event $A_2$ is

$$F_{x1,x2}(a_1|A_2) = \frac{P\{x_1 \leqq a_1, A_2\}}{P(A_2)} = \frac{\int_{-\infty}^{a_1}\int_{A_2} p_{x1,x2}(b_1, b_2)\, db_1\, db_2}{\int_{A_2} p_{x2}(b_2)\, db_2} \tag{1.6.11}$$

and the pdf of $x_1$ conditioned on event $A_2$ is the derivative with respect to $a_1$

$$p_{x1,x2}(a_1|A_2) = \frac{\int_{A_2} p_{x1,x2}(a_1, b_2)\, db_2}{\int_{A_2} p_{x2}(b_2)\, db_2} \tag{1.6.12}$$

Particularly if $A_2 = \{x_2 \leqq a_2\}$, we can write

$$F_{x1,x2}(a_1|A_2) = F_{x1,x2}(a_1|a_2) = \frac{F_{x1,x2}(a_1, a_2)}{F_{x2}(a_2)} \tag{1.6.13}$$

If, on the other hand

$$A_2 = \{a_2 \leqq x_2 \leqq a_2 + \Delta\}$$

then

$$p_{x1,x2}(a_1|a_2) = \lim_{\Delta \to 0} p_{x1|x2}(a_1|A_2) = \frac{p_{x1,x2}(a_1, a_2)}{p_{x2}(a_2)} \tag{1.6.14}$$

From the last equation we obtain Bayes' rule for rvs

$$p_{x1|x2}(a_1|a_2)p_{x2}(a_2) = p_{x2|x1}(a_2|a_1)p_{x1}(a_1) \tag{1.6.15}$$

since

$$p_{x1}(a_1) = \int_{-\infty}^{\infty} p_{x1,x2}(a_1, a_2)\, da_2 = \int_{-\infty}^{\infty} p_{x2|x1}(a_2|a_1)p_{x1}(a_1)\, da_1 \tag{1.6.16}$$

we obtain

$$p_{x1,x2}(a_1|a_2) = \frac{p_{x2|x1}(a_2|a_1)p_{x1}(a_1)}{\displaystyle\int_{-\infty}^{\infty} p_{x2|x1}(a_2|a_1)p_{x1}(a_1)\,da_1} \tag{1.6.17}$$

When one of the rvs is discrete, the pdf for this rv may be replaced by probabilities.

*Example* 1.6.3 Binary communication system
Let $x_1 = \pm a$ be a drv with $P(x_1 = a) = P_1$ and $P(x_1 = -a) = P_2 = 1 - P_1$. Let

$$p_{x2|x1}(a_2|a_1) = (2\pi\sigma^2)^{-1/2} \exp\left(-\frac{1}{2}\frac{(a_2 - a_1)^2}{\sigma^2}\right)$$

To compute $P(x_1 = a|x_2 = a_2)$, we write

$$P(x_1 = a|x_2 = a_2) = \frac{p_{x2|x1}(a_2|a)P(x_1 = a)}{p_{x2|x1}(a_2|a)P(x_1 = a) + p_{x2|x1}(a_2|-a)P(x_1 = -a)}$$

$$= \frac{P_1 \exp\left(-\frac{1}{2}\frac{(a_2 - a)^2}{\sigma^2}\right)}{P_1 \exp\left(-\frac{1}{2}\frac{(a_2 - a)^2}{\sigma^2}\right) + P_2 \exp\left(-\frac{1}{2}\frac{(a_2 + a)^2}{\sigma^2}\right)}$$

$$= \frac{P_1 \exp(aa_2/\sigma^2)}{P_1 \exp(aa_2/\sigma^2) + P_2 \exp(-aa_2/\sigma^2)}$$

Particularly when $P_1 = P_2 = 1/2$, the result is

$$P(x_1 = a|x_2 = a_2) = (1 + \exp(-2\,aa_2/\sigma^2)^{-1})$$

In many cases it is inconvenient to have one symbol for the name of the rv, say $x_2$, and another symbol for its values, say $a_2$. If there is no confusion, we shall use the same symbol for both. Thus in the last example we would write

$$P(x_1 = a|x_2) = \{1 + \exp(-2\,ax_2/\sigma^2)\}^{-1}$$

and we emphasize the fact here that the conditional probability is a rv, because it depends on $x_2$.

$x_1$ and $x_2$ are *independent random variables* if

$$p_{x1,x2}(a_1, a_2) = p_{x1}(a_1)p_{x2}(a_2) \tag{1.6.18}$$

This implies that

$$P(A_1, A_2) = P(A_1)P(A_2) \tag{1.6.19}$$

hence

$$F_{x1,x2}(a_1, a_2) = F_{x1}(a_1)F_{x2}(a_2) \tag{1.6.20}$$

and from (1.6.14)

$$p_{x1|x2}(a_1|a_2) = p_{x1}(a_1) \tag{1.6.21}$$

The rvs in example 1.6.1 are dependent, but if we substitute $\rho = 0$ they become independent.

### 1.6.2 Averages

Let $f(x_1, x_2)$ be a function of $x_1, x_2$. The average of the function is denoted by $E\{f(x_1, x_2)\}$ or by $\overline{f(x_1, x_2)}$ and is defined by

$$\overline{f(x_1, x_2)} = \int_{-\infty}^{\infty}\int_{-\infty}^{\infty} f(a_1, a_2)p_{x1,x2}(a_1, a_2)\, da_1\, da_2 \tag{1.6.22}$$

The joint $k$, $r$ moment is defined as

$$m_{k,r} = \overline{x^k{}_1 x^r{}_2} \tag{1.6.23}$$

The joint $k$, $r$ central moment is defined as

$$\mu_{k,r} = E\{(x_i - m_i)^k(x_2 - m_2)^r\} \tag{1.6.24}$$

where

$$m_i = E(x_i) \qquad i = 1, 2 \tag{1.6.25}$$

$m_{1,1}$ is called the *correlation*. $\mu_{1,1}$ is called the *covariance*. When the averages are zero $\mu_{1,1} = m_{1,1}$. In Example 1.6.1 the correlation is $\rho$.

Note that if $f(x_1, x_2) = f_1(x_1)f_2(x_2)$ and the rvs are independent, then

$$\overline{f_1(x)f_2(x_2)} = \overline{f_1(x_1)}\;\overline{f_2(x_2)} \tag{1.6.26}$$

Thus for independent rvs

$$m_{k,r} = \overline{x_1^k}\,\overline{x_2^r} \tag{1.6.27}$$

$$\mu_{k,r} = \overline{(x_1 - m_1)^k}\,\overline{(x_2 - m_2)^r} \tag{1.6.28}$$

and particularly

$$m_{1,1} = \overline{x_1}\,\overline{x_2} = m_1 m_2 \tag{1.6.29}$$

$$\mu_{1,1} = \overline{(x_1 - m_1)}\,\overline{(x_2 - m_2)} = 0 \tag{1.6.30}$$

thus the covariance of independent rvs is zero. $x_1$ and $x_2$ are *uncorrelated* if

$$E(x_1 x_2) = m_1 m_2 \tag{1.6.31}$$

For uncorrelated rvs

$$\mu_{1,1} = \overline{(x_1 - m_1)(x_2 - m_2)} = \overline{x_1 x_2} - m_1 m_2 = 0 \tag{1.6.32}$$

Independence of $x_1$, $x_2$ implies that they are uncorrelated; however, if $x_1$, $x_2$ are uncorrelated, they are not necessarily independent. The only exception is when $x_1$, $x_2$ are jointly Gaussian, as in Example 1.6.1. There $\mu_{1,1} = \rho$, and if $\rho = 0$ they are independent.

Note that the average is a linear operation, i.e., if

$$f(x_1, x_2) = \sum_{i=1}^{N} f_i(x_1, x_2) \tag{1.6.33}$$

then

$$\overline{f(x_1, x_2)} = \sum_{i=1}^{N} \overline{f_i(x_1, x_2)} \tag{1.6.34}$$

particularly

$$E(x_1 + x_2) = m_1 + m_2 \tag{1.6.35}$$

The conditional average of $x_2$, given that $x_1 = a_1$, is

$$E(x_2|a_1) = \int_{-\infty}^{\infty} a_2 p_{x2|x1}\,(a_2|a_1)\,da_2 \tag{1.6.36}$$

and the conditional average of $x_2$, given the event $x_1 \in A_1$ is

$$E(x_2|A_1) = \int_{-\infty}^{\infty} a_2 p_{x2|x1}(a_2|A_1)\, da_2 \tag{1.6.37}$$

The conditional averages of $f(x_2)$, given that $x_1 = a_1$ or $x_1 \in A_1$, are

$$E(f(x_2)|a_1) = \int_{-\infty}^{\infty} f(a_2) p_{x2|x1}(a_2|a_1)\, da_2 \tag{1.6.38}$$

and

$$E(f(x_2)|A_1) = \int_{-\infty}^{\infty} f(a_2) p_{x2|x1}(a_2|A_1)\, da_2 \tag{1.6.39}$$

The joint *characteristic function* is

$$C_{x1,x2}(v_1, v_2) = \overline{\exp(j\{v_1 x_1 + v_2 x_2\})} \tag{1.6.40}$$

and we can obtain the $k$, $r$ moment by

$$m_{k,r} = \frac{\partial^{k+r} C_{x1,x2}(0,0)}{\partial v_1^k \partial v_2^r} j^{-k-r} \tag{1.6.41}$$

### 1.6.3 Transformations

Let $y_1 = f_1(x_1, x_2)$, $y_2 = f_2(x_1, x_2)$; then the pair $y_1, y_2$ are rvs, provided $\{y_1 \leqq b_1, y_2 \leqq b_2\}$ are events and the joint pdf of $y_1, y_2$ is $p_{y1,y2}(b_1, b_2)$. To find $p_{y1,y2}(b_1, b_2)$, we first compute the PDF

$$F_{y1,y2}(b_1, b_2) = P(y_1 \leqq b_1, y_2 \leqq b_2) = P\{(x_1, x_2): f_1(x_1, x_2) \leqq b_1$$

$$f_2(x_1, x_2) \leqq b_2\} = \iint_{X_b} p_{x1,x2}(a_1, a_2)\, da_1\, da_2 \tag{1.6.42}$$

where

$$X_b = \{(x_1, x_2): f_1(x_1, x_2) \leqq b_1, f_2(x_1, x_2) \leqq b_2\}$$

and then take the derivative.

When the transformation is one to one, the infinitesimal area $dy_1\, dy_2$ around the point $y_1 = b_1, y_2 = b_2$ is a mapping of the infinitesimal area $dx_1$

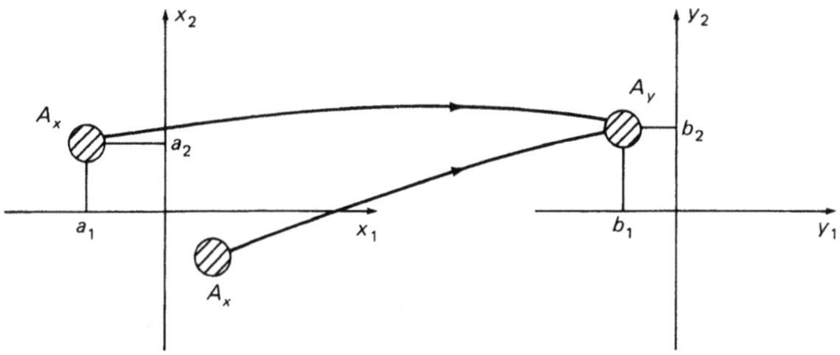


Fig. 1.24. Transformation of random variables.

$dx_2$ around the point $x_1 = a_1, x_2 = a_2$, such that $f_1(a_1, a_2) = b_1, f_2(a_1, a_2) = b_2$, as shown in Fig. 1.24. The mapping of the areas is through the Jacobian

$$dy_1\, dy_2 = |J_y(x_1, x_2)| dx_1\, dx_2 \tag{1.6.43}$$

where the Jacobian is the matrix of partial derivatives

$$J_y(x_1, x_2) = \begin{pmatrix} \dfrac{\partial f_1}{\partial x_1}(x_1, x_2) & \dfrac{\partial f_1}{\partial x_2}(x_1, x_2) \\ \\ \dfrac{\partial f_2}{\partial x_1}(x_1, x_2) & \dfrac{\partial f_2}{\partial x_2}(x_1, x_2) \end{pmatrix} \tag{1.6.44}$$

and $|\ |$ denotes here the determinant.

Because the probabilities of the areas are the same, we obtain

$$p_{y1,y2}(b_1, b_2) = \left. \frac{p_{x1,x2}(a_1, a_2)}{|J_y(a_1, a_2)|} \right|_{\substack{f_1(a_1, a_2) = b_1 \\ f_2(a_1, a_2) = b_2}} \tag{1.6.45}$$

*Example* 1.6.4 Rayleigh pdf

Let

$$y_1 = A_x = (x_1^2 + x_2^2)^{1/2} = f_1(x_1, x_2)$$

$$y_2 = \phi_x = \tan^{-1}(x_2/x_1) = f_2(x_1, x_2)$$

Note that $y_1$ and $y_2$ are restricted to $y_1 \geqq 0$ $0 \leqq y_2 \leqq 2\pi$. Thus

$$|J_y(x_1, x_2)| = \begin{vmatrix} \dfrac{x_1}{A_x} & \dfrac{x_2}{A_x} \\ \\ \dfrac{-x_2}{A_x^2} & \dfrac{x_1}{A_x^2} \end{vmatrix} = A_x^{-1} = (x_1^2 + x_2^2)^{-1/2}$$

If we assume that $p_{x1,x2}(a_1, a_2)$ is Gaussian

$$p_{x1,x2}(a_1, a_2) = (2\pi\sigma^2)^{-1} \exp\left(-\frac{1}{2}\frac{a_1^2 + a_2^2}{\sigma^2}\right)$$

i.e., $x_1, x_2$ are independent, zero mean Gaussian rvs with the same variance $\sigma^2$, then from (1.6.45)

$$p_{y1,y2}(b_1, b_2) = (2\pi\sigma^2)^{-1}(a_1^2 + a_2^2)^{1/2} \exp\left(-\frac{1}{2}\frac{a_1^2 + a_2^2}{\sigma^2}\right)$$

$$= (2\pi)^{-1}(b_1/\sigma^2) \exp(-b_1^2/2\sigma^2) = p_{y1}(b_1)p_{y2}(b_2)$$

where

$$p_{y1}(b_1) = (b_1/\sigma^2) \exp(-b_1^2/2\sigma^2)u(b_1)$$

$$p_{y2}(b_2) = (2\pi)^{-1}\{u(b_2) - u(b_2 - 2\pi)\}$$

i.e., $y_1$ has the Rayleigh pdf, while $y_2$ is uniformly distributed in 0–2 $\pi$.

If the transformation is many to one, as indicated in Fig. 1.24, the right-hand side of (1.6.45) will contain an additional term for each $A_x$ area mapped into the same $A_y$ area.

If there is only one function $y = f(x_1, x_2)$ and the pdf of $y$ is required, we can always consider $y$ as $y_1$, $f(x_1, x_2)$ as $f_1(x_1, x_2)$, and we can arbitrarily add $y_2 = f_2(x_1, x_2) = x_2$, so that the Jacobian is

$$|J_y(x_1, x_2)| = \begin{vmatrix} \dfrac{\partial f_1(x_1, x_1)}{\partial x_1} & \dfrac{\partial f_1(x_2, x_2)}{\partial x_2} \\ 0 & 1 \end{vmatrix} = \left|\frac{\partial f_1(x_1, x_2)}{\partial x_1}\right| \tag{1.6.46}$$

and after $p_{y1,y2}(b_1, b_2)$ is available, we integrate to obtain

$$p_y(b) = \int_{-\infty}^{\infty} p_{y1,y2}(b_1, b_2)\, db_2 \tag{1.6.47}$$

*Example* 1.6.5 Sum of rvs

Let $y = x_1 + x_2$, and we add $y_2 = x_2$. Thus

$$|J_y(x_1, x_2)| = 1$$

and

$$p_{y1,y2}(b, b_2) = p_{x1,x2}(b - b_2, b_2)$$

thus

$$p_y(b) = \int_{-\infty}^{\infty} p_{x1,x2}(b - b_2, b_2)\, db_2$$

If $x_1$, $x_2$ are independent, we obtain

$$p_y(b) = \int_{-\infty}^{\infty} p_{x1}(b - b_2)p_{x2}(b_2)\, db_2 = p_{x1}(b) * p_{x2}(b) \qquad (1.6.48)$$

i.e., the pdf of the sum of independent rvs is the convolution of their pdfs.

*Example* 1.6.6 Product of rvs
Let $y = x_1 x_2$, an we add $y_2 = x_2$. Therefore

$$|J_y(x_1, x_2)| = \begin{vmatrix} x_2 & x_1 \\ 0 & 1 \end{vmatrix} = |x_2|$$

thus

$$p_{y1,y2}(b, b_2) = p_{x1,x2}(b/b_2, b_2)/|b_2|$$

and

$$p_y(b) = \int_{-\infty}^{\infty} p_{x1,x2}(b/b_2, b_2)|b_2|^{-1}\, db_2$$

If $x_1$, $x_2$ are independent

$$p_y(b) = \int_{-\infty}^{\infty} p_{x1}(b/b_2)p_{x2}(b_2)|b_2|^{-1}\, db_2$$

### 1.6.4 Complex random variables

In many cases it is more convenient to consider two real rvs $x_1$, $x_2$ as a single complex random variable

$$x = x_1 + jx_2 \qquad (1.6.49)$$

the average of which is

$$m_x = m_1 + jm_2 \tag{1.6.50}$$

The variance is defined as

$$\begin{aligned}\sigma_x^2 &= \overline{(x - m_x)(x - m_x)^*} = \overline{xx^*} - |m_x|^2 \\ &= \overline{x_1^2} + \overline{x_2^2} - m_1^2 - m_2^2 = \sigma_{x1}^2 + \sigma_{x2}^2\end{aligned} \tag{1.6.51}$$

The covariance of two complex rvs

$$x = x_1 + jx_2, \qquad y = y_1 + jy_2 \tag{1.6.52}$$

is

$$E(x - m_x)(y - m_y)^* = E(xy^*) - m_x m_y^* \tag{1.6.53}$$

They are uncorrelated if

$$E(xy^*) = m_x m_y^* \tag{1.6.54}$$

and in this case the covariance is zero.

## 1.7 RANDOM VECTORS

### 1.7.1 Definition and probabilities

In Section 1.6 we considered two rvs. Similarly, we can define a sequence of $N$ rvs $x_1(\omega)$, $x_2(\omega)$, $\ldots$, $x_N(\omega)$, and for conciseness we may consider the sequence as a random $N$-dimensional row vector

$$\mathbf{x}(\omega) = \{x_1(\omega), \ldots, x_N(\omega)\} \tag{1.7.1}$$

Let $A$ be the event

$$A = \prod_{i=1}^{N} A_i = \{\omega: \omega \in A_1, \omega \in A_2, \ldots, \omega \in A_N\} \tag{1.7.2}$$

where $A_i$ is as in (1.6.1). The probability of this event is

$$P(A) = P(A_1, \ldots, A_N) \tag{1.7.3}$$

We may consider $\mathbf{x}$ as made up of two lower dimensional vectors, say

$$\mathbf{y}(\omega) = (y_1, y_2, \ldots, y_k) = (x_1, x_2, \ldots, x_k) \tag{1.7.4}$$

and

$$\mathbf{z}(\omega) = (z_1, z_2, \ldots, z_{N-k}) = (x_{k+1}, \ldots, x_N) \tag{1.7.5}$$

and write

$$\mathbf{x} = (\mathbf{y}, \mathbf{z}) \tag{1.7.6}$$

The joint PDF is

$$F_{\mathbf{x}}(\mathbf{a}) = F_{x1,x2,\ldots,xN}(a_1, a_2, \ldots, a_N) = P\{\omega\colon \mathbf{x}(\omega) \leqq \mathbf{a})\} \tag{1.7.7}$$

and the joint pdf is

$$p_{\mathbf{x}}(\mathbf{a}) = \frac{\partial^N F_{\mathbf{x}}(\mathbf{a})}{\partial a_1 \partial a_2, \ldots, \partial a_N} \tag{1.7.8}$$

The PDF and pdf have the following properties

a. $0 \leqq F_{\mathbf{x}}(\mathbf{a}) \leqq 1, \qquad 0 \leqq p_{\mathbf{x}}(\mathbf{a})$

b. $F_{\mathbf{x}}(\mathbf{a}) = \int_{-\infty}^{a} p_{\mathbf{x}}(\mathbf{b})\, d\mathbf{b} = \int_{-\infty}^{a_1} \cdots \int_{-\infty}^{a_N} p_{\mathbf{x}}(\mathbf{b})\, db_1 \ldots db_N$

c. $F_{\mathbf{x}}(\infty) = 1, \qquad \int_{-\infty}^{\infty} p_{\mathbf{x}}(\mathbf{a})\, d\mathbf{a} = 1$ (1.7.9)

d. $F_{\mathbf{x}}(\mathbf{a}) = 0$ if at least one component of $\mathbf{a}$ is $-\infty$.

e. If $\mathbf{a} \geqq \mathbf{b}$ (i.e., $a_i > b_i \quad i = 1, \ldots, N$), then

$$F_{\mathbf{x}}(\mathbf{a}) \geqq F_{\mathbf{x}}(\mathbf{b})$$

f. $F_{\mathbf{y}}(\mathbf{b}) = F_{\mathbf{y},\mathbf{z}}(\mathbf{b}, \infty), \qquad p_{\mathbf{y}}(\mathbf{b}) = \int_{-\infty}^{\infty} p_{\mathbf{y},\mathbf{z}}(\mathbf{b}, \mathbf{c})\, d\mathbf{c}$

Because a scalar is a one-dimensional vector, all results that are obtained here for vectors apply also for scalars. In fact Section 1.6 can be considered as a special case of this section, i.e., a two-dimensional vector.

*Example* 1.7.1 Gaussian vector

$$p_{\mathbf{x}}(\mathbf{a}) = \{(2\pi)^N|\Lambda_x|\}^{-1/2} \exp\{(-1/2)(\mathbf{a} - \mathbf{m}_x)\Lambda_x^{-1}(\mathbf{a} - \mathbf{m}_x)^T\} \tag{1.7.10}$$

where $T$ denotes transpose $\mathbf{m}_x$ is a vector, the $i$th element of which is

$$m_i = E(x_i)$$

and $\Lambda_x$ is an $N \times N$ matrix, the covariance matrix, the $i$, $j$th element of which is

$$\lambda_{ij} = \overline{(x_i - m_i)(x_j - m_j)}$$

We can obtain the marginal pdf of, say, $y = x_i$ by integrating over all other rvs denoted by $\mathbf{z}$

$$p_{xi}(a_i) = p_y(a_i) = \int_{-\infty}^{\infty} p_{y,\mathbf{z}}(a_i, \mathbf{c})\, d\mathbf{c}$$

$$= (2\pi\sigma_i^2)^{-1/2} \exp(-(1/2)(a_i - m_i)^2/\sigma_i^2) \tag{1.7.11}$$

where

$$\sigma_i^2 = \lambda_{ii}$$

Each of the rvs may be discrete, continuous, or mixed. If all rvs are discrete (continuous), then the joint pdf is also discrete (continuous); otherwise it is mixed. For discrete rvs it is more convenient to write probabilities.

*Example* 1.7.2 Discrete rvs

$$p_{x1,x2,x3}(a_1, a_2, a_3) = \sum_{i=1}^{K_1}\sum_{j=1}^{K_2}\sum_{k=1}^{K_3} P_{ijk}\delta(a_1 - a_{1i})\delta(a_2 - a_{2j})\delta(a_3 - a_{3k})$$

The probabilities are

$$P(x_1 = a_{1i}, x_2 = a_{2j}, x_3 = a_{3k}) = P_{ijk}$$

$$P(x_2 = a_{2j}) = \sum_{i=1}^{K_1}\sum_{k=1}^{K_3} P_{ijk}, \quad \sum_{i=1}^{K_1}\sum_{j=1}^{K_2}\sum_{k=1}^{K_1} P_{ijk} = 1$$

The rvs are independent if

$$p_x(a) = \prod_{i=1}^{N} p_{xi}(a_i) \tag{1.7.12}$$

Two random vectors are independent if

$$p_{\mathbf{y},\mathbf{z}}(\mathbf{b}, \mathbf{c}) = p_{\mathbf{y}}(\mathbf{b})p_{\mathbf{z}}(\mathbf{c}) \tag{1.7.13}$$

*Example* 1.7.3 Independent Gaussian rvs
If in Example 1.7.1 (Eq. (1.7.10)), we assume that $\lambda_{ij} = 0$ for $i \neq j$, then (1.7.12) is satisfied with $p_{xi}(a_i)$ as in (1.7.11).

This example shows that if Gaussian rvs are uncorrelated they are also independent.

The conditional pdf of $\mathbf{y}$ conditioned on $\mathbf{z} = \mathbf{c}$ is

$$p_{\mathbf{y}|\mathbf{z}}(\mathbf{b}|\mathbf{c}) = \frac{p_{\mathbf{y},\mathbf{z}}(\mathbf{b}, \mathbf{c})}{p_{\mathbf{z}}(\mathbf{c})} \tag{1.7.14}$$

hence if they are independent

$$p_{\mathbf{y}|\mathbf{z}}(\mathbf{b}|\mathbf{c}) = p_{\mathbf{y}}(\mathbf{b}) \tag{1.7.15}$$

The conditional pdf of $y$ conditioned on the event

$$A_z = \{\mathbf{c}: \mathbf{c}_1 \leqq \mathbf{c} \leqq \mathbf{c}_2\} \tag{1.7.16}$$

is

$$p_{\mathbf{y}|\mathbf{z}}(\mathbf{b}|A_z) = \int_{A_z} p_{\mathbf{y},\mathbf{z}}(\mathbf{b}, \mathbf{c})\, d\mathbf{c} \Big/ \int_{A_z} p_{\mathbf{z}}(\mathbf{c})\, d\mathbf{c} \tag{1.7.17}$$

Bayers' rule has the form

$$p_{\mathbf{y}|\mathbf{z}}(\mathbf{b}|\mathbf{c})p_{\mathbf{z}}(\mathbf{c}) = p_{\mathbf{z}|\mathbf{y}}(\mathbf{c}|\mathbf{b})p_{\mathbf{y}}(\mathbf{b}) \tag{1.7.18}$$

and

$$p_{\mathbf{y}|\mathbf{z}}(\mathbf{b}|\mathbf{c}) = \frac{p_{\mathbf{z}|\mathbf{y}}(\mathbf{c}|\mathbf{b})p_{\mathbf{y}}(\mathbf{b})}{\int_{-\infty}^{\infty} p_{\mathbf{z}|\mathbf{y}}(\mathbf{c}|\mathbf{b})p_{\mathbf{y}}(\mathbf{b})\, d\mathbf{b}} \tag{1.7.19}$$

### 1.7.2 Transformation and averages

Let $\mathbf{x}$ and $\mathbf{y}$ be two $N$-dimensional random vectors functionally related by

$$\mathbf{y} = \mathbf{f}(\mathbf{x}) \tag{1.7.20}$$

$$y_i = f_i(\mathbf{x}) = f_i(x_1, x_2, \ldots, x_N) \qquad i = 1, 2, \ldots, N \tag{1.7.21}$$

If $p_{\mathbf{x}}(\mathbf{a})$ is known, we can find $p_{\mathbf{y}}(\mathbf{b})$ by first computing

$$F_{\mathbf{y}}(\mathbf{b}) = P(\mathbf{y} \leqq \mathbf{b}) = P\{\mathbf{x}: \mathbf{f}(\mathbf{x}) \leqq \mathbf{b}\}$$

$$= \int_{X_b} p_{\mathbf{x}}(\mathbf{a})\, d\mathbf{a} \qquad (1.7.22)$$

where

$$X_b = \{\mathbf{x}: \mathbf{f}(\mathbf{x}) \leqq \mathbf{b})\} \qquad (1.7.23)$$

If the transformation is one to one, then the infinitesimal volume $d\mathbf{x} = dx_1\, dx_2 \ldots dx_N$ is transformed into the infinitesimal volume $d\mathbf{y} = dy_1\, dy_2 \ldots dy_N$, related by the Jacobian

$$d\mathbf{y} = |J_y(\mathbf{x})|\, d\mathbf{x},\ d\mathbf{x} = |J_x(\mathbf{y})| d\mathbf{y} \qquad (1.7.24)$$

where the $i, j$ element of $J_y(\mathbf{x})$ is $\partial f_i/\partial x_j$, and the $i, j$ element of $J_x(\mathbf{y})$ is $\partial g_i/\partial y_j$, and $\mathbf{g}(\mathbf{y}) = f^{-1}(\mathbf{y})$ is the inverse transformation. Because the probabilities of the infinitesimal volumes are the same

$$p_{\mathbf{y}}(\mathbf{b})\, d\mathbf{b} = p_{\mathbf{x}}(\mathbf{a})\, d\mathbf{a} \qquad (1.7.25)$$

we obtain

$$p_{\mathbf{y}}(\mathbf{b}) = \left. \frac{p_{\mathbf{x}}(\mathbf{a})}{|J_x(\mathbf{a})|} \right|_{\mathbf{f}(\mathbf{a}) = \mathbf{b}} \qquad (1.7.26)$$

If the transformation is many to one, the right-hand side of (1.7.26) contains more terms, one term for each value of **a**, such that $\mathbf{f}(\mathbf{a}) = \mathbf{b}$.

*Example* 1.7.4 Linear transformation of Gaussian vector
Let **x** be a Gaussian vector with joint pdf as in (1.7.10). Let

$$\mathbf{y} = \mathbf{x}A + \mathbf{c} = \mathbf{f}(\mathbf{x}) \qquad (1.7.27)$$

The Jacobian here is the constant matrix

$$J_y(\mathbf{a}) = A \qquad (1.7.28)$$

and, assuming that $A$ has an inverse $A^{-1}$

$$\mathbf{x} = (\mathbf{y} - \mathbf{c})A^{-1} = \mathbf{g}(\mathbf{y}) \qquad (1.7.29)$$

Thus from (1.7.10), (1.7.26), (1.7.28), and (1.7.29), we obtain

$$p_{\mathbf{y}}(\mathbf{b}) = \{(2\pi)^N|\Lambda_x||A|^2\}^{-1/2} \exp\{(-1/2)(\mathbf{b} - \mathbf{c} - \mathbf{m}_x A)\} \\ A^{-1}\Lambda_x^{-1}A^{-1T}(\mathbf{b} - \mathbf{c} - \mathbf{m}_x A)^T \tag{1.7.30}$$

Now note that

$$\mathbf{m}_y = E(\mathbf{x}A + \mathbf{c}) = E(\mathbf{x})A + \mathbf{c} = \mathbf{m}_x A + \mathbf{c}$$

and

$$\Lambda_y = E((\mathbf{y} - \mathbf{m}_y)^T(\mathbf{y} - \mathbf{m}_y)) = E\{A^T(\mathbf{x} - \mathbf{m}_x)^T(\mathbf{x} - \mathbf{m}_x)A\} \\ = A^T E\{(\mathbf{x} - \mathbf{m}_x)^T(\mathbf{x} - \mathbf{m}_x)\}A = A^T\Lambda_x A$$

Thus

$$|\Lambda_y| = |A^T||\Lambda_x||A| = |\Lambda_x||A|^2$$

and

$$\Lambda_y^{-1} = A^{-1}\Lambda_x^{-1}A^{-1T}$$

With these results we can write (1.7.30) as

$$p_{\mathbf{y}}(\mathbf{b}) = \{(2\pi)^N\Lambda_Y\}^{-1/2} \exp\{(-1/2)(b - m_y)\Lambda_Y^{-1}(b - m_y)^T\}$$

This example shows that a linear transformation of a Gaussian vector is also a Gaussian random vector. If $\mathbf{y} = f(\mathbf{x})$ is a $K < N$-dimensional random vector, we can add artificially the variables

$$y_{K+1} = x_{K+1}, \ldots, y_N = x_N$$

to obtain first the vector

$$\mathbf{z} = (\mathbf{y}, x_{K+1}, \ldots, x_N) \tag{1.7.31}$$

and then the pdf of $\mathbf{y}$ by

$$p_{\mathbf{y}}(\mathbf{b}) = \int_{-\infty}^{\infty} \cdots \int_{-\infty}^{\infty} p_{\mathbf{z}}(\mathbf{b}, a_{K+1}, \ldots, a_N)\, da_{K+1}\, da_N \tag{1.7.32}$$

*Example* 1.7.5 Sum of rvs
Let

$$y = y_1 = x_1 + x_2 \ldots x_N = f_1(\mathbf{x})$$

To find the pdf of $y$, we assume first

$$y_i = x_i \qquad i = 2, \ldots, N$$

Now

$$|J_y(\mathbf{x})| = 1$$

Hence

$$p_y(b) = \int_{-\infty}^{\infty} \cdots \int_{-\infty}^{\infty} p_{x_1,\ldots,x_N}\left(b - \sum_2^N a_i, a_2, \ldots, a_N\right) da_2, \ldots, a_N$$

If $\{x_i\}$ are independent, then

$$p_y(b) = \int_{-\infty}^{\infty}\int_{-\infty}^{\infty} p_{x1}\left(b - \sum_2^N a_i\right) \prod_2^N p_{xi}(a_i)\, da_2, \ldots, da_N$$

$$= p_{x1}(b) * p_{x2}(b) * \ldots * p_{xN}(b)$$

This shows that the pdf of the sum of independent rvs is the convolution of the pdfs.

The average value of $\mathbf{y} = \mathbf{f}(\mathbf{x})$ is

$$E(\mathbf{y}) = \int_{-\infty}^{\infty} \mathbf{b} p_y(\mathbf{b})\, d\mathbf{b} = \int_{-\infty}^{\infty} \mathbf{f}(\mathbf{a}) p_{\mathbf{x}}(\mathbf{a})\, d\mathbf{a} \tag{1.7.33}$$

This follows from the fact that infinitesimal volume $d\mathbf{a}$ around $\mathbf{a}$ is mapped into $d\mathbf{b}$ around $\mathbf{b} = \mathbf{f}(\mathbf{a})$ and has the same probability. The conditional average of $\mathbf{y}$, given $\mathbf{z} = \mathbf{c}$, is

$$E(\mathbf{y}|\mathbf{z} = \mathbf{c}) = \int_{-\infty}^{\infty} \mathbf{b} p_{\mathbf{y}|\mathbf{z}}(\mathbf{b}|\mathbf{c})\, d\mathbf{b} \tag{1.7.34}$$

The conditional average of $\mathbf{y}$, given the event $A_z$, is

$$E(\mathbf{y}|\mathbf{z} \in A_z) = \int_{-\infty}^{\infty} \mathbf{b} p_y(\mathbf{b}|\mathbf{A}_z)\, d\mathbf{b} \tag{1.7.35}$$

Particularly let

$$y = f(\mathbf{x}) = \prod_{i=1}^{N} f_i(x_i) \tag{1.7.36}$$

then

$$E(y) = \int_{-\infty}^{\infty} \cdots \int_{-\infty}^{\infty} \prod_{i=1}^{N} f_i(a_i) p_{x1,\ldots,xN}(a_1, \ldots, a_N)\, da_1 \ldots da_N \tag{1.7.37}$$

and if the rvs $x_i$ are independent

$$E(y) = \prod_{i=1}^{N} E(f_i(a_i)) \tag{1.7.38}$$

For example, if

$$y = \prod_{i=1}^{N} x_i \tag{1.7.39}$$

$$E(y) = \prod_{i=1}^{N} E(x_i) \tag{1.7.40}$$

The average of the sum

$$y = \sum_{i=1}^{N} f_i(x_i) \tag{1.7.41}$$

is

$$E(y) = \sum_{i=1}^{N} E(f_i(x_i)) \tag{1.7.42}$$

particularly if

$$y = \sum_{i=1}^{N} x_i \tag{1.7.43}$$

$$E(y) = \sum_{1}^{N} E(x_i) \tag{1.7.44}$$

The covariance matrix of two $N$-dimensional vectors $\mathbf{x}$, $\mathbf{y}$ is

$$\Lambda_{x,y} = \overline{(\mathbf{x} - \mathbf{m}_x)^T(\mathbf{y} - \mathbf{m}_y)} = \overline{(\mathbf{y} - \mathbf{m}_y)^T(\mathbf{x} - \mathbf{m}_x)} \tag{1.7.45}$$

whose $i, j$ element is

$$\overline{(x_i - m_{xi})(y_j - m_{yj})} = E(x_i y_i) - m_{xi} m_{yj} \tag{1.7.46}$$

and

$$m_{xi} = E(x_i),\ m_{yj} = E(y_i) \tag{1.7.47}$$

If

$$E(x_i y_j) = E(x_i) E(y_j) = m_{xi} m_{yj} \tag{1.7.48}$$

for all $i, j = 1, \ldots, N$, we say that $x$, $y$ are *uncorrelated* and $\Lambda_{x,y}$ is a zero matrix. If

$$E(\mathbf{x}\mathbf{y}^T) = \sum_{i=1}^{N} E(x_i y_i) = 0 \tag{1.7.49}$$

we say that **x**, **y** are *orthogonal*.

The characteristic function of **x** is

$$C_{\mathbf{x}}(\mathbf{v}) = \overline{\exp(j\mathbf{v}^T\mathbf{x})} = \int_{-\infty}^{\infty} \prod_{i=1}^{N} \exp(ja_i v_i)\, p_{\mathbf{x}}(\mathbf{a})\, d\mathbf{a} \tag{1.7.50}$$

hence, if the $\{x_i\}$ are independent

$$C_{\mathbf{x}}(\mathbf{v}) = \prod_{i=1}^{N} C_{xi}(v_i) \tag{1.7.51}$$

$$C_{xi}(v_i) = \overline{\exp(jx_i v_i)} \tag{1.7.52}$$

For Gaussian random vector

$$\begin{aligned} C_{\mathbf{x}}(\mathbf{v}) &= \exp\{(-1/2)\mathbf{v}\Lambda_x\mathbf{v}^T + j\mathbf{v}\mathbf{m}^T{}_x\} \\ &= \exp\left(-\frac{1}{2}\sum_{i=1}^{N}\sum_{i=1}^{N} v_i v_j \lambda_{ij} + j\sum_{i=1}^{N} v_i m_i\right) \end{aligned} \tag{1.7.53}$$

## 1.8 RANDOM PROCESS

### 1.8.1 Definitions

While a random vector associates with each $\omega \in \Omega$, a sequence of $N$ numbers $x_1(\omega), \ldots, x_N(\omega)$, a *random process* (rp) associates with $\omega \in \Omega$ a function $x(t,$

$\omega$) defined for all $-\infty < t < \infty$ or for a subset of the real line. In fact if $t$ is taken from a subset with a finite number of terms, say, $t \in \mathbf{t} = \{t_1, t_2, \ldots, t_N\}$ the process is reduced to a vector $\mathbf{x} = (x_1, \ldots, x_N)$ where

$$x_i = x(t_i, \omega) \tag{1.8.1}$$

For a single value of $t$, say $t = t_1$, $x(t, \omega)$ is a random variable. For convenience we shall drop the $\omega$ dependence of the rp $x(t, \omega)$.

*Example* 1.8.1 Random sinusoid
Let $A$ and $\phi$ be rvs $A \geqq 0$ and $0 \leqq \phi \leqq 2\pi$. Let

$$x(t) = A \cos (2\pi f t + \phi)$$

$$y(t) = A \sin (2\pi f t + \phi)$$

Both $x(t)$ and $y(t)$ are random process.

*Example* 1.8.2 Digital signal
Let $\{a_i\}$ $-\infty < i < \infty$ be a sequence of independent, identically distributed, discrete rvs taking values in the set $\hat{A}_{\pm} = \{\pm 1, \pm 3, \ldots, \pm M\}$ with equal probability. Let $h(t)$ be a function that is nonzero for $0 \leqq t \leqq T$. Let

$$x(t) = \sum_i a_i h(t - iT)$$

$x(t)$ is a rp that represents a digital signal.

*Example* 1.8.3 Gaussian random processes
Let $x(t)$ be a rp such that for any $N$, and any set $\{t_1, t_2, \ldots, t_N\}$ the resulting random vector $\mathbf{x}$ has a Gaussian pdf. Such a process is called a *Gaussian process.*
Noise generated in electronic devices is often modeled as a zero mean, Gaussian process.
Let

$$\mathbf{x}(t) = (x(t_1), x(t_2), \ldots, x(t_N)) \tag{1.8.2}$$

and

$$\mathbf{x}(t + \Delta) = (x(t_1 + \Delta), x(t_2 + \Delta), \ldots, x(t_N + \Delta)) \tag{1.8.3}$$

be the vectors associated with the rp, taken $\Delta$ seconds apart. The process is called *stationary* (or *strictly stationary*) if for all $N$ and all $\{t_i\}$ the pdf is independent of the time shift $\Delta$, i.e.

$$p_{\mathbf{x}(t)}(\mathbf{a}) = p_{\mathbf{x}(t+\Delta)}(\mathbf{a}) \tag{1.8.4}$$

A process is called *stationary of order K* if (1.8.4) is true only if the dimension of the vector is less then $K + 1$, i.e., $N \leq K$. Particularly a stationary process of order two has the following properties

a. The pdf of $x(t)$ is independent of time

$$p_{x(t)}(a) = p_{x(t+\Delta)}(a) = p_{x(0)}(a) \tag{1.8.5}$$

because we can take $t = t_1$ and $\Delta = -t_1$.

b. The joint probability density of $x(t)$ and $x(t + \tau)$ (here $t = t_1$ and $t + \tau = t_2$) is a function of the time difference, $t_2 - t_1 = \tau$, only

$$p_{x(t+\tau),x(t)}(a_2, a_1) = p_{x(\tau),x(0)}(a_2, a_1) \tag{1.8.6}$$

because we can select $\Delta = -t$.

### 1.8.2 Correlation

The average of a rp is

$$\overline{x(t)} = E(x(t)) = \int_{-\infty}^{\infty} a p_{x(t)}(a)\, da \tag{1.8.7}$$

and in general is a function of time. The autocorrelation of a rp is

$$R_x(t + \tau, t) = \overline{x(t + \tau)x(t)} = \int_{-\infty}^{\infty}\int_{-\infty}^{\infty} a_1 a_2 p_{x(t+\tau),x(t)}(a_2, a_1)\, da_1\, da_2 \tag{1.8.8}$$

and in general is both a function of $t$ and $\tau$. If the process is stationary of order two or more, then $\overline{x(t)}$ is a constant $m_x$, and the autocorrelation depends only on $\tau$

$$R_x(t + \tau, t) = R_x(\tau) = \int_{-\infty}^{\infty}\int_{-\infty}^{\infty} a_1 a_2 p_{x(\tau),x(0)}(a_2, a_1)\, da_2\, da_1 \tag{1.8.9}$$

A process is called *wide-sense stationary* (wss) if

$$E(x(t)) = m_x,\ R_x(t + \tau, t) = R_x(\tau) \tag{1.8.10}$$

Thus a stationary rp is also wss, but the reverse is true only for a Gaussian process, because the pdf of a Gaussian process depends only on the average and the autocorrelation. A wssp has the following properties

a. $R_x(\tau)$ is an even function

$$R_x(\tau) = R_x(-\tau) \tag{1.8.11}$$

b. $R_x(0)$ is the average power

$$\overline{R_x(0)} = x^2(t) \geqq R_x(\tau) \tag{1.8.12}$$

The *cross-correlation* between two rps $x(t)$ and $y(t)$ is

$$R_{x,y}(t_1, t_2) = \overline{x(t_1)y(t_2)} = R_{y,x}(t_2, t_1) \tag{1.8.13}$$

$x(t)$ and $y(t)$ are jointly wss if they are wss individually, and

$$R_{x,y}(t + \tau, t) = R_{x,y}(\tau) = R_{y,x}(-\tau) \tag{1.8.14}$$

In fact if we set $y(t) = x(t)$, we obtain the autocorrelation

$$R_{x,x}(\tau) = R_x(\tau) \tag{1.8.15}$$

### 1.8.3 Effect of linear systems on random processes

Let $x(t)$ be a rp, and let $h(t, \tau)$ be the response at time $t$ to an impulse applied at time $t - \tau$. The output is

$$y(t) = \int_{-\infty}^{\infty} x(\tau)h(t, \tau)\, d\tau = \lim_{\Delta \to 0} \sum_i x(\tau_i)h(t, \tau_i)\, \Delta \tag{1.8.16}$$

with $\tau_i = \tau_{i-1} + \Delta$, i.e, a linear combination of $x(\tau_i)$. Thus $y(t)$ is a rp and if $x(t)$ is Gaussian, so is $y(t)$.

Although we can continue with general linear systems in this book, we are mainly interested in linear time-invariant systems. Therefore from now on we shall assume that this is the case. The average and atuocorrelation of the output are thus

$$E(y(t)) = \int_{-\infty}^{\infty} h(t_1)\overline{x(t - t_1)}\, dt_1 \tag{1.8.17}$$

$$R_y(t + \tau, t) = \int_{-\infty}^{\infty}\int_{-\infty}^{\infty} \overline{x(t + \tau - t_1)x(t - t_2)}h(t_1)h(t_2)\, dt_1\, dt_2$$

$$= \int_{-\infty}^{\infty}\int_{-\infty}^{\infty} R_x(t + \tau - t_1, t - t_2)h(t_1)h(t_2)\, dt_1\, dt_2 \qquad (1.8.18)$$

If $x(t)$ is wss, so is $y(t)$, because

$$E(y(t)) = m_x \int_{-\infty}^{\infty} h(t_1)\, dt_1 = m_x H(0) = m_y$$

$$R_y(t + \tau, t) = \int_{-\infty}^{\infty}\int_{-\infty}^{\infty} R_x(\tau + t_2 - t_1)h(t_1)h(t_2)\, dt_1\, dt_2 = R_y(\tau) \quad (1.8.19)$$

The *power spectral density* of a rp is the FT of the autocorrelation. Thus the PSD of the output, $y(t)$, is

$$S_y(f) = \int_{-\infty}^{\infty} R_y(\tau) \exp(-j\, 2\, \pi f \tau)\, d\tau$$

$$= \int_{-\infty}^{\infty}\int_{-\infty}^{\infty}\int_{-\infty}^{\infty} R_x(\tau + t_2 - t_1)h(t_1)h(t_2) \exp(-j\, 2\, \pi f(\tau + t_2 - t_1))$$

$$\exp(-j\, 2\, \pi f t_1) \exp(j\, 2\, \pi f t_2)\, dt_1\, dt_2\, d\tau \qquad (1.8.20)$$

Changing variables from $\tau$ to

$$\tau_1 = \tau + t_2 - t_1 \qquad (1.8.21)$$

and performing the integration first with respect to $\tau_1$ (thus keeping $t_1$, $t_2$ constant), we obtain

$$S_y(f) = S_x(f)H(f)H^*(f) = S_x(f)|H(f)|^2 \qquad (1.8.22)$$

The PSD has the following properties

a. $S_x(f)$ is an even function of $f$ because $R_x(\tau)$ is even

$$S_x(f) = S_x(-f) \qquad (1.8.23)$$

b. The integral of $S_x(f)$ is the average power in $x(t)$

$$\int_{-\infty}^{\infty} S_x(f)\, df = R_x(0) = \overline{x^2(t)} \tag{1.8.24}$$

c. The average power of $x(t)$ within the frequency band $|f \pm f_1| \leqq \Delta f/2$ is $2\ S_x(f_1)\ \Delta f \geqq 0$, thus justifying the name *power spectral density*. This statement can be proved as follows: let us apply $x(t)$ to an ideal bandpass filter with transfer function

$$H(f) = \begin{cases} 1 & |f \pm f_1| \leqq \Delta f/2 \\ 0 & \text{otherwise} \end{cases} \tag{1.8.25}$$

hence the output, $y(t)$, is identical to the input for these frequencies and has an average power

$$\overline{y^2(t)} = \int_{-\infty}^{\infty} S_x(f)|H(f)|^2\, df = 2\ S_x(f_1)\ \Delta f \geqq 0 \tag{1.8.26}$$

A rp is called *white* if

$$S_x(f) = N_0/2 \tag{1.8.27}$$

i.e., the PSD is constant for all frequencies. If not white, the process is called *coloured*. The power in a white process is infinite, and the autocorrelation is

$$R_x(\tau) = (1/2)N_0\delta(\tau) \tag{1.8.28}$$

Because no physical process has infinite power, white noise is a model of a process whose PSD declines at frequencies beyond the bandwidth of the system of interest.

*Example* 1.8.1 Baseband noise
Let $x(t)$ be a white wssp, and let $h(t)$ be an ideal lowpass filter, i.e.

$$H(f) = \begin{cases} 1 & |f| \leqq B \\ 0 & |f| > B \end{cases}$$

The PSD and autocorrelation of the output is

$$S_y(f) = \begin{cases} (1/2)N_0 & |f| \leqq B \\ 0 & |f| > B \end{cases}$$

$$R_y(\tau) = N_0 B \sin(2\ \pi B\tau)/(2\ \pi B\tau) \tag{1.8.29}$$

Note that if

$$\tau = (2\,B)^{-1}\,k = \tau_k$$

where $k$ is an integer

$$R_y(\tau_k) = 0$$

Hence $\{y(\tau_k)\}$ are uncorrelated rvs, and if $x(t)$ is Gaussian they are independent. The input and output PSD and autocorrelation are show in Fig. 1.25.

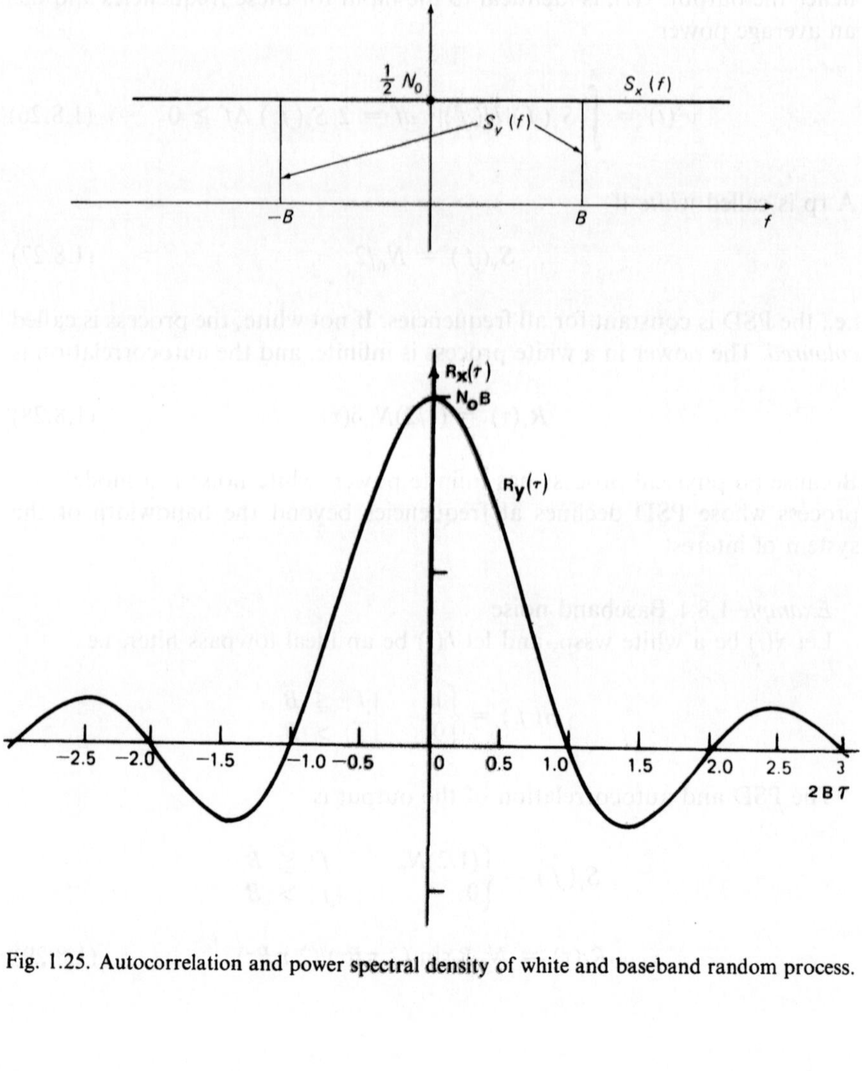


Fig. 1.25. Autocorrelation and power spectral density of white and baseband random process.

The *cross-spectral density* is the FT of cross-correlation

$$S_{x,y}(f) = \int_{-\infty}^{\infty} R_{x,y}(\tau) \exp(-j\,2\,\pi f\tau)\,d\tau \tag{1.8.30}$$

and again when $y(t) = x(t)$, we obtain the PSD of $x(t)$

$$S_{x,x}(f) = S_x(f) \tag{1.8.31}$$

Next let us consider the system in Fig. 1.26. The inputs are $x_1(t)$, $x_2(t)$, with cross-correlation $R_{x1,x2}(\tau)$. The cross-correlation of the output is

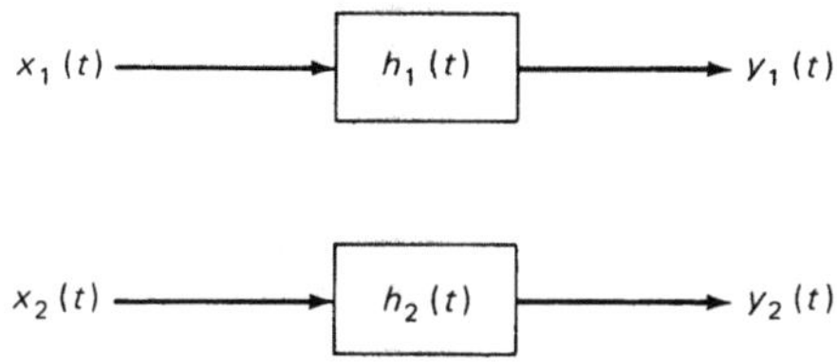


Fig. 1.26. Linear systems and random signals.

$$R_{y1,y2}(t+\tau, t) = \overline{y_1(t+\tau)y_2(t)} = \int_{-\infty}^{\infty}\int_{-\infty}^{\infty} \overline{x_1(t+\tau-t_1)x_2(t-t_2)h_1(t_1)h_2(t_2)}$$

$$dt_1 dt_2 = \int_{-\infty}^{\infty}\int_{-\infty}^{\infty} R_{x1,x2}(\tau+t_2-t_1)h_1(t_1)h_2(t_2)\,dt_1\,dt_2$$

$$= R_{y1,y2}(\tau) \tag{1.8.32}$$

When we take the FT, we obtain as in (1.8.20)

$$S_{y1,y2}(f) = S_{x1,x2}(f)H_1(f)H_2^*(f) \tag{1.8.33}$$

From (1.8.33) we can draw the following important corrollaries

a. If $x_1(t) = x_2(t) = x(t)$ and $h_1(t) = h_2(t) = h(t)$, we obtain $y_1(t) = y_2(t) = y(t)$, and

$$S_y(f) = S_x(f)|H(f)|^2 \tag{1.8.34}$$

b. Let

$$H_1(f) = H_2(f) = j\,2\,\pi f$$

i.e.,

$$y_i(t) = \frac{dx_i(t)}{dt} = \dot{x}_i(t), \qquad i = 1, 2$$

then

$$S_{y1,y2}(f) = (2\,\pi f)^2\, S_{x1,x2}(f) \tag{1.8.35}$$

and particularly when $x_1(t) = x_2(t) = x(t)$

$$S_y(f) = (2\,\pi f)^2\, S_x(f) \tag{1.8.36}$$

c. Let

$$H_2(f) = 1, \qquad H_1(f) = j\,2\,\pi f$$

i.e.

$$y_2(t) = x_2(t), \qquad y_1(t) = \dot{x}_1(t)$$

then

$$S_{\dot{x}1,x2}(f) = j\,2\,\pi f S_{x1,x2}(f) \tag{1.8.37}$$

Particularly when $x_1(t) = x_2(t) = x(t)$

$$S_{\dot{x},x}(f) = j\,2\,\pi f S_x(f) \tag{1.8.38}$$

Because this is an odd function

$$R_{\dot{x},x}(0) = \overline{\dot{x}(t)x(t)} = \int_{-\infty}^{\infty} S_{\dot{x},x}(f)\, df = 0 \tag{1.8.39}$$

which means that at any time, $t$, the random process and its derivative are uncorrelated, and if $x(t)$ is Gaussian they are independent rvs.

d. Let

$$x_1(t) = x_2(t) = x(t), \text{ and let } H_2(f) = 1$$

Hence

$$y_2(t) = x(t)$$

Then

$$S_{y1,x}(f) = S_x(f)H_1(f) \tag{1.8.40}$$

### 1.8.4 Complex random process

A *complex random process* is defined by

$$x(t) = x_I(t) + jx_Q(t) \tag{1.8.41}$$

where $x_I(t)$ and $x_Q(t)$ are real rps. Their cross-correlation is defined by

$$R_{x,y}(t + \tau, t) = (1/2)\overline{x(t + \tau)y^*(t)} \tag{1.8.42}$$

and if $y(t) = x(t)$

$$R_x(t + \tau, t) = (1/2)\overline{x(t + \tau)x^*(t)} \tag{1.8.43}$$

The processes are wss if

$$R_{x,y}(t + \tau, t) = R_{x,y}(\tau) \tag{1.8.44}$$

In terms of the real and imaginary parts we have

$$\begin{aligned} R_{x,y}(\tau) &= (1/2)\overline{\{x_I(t + \tau) + jx_Q(t + \tau)\}\{y_I(t) - jy_Q(t)\}} \\ &= (1/2)\{R_{xI,yI}(\tau) + R_{xQ,yQ}(\tau) + j(R_{xQ,yI}(\tau) - R_{xI,yQ}(\tau)\} \end{aligned} \tag{1.8.45}$$

Particularly the autocorrelation is

$$R_x(\tau) = (1/2)\{R_{xI}(\tau) + R_{xQ}(\tau) + j(R_{xQ,xI}(\tau) - R_{xI,xQ}(\tau))\} \tag{1.8.46}$$

Because

$$R_{xI,xQ}(\tau) = R_{xQ,xI}(-\tau) \tag{1.8.47}$$

we obtain

$$\begin{aligned} R_x(\tau) &= (1/2)\{R_{xI}(\tau) + R_{xQ}(\tau) + j(R_{xQ,yI}(\tau) - R_{xQ,yI}(-\tau))\} \\ &= R_{xe}(\tau) + jR_{xo}(\tau) \end{aligned} \tag{1.8.48}$$

where

$$R_{xe}(\tau) = \text{Re}\,\{R_x(\tau)\} = (1/2)\{R_{xI}(\tau) + R_{xQ}(\tau)\} \tag{1.8.49}$$

$$R_{xo}(\tau) = \text{Im}\,\{R_x(\tau)\} = (1/2)\{R_{xQ,xI}(\tau) - R_{xQ,xI}(-\tau)\} \tag{1.8.50}$$

Note that $R_{xe}(\tau)$ is an even function, and $R_{xo}(\tau)$ is an odd function; therefore when we take the FT

$$S_x(f) = \int_{-\infty}^{\infty} R_{xe}(\tau)\cos(2\pi f\tau)\,d\tau + \int_{-\infty}^{\infty} R_{xo}(\tau)\sin(2\pi f\tau)\,d\tau$$

$$= S_{xe}(f) + S_{xo}(f) \tag{1.8.51}$$

where $S_{xe}(f)$ is an even function, and $S_{xo}(f)$ is an odd function; thus $S_x(f)$ is real, although $x(t)$ and $R_x(\tau)$ are complex.

If $x_Q(t + \tau)$ and $x_I(t)$ are uncorrelated for all $t$ and $\tau$ (not only for $\tau = 0$), then $R_{xQ,xI}(\tau) = 0$, $R_{xo}(\tau) = 0$, $R_x(\tau)$ is even, and

$$S_x(f) = S_{xe}(f) \tag{1.8.52}$$

On the other hand, if $S_x(f)$ is even, that means that $S_{xo}(f) = 0$, $R_x(\tau)$ is real and even, and $x_Q(t + \tau)$ and $x_I(t)$ are uncorrelated.

### 1.8.5 Equivalence of bandpass and baseband noise

$n(t)$ is a *baseband wssp* if $S_n(f) = 0$ for $|f| \geqq B$. $n_M(t)$ is a *bandpass wssp* if $S_n(f) = 0$ for $|f \pm f_c| > B$, $B < f_c$. $n_M(t)$ is *narrowband* if $n_M(t)$ is bandpass and $B \ll f_c$. If bandpass noise passes an ideal bandpass filter.

$$H(f) = \begin{cases} 1 & |f \pm f_c| \leqq W \\ 0 & \text{otherwise} \end{cases} \tag{1.8.53}$$

where $B \leqq W \leqq f_c$ the output is identical to the input. The scheme in Fig. 1.11 is a realization of such a filter, provided $h_{\text{id}}(t)$ has bandwidth $W$, i.e., the FT of $h_{\text{id}}(t)$ is from (1.7.11)

$$H_{\text{id}}(f) = u_{2W}(f + W) = \begin{cases} 1 & |f| < W \\ 0 & \text{otherwise} \end{cases} \tag{1.8.54}$$

This filter does not change if the number, 2, is attached to the first pair multipliers rather then to the second pair. Thus we obtain the representation of bandpass noise as in Fig. 1.27, i.e.

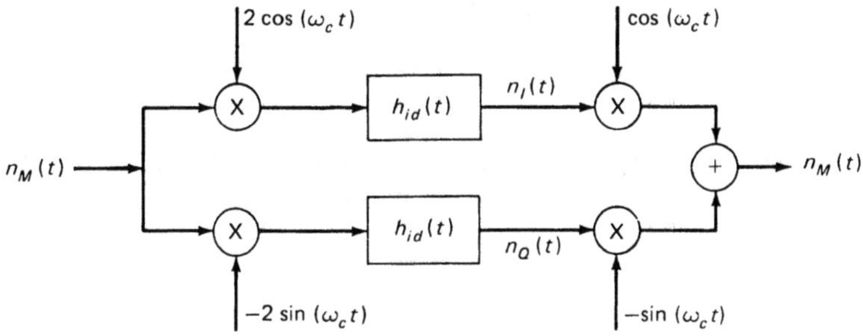


Fig. 1.27. Representation of bandpass noise.

$$\begin{aligned} n_M(t) &= n_I(t) \cos(\omega_c t) - n_Q(t) \sin(\omega_c t) \\ &= \text{Re}\{n(t) \exp(j\omega_c t)\} \end{aligned} \tag{1.8.55}$$

where

$$n(t) = n_I(t) + jn_Q(t) \tag{1.8.56}$$

is complex baseband noise because its components have passed an ideal baseband filter

$$n_I(t) = 2n_M(t) \cos(\omega_c t) * h_{\text{id}}(t) \tag{1.8.57}$$

$$n_Q(t) = -2\, n_M(t) \sin(\omega_c t) * h_{\text{id}}(t) \tag{1.8.58}$$

i.e.

$$n(t) = 2n_M(t) \exp(-j\omega_c t) * h_{\text{id}}(t) \tag{1.8.59}$$

We can see from Fig. 1.27 or Eqs. (1.8.55) and (1.8.59) that the bandpass noise $n_M(t)$ and baseband noise $n(t)$ are simply related to each other. We shall call $n(t)$ the baseband equivalent noise of $n_M(t)$. In this section we shall determine the PSD of $n(t)$, $n_I(t)$, and $n_Q(t)$ in terms of the PSD of $n_M(t)$. Let

$$x(t) = 2\, n_M(t) \exp(-j\omega_c t) \tag{1.8.60}$$

hence

$$R_x(\tau) = (1/2)x(t + \tau)x^*(t) = 2\, R_{nM}(\tau) \exp(-j\omega_c \tau) \tag{1.8.61}$$

and

$$S_x(f) = 2\, S_{nM}(f + f_c) \tag{1.8.62}$$

It follows from (1.8.59) and (1.8.60) that

$$S_n(f) = 2\, S_{nM}(f + f_c)H_{\text{id}}(f) \tag{1.8.63}$$

This can be illustrated as in Fig. 1.10, with $H$ *replaced by* $S_n$. We can decompose (1.8.63) into odd and even parts

$$S_n(f) = S_{ne}(f) + S_{no}(f) \tag{1.8.64}$$

where

$$S_{ne}(f) = (1/2)\{S_n(f) + S_n(-f)\} \tag{1.8.65}$$

$$S_{no}(f) = (1/2)\{S_n(f) - S_n(-f)\} \tag{1.8.66}$$

and comparing with (1.8.49)–(1.8.50)

$$S_{ne}(f) = (1/2)\{S_{nI}(f) + S_{nQ}(f)\} \tag{1.8.67}$$

$$S_{no}(f) = (1/2)\{S_{nQ,nI}(f) - S_{nI,nQ}(f)\} \tag{1.8.68}$$

Let us also compute

$$V_n(t, \tau) = (1/2)\overline{n(t + \tau)n(t)} \tag{1.8.69}$$

When we substitute (1.8.56) we obtain

$$V_n(t, \tau) = (1/2)\{R_{nI}(\tau) - R_{nQ}(\tau)\} - (1/2)j\{R_{nI,nQ}(\tau) + R_{nQ,nI}(\tau)\} = V_n(\tau) \tag{1.8.70}$$

which is not a function of $t$. On the other hand, when we substitute (1.8.59), $V_n(t, \tau)$ is proportional to $\exp(-j\, 2\, \omega_c t)$. The only way to reconcile this contradiction is that the part that is independent of $t$ is zero (this can be proved directly). Hence from (1.8.70)

$$R_{nI}(\tau) = R_{nQ}(\tau) \tag{1.8.71}$$

$$R_{nI,nQ}(\tau) = -R_{nQ,nI}(\tau) \tag{1.8.72}$$

We thus obtain in (1.8.46) and (1.8.47), with $x$ replaced by $n$

$$R_n(\tau) = R_{nI}(\tau) + jR_{nQ,nI}(\tau) = R_{ne}(\tau) + jR_{no}(\tau) \tag{1.8.73}$$

We also obtain from (1.8.67) and (1.8.68)

$$S_{nI}(f) = S_{nQ}(f) = S_{ne}(f) = \{S_{nM}(f + f_c) + S_{nM}(-f + f_c)\}H_{id}(f) \quad (1.8.74)$$

$$S_{nQ,nI}(f) = S_{no}(f) = \{S_{nM}(f + f_c) - S_{nM}(-f + f_c)\}H_{id}(f) \quad (1.8.75)$$

We thus conclude that if $S_{nM}(f)$ is an even function around $f_c$ for $f > 0$, then

$$S_{nM}(f + f_c) = S_{nM}(-f + f_c) = S_{nM}(f - f_c) \quad (1.8.76)$$

hence

$$S_{no}(f) = S_{nQ,n1}(f) = 0 \quad (1.8.77)$$

and

$$S_n(f) = S_{ne}(f) = S_{nQ}(f) = S_{nI}(f) = 2\, S_{nM}(f + f_c)H_{id}(f) \quad (1.8.78)$$

The average power in $n(t)$ is from (1.8.64) and (1.8.74)

$$\overline{n^2(t)} = \int_{-\infty}^{\infty} S_{ne}(f)\, df = \overline{n_I^2(t)} = \overline{n_Q^2(t)} = \overline{n_M^2(t)} \quad (1.8.79)$$

i.e., the same as in the bandpass noise. We also see from (1.8.79) that the average power in the components is the same as in the bandpass noise.

We also conclude that if $S_n(f)$ is even, $n_Q(t)$ and $n_I(t)$ are uncorrelated processes (not only for the same $t$), and if they are Gaussian they are independent.

Bandpass noise has the following additional properties

a. Let $n(t)$ be a zero mean complex process, and let

$$n_1(t) = n(t) \exp(j\phi(t)) \quad (1.8.80)$$

Then the variance of $n_1(t)$ is

$$\sigma_{n1}^2 = R_{n1}(0) = (1/2)\overline{n_1(t)n_1^*(t)} = R_n(0) = \sigma_n^2 \quad (1.8.81)$$

i.e., the variance is the same as for $n(t)$. $n_1(t)$ is also zero mean.

b. With the same condition as in (a)

$$R_{n1}(\tau) = R_n(\tau) \exp\{j(\phi(t + \tau) - \phi(t))\} \quad (1.8.82)$$

Thus whenever $n(t)$ and $n(t + \tau)$ are uncorrelated, ($R_n(\tau) = 0$) also $n_1(t)$ and $n_1(t + \tau)$ are uncorrelated. Particularly, if $\phi$ is a constant, then

$$R_{n1}(\tau) = R_n(\tau) \tag{1.8.83}$$

Because a Gaussian process is determined by its average, which is here zero, and the autocorrelation, $n_1(t)$ and $n(t)$ have identical pdf. This implies that for a Gaussian process we can in (1.8.55) and (1.8.59) (and also in Fig. 1.27) add an arbitrary constant phase without affecting the properties of the noise.

c. Let $n_c(t)$ be white, Gaussian noise, and let $H_{RM}(f)$ be a bandpass filter. The output of this filter will be bandpass noise $n_M(t)$ with PSD

$$S_{nM}(f) = (1/2)N_0|H_{RM}(f)|^2 \tag{1.8.84}$$

The baseband equivalent noise will have a PSD

$$S_n(f) = (1/2)N_0|H_{RM}(f + f_c)H_{id}(f)|^2 = (1/2)N_0|H_R(f)|^2 \tag{1.8.85}$$

where $H_R(f)$ is the baseband equivalent transfer function of the bandpass filter. It follows that the bandpass and baseband systems in Fig. 1.28 are equivalent so far as noise is concerned. In Fig. 1.28(b), we have omitted the block $h_{id}(t)$, because it does not affect $h_R(t)$ (the bandwidth $W \geq B$).

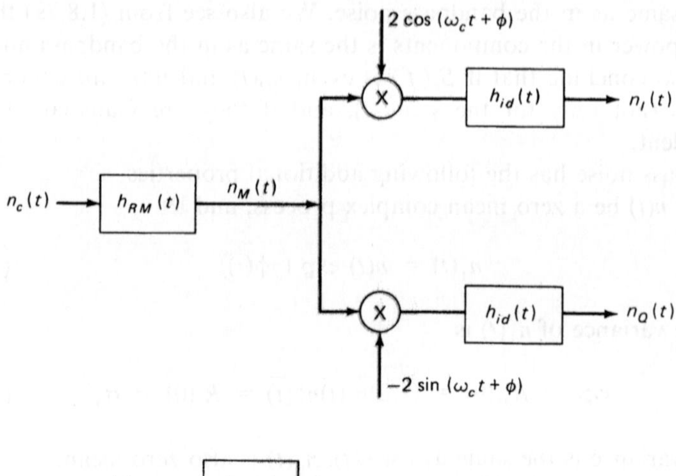


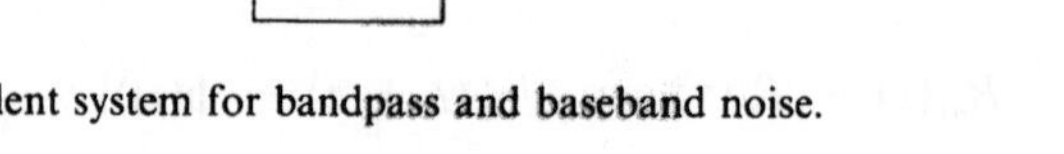


Fig. 1.28. Equivalent system for bandpass and baseband noise.

Up till now we have assumed that $S_{nM}(f) = 0$ for $|f \pm f_c| \geqq f_c$. If this is not true we have to use Hilbert transforms as we have done in Section 1.4.6. We can define a complex envelope for the noise, $n(t)$ with PSD $S_n(f)$ as follows. Instead of (1.8.59) let

$$n(t) = 2\, n_M(t) \exp(-j\omega_c t) * h_a(t) \tag{1.8.86}$$

where, as in (1.4.51), $h_a(t)$ is the IFT of $u(f + f_c)$. Since

$$|u(f + f_c)|^2 = u(f + f_c) \tag{1.8.87}$$

we obtain from (1.8.86)

$$S_n(f) = 2\, S_{nM}(f + f_c) u(f + f_c) \tag{1.8.88}$$

$$R_n(\tau) = 2\, R_{nM}(\tau) \exp(-j\omega_c \tau) * h_a(t) \tag{1.8.89}$$

The analytic signal obtained from $S_{nM}(f)$ is

$$S_{nMa}(f) = 2\, S_{nM}(f) u(f) = S_{nM}(f) + jS_{nMH}(f)$$

where $S_{nMH}(f)$ is the HT of $S_{nM}(f)$. Thus

$$S_n(f) = S_{nMa}(f + f_c) \tag{1.8.90}$$

All derivations in this subsection remain valid provided we replace $h_{\mathrm{id}}(t)$ by $h_a(t)$. When the noise is bandpass, we can replace $h_a(t)$ by $h_{\mathrm{id}}(t)$.

## 1.9 SUMMARY

In this chapter I have presented a brief review of the interaction of deterministic and random signals with linear filters. I presented and analysed various mathematical tools (correlation, orthogonal series, Fourier series, Fourier transforms, Laplace transforms, Hilbert transforms, auto and cross-correlation, power spectral density) needed in the understanding, analysis, and design of digital communications systems. I have treated in some depth the problem of equivalence between bandpass and baseband signals, filters, and stochastic processes. It is hoped that the reader is in fact familiar with most or all of the material presented in this chapter and that the chapter is required only as a refreshment of the memory and as an introduction to the notation used in the book. Although most chapters of the book are self-contained, it was necessary in some instances to refer to the material of this chapter.

## 1.10 PROBLEMS

1.2.1 Show that the energy of a periodic signal is infinite.

1.2.2

a. Show that

$$x(t) * y(t) = y(t) * x(t)$$

b. Show that if $x(t)$ and $y(t)$ are causal, then

$$x(t) * y(t) = \int_0^t x(t - \tau)y(\tau)\, d\tau$$

1.2.3

a. Show that

$$R_{x,y}(\tau) = R^*_{y,x}(-\tau)$$

b. Show that the autocorrelation of

$$z(t) = x(t) + y(t)$$

is

$$R_z(\tau) = R_x(\tau) + R_y(\tau) + R_{x,y}(\tau) + R_{y,x}(\tau)$$

c. Show that $R_x(\tau)$ is even when $x(t)$ is real.
d. Show that if $x(t) = x_I(t) + jx_Q(t)$, then

$$R_x(\tau) = R_{xI}(\tau) + R_{xQ}(\tau) + j(R_{xQ,xI}(\tau) - R_{xQ,xI}(-\tau))$$

1.2.4

a. Show that $\{\cos(2\pi kt/T)\}$ and $\{\sin(2\pi kt/T)\}$ are sets of orthogonal functions in any interval of length $T$.

b. Show that the periodic function

$$x(t) = x(t + T)$$

can be expanded into Fourier series

$$x(t) = c_0 + \sum_i c_n \cos(2\pi nt/T) + s_n \sin(2\pi nt/T)$$

where

$$c_0 = \int_{-T/2}^{T/2} x(t)\, dt/T$$

$$c_n = \frac{1}{2}\int_{-T/2}^{T/2} x(t) \cos (2\, \pi n t/T)\, dt/T$$

c. Show that $\{s_n = 0\}$ if $x(t)$ is even and $\{c_n = 0\}$ if $x(t)$ is odd.
d. Express $\{c_n\}$ and $\{s_n\}$ as a function of $\{x_n\}$.

1.2.5 Derive the Fourier transforms in Table 1.1.

1.2.6 Prove the properties of Fourier transforms in Table 1.2.

1.2.7 Compute and sketch the Fourier series and Fourier transforms of

$$x(t) = \sum_i h(t - iT)$$

where (a) $h(t) = \cos (\pi t/T) u_T(t + T/2)$; (b) $h(t) = \sin (\pi t/T) u_T(t)$.

1.2.8

a. Compute and sketch the energy spectral density of

$$x(t) = \sin (\pi t/T) u_T(t)$$

b. Compute the energy of this signal.

1.2.9

a. Show that if $x_1(t)$ and $x_2(t)$ are causal, then

$$\int_{-\infty}^{\infty} X_1(f) X_2(f) = 0$$

b. Show that (a) is true if $x_1(t)$, $x_2(t)$ are real and one of the functions is even while the other is odd.

1.2.10 Compute and sketch the FT of

$$y(t) = x(t) \cos (2\, \pi f_c t + \phi)$$

if $X(f)$ is as in Fig. 1.4 and $f_c > B$.

1.2.11 Compute the Laplace transforms of Table 1.3

1.2.12 Prove the properties of Laplace transforms in Table 1.4.

1.2.13 Compute $h(t)$ if

$$H'(s) = \frac{s^2 + 1}{s^3 + 3s^2 + 7s + 5}$$

1.3.1 Compute the response of a filter with LT

$$H'(s) = \frac{1}{s + a}$$

to the sinusoid

$$x(t) = A \sin (2\pi ft + \phi)$$

1.3.2

a. Show that a filter with LT

$$H'(s) = \frac{1}{(s + 1)(s^2 + s + 1)}$$

is a Butterworth filter of order 3.

b. Compute the 3-dB bandwidth of this filter.

c. Compute the response of this filter to a rectangular pulse $u_T(t)$.

1.3.3

a. Show that all poles of an $n$th. order Butterworth filter are on a circle of radius $2\pi f_0$.

b. Compute the Laplace transform of a Butterworth filter of order $n = 1$, 2, 3, 4, 5.

1.3.4

a. Show that the energy in $x(t)$ and in its Hilbert transform $x_h(t)$ is the same.

b. Show that

$$\int_{-\infty}^{\infty} x(t)x_h(t)\, dt = 0$$

1.3.5 Compute the Hilbert transform of Table 1.5.

1.3.6 Show that bandlimiting filters with finite $f_H$ are not causal.

1.4.1 Let

$$x_M(t) = x(t) \cos (2 \pi f_c t)$$

where

$$x(t) = \sin (\pi t/T) u_T(t)$$

and $1/T \ll f_c$.

This signal is applied to a bandpass filter whose transfer function for $f > 0$ is ($Q$ is a constant)

$$H_M(f) = \{1 + j 2 Q(f - f_c)/f_c\}^{-1}$$

Compute the output of the filter.

1.4.2 Let

$$x_M(t) = x(t) \cos (2 \pi f_T t)$$

where

$$X(f) = \cos (\pi f/F) u_F(f + F/2)$$

and $F = f_T/2$.

Compute and sketch the complex envelope of this signal with respect to $f_R = f_T - F$.

1.4.3 Compute the analytic signal of

$$x_M(t) = x(t) \cos (2 \pi f_c t)$$

$$x(t) = \exp (-\lambda t) u(t)$$

1.4.4 Let $x(t)$ be the complex envelope with respect to frequency $f_T$ and phase $\phi_T$. Show that the complex envelope with respect to frequency $f_R = f_T - \Delta f$ and $\phi_R = \phi_T - \Delta\phi$ is

$$x(t, \Delta f, \Delta\phi) = x(t) \exp (j(2 \pi \Delta f t + \Delta\phi))$$

1.4.5 In the system of Fig. P1.4.5a, $h_{TM}(t)$ is the impulse response of a bandpass filter with center frequency $f_T$ and complex envelope $h_T(t)$ with respect to $f_T$, while $h_{CM}(t)$ and $h_{RM}(t)$ have center frequency $f_R$ and complex

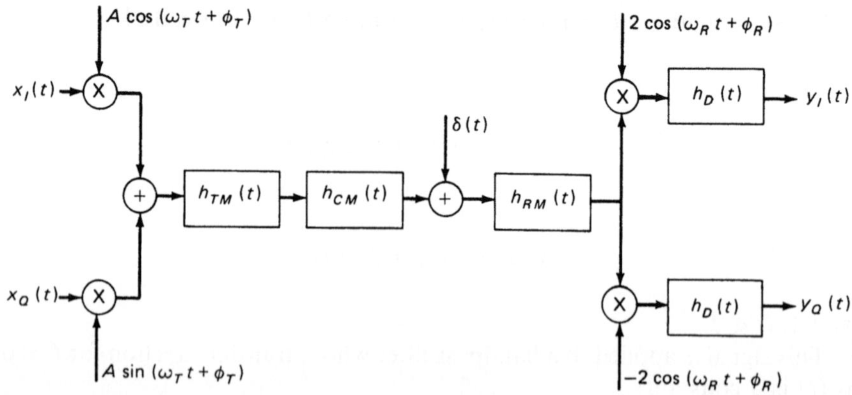


Fig. P1.4.5a.

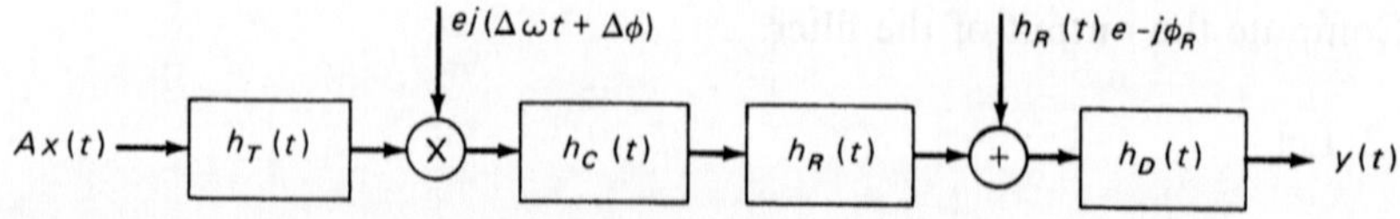


Fig. P1.4.5b.

envelopes $h_C(t)$ and $h_R(t)$, respectively, with respect to $f_R$. $h_D(t)$ is the impulse response of a baseband filter. All filters are real:

a. Show that Fig. P1.4.5b represents the baseband equivalent system and $x(t) = x_I(t) + jx_Q(t)$, $y(t) = y_I(t) + jy_Q(t)$.

b. Show that $y_I(t)$ is not a function of $x_Q(t)$ if

$$h(t) = h_T(t) \exp(j(\Delta\omega t + \Delta\phi)) * h_C(t) * h_R(t)$$

is real, i.e.

$$H(f) = H_T(f - \Delta f)H_C(f)H_R(f) \exp(j\Delta\phi)$$

is symmetric.

c. Show that if (b) is satisfied, then $y_Q(t)$ is not a function of $x_I(t)$.

d. Show that if $h_{TM}(t)$, $h_{CM}(t)$, $h_{RM}(t)$ are symmetric around their center frequencies, (b) is satisfied only if

$$\Delta f = \Delta\phi = 0$$

1.5.1 Prove the properties of sets in eq. (1.5.8).

1.5.2 Prove the properties of probabilities in eq. (1.5.10).

1.5.3 In a binary communications system the transmitted symbols are $a_1 = 1, a_2 = -1$, and the received symbols are $b_1 = 1, b_2 = -1, b_3 = 0$. The transmitted symbols have probabilities $P(a_1) = P_+, P(a_2) = P_-, P_+ + P_- = 1$. It is given that

$$\begin{aligned} P(b_1|a_1) &= P(b_2|a_2) = 0.8 \\ P(b_1|a_2) &= P(b_2|a_1) = 0.05 \\ P(b_2|a_1) &= P(b_3|a_2) = 0.15 \end{aligned}$$

Let $a$ be either $a_1$ or $a_2$ and $b$ be either $b_1$, $b_2$, or $b_3$. Compute

a. The probability of error

$$P(b \neq a)$$

b. The probability of erasure

$$P(b = b_3)$$

c. The conditional probability

$$P(a_1|b_2)$$

1.5.4

a. Using integration by parts, prove the bounds to $Q(a)$ in (1.5.38).

b. Show that $Q(a)$ can be approximated by $Q(a) = (2\pi a^2)^{-1/2} \exp(-a^2/2) \{1 - x^{-2} + 3x^{-4} - 15x^{-6} + 105x^{-8} \ldots\}$.

1.5.5 Prove the properties of PDF and pdf in (1.5.28) and (1.5.32).

1.5.6 $x$ is a zero-mean, Gaussian rv. Compute the pdf of

a. $y = x^n$, $n > 0$, $n$ integer.

b. $y = x^\alpha u(x) \qquad \alpha > 0.$

c. Compute the conditional pdf

$$p_x(a|\,|x| < \sigma)$$

1.5.7 Let $x$ have pdf

$$p_x(a) = \lambda \exp(-\lambda a)u(a)$$

a. Compute the pdf of $y = cx + d$.

b. Compute the *pdf* of $y = cx^2$.

1.5.8

a. Let $x$ be a drv with equiprobable values $x_i$, $i = 1, \ldots, M$, i.e., $P(x = x_i) = 1/M$. Let $y = -\ln P(x)$. Compute $\bar{y}$.

b. Let $x$ be a zero-mean, Gaussian rv. Compute the average of $y = -\ln p_x(a)$.

1.5.9 Let $x$ be a drv with $M$ values $\{\pm 1, \pm 3, \pm 5, \pm(1 + M)\}$. Compute $\bar{x}$ and $\overline{x^2}$.

1.6.1 Let $x_1$ and $x_2$ have a joint pdf as in Example 1.6.1. Compute $\overline{x_1 x_2}$.

1.6.2 Let $x$ and $n$ be independent rvs. $x$ is discrete with equiprobable values $\pm 1$, while $n$ has a zero-mean Gaussian pdf.

a. Compute the pdf of $y = Ax + n$.

b. Let $\hat{x} = \text{sign } y$. Compute

$$P(\hat{x} = 1|x = 1), \; P(\hat{x} = -1|x = 1)$$

1.6.3 Let $x_1$ and $x_2$ be independent rvs. Let $x_1$ have a uniform pdf in 0—$A$, and let $x_2$ have an arbitrary pdf.

a. Show that the pdf of

$$y = x_1 + x_2$$

is

$$p_y(b) = A^{-1} \int_{b-A}^{b} p_{x2}(a)\, da$$

b. Let

$$y_m = y \qquad \text{(modulo A)}$$

i.e., if $kA \leq y \leq (k + 1)A$, then $y_m = y - kA$ for all integer $k$. Show first that

$$p_{y_m}(b) = \sum_k p_y(b + kA)$$

and next that $y$ is uniformly distributed in 0—$A$.

1.6.4 Let $n_I$ and $n_Q$ be independent, zero-mean, Gaussian rvs with the same variance. Let $A_c$ be a constant. Let

$$A^2 = (n_I + A_c)^2 + n_Q^2$$

$$\theta = \tan^{-1}\{n_Q(n_I + \text{A})^{-1}\}$$

a. Compute the joint pdf of $p_{A,\theta}(a, b)$.
b. Show that the pdf of $A$ is

$$p_A(a) = (A/\sigma^2) \exp(-(a^2 + A_c^2))I_0(aA_c/\sigma)$$

where

$$I_0(x) = (2\pi)^{-1}\int_0^{2\pi} \exp(x \cos\theta)\, d\theta$$

is the modified Bessel function of the first kind and zero order.

1.7.1 Show by induction that the pdf of the sum of $N$ independent rv is the convolution of the pdfs.

1.7.2 Let $x_i$ $i = 1, \ldots, N$ be Gaussian rvs. Let

$$y = \sum_{i=1}^{N} a_i x_i$$

a. Compute $\bar{y}$.
b. Compute $\sigma_y^2$.
c. Show that the characteristic function of a Gaussian vector $\mathbf{x} = (x_1, \ldots, x_N)$ is

$$M_{\mathbf{x}}(\mathbf{v}) = \exp(-\mathbf{v}\Lambda\mathbf{v}^T/2 + j\mathbf{v}\mathbf{m}^T{}_x)$$

$$= \exp\left(-\frac{1}{2}\sum_{i=1}^{N}\sum_{j=1}^{N} v_i\lambda_{ij}v_j + j\sum_{i=1}^{N} v_i m_i\right)$$

where

$$m_i = \overline{x_i},\ \lambda_{ij} = \overline{(x_i - m_i)(x_j - m_j)}$$

1.7.3 Using Problem 1.7.2, show that if $\mathbf{y}$ is a vector that contains a subset of the components of $\mathbf{x}$, then $\mathbf{y}$ is also Gaussian. Particularly, show that if

$$y_1 = \sum_{i=1}^{N} a_i x_i$$

$y_i$ is Gaussian.

1.8.1 Let

$$x(t) = A \cos(2\pi f t + \phi)$$

where $A$ and $\phi$ are independent rvs. Assume that $A$ is a symmetric rv and $\phi$ is uniformly distributed in 0—2 $\pi$. Compute the average, the variance, and the autocorrelation of $x(t)$.

1.8.2 Let

$$x(t) = \sum_i a_i h(t - iT - \tau)$$

where $a_i$ are uncorrelated, identically distributed rvs, and $\tau$ is uniformly distributed in 0—$T$. Compute the average, the variance, and the autocorrelation of $x(t)$.

1.8.3 Let

$$y = \int_0^T x(t)\, dt$$

where $x(t)$ is a Gaussian, zero-mean random process. Compute the average and variance of $y$ if the autocorrelation of $x(t)$ is

$$R_x(\tau) = \exp(-\lambda|\tau|)$$

1.8.4 Let

$$y(t) = \int_{t-T}^{t} x(t)\, dt$$

where $x(t)$ is zero-mean, Gaussian process with

$$R_x(\tau) = \exp(-\lambda|\tau|)$$

a. Compute the average and autocorrelation of $y(t)$.
b. Compute the PSD of $x(t)$ and $y(t)$.

1.8.5 Let $x(t)$ be a random process applied to a linear system with impulse response $h(t)$, and let $y(t)$ be the output process. Show that

$$R_y(\tau) = R_x(\tau) * R_h(\tau)$$

1.8.6 Let $H(f)$ in Fig. 1.12(a) and Fig. 1.13(a) represent $S_n(f)$, the baseband equivalent noise. Sketch the even and odd components of the PSD in both cases.

1.8.7 Let

$$n(t) = n_I(t) + jn_Q(t)$$

a. Show that

$$\overline{\dot{n}_I(t)n_I(t)} = \overline{\dot{n}_Q(t)n_Q(t)} = 0 = \overline{\dot{n}_I(t)\dot{n}_Q(t)}$$

b. Show that if $S_n(f)$ is a symmetric function, then

$$\overline{n_I(t + \tau)n_Q(t)} = 0$$

c. Show that if $S_n(f)$ is a symmetric function, then

$$\overline{\dot{n}_I(t + \tau)\dot{n}_Q(t)} = 0$$

1.8.8 Let $x_M(t)$ be a bandpass random process

$$x_M(t) = Re\,\{x(t)\exp(j\omega_c t)\}$$

and let $h_M(t)$ be the impulse response of a bandpass filter with complex envelope $h(t)$.

a. Show that the output process is

$$y_M(t) = Re\,\{y(t)\exp(j\omega_c t)\}$$

where

$$y(t) = x(t) * h(t)$$

1.8.9 Let in Fig. P1.4.5a of Problem 1.4.5 $\delta(t)$ be replaced by $n_c(t)$, white Gaussian noise with PSD $N_0/2$. Show that Fig. P1.4.5b is a baseband equivalent model for this system if $h_R(t)\exp(-j\phi_R)$ is replaced by $n_R(t)$ with PSD

$$S_n(f) = \tfrac{1}{2}N_0|H_R(f)|^2$$

## 1.11 REFERENCES

1.1 D. K. Frederick and A. B. Carlson, *Linear Systems in Communication and Control*, John Wiley & Sons, Inc., New York, 1971.

1.2 A. Papoulis, *Signal Analysis*, McGraw-Hill Book Company, New York, 1977.

1.3 A. Papoulis, *Probability, Random Variables and Stochastic Processes*, McGraw-Hill Book Company, New York, 1965.

1.4 W. B. Davenport, *Probability and Random Processes*, McGraw-Hill Book Company, New York, 1970.

# 2 BASEBAND AND MODULATED SIGNALS

## 2.1 INTRODUCTION

A model of a digital communications system is presented in Fig. 2.1. It is composed of a communication channel, a source-destination pair, and matching devices: a transmitter between source and channel and a receiver between channel and destination.

The *communication channel* is able to carry electromagnetic signals (voltages and currents) within a certain frequency band. These signals are either *baseband* (i.e., lowpass) signals or *bandpass* signals. Baseband signals are essentially confined to a frequency band $0-B$, while bandpass signals are essentially confined to a frequency band $F_1 - F_2$ with $F_1 > 0$. Normally the bandwidth, $B$

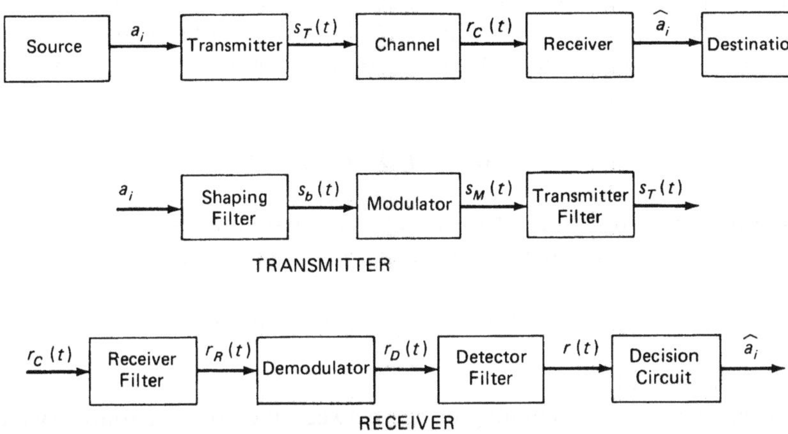


Fig. 2.1. Model of digital communications system.

$$B = F_2 - F_1 \tag{2.1.1}$$

of the channel is much smaller then the center frequency, $f_c$

$$f_c = 0.5\,\{F_1 + F_2\} \tag{2.1.2}$$

A pair of metallic wires (for example, copper wires in a telephone cable) is a typical baseband channel, while a coaxial cable, waveguide, optical fiber, atmosphere, and free space are typical bandpass channels. The details of models for some of these channels will be presented in later chapters.

The *source* produces every $T$ seconds a random symbol from a set of $M$ symbols. Let the set be denoted by

$$\mathring{A} = \{a(1), a(2), \ldots, a(M)\} \tag{2.1.3}$$

and the symbols are $a(m)$, $m = 1, 2, \ldots M$. Typical symbol sets are

$$\mathring{A}_1 = \{1, 2, \ldots, M\} \tag{2.1.4}$$

$$\mathring{A}_\pm = \{\pm 1, \pm 3, \ldots, \pm(M-1)\} \tag{2.1.5}$$

Thus at time $iT$, the source generates the symbol $a_i \in \mathring{A}$. At the destination a symbol is delivered at time

$$t_i = iT + t_d \tag{2.1.6}$$

where $t_d$ is the time delay introduced by the communications system. The delivered symbol is $\hat{a}_i \in \mathring{A}$, which is an estimate of the source symbol $a_i$. When symbol $\hat{a}_i$ differs from $a_i$ an error occurs. The symbol error probability is the probability that the symbol delivered to destination differs from the symbol emitted by source, i.e.

$$P(e) = P(\hat{a}_i \neq a_i) \tag{2.1.7}$$

$P(\ )$ means the probability of the event in the parentheses.

The *symbol rate*, i.e., the rate of generating the symbols, is

$$R = 1/T \qquad \text{symbols/sec \{bauds\}} \tag{2.1.8}$$

and has the unit of baud.

The *transmitter* is a matching device between the abstract source (which generates random numbers $\{a_i\}$) and the physical channel (which carries only signals). Thus when symbol $a_i$ is generated at time $iT$, the first stage of the transmitter produces the baseband signal $h_s(t - iT, a_i)$, which is a time-shifted version of $h_s(t, a_i)$. Because there are $M$ symbols, the transmitter associates with symbol $a_i = a(m)$, $m = 1, 2 \ldots M$ the signal $h_s(t, m)$. All signals in the set $\{h_s(t, m)\ m = 1, 2, \ldots, M\}$ are baseband. When the source produces the sequence of symbols $\{a_i\}$, $-\infty < i < \infty$ the first stage of the transmitter produces the sequence of signals $\{h_s(t - iT, a_i)\}$ or, in a concise form, the resulting baseband signal, $s_b(t)$

$$s_b(t) = \sum_i h_s(t - iT, a_i) \tag{2.1.9}$$

where the summation is over all $i$. If the channel is a baseband channel, the signal of (2.1.9) can be either directly delivered to the channel or may first be filtered by a baseband transmitter filter and then delivered to the channel. Such a filter will change the temporal and spectral properties of the baseband signal. If the channel is a bandpass channel, a *modulator*, which is part of the transmitter, produces a modulated signal from the baseband signal and a carrier signal

$$c(t) = A \cos (2 \pi f_c t + \phi_T) \tag{2.1.10}$$

where $A, f_c$, and $\phi_T$ are, respectively, the amplitude, carrier frequency, and phase, so that a bandpass signal with center frequency $f_c$ is generated. This bandpass signal may be directly delivered to the channel or may first be filtered by a bandpass transmitter filter, so that the power spectral density (which is defined precisely in Chapter 3) of the transmitted signal complies with international and national regulations.

The *receiver* is a matching device between the physical channel and abstract destination. The receiver is reached by an attenuated, distorted, and noise-corrupted version of the transmitted baseband or bandpass signal. This signal is first filtered by a baseband (if the channel is baseband) or bandpass (if the channel is bandpass) receiver filter, which reduces the effect of noise. If the signal is bandpass, the *demodulator*, which is part of the receiver, converts the signal from bandpass to baseband, and the resulting baseband signal may again be filtered by a baseband demodulator filter. The output of the last filter is sampled every $T$ seconds and a decision is made about the value of the transmitted symbol. At time $t_i = iT + t_d$, the decision is $\hat{a}_i$, and this symbol is delivered to destination.

The signals $\{h_s(t, m), m = 1, 2, \ldots, M)\}$ will be called here *shaping functions*. Various shaping functions are used in communications systems, and these are presented in later sections of this chapter. A shaping function is called *nonoverlapping* or of *full response* if its duration is not greater then $T$. Mathematically such a function is defined by

$$h_s(t, a_i) = h_s(t, a_i) u_T(t) \tag{2.1.11}$$

where $u_T(t)$ is a rectangular pulse of duration $T$ and amplitude 1

$$u_T(t) = u(t) - u(t - T) \tag{2.1.12}$$

and $u(t)$ is the unit step function

$$u(t) = \begin{cases} 1 & t \geqq 0 \\ 0 & t < 0 \end{cases} \tag{2.1.13}$$

If all shaping functions are identical except for the amplitude that depends on $a_i$, i.e.

$$h_s(t, a_i) = a_i h_s(t) \tag{2.1.14}$$

then $h_s(t)$ is called the *common shaping function.* The common shaping function is nonoverlapping if

$$h_s(t) = h_s(t)u_T(t) \tag{2.1.15}$$

In practical communications systems, most shaping functions are common and in the majority of cases also of full response. *Overlapping*, or *partial response*, shaping functions are also used in many communications systems because they require a reduced bandwidth (see Chapter 3 for details).

If the number of symbols, $M$, is an integer power of 2, i.e.

$$M = 2^\mu \tag{2.1.16}$$

then we can visualize the symbol generation as the following process. A *binary source* produces every $T_b$ seconds

$$T_b = T/\mu \tag{2.1.17}$$

a *binary symbol* (say 0 or 1, or $\pm 1$). A binary symbol will be called a *bit*. $\mu$ consecutive binary symbols are encoded into an $M$-ary symbol. Thus a symbol rate of $R$ bauds is equivalent to a bit rate of

$$R_b = 1/T_b = R \log_2 M \text{ (bps)} \tag{2.1.18}$$

where bps stands for bits per second. We shall use (2.1.18) even where $\log_2 M$ is not an integer. Various mappings or codes exist between the $\mu$-tuples of binary symbols and the $M$-ary symbols. A useful mapping is the *Gray code*, which has the following useful property: an error in the $M$-ary symbol will usually mean that only one of the $\mu$ bits is in error. Thus the *bit error rate* (BER), $P_b(e)$ is related to the symbol error rate by

$$P_b(e) = P(e)/\log_2 M \tag{2.1.19}$$

Details about Gray codes will be presented in Chapter 4.

Various methods of modulation are employed in digital communications, Generally speaking we can modulate the amplitude, the phase, or the frequency of the carrier signal. In many systems both the amplitude and phase are modulated simultaneously. In theory it is possible to modulate simultaneously any two or even all three of these parameters. The various types of modulation will be presented in the next sections of this chapter. The main aim of this chapter is to present a single formula for all types of modulation. Thus, whatever the modulation method, the modulated signal has the form

$$s_M(t) = Re\,\{s(t)\exp\,(j(2\,\pi f_c t + \phi))\} \tag{2.1.20}$$

where $Re\,\{\ \}$ denotes the real part of the term in the bracket, and $s(t)$, called the *complex envelope* of the modulated signal, has the form

$$s(t) = A\sum_i b(t - iT, \mathbf{a}_i) \tag{2.1.21}$$

where $b(t, \mathbf{a}_i)$ is in general a complex baseband signal, in most cases nonoverlapping, and $\mathbf{a}_i$ denotes the sequence of symbols $\{a_{i-k}, k = 0, 1, \ldots, K\}$ with $K$ infinite, finite, or zero. The *equivalent shaping function* $b(t, \mathbf{a}_i)$ depends on the original shaping function $h_s(t, a_i)$ and the method of modulation, while the memory length $K$ depends on the modulation method and the time duration of $h_s(t, a_i)$.

The fact that all modulated signals have the form (2.1.20), (2.1.21) enables a unified derivation of the *power spectral density* (a precise definition of which is presented in Chapter 3) by first deriving the power spectral density of the complex envelope $s(t)$.

In Section 2.2, we present $s(t)$, assuming a common, nonoverlapping function $h_s(t)$. In Section 2.3, we present $s(t)$, assuming that $\{h_s(t, a_i)\}$ are nonoverlapping. In Section 2.4, we present $s(t)$ in the case when $\{h_s(t, a_i)\}$ or the common shaping function $h_s(t)$ are overlapping. In Section 2.5, we summarize this chapter. Problems are presented in Section 2.6, followed by a list of references in Section 2.7.

## 2.2 Common, full-response, shaping function

In this section we assume that the shaping function is common to all symbols, i.e.

$$h_s(t, a_i) = a_i h_s(t) \tag{2.2.1}$$

and $h_s(t)$ has duration $T$, i.e.

$$h_s(t) = h_s(t)u_T(t) \tag{2.2.2}$$

Typical shaping functions are shown in Fig. 2.2. These functions can be described mathematically by

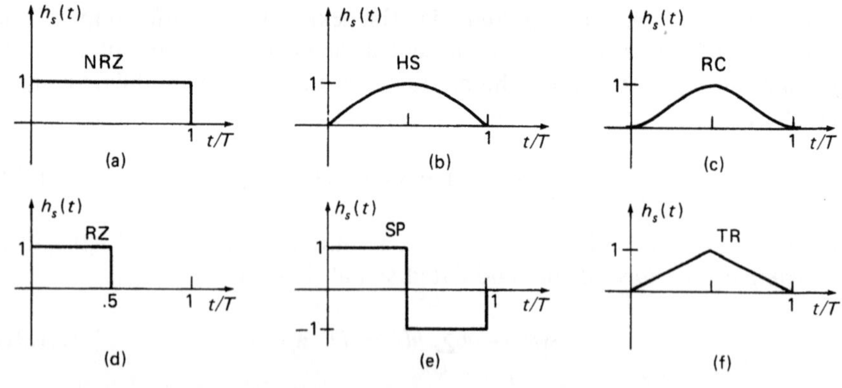


Fig. 2.2. Examples of full response (nonoverlapping) shaping functions.

$$h_s(t) = \begin{cases} u_T(t) & \text{NRZ} \\ \sin(\pi t/T) u_T(t) & \text{HS} \\ 0.5\,\{1 - \cos(2\,\pi t/T)\} u_T(t) & \text{RC} \\ u_{0.5T}(t) & \text{RZ} \\ u_{0.5T}(t) - u_{0.5T}(t - 0.5T) & \text{SP, BP} \\ 2\,(t/T) u_{0.5T}(t) + 2\,(1 - (t/T)) u_{0.5T}(t - 0.5T) & \text{TR} \end{cases} \tag{2.2.3}$$

where the initials stand for

NRZ—non return to zero
HS—half cycle of a sinusoid
RC—raised cosine
RZ—return to zero
SP(BP)—split phase (biphase)
TR—triangle

The RZ shaping function returns to zero in the middle of the symbol interval, a fact that is useful in the determination of symbol timing by the synchronization circuits of the receiver. The NRZ shaping function does not have this property, and in fact a long sequence of indentical signals will result in a DC signal. Thus an NRZ shaping function can be used for synchronization purposes only if certain rules are established to eliminate long strings of identical symbols (see, for details, Chapter 12 on line coding). Chapter 3 shows that the power spectral density of the baseband signal is proportional to $|H_s(f)|^2$, where $H_s(f)$ is the Fourier transform of $h_s(t)$. The bandwidth of the signal depends on the duration and the smoothness of the shaping function. Thus the bandwidth of RZ and SP is greater than the bandwidth of NRZ, and the bandwidth of NRZ is greater than the bandwidth of HS, TR, or RC. The exact definition of bandwidth is given in Chapter 3. Only the SP shaping function (also known as *Manchester code*) has a zero DC term, i.e., $H_s(0) = 0$, and hence can be used directly on a channel that blocks DC, for example, the telephone channel. When other shaping functions are used on such channels, either DC-restoration circuits are required in the receiver or long strings of identical symbols must be prevented from appearance. These are some of the reasons so many shaping functions have been considered for digital communications.

## 2.2.1 Baseband signal

It follows from (2.1.9) and (2.2.1) that the baseband signal has the form

$$s_b(t) = \sum_i a_i h_s(t - iT) \tag{2.2.4}$$

*Example* 2.2.1 Binary and quaternary symbols with RZ and TR shaping functions

a. Sketch the baseband signal, assuming the sequence is

$$a_0 a_1 a_2 a_3 a_4 a_5 = +1 + 1 - 3 + 3 - 1 + 1$$

(the symbols are quaternary from the set $\mathring{A}_\pm = \{\pm 1, \pm 3\}$), and the shaping function is RZ (return to zero)

b. Sketch the baseband signal, assuming the symbol sequence is $-1 + 1 - 1 - 1 + 1 + 1$ (the symbols are binary from the set $\{\mathring{A}_\pm = \pm 1\}$), and the shaping function is TR (triangle).

Based on Fig. 2.2 and eq. (2.2.4), the signals are shown in Fig. 2.3.

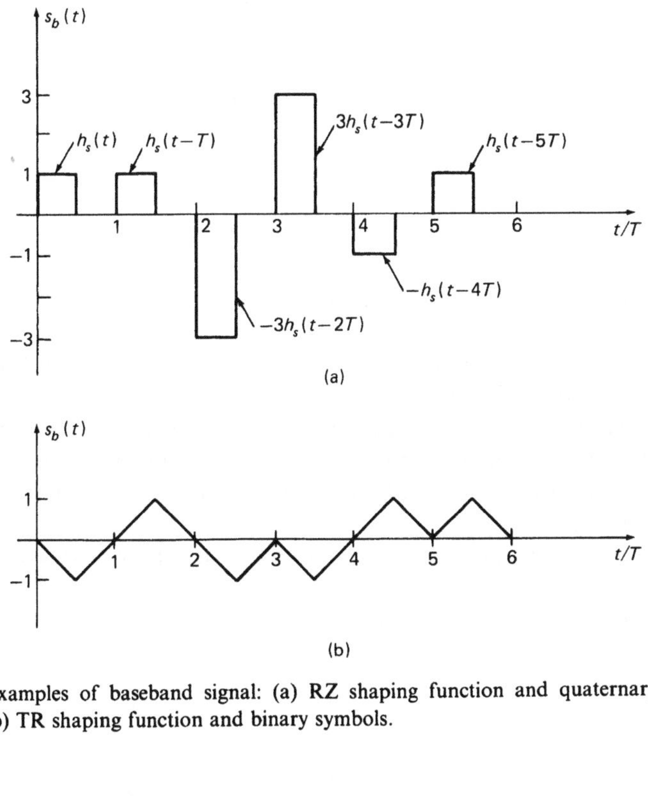


Fig. 2.3. Examples of baseband signal: (a) RZ shaping function and quaternary symbols, (b) TR shaping function and binary symbols.

The signal (2.2.4) is a random process because the sequence $\{a_i\}$ is a sequence of random symbols. The marginal and joint probabilities of these symbols are

$$P_m = P(a_i = a(m)) \qquad m = 1, 2, \ldots, M \tag{2.2.5}$$

$$P_{k,q}(n) = P(a_i = a(q), a_{i+n} = a(k)) \qquad k, q = 1, 2, \ldots, M \tag{2.2.6}$$

It is assumed that the sequence of symbols is a stationary process (in many cases wide sense stationarity is sufficient); hence $P_m$ and $P_{k,q}(n)$ are independent of the time index $i$. Unless specified otherwise, it will be assumed that the symbols are equiprobable, i.e.

$$P_m = 1/M \tag{2.2.7}$$

and independent, i.e.

$$P_{k,q}(n) = 1/M^2 \qquad n \neq 0 \tag{2.2.8}$$

The average and the mean square value of the symbols are

$$E(a) = \sum_{i}^{M} a(m)P_m \tag{2.2.9}$$

$$E(a^2) = \sum_{i}^{M} a^2(m)P_m \tag{2.2.10}$$

In most cases under consideration the average is zero.

### 2.2.2 Modulated signal

There are many reasons for modulation. One of them was already mentioned. Some others are

1. The channel is bandpass while the signal is baseband; hence the signal must be shifted in frequency.
2. Several baseband signals that occupy the same frequency band can be transmitted through a single broadband channel if they are separated in frequency, by modulating each signal on a separate carrier frequency.
3. The complexity and cost of a bandpass system may be less than a brute force baseband system.

There are essentially three methods of modulation

1. linear shift keying (LSK)

2. phase shift keying (PSK)
3. frequency shift keying (FSK)

In LSK the modulated signal $s_M(t)$ is a linear function of the modulating signal, $s_b(t)$, namely the amplitude of the carrier varies linearly with the baseband signal. In PSK the phase of the carrier is a linear function of the modulating signal. In FSK the instantanous frequency of the carrier is a linear function of the modulating signal.

### 2.2.3 Linear shift keying[2.1–2.4, 2.15–2.25]

LSK is sometimes called in the literature APSK (amplitude phase shift keying), but, in fact, in view of the definition of LSK in Sections 2.3 and 2.4 LSK is more general. Within LSK there are several methods of modulation.

#### 2.2.3.1 Amplitude shift keying-double side band (ASK-DSB)[2.1]

The relation between the modulated signal $s_M(t)$ and modulating signal $s_b(t)$ is

$$s_M(t) = As_b(t) \cos (2 \pi f_c t + \phi_T) \tag{2.2.11}$$

which can be written in the form

$$s_M(t) = \text{Re} \{s(t) \exp (j(2 \pi f_c t + \phi_T))\} \tag{2.2.12}$$

with

$$s(t) = As_b(t) = A \sum_i a_i h_s(t - iT) \tag{2.2.13}$$

which is in this case a real signal. For any specific symbol sequence, we can take the Fourier transform of (2.2.11), resulting in

$$S_M(f) = 0.5\, A\{S_b(f - f_c) \exp (j\phi_T) + S_b(f + f_c) \exp (-j\phi_t)\} \tag{2.2.14}$$

where $S_M(f)(S_b(f))$ is the Fourier transform of $s_M(t)(s_b(t))$. Equation (2.2.11) is illustrated in Fig. 2.4 for the baseband signal in Fig. 2.3(b). Equation (2.2.14) is illustrated in Fig. 2.5. As can be seen in this figure, both sidebands (the lower ($L$) and upper ($U$)) of the modulating signal are represented; hence the bandwidth of the modulated signal is twice the bandwidth of the modulating signal. The bandwidth is reduced if we eliminate completely or reduce considerably one of the sidebands by shaping the modulated signal with a single sideband or vestigial sideband filter, as shown in Fig. 2.6.

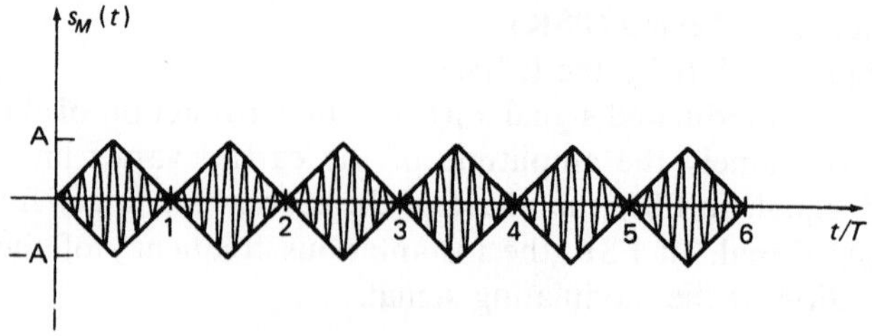


Fig. 2.4. Example of ASK-DSB modulated signal.

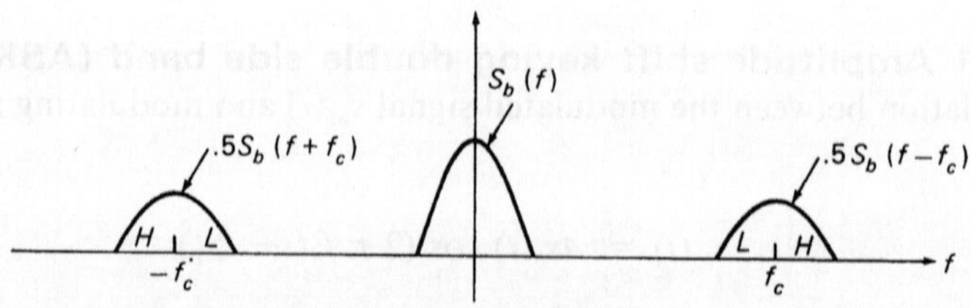


Fig. 2.5. Fourier transform of baseband and modulated signal.

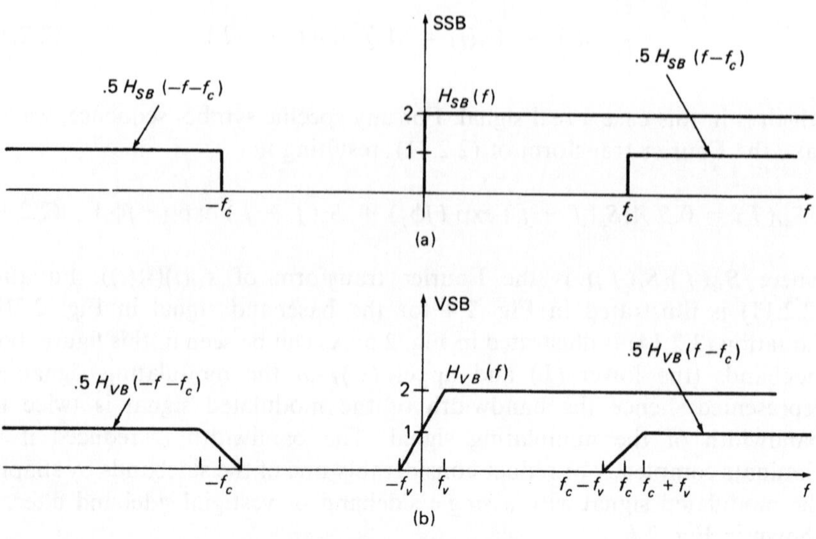


Fig. 2.6. Filters that generate: (a) SSB and (b) VSB signals.

**2.2.3.2 ASK-single side band (ASK-SSB)** Filtering of the bandpass signal is equivalent to filtering of the baseband signal. It is shown in Sections 1.4.2 and 1.4.6 that we obtain an SSB signal if we multiply $S_b(f)$ by

$$H_{\mathrm{SB}}(f) = 1 \pm jH_{\mathrm{SSB}}(f) \tag{2.2.15}$$

where

$$H_{\mathrm{SSB}}(f) = -j \operatorname{sign}(f) = \begin{cases} -j & f \geqq 0 \\ j & f < 0 \end{cases} \tag{2.2.16}$$

and the + sign corresponds to upper sideband SSB, while the − sign corresponds to lower sideband SSB. $H_{SB}(f)$ is illustrated in Fig. 2.6(a). The resulting modulated signal is as in (2.2.12) with

$$s(t) = A \sum_i a_i b(t - iT) \tag{2.2.17}$$

where $b(t)$ is a complex shaping function

$$b(t) = h_s(t) * \{\delta(t) \pm jh_{\mathrm{SBB}}(t)\} \tag{2.2.18}$$

* denotes convolution and $\delta(t)$ is the impulse function. Taking the inverse Fourier transform of (2.2.16), we obtain in the time domain

$$h_{\mathrm{SSB}}(t) = 1/(\pi t) \tag{2.2.19}$$

When we substitute (2.2.18) and (2.2.19) into (2.2.12), we see that in the time domain the SSB signal has the form

$$s_M(t) = A\left\{\sum_i a_i b_I(t - iT) \cos(2\pi f_c t + \phi_t) + \sum_i a_i b_Q(t - iT) \sin(2\pi f_c t + \phi_T)\right\} \tag{2.2.20}$$

with

$$b_I(t) = h_s(t),\ b_Q(t) = h_s(t) * 1/(\pi t) \tag{2.2.21}$$

From (2.2.18) and (2.2.16), the FT of $b(t)$ is

$$B(f) = H_s(f)u(f) \tag{2.2.22}$$

where $u(f)$ is the unit step function.

**2.2.3.3 ASK-vestigial side band (ASK-VSB)** To obtain a vestigial side band signal, we operate on $H_s(f)$ with a filter (see Sections 1.4.2 and 1.4.6)

$$H_{VB}(f) = 1 \pm jH_{VSB}(f) \tag{2.2.23}$$

where

$$H_{VSB}(f) = \begin{cases} -jH_{od}(f) & |f| \leq f_v \\ -j \text{ sign } (f) & |f| \geq f_v \end{cases} \tag{2.2.24}$$

with $H_{od}(f)$ an odd function of $f$, such that $H_{od}(f_v) = 1$, and $f_v$ is a fixed frequency. $H_{VSB}(f)$ is illustrated in Fig. 2.6(b).

The resulting modulated signal has the form of eq. (2.2.13) with

$$s(t) = A \sum_i a_i b(t - iT) \tag{2.2.25}$$

$$b(t) = h_s(t) * \{\delta(t) \pm jh_{VSB}(t)\} \tag{2.2.26}$$

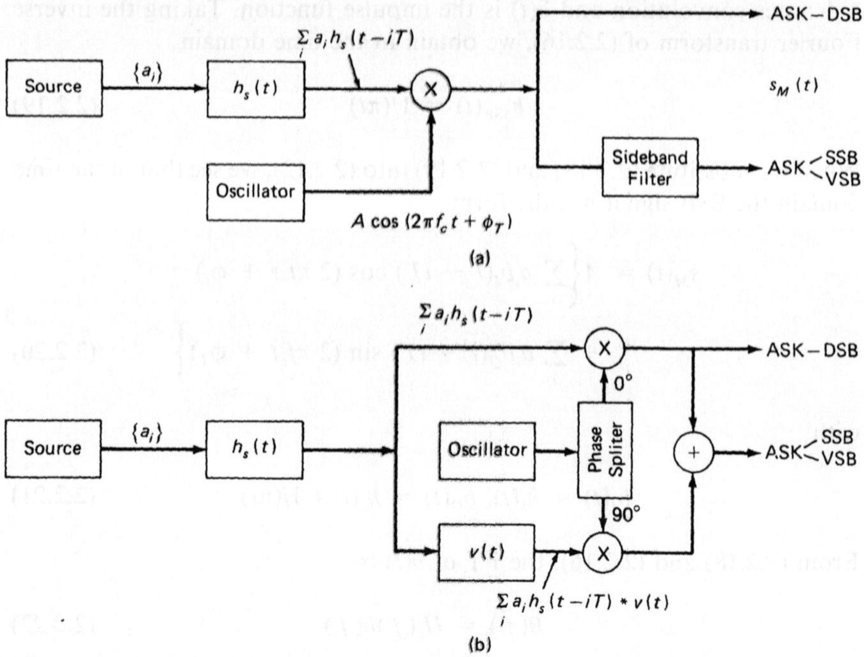


Fig. 2.7. Generation of ASK-DSB, SSB, and VSB: (a) bandpass filters (b) lowpass filters.

ASK-SSB and ASK-VSB are rarely used in modern digital communications systems, because another method, quadrature amplitude shift keying (QASK), presented next, uses the available bandwidth as efficiently as SSB, but can be generated without complicated filters. In the future we shall refer to ASK-DSB as ASK. In Fig. 2.7 we present a model of a transmitter that generates ASK (DSB, SSB, and VSB) using (a) a bandpass filter or (b) a lowpass filter.

**2.2.3.4 Quadrature amplitude shift keying (QASK)**[2.2–2.4, 2.2.5] Assume that one source generates symbols $a_{Ii} \in \mathring{A}_I$ while another source generates simultaneously $a_{Qi} \in \mathring{A}_Q$, where $\mathring{A}_Q$ and $\mathring{A}_I$ may be identical. We associate with $a_{Ii}$ the shaping function $h_{sI}(t)$ and with $a_{Qi}$ the shaping function $h_{sQ}(t)$. We form two baseband signals

$$s_{bI}(t) = \sum_i a_{Ii} h_{sI}(T - iT) \tag{2.2.27}$$

$$s_{bQ}(t) = \sum_i a_{Qi} h_{sQ}(t - iT) \tag{2.2.28}$$

The signal $s_{bI}(t)$ modulates $A_I \cos(2\pi f_c t + \phi_T)$, and $s_{bQ}(t)$ modulates the orthogonal carrier $A_Q \sin(2\pi f_c + \phi_T)$. The two carriers are in quadrature with each other. The final modulated signal is

$$s_M(t) = A_I \sum_i a_{Ii} h_{sI}(t - iT) \cos(2\pi f_c t + \phi_T)$$

$$+ A_Q \sum_i a_{Qi} h_{sQ}(t - iT) \sin(2\pi f_c t + \phi_T) \tag{2.2.29}$$

which can also be written, as in (2.2.12), with

$$s(t) = A_I \sum_i a_{Ii} h_{sI}(t - iT) + jA_Q \sum_i a_{Qi} h_{sQ}(t - iT) \tag{2.2.30}$$

In all practical systems $A_I = A_Q = A$, the two shaping functions are identical

$$h_{sI}(t) = h_{sQ}(t) = h_s(t) \tag{2.2.31}$$

hence

$$s(t) = A \sum_i a_i h_s(t - iT) \tag{2.2.32}$$

where $a_i$ is a complex (or two-dimensional) symbol

$$a_i = a_{Ii} + ja_{Qi} \tag{2.2.33}$$

This method of modulation is also called in the literature *quadrature amplitude modulation* (QAM).

The complex symbols belong to the set of pairs generated by the sets $\mathring{A}_I$ and $\mathring{A}_Q$, which can be considered as a single set of complex symbols. The set of complex symbols defines a symbol *constellation*. Several symbol constellations are presented in Fig. 2.8 for $M = 4$, 8, and 16. When we substitute eq. (2.2.32) into (2.2.12), we obtain

$$s_M(t) = A \sum_i |a_i| h_s(t - iT) \cos(2\pi f_c t + \phi_T + \arg(a_i)) \quad (2.2.34)$$

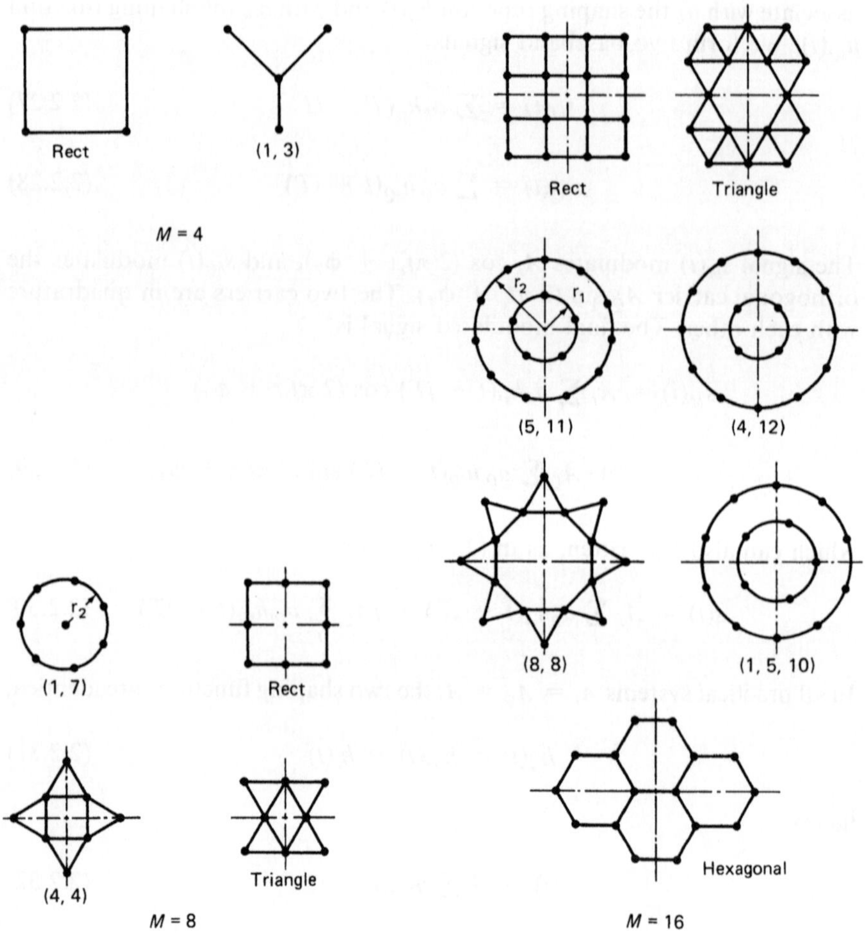


Fig. 2.8. Symbol constellations (C. M. Thomas, M. Y. Weidner, and S. H. Durrani, "Digital Amplitude Phase Shift Keying M-ary Alphabets," *IEEE Tr. Comm.*, Vol. COM-22, Feb. 1974, pp. 168–180. Copyright © 1974 IEEE).

where we assume that $h_s(t)$ is nonnegative and

$$|a_i| = \{a_{Ii}^2 + a_{Qi}^2\}^{1/2}, \arg(a_i) = \tan^{-1}(a_{Qi}/a_{Ii}) \qquad (2.2.35)$$

thus both the phase and amplitude depend on the symbol. For this reason this method of modulation is also called amplitude phase keying (APK). If all symbols are located on a single circle, the constellation is called *circular*, and the symbols can be described by

$$a_i = \exp(jK_p a_i') \qquad (2.2.36)$$

where $K_p$ is constant, $a_i'$ is real, and $a_i$ is complex. Therefore, from (2.2.34)

$$s_M(t) = A \sum_i h_s(t - iT) \cos(2\pi f_c t + \phi_T + K_p a_i') \qquad (2.2.37)$$

which is a special case of phase shift keying (see Section 2.2.4 for definition) provided $h_s(t)$ is the NRZ shaping function. Thus QASK with a circular constellation and NRZ shaping function is identical to PSK with the same shaping function. When the shaping function is not NRZ, these two modulation methods are definitely different. Most of the literature considers PSK with the NRZ shaping function only. Practical PSK systems are also of this kind; hence they can be treated as special cases of QASK. In Fig. 2.9 we illustrate the complex envelope (2.2.32) in the case of quaternary symbols $\{\pm 1 \pm j\}$ and HS shaping function. Note that the magnitude (or the envelope) is not a constant.

We mentioned before that the symbols $\{a_i\}$ are pairs of symbols from the sets $\mathring{A}_I$ and $\mathring{A}_Q$, which may contain identical symbols. In practice there may be a single source of binary symbols. We may collect $\mu/2$-tuples of these symbols and identify them with $a_{Ii}$ and $a_{Qi}$, respectively, after a proper coding.

*Example* 2.2.2 Generation of quaternary QASK from a binary source.
We illustrate generation of quaternary QASK from a binary source. We identify the even indexed bits with $a_{Ii}$, i.e., $a_{Ii} = a_{2i}$ and the odd indexed bits with $a_{Qi}$, i.e., $a_{Qi} = a_{2i+1}$. The resulting scheme is shown in Fig. 2.10.

*Example* 2.2.3 Generation of 16-ary QASK from a binary source.
We illustrate generation of 16-ary QASK with a rectangular constellation ($a_{Ii} = \pm 1, \pm 3$, $a_{Qi} = \pm 1, \pm 3$) from a binary source.

We collect sequences of four bits. Each pair of two bits is encoded into a quaternary symbol (for example, $+1+1 \rightarrow 3$, $+1-1 \rightarrow 1$, $-1+1 \rightarrow -1$, $-1-1 \rightarrow -3$). The first pair of the sequence is named $a_{Ii}$ after encoding, while the second pair is called $a_{Qi}$. The resulting scheme is shown in Fig. 2.11.

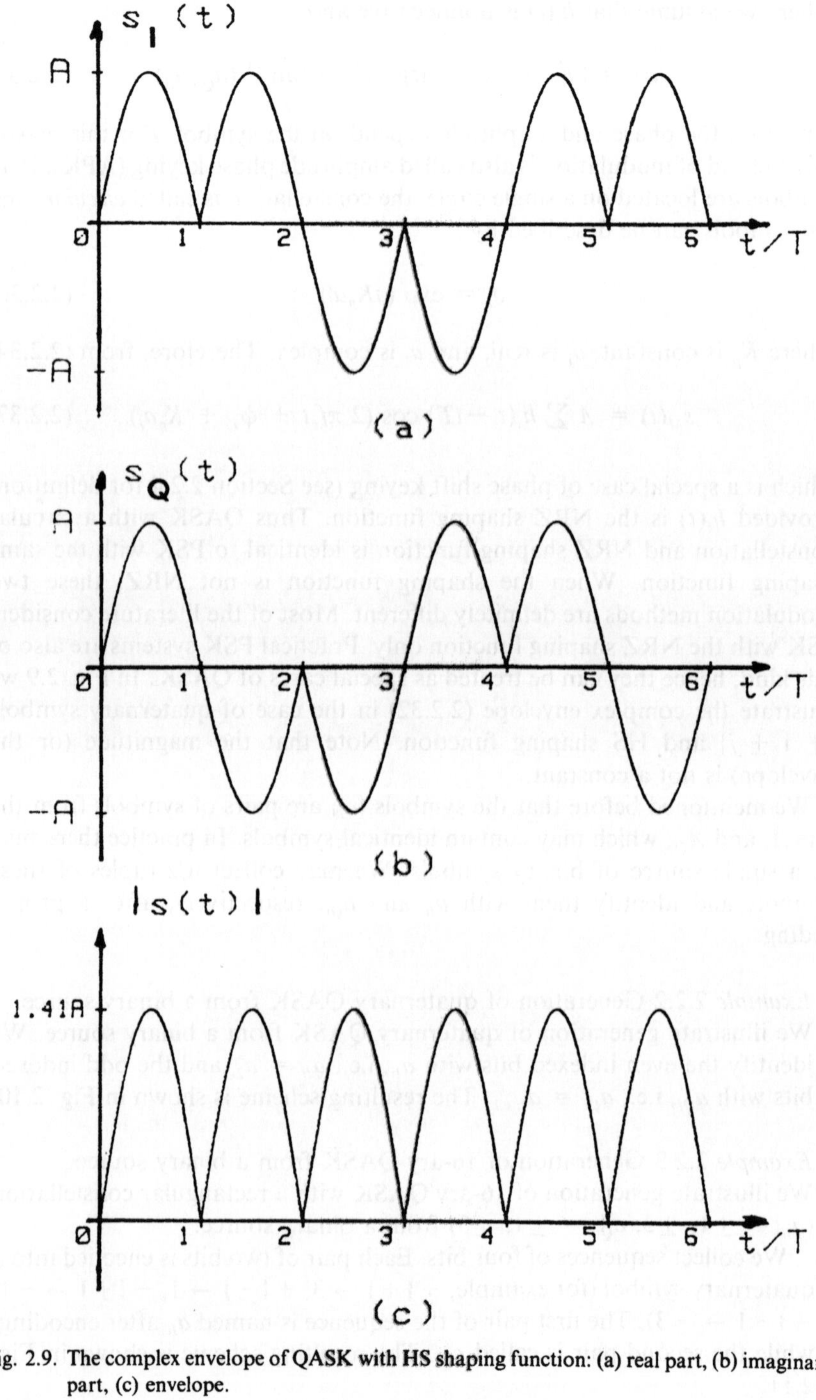


Fig. 2.9. The complex envelope of QASK with HS shaping function: (a) real part, (b) imaginary part, (c) envelope.

**2.2.3.5 Offset quadrature amplitude shift keying (OQASK)**[2.16, 2.17, 2.19, 2.20, 2.24] In this method of modulation, $s_{bQ}(t)$ is shifted with respect to $s_{bI}(t)$ by $\varepsilon T$ where $\varepsilon$ is normally 0.5. Thus the complex envelope in the general case is

$$s(t) = A_I \sum_i a_{Ii} h_{sI}(t - iT) + jA_Q \sum_i a_{Qi} h_{sQ}(t - iT - 0.5\,T) \quad (2.2.38)$$

and when $A_I = A_Q = A$, $h_{sI}(t) = h_{sQ}(t) = h_s(t)$, we obtain

$$s(t) = A \sum_i a_{Ii} h_s(t - iT) + j a_{Qi} h_s(t - iT - 0.5\,T) \quad (2.2.39)$$

OQASK generation is also illustrated in Figs. 2.10 and 2.11. The only difference is that the symbols in the quadrature channel need not be delayed by 0.5 $T$ when they are emitted by the binary source because they are already delayed by that amount.

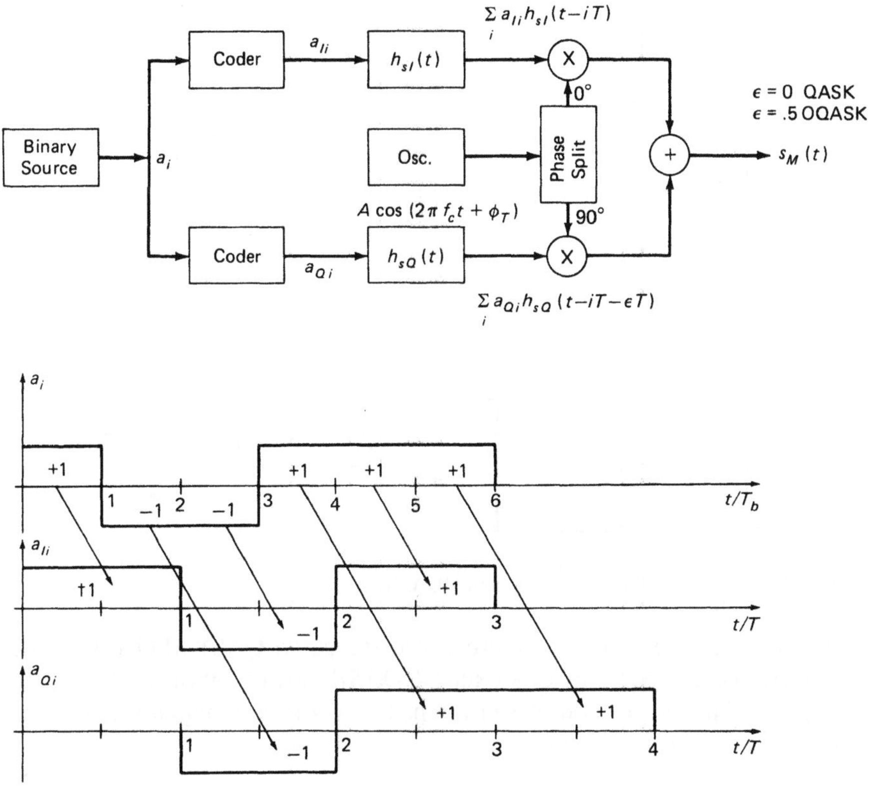


Fig. 2.10. Generation of quaternary QASK and OQASK.

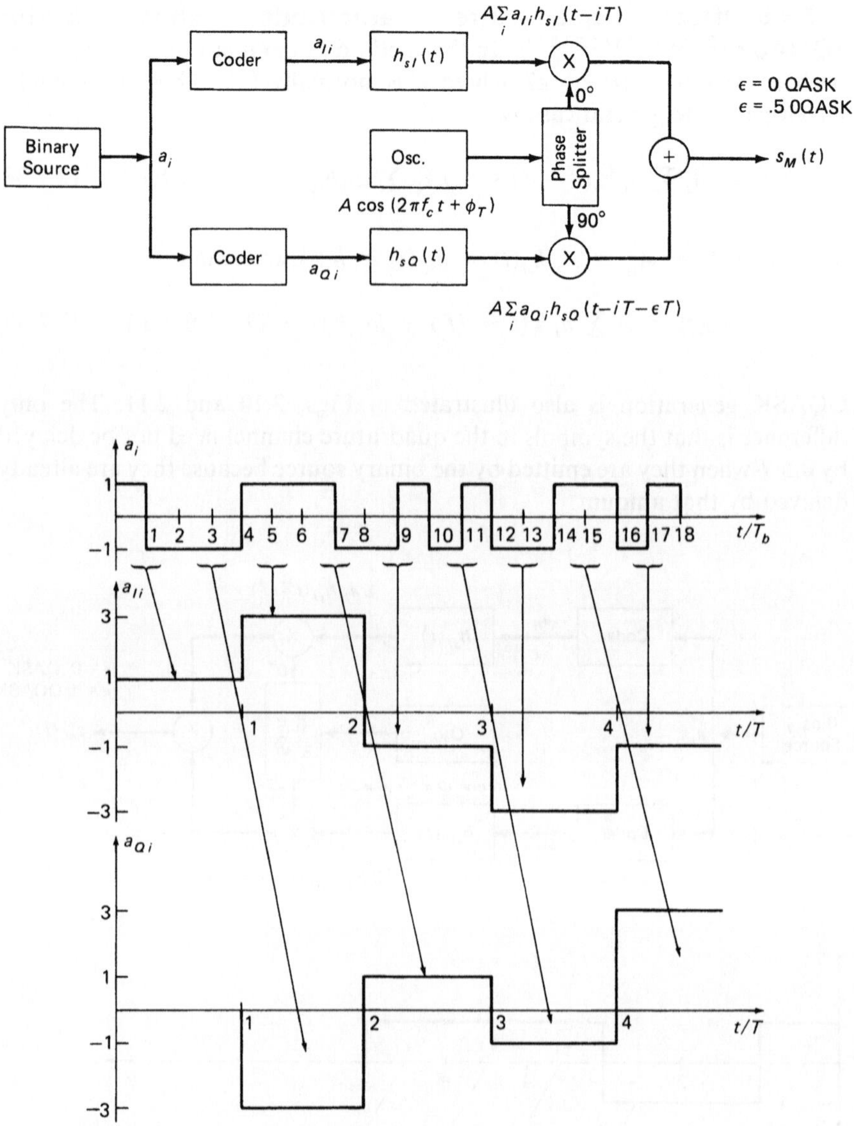


Fig. 2.11. Generation of 16-ary QASK and OQASK.

In the literature OQASK is also called staggered QASK (SQASK). The literature considers mainly quaternary OQASK, with symbols $\{\pm 1 \pm j\}$. In this particular case the complex envelope has a constant magnitude (i.e., the envelope is constant) whenever

$$h_s^2(t) + h_s^2(t - 0.5\,T) = 1 \tag{2.2.40}$$

(on the RHS we can have any other constant). This will happen if we can express

$$h_s(t) = \sin \theta(t)u_T(t),\ h_s(t - 0.5\ T) = \cos \theta(t)u_t(t - 0.5\ T) \quad (2.2.41)$$

with an arbitrary $\theta(t)$. Many shaping functions proposed in the literature satisfy (2.2.41).

*Example* 2.2.4 Constant envelope shaping functions.
We give examples of shaping functions that satisfy (2.2.41)
The first example is

$$\theta(t) = \{\pi t/T\}u_T(t) \quad (2.2.42)$$

The shaping function is

$$h_s(t) = \sin(\pi t/T) = \sin \theta(t)$$

and indeed

$$h_s(t - 0.5\ T) = \sin(\pi t/T - 0.5\ \pi) = \cos \theta(t)$$

The resulting shaping function is the same as HS in Fig. 2.2. The complex envelope of OQASK with this shaping function is illustrated in Fig. 2.12. OQASK with the HS shaping function is also known as *minimum shift keying* (MSK), which will be presented in the section about *frequency shift keying* (FSK).

Another example is

$$\theta(t) = \{\pi t/T - 0.5 \sin(2\ \pi t/T)\}u_T(t) \quad (2.2.43)$$

which is also known as *sinusoidal frequency shift keying* (SFSK), because the frequency is a sinusoidal function.

A complex envelope with a constant amplitude implies a constant envelope of the modulated signal, because

$$s_M(t) = |s(t)| \cos(2\ \pi f_c t + \phi_T + \arg(s(t)) \quad (2.2.44)$$

Signals with this property are power efficient in systems with nonlinear amplifiers. In digital satellite communications the power amplifiers are traveling wave tubes (TWT), which are used in a nonlinear mode; hence modulation methods with constant envelopes are suitable candidates.

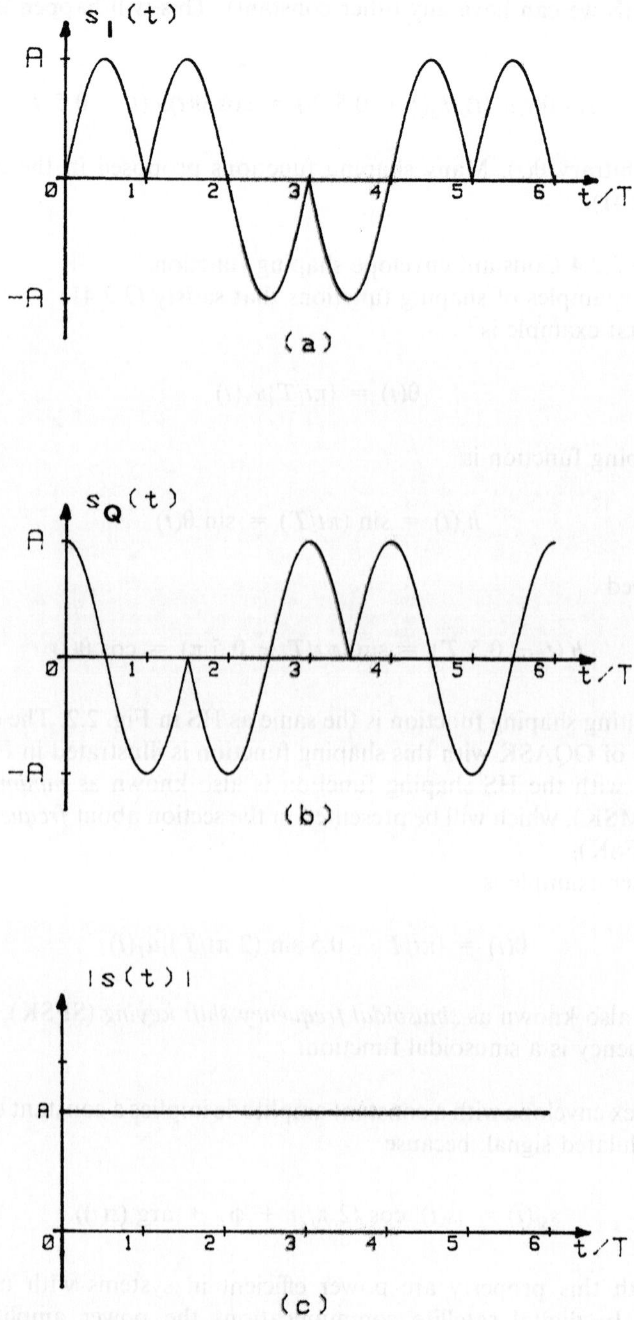


Fig. 2.12. The complex envelope of OQASK with HS shaping function: (a) real part, (b) imaginary part, (c) envelope.

### 2.2.4 Phase shift keying (PSK)[2.1,2.5,2.8]

In *phase shift keying* (PSK), the baseband signal modulates the phase of the carrier; hence the modulated signal is

$$s_M(t) = A \cos (2 \pi f_c t + \phi_T + K_p s_b(t)) \tag{2.2.45}$$

where $K_p$ is a constant. The symbol-dependent part of the phase is

$$\phi(t) = K_p s_b(t) = K_p \sum_i a_i h_s(t - iT) \tag{2.2.46}$$

where $a_i = a_{Ii}$ is real.

If we sample $\phi(t)$ in the middle of the time interval, i.e., at times $t_k = kT + 0.5\ T$ ($k$ is an integer), we obtain

$$\phi(t_k) = K_p a_k \tag{2.2.47}$$

for all shaping function in Fig. 2.2 (except for SP). Because the phase is modulo $2\ \pi$, all values of $\phi(t_k)$ lie on a circle. If we assume that all the values are unfirmly distributed on the circle according to the symbol value, we obtain

$$k_p = \pi/M \tag{2.2.48}$$

for symbols in the set $\mathring{A}_\pm = \{\pm 1, \pm 3, \ldots \pm(m - 1)\}$ (an equivalent set here is $\{2\ k - 1, k = 1, 2, \ldots, M\}$) or

$$K_p = 2\ \pi/M \tag{2.2.49}$$

for symbols in the set $\mathring{A}_0$ or $\mathring{A}_1$.

Equation (2.2.45) can be rewritten in the form of (2.2.12) with

$$s(t) = A \exp (jK_p \sum_i a_i h_s(t - iT) \tag{2.2.50}$$

The following statement, although trivial, seems to be a hard nut for some students. Because $h_s(t)$ is nonzero for $0 \leqq t \leqq T$ only, the value of $s(t)$ at time $kT \leqq t \leqq (k + 1)T$ is given by

$$s(t) = A \exp \{jK_p a_k h_s(t - kT)\} u_T(t - kT) \tag{2.2.51}$$

Denote

$$b(t, a_k) = \exp \{jK_p a_k h_s(t)\} u_T(t) \tag{2.2.52}$$

then for $kT \leqq t \leqq (k + 1)T$

$$s(t) = Ab(t - kT, a_k) \tag{2.2.53}$$

and thus for all times

$$s(t) = A \sum_i b(t - iT, a_i) \tag{2.2.54}$$

This form is very similar to QASK (eq. (2.2.32)), the difference being that the shaping function in (2.2.54) is not any more common as in (2.2.32). There is only one exception to this statement: if $h_s(t)$ is the NRZ pulse, then

$$b(t, a_k) = \exp(jK_p a_k) u_T(T) \tag{2.2.55}$$

and defining the complex symbol on a circle

$$\tilde{a}_k = \exp(jK_p a_k) \tag{2.2.56}$$

we obtain

$$s(t) = A \sum_i \tilde{a}_i h_s(t - iT) \tag{2.2.57}$$

with

$$h_s(t) = u_T(t) \tag{2.2.58}$$

i.e., the NRZ shaping function. The conclusion from this derivation has already been stated before, namely: PSK and QASK with a circular constellation are mathematically identical methods of modulation, provided the shaping function is NRZ. The implication of this statement is that we can study PSK with NRZ shaping functions within the frame of QASK. As PSK is a nonlinear method of modulation, and QASK is linear, we significantly simplify the computation of error probability of PSK in the presence of various interferences and noise.

A PSK modulated signal with an NRZ shaping function and quaternary symbols {1, 2, 3, 4} (hence $K_p = 0.5\,\pi$) is shown in Fig. 2.13. In this figure we have assumed $\phi_T = -0.5\,\pi$ and $f_c = 1/T$. Note that in this case both $\phi(t)$ (hence also $s(t)$) are not continuous functions of time. For example at $t = T$, there is an abrupt change of $0.5\,\pi$ in $\phi(t)$, and $s(t)$ changes from one to zero. Generation of 8-ary PSK from binary symbols is illustrated in Fig. 2.14.

PSK with four symbols is called (naturally) *quaternary PSK* (QPSK). If we use an NRZ shaping function, we can also have *offset QPSK* (OQPSK), which is the same as OQASK with four symbols on a square (or circle). In OQPSK a phase transition occurs every $0.5\,T$ second, and the magnitude of phase change does not exceed $0.5\,\pi$.

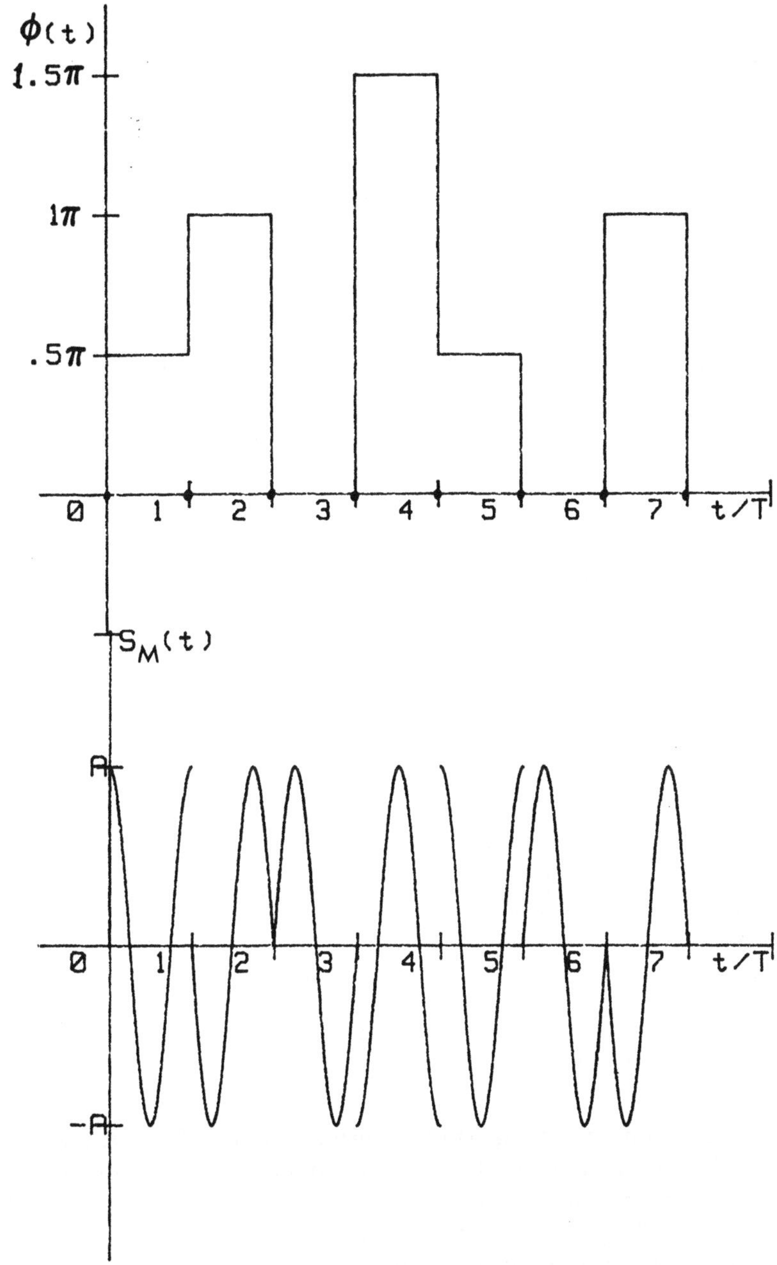


Fig. 2.13. (a) The phase and (b) modulated signal of quaternary PSK with NRZ shaping function.

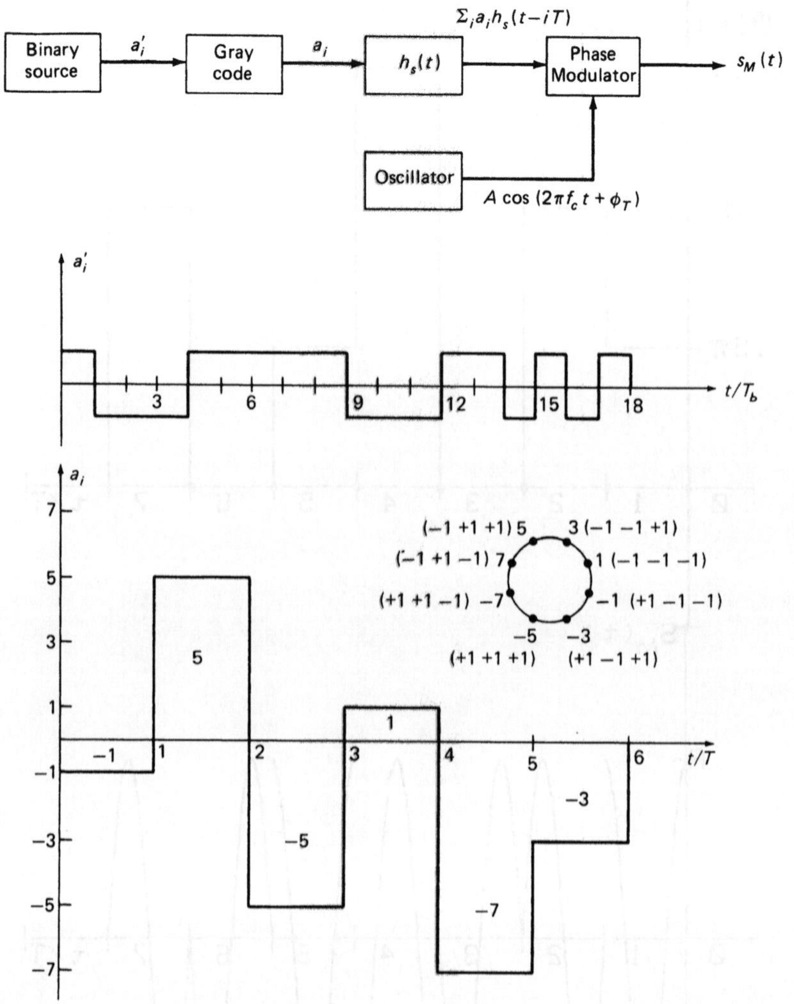


Fig. 2.14. Generation of 8-ary PSK.

**2.2.4.1 Differential phase shift keying (DPSK)[2.6,2.7]** A main difficulty in the implementation of PSK is the randomness of $\phi_T$, the phase of transmitted carrier, which is unknown to the receiver. In order to demodulate the baseband signal from the bandpass signal, the receiver generates a local carrier that must be identical both in frequency and phase to the transmitter carrier for efficient detection of the transmitted symbols. The complexity of the receiver can be substantially reduced if we can relax this demand on phase coherence. This is achieved in *differential PSK* (DPSK), where the symbols are represented as phase differences rather than phases.

Hence in the receiver the phase difference at successive $T$ intervals is required and not the absolute phase. The transmitted signal in DPSK is

$$s_M(t) = A \cos\left(2\pi f_c t + \phi_T + K_p \sum_i a_i' h_s(T - iT)\right) \tag{2.2.59}$$

where the symbols $\{a_i'\}$ are related to the source symbols by

$$a_i' = a_{i-1}' + a_i \tag{2.2.60}$$

Thus the phase difference at two successive time intervals is

$$\begin{aligned} \phi(kT + 0.5\,T) - \phi(kT - 0.5) &= K_p a_k' h_s(0.5\,T) - K_p a_{k-1}' h_s(0.5\,T) \\ &= a_k K_p \end{aligned} \tag{2.2.61}$$

because $h_s(0.5\,T) = 1$. Thus, here also, eq. (2.2.59) has the form of (2.2.12) with

$$s(t) = A \exp\left\{jK_p \sum_i a_i' h_s(t - iT)\right\} \tag{2.2.62}$$

which can also be expressed as

$$s(t) = A \sum_i b(t - iT, a_i') \tag{2.2.63}$$

with

$$b(t, a_i') = \exp\left(jK_p a_i' h_s(t)\right) u_T(t) \tag{2.2.64}$$

In the case of an NRZ shaping function (and this is the only shaping function mentioned in the literature for DPSK), we obtain

$$b(t, a_i') = \tilde{a}_i u_T(t) \tag{2.2.65}$$

where

$$\tilde{a}_i = \exp\left(jK_p a_i'\right) \tag{2.2.66}$$

Assume without any loss in generality that the symbols are from the set $\mathring{A}_0 = \{0, 1, \ldots, M - 1\}$; hence $K_p = 2\pi/M$. Because the phase $\phi(t)$ is invariant to modulo $2\pi$ operation, i.e.

$$\phi(t) = \phi(t) + k\,2\pi \qquad (k \text{ integer}) \tag{2.2.67}$$

we can select the symbols in (2.2.60) using the modulo $M$ operation

$$a_i' = (a'_{i-1} + a_i) \bmod M, \; a_i, a_i' \in \mathring{A}_0 \tag{2.2.68}$$

so that $\phi(t)$ remains in the principle range 0–2 $\pi$.

*Example* 2.2.5 Generation of quaternary DPSK.
We show the generation of quaternary symbols assuming $a'_{-1} = 0$ and $a_0a_1a_2a_3a_4a_5a_6 = 3203102$

The symbols $a_i$ and $a_i'$ are shown in Table 2.1.

**Table 2.1 DPSK symbol generation**

| | | | | | | | |
|---|---|---|---|---|---|---|---|
| $i$ | 0 | 1 | 2 | 3 | 4 | 5 | 6 |
| $a_i$ | 3 | 2 | 0 | 3 | 1 | 0 | 2 |
| $a_i'$ | 3 | 1 | 1 | 0 | 1 | 1 | 3 |

### 2.2.5 Frequency shift keying (FSK)

**2.2.5.1 Continuous phase frequency shift keying (CPFSK)** In *frequency shift keying* the instantaneous frequency of the carrier is a linear function of the baseband signal, i.e.

$$f_{\text{inst}}(t) = (2\,\pi)^{-1}\frac{d\phi_{\text{in}}(t)}{dt} = f_c + f_d s_b(t) = f_c + f_d \sum_i a_i h_s(t - iT) \tag{2.2.69}$$

where $\phi_{\text{in}}(t)$ is the instantaneous phase of the carrier

$$\phi_{\text{in}}(t) = 2\,\pi f_c t + \phi_T + K_F \int_{-\infty}^{t} \sum_i a_i h_s(t' - iT)\, dt' \tag{2.2.70}$$

$K_F$ and $f_d$ are related constants

$$K_F = 2\,\pi f_d \tag{2.2.71}$$

The instantaneous frequency deviation from the carrier frequency is

$$f_{\text{dev}}(t) = f_d \sum_i a_i h_s(t - iT) \tag{2.2.72}$$

If $h_s(t)$ is the NRZ shaping function, then

$$f_{\text{dev}}(t) = f_d \sum_i a_i u_T(t - iT) \tag{2.2.73}$$

and at any given time

$$f_{\text{dev}} = \pm f_d, \pm 3 f_d, \ldots, \pm(M - 1)f_d \tag{2.2.74}$$

if the symbols belong to the set $\mathring{A}_{\pm} = \{\pm 1, \pm 3, \ldots \pm(M - 1)\}$. Thus in the binary case only two frequencies are transmitted, namely

$$f_H = f_c + f_d, f_L = f_c - f_d \tag{2.2.75}$$

and $f_d$ is justifiably called the *frequency deviation from the carrier*.

The modulated signal has the form of (2.2.12) with

$$s(t) = A \exp(j\phi(t)) = A \exp\{jK_F \int_{-\infty}^{t} \sum_i a_i h_s(t' - iT)\, dt'\} \tag{2.2.76}$$

The phase $\phi(t)$ is a continuous function of time, unless $h_s(t)$ contains impulses. For this reason this FSK is called *continuous phase FSK*.

Although eq. (2.2.74) was written only for an NRZ shaping function, it remains valid for other shaping functions in Fig. 2.2, provided the samples are taken in the middle of the time interval $T$. For the other shaping functions, $f_d$ is the maximal frequency deviation from the carrier (in the binary case).

*Example* 2.2.6 Quaternary FSK
In Fig. 2.15 we show a CPFSK signal assuming quaternary symbols and NRZ shaping function. We have selected for convenience $f_d = 1/T$ and $f_c = 4 f_d$, so that the instantaneous frequencies are $f_d$, $3 f_d$, $5 f_d$, and $7 f_d$. Note that, although the baseband signal is not continuous, the modulated signal is continuous.

Generation of CPFSK is illustrated in Fig. 2.16.

The phase $\phi(t)$ in (2.2.76) can be expressed in the time interval $kT \leqq t \leqq (k + 1)T$ by

$$\phi(t) = K_F \int_{-\infty}^{kT} \sum_i a_i h_s(t' - iT)\, dt' + K_F \int_{kT}^{t} a_k h_s(t' - kT)\, dt'$$

$$= \{\beta(T) \sum_{-\infty}^{k-1} a_i + a_k \beta(t - kT)\} u_T(t - kT) \tag{2.2.77}$$

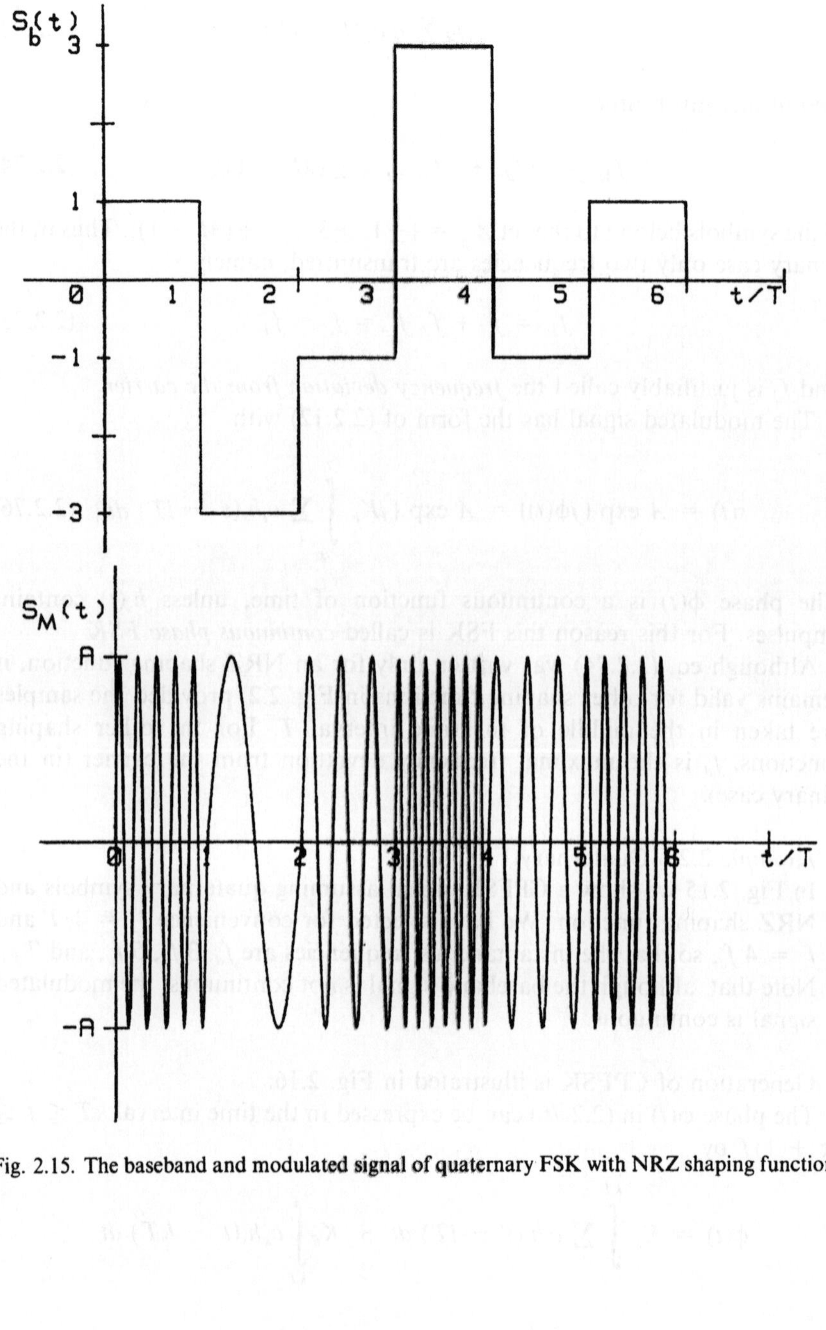


Fig. 2.15. The baseband and modulated signal of quaternary FSK with NRZ shaping function.

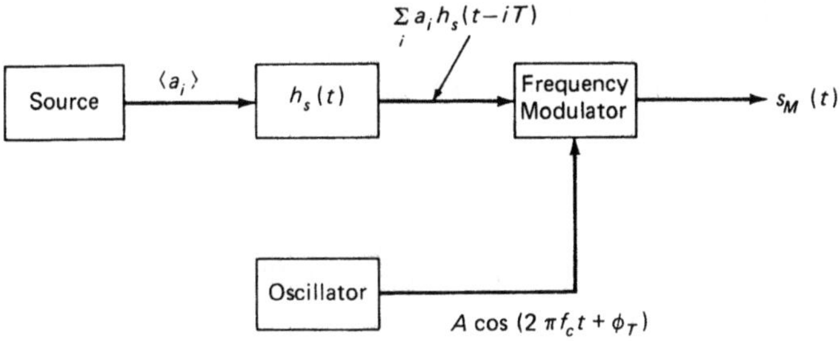


Fig. 2.16. Generation of continuous phase FSK.

where $\beta(t)$ is the integral of the shaping function

$$\beta(t) = \begin{cases} 0 & t < 0 \\ K_F \int_0^t h_s(t')\,dt' & 0 \leqq t \leqq T \\ \beta(T) & T \leqq t \end{cases} \tag{2.2.78}$$

The normalized frequency deviation is defined as

$$h = \beta(T)/\pi = 2\bar{f}_d/R \tag{2.2.79}$$

where the average frequency deviation is

$$\bar{f}_d = f_d \int_0^T h_s(t)\,dt/T \tag{2.2.80}$$

and $R = 1/T$ is the symbol rate. In the case of NRZ shaping function, the average frequency deviation is the same as the frequency deviation $f_d$. The normalized frequency deviation is normalized with respect to the symbol rate.

We obtain from (2.2.77) and (2.2.76) that in the interval $kT \leqq t \leqq (k+1)T$

$$s(t) = A\exp\{j(\phi_k + a_k\beta(t-kT))\}u_T(t-kT) \tag{2.2.81}$$

where

$$\phi_k = \phi(kT) = \beta(T)\sum_{-\infty}^{k-1} a_i \tag{2.2.82}$$

hence for all times we can write

$$s(t) = A\sum_k b(t - kT, \mathbf{a}_k) \tag{2.2.83}$$

where

$$b(t, \mathbf{a}_k) = \exp\{j(\phi_k + a_k\beta(t))\}u_T(t) \tag{2.2.84}$$

and the vector

$$\mathbf{a}_k = (a_k, a_{k-1}, \ldots) \tag{2.2.85}$$

depends on present symbol $a_k$, as well as on all past symbols through $\phi_k$.

If we assume $\phi_k = 0$ for all $k$, then we note from (2.2.77) that

$$\phi(t) = \sum_k a_k\beta(t - kT)u_T(t - kT) \tag{2.2.86}$$

which is the same as PSK with $\beta(t)$ replacing $K_p h_s(t)$ (see eq. (2.2.46)). For example when the shaping function is the SP from Fig. 2.2, the condition $\beta(T) = 0$ is satisfied; hence $\phi_k = 0$. Thus FSK with a shaping function that satisfies $\beta(T) = 0$ is equivalent to PSK and can be analyzed using PSK methods.

The path (or trajectory) of the phase $\phi(t)$ as a function of time and various symbol sequences is of great importance in investigating modern CPFSK systems.[2.11–2.14]

*Example* 2.2.7 The phase tree of binary FSK
In Fig. 2.17 we show a diagram of possible phase paths assuming binary symbols and a triangular shaping function (hence $\beta(T) = 0.5\,TK_F = \pi f_d T$). We assume that $\phi_0 = 0$. When the symbol is $+1$ the phase increases by $\beta(T)$, while when the symbol is $-1$ the phase decreases by $\beta(T)$. The heavy line path corresponds to the sequence of symbols $+1\ +1\ -1\ -1\ +1\ -1\ -1\ -1\ +1\ +1$. Such a collection of paths is called a *phase tree*.

**2.2.5.2 FSK with noncontinuous phase** In some practical systems the modulated signal can be viewed as being generated by $M$ oscillators, an oscillator for each symbol value, with frequency $f_m$ and phase $\phi_m$, $m = 1, 2, \ldots, M$. This is illustrated for the binary case in Fig. 2.18, where the position of the switch that connects the line to the oscillators depends on the symbol value. If the symbol value is $+1$, the line is connected to the oscillator with frequency $f_{+1} = f_H$, but if the symbol is $-1$, the line is connected to the

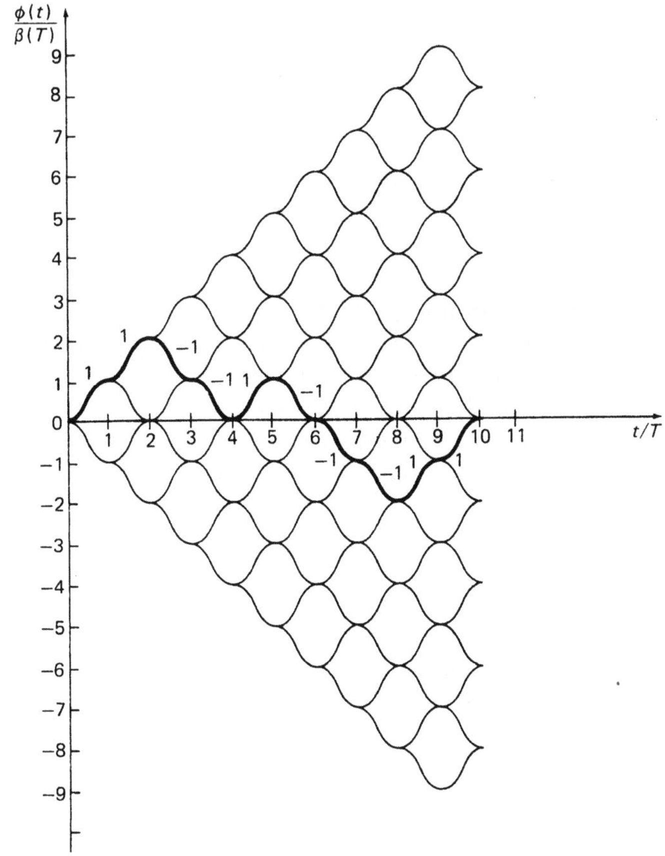


Fig. 2.17. Phase tree of binary CPFSK with triangular shaping.

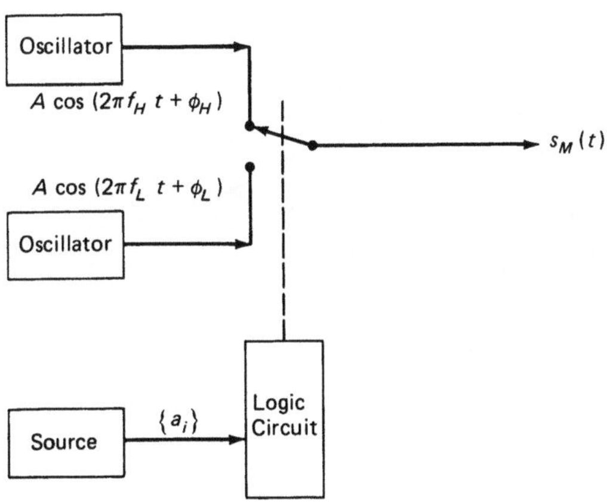


Fig. 2.18. Generation of binary FSK with noncontinuous phase.

oscillator with carrier frequency $f_{-1} = f_L$. The modulated signal can still be described as in (2.2.12) and (2.2.83) provided $b(t, \mathbf{a}_k)$ is replaced by

$$b(t, \mathbf{a}_k) = \exp\{j(\phi(a_k) + a_k\beta(t))\}u_T(t) \tag{2.2.87}$$

where $\phi(a_k)$ is the phase of the oscillator $m$ when $a_k = m$ and

$$\beta(t) = 2\pi f_d t \tag{2.2.88}$$

**2.2.5.3 Multi-*h* frequency shift keying**[2.14] In Section 2.2.5.1 we assumed that $f_d$ and thus $h$ were constants. The efficiency of the system may be improved (by efficiency we mean either reduced bandwidth or reduced error probability or both) if instead of a constant $h$ we select $h$ cyclically from the set $\{h_1, h_2, \ldots, h_H\}$ of $H$ rational numbers. Thus we associate with symbol $a_i$ the frequency deviation $f_{di}$ and $h_i$, which are cyclic, i.e.

$$f_{di+nH} = f_{di} \tag{2.2.89}$$

$$h_{i+nH} = h_i \tag{2.2.90}$$

where $n$ is an integer. If we assume the NRZ shaping function and restrict the $h_i$ to be a multiple of $1/q$, ($q$ is a positive integer), then the phase transition during any $T$ interval is a multiple of $\pi/q$.

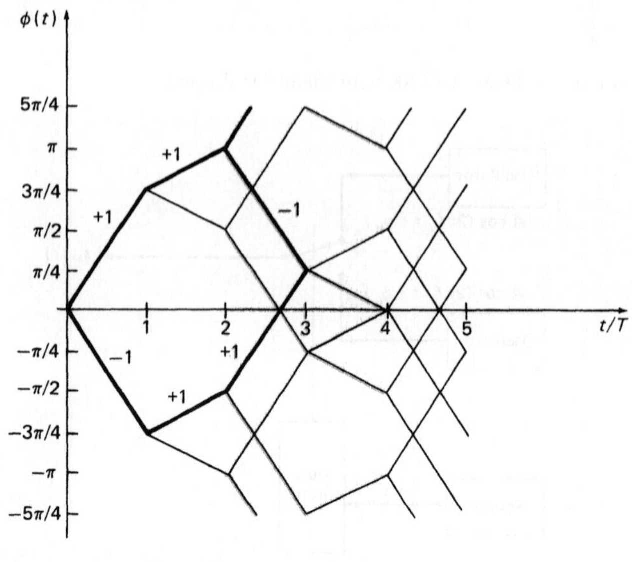


Fig. 2.19. Phase tree of multi-*h* FSK.

*Example* 2.2.8 Multi-$h$ FSK
For binary symbols and NRZ shaping function, select $q = 4$ and $h_i = 1/4$, $h_2 = 3/4$. The phase transitions are thus $\pm 0.25\ \pi$ in the odd indexed intervals and $\pm 0.75\ \pi$ in the even indexed time intervals. This is illustrated in Fig. 2.19. The two paths correspond to symbol sequences $+1+1-1$ and $-1+1+1$ and merge after 3 $T$.

**2.2.5.4 Minimum shift keying (MSK)**[2.15–2.25] *Minimum shift keying* (MSK) (also called fast FSK (FFSK)) is a special case of CPFSK with normalized frequency deviation $h = 0.5$ (i.e., $\beta(T) = 0.5\ \pi$). Using this condition and also assuming $\phi_0 = 0$, we obtain from (2.2.82)

$$\phi_k = 0.5\ \pi \sum_0^{k-1} a_i, \qquad \phi_0 = 0 \tag{2.2.91}$$

and the phase transition during a $T$ interval is

$$\Delta\phi_k = \phi_{k+1} - \phi_k = 0.5\ \pi a_k \tag{2.2.92}$$

i.e., an odd multiple of 0.5 $\pi$ for $a_k \in \mathring{A}_{\pm}$. Thus

$$\phi_k = \begin{cases} \text{odd multiple of } 0.5\ \pi & k = \text{odd} \\ \text{even multiple of } 0.5\ \pi & k = \text{even} \end{cases} \tag{2.2.93}$$

i.e.

$$\sin\phi_k = \begin{cases} 0 & k = \text{even} \\ \pm 1 & k = \text{odd} \end{cases} \tag{2.2.94}$$

$$\cos\phi_k = \begin{cases} 0 & k = \text{odd} \\ \pm 1 & k = \text{even} \end{cases} \tag{2.2.95}$$

*Example* 2.2.9 The phase tree and trellis of MSK
The phase tree for MSK with binary symbols and NRZ shaping function is shown in Fig. 2.20(a). The heavy line path corresponds to the sequence of symbols $+1+1-1-1+1-1-1-1+1$. Because the phase $\phi(t)$ appears only as an argument of $\exp\{j\phi(t)\}$, it has circular symmetry, i.e.

$$\phi(t) = \phi(t) + 2\ n\pi \tag{2.2.96}$$

where $n$ is an integer, or, in other words, $\phi(t)$ is taken modulo 2 $\pi$. Denoting

$$\phi_{\text{mod}}(t) = \phi(t) \qquad (\text{modulo } 2\ \pi) \tag{2.2.97}$$

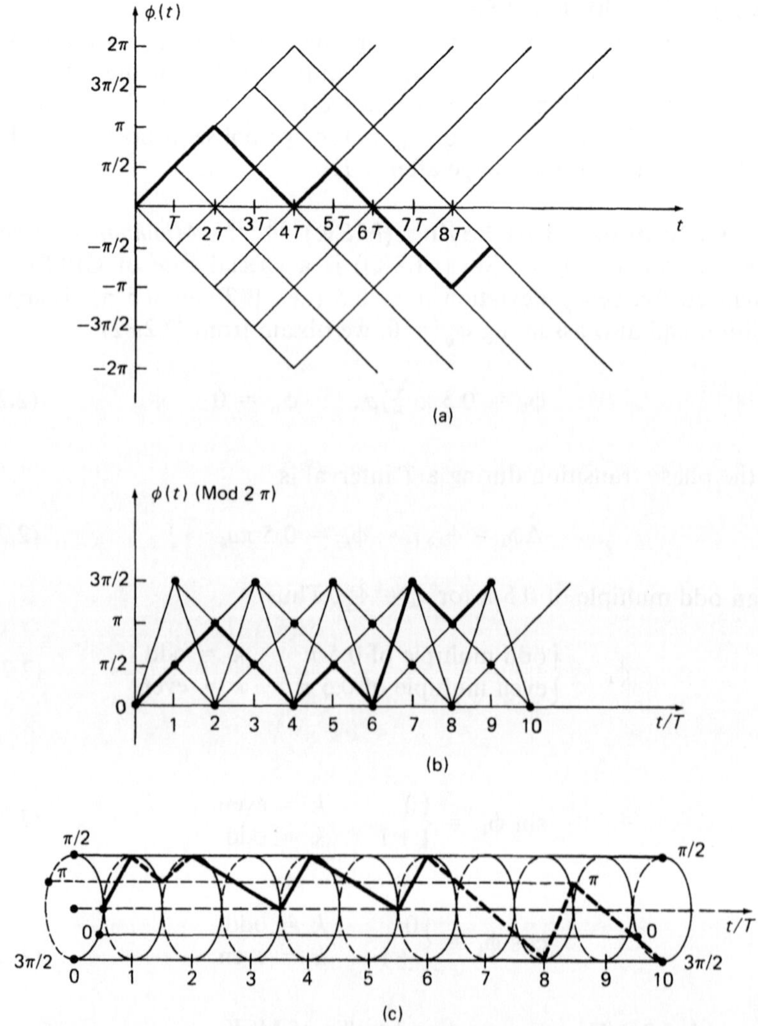


Fig. 2.20. Binary MSK with NRZ shaping function: (a) phase tree, (b) trellis, (c) cylinder.

and confining $\phi_{\text{mod}}(t)$ to its principle range 0–2 π (or $-\pi$—π) the tree of Fig. 2.20(a) collapses into a *trellis*, shown in Fig. 2.20(b). The circular symmetry of the trellis is shown in Fig. 2.20(c), in which the heavy line path is enscribed on the surface of the cylinder.

**2.2.5.5 Equivalence of binary MSK and quaternary OQASK** We intend to show here that the complex envelope of binary MSK is identical to the complex envelope of OQASK. We start with general *M*-ary MSK, to be useful in Section 2.2.5.7, but with the binary assumption only, in eq.

(2.2.108). The starting point is eq. (2.2.83) and (2.2.84), where $\phi_k$ is from (2.2.92)

$$\phi_k = \phi_{k+1} - 0.5\,\pi a_k \tag{2.2.98}$$

Combining odd and even indexed terms of (2.2.83), we obtain either

$$\begin{aligned} s(t) = A \sum_i \exp\{j(\phi_{2i-1} + a_{2i-1}\beta(t-(2\,i-1)T))\}u_T(t-(2\,i-1)T) \\ + \exp\{j(\phi_{2i} + a_{2i}\beta(t-2\,iT))\}u_T(t-2\,iT) \end{aligned} \tag{2.2.99}$$

or

$$\begin{aligned} s(t) = A \sum_i \exp\{j(\phi_{2i} + a_{2i}\beta(t-2\,iT))\}u_T(t-2\,iT) \\ + \exp\{j(\phi_{2i+1} + a_{2i+1}\beta(t-(2\cdot i+1)T))\}u_T(t-2\,(i+1)T) \end{aligned} \tag{2.2.100}$$

Substitute into (2.2.99) using (2.2.98)

$$\phi_{2i-1} = \phi_{2i} - 0.5\,\pi a_{2i-1} \tag{2.2.101}$$

thus

$$\begin{aligned} s(t) = A \sum_i \exp(j\phi_{2i})\{\exp\{j(a_{2i-1}\beta(t-(2i-1)T)) - 0.5\,\pi a_{2i-1})\} \\ u_T(t-(2i-1)T) + \exp\{ja_{2i}\beta(t-2iT)\}u_T(t-2iT)\} \end{aligned} \tag{2.2.102}$$

Denote

$$d_k = \exp(j\phi_k) \tag{2.2.103}$$

$$m_k = \sin(0.5\,\pi a_k) \tag{2.2.104}$$

Substitute (2.2.91) into (2.2.103), and note that $\cos(0.5\,\pi a_k) = 0$ for all $a_k \in \mathring{A}_{\pm}$. The result is

$$d_k = \prod_0^{k-1} \exp(j\,0.5\,\pi a_i) = j^k \prod_0^{k-1} m_i \tag{2.2.105}$$

Note that $d_k$ is real for even $k$ and imaginary for odd $k$. In the binary case

$$m_k = a_k = \pm 1 \tag{2.2.106}$$

hence

$$d_k = j^k \prod_0^{k-1} a_i \tag{2.2.107}$$

We substitute (2.2.105) into (2.2.102) and take the real part

$$\operatorname{Re}\{s(t)\} = A \sum_i d_{2i}\{m_{2i-1} \sin(a_{2i-1}\beta(t - (2i-1)T))u_T(t - (2i-1)T) + \cos(a_{2i}\beta(t - 2iT))u_T(t - 2iT)\} \tag{2.2.108}$$

In the binary case

$$m_{2i-1} \sin(a_{2i-1}\beta) = \sin\beta \tag{2.2.109}$$

$$\cos(a_{2i}\beta) = \cos\beta \tag{2.2.110}$$

hence

$$\operatorname{Re}\{s(t)\} = A \sum_i d_{2i}\{\sin\beta(t - (2i-1)T)u_T(t - (2i-1)T) + \cos\beta(t - 2iT)\, u_T(t - 2iT)\} \tag{2.2.111}$$

Similarly if we substitute

$$\phi_{2i} = \phi_{2i+1} - 0.5\,\pi a_{2i} \tag{2.2.112}$$

into (2.2.100), we obtain first

$$s(t) = A \sum_i d_{2i+1}\{\exp\{j(a_{2i}\beta(t - 2iT) - 0.5\,\pi a_{2i})\}u_T(t - 2iT) + \exp\{j(a_{2i+1}\beta(t - (2i+1)T)\}u_T(t - (2i+1)T)\} \tag{2.2.113}$$

Now we substitute (2.2.105) and take the imaginary part (note that $d_{2i+1}$ is imaginary and in the binary case $a_i = m_i = \pm 1$)

$$\operatorname{Im}\{s(t)\} = A \sum_i (d_{2i+1}/j)\{\sin\beta(t - 2iT)u_T(t - 2iT) + \cos(\beta(t - (2i+1)T)u_T(t - (2i+1)T)\} \tag{2.2.114}$$

We combine the real and imaginary part of $s(t)$ and obtain from (2.2.111) and (2.2.114)

$$s(t) = A \sum_i a_{Ii}(b(t - i\,2\,T) + ja_{Qi}b(t - i\,2\,T - T) \tag{2.2.115}$$

where

$$a_{Ii} = d_{2i} = (-1)^i \prod_0^{2i-1} a_k = -a_{Qi-1}a_{2i-1} \tag{2.2.116}$$

$$a_{Qi} = (d_{2i+1}/j) = (-1)^i \prod_0^{2i} a_k = a_{Ii}a_{2i} \tag{2.2.117}$$

and

$$b(t) = \sin \beta(t + T)u_T(t + T) + \cos \beta(t)u_T(t) \qquad (2.2.118)$$

Note that the duration of $b(t)$ is $2\,T$. Because we are concerned here with the binary case, we should in fact use $T = T_b$, hence we have from (2.2.115) and (2.2.118)

$$s(t) = A \sum_i a_{Ii}(b(t - i\,2\,T_b) + ja_{Qi}b(t - i\,2\,T_b - T_b) \qquad (2.2.119)$$

$$b(t) = \sin \beta(t + T_b)u_{Tb}(t + T_b) + \cos \beta(t)u_{Tb}(t) \qquad (2.2.120)$$

Comparing (2.2.119) to (2.2.39), we see indeed that binary MSK has the same form as quaternary OQASK ($T = 2\,T_b$), with the equivalent shaping function $b(t)$ related to the original shaping function $h_s(t)$ through (2.2.120) and

$$\beta(t) = 0.5\,\pi \int_0^t h_s(t')\,dt' u_{Tb}(t) \Big/ \int_0^{Tb} h_s(t)\,dt \qquad (2.2.121)$$

Note that the symbols $\{a_{Ii}, a_{Qi}\}$ are independent, equiprobable, and binary random variables ($\pm 1$), whenever $\{a_i\}$ have the same properties.

*Example* 2.2.10 Equivalence of binary MSK and OQASK
Assume that $h_s(t)$ is the NRZ shaping function. Hence from (2.2.121)

$$\beta(t) = 0.5\,\pi t/T_b \qquad (2.2.122)$$

and from (2.2.120)

$$\begin{aligned} b(t) &= \sin(0.5\,\pi t/T_b + 0.5\,\pi)u_{Tb}(t + T_b) + \cos(0.5\,\pi t/T_b)u_{Tb}(t) \\ &= \cos(0.5\,\pi t/T_b)u_{2Tb}(t + T_b) \qquad (2.2.123) \end{aligned}$$

Both $h_s(t)$ and $b(t)$ are illustrated in Fig. 2.21. We see from this figure that binary MSK with an NRZ shaping function is equivalent to OQASK with the HS shaping function.

To recover the original binary symbols $\{a_i\}$ from $\{a_{Ii}, a_{Qi}\}$, we can perform the following operations (see (2.2.116) and (2.2.117), and remember that $a_{Ii}^2 = 1 = a_{Qi}^2$)

$$a_{2i} = a_{Qi}a_{Ii} \qquad (2.2.124)$$

$$a_{2i-1} = -a_{Ii}a_{Qi-1} \qquad (2.2.125)$$

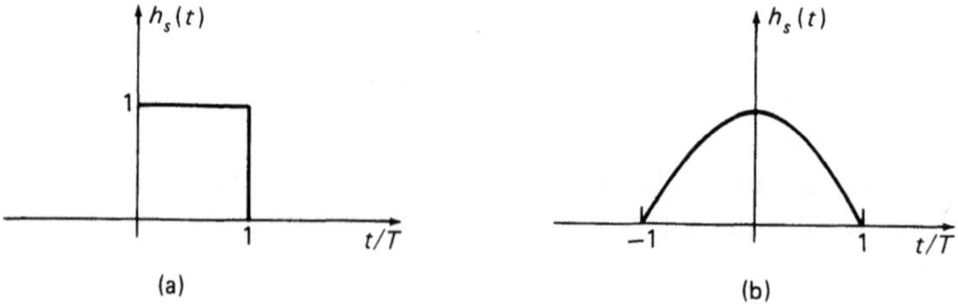


Fig. 2.21. (a) NRZ shaping function of binary MSK and (b) its equivalent OQASK shaping function.

If $a_{Ii}$ is in error, both $a_{2i-1}$ and $a_{2i}$ will be in error. The same happens when $a_{Qi}$ is in error. This should be remembered when the error probability is computed for MSK in the equivalent OQASK form.

**2.2.5.6 Binary MSK as a form of DPSK** We note from (2.2.98) that the phase difference during a $T$ interval is

$$\phi_{k+1} - \phi_k = 0.5\ \pi a_k \tag{2.2.126}$$

which is the same as (2.2.61) for DPSK, because for binary symbols $\{\pm 1\}$, $K_P = 0.5\ \pi$. Thus for the recovery of the binary symbols in MSK, we do not need the absolute phase of the carrier; we need only the phase difference.

**2.2.5.7 Equivalence of *M*-ary MSK and a modified OQASK** For nonbinary symbols we can also represent MSK in a form similar to OQASK, but the equivalent shaping function is symbol-dependent. The derivation of the equivalence is quite similar to the procedure in the binary case. The starting point is eq. (2.2.113). Denote

$$b(t, \mathbf{a}_k) = \sin(0.5\ \pi a_{k-1}) \sin(a_{k-1}\beta(t + T))u_T(t + T) + \cos(a_k\beta(t))u_T(t) \tag{2.2.127}$$

With this notation we obtain

$$s(t) = A \sum_i a_{Ii} b(t - i\,2\,T, \mathbf{a}_{2i}) + j a_{Qi} b(t - i\,2\,T - T, \mathbf{a}_{2i+1}) \tag{2.2.128}$$

where

$$a_{Ii} = (-1)^i \prod_0^{2i-1} m_k = -a_{Qi} m_{2i-1} \tag{2.2.129}$$

$$a_{Qi} = (-1)^i \prod_0^{2i} m_k = a_{Ii} m_{2i} \tag{2.2.130}$$

and $m_k$ is defined in (2.2.104). Equation (2.2.127) can be simplified to

$$b(t, \mathbf{a}_k) = \sin(0.5\,\pi|a_{k-1}|)\sin(|a_{k-1}|\beta(t+T))u_T(t+T) + \cos(|a_k|\beta(t))u_T(t) \quad (2.2.131)$$

When $a_k$ are binary ($\pm 1$), eq. (2.2.131) is identical to (2.2.118). When $a_k$ are $M$-ary symbols, the number of equivalent shaping functions, $b(t, \mathbf{a}_k)$, is in general $(0.5\,M)^2$.

*Example* 2.2.11 Equivalence of MSK and OQASK
Assume quaternary symbols $\{\pm 1, \pm 3\}$ and an NRZ shaping function. Thus

$$\beta(t) = 0.5\,\pi t/T$$

Substitution into (2.2.131) gives

$$b(t, 1, 1) = b(t, -1, -1) = \cos(0.5\,\pi t/T)u_{2T}(t)$$
$$b(t, 3, 3) = b(t, -3, -3) = \cos(1.5\,\pi t/T)u_{2T}(t)$$
$$b(t, 1, 3) = b(t, -1, -3) = \cos(0.5\,\pi t/T)u_T(t+T) + \cos(1.5\,\pi t/T)u_T(t)$$
$$b(t, 3, 1) = b(t, -3, -1) = \cos(1.5\,\pi t/T)u_T(t+T) + \cos(0.5\,\pi t/T)u_T(t)$$
$$b(t, 1, 1) = b(t, -1, -1) = b(t, -1, 1) = b(t, 1, -1)$$
$$b(t, 3, 3) = b(t, -3, -3) = b(t, -3, 3) = b(t, 3, -3)$$
$$b(t, 1, 3) = b(t, -1, -3) = b(t, -3, 1) = b(t, 3, -1)$$
$$b(t, 3, 1) = b(t, -3, -1) = b(t, -3, 1) = b(t, 3, -1)$$

These shaping functions are illustrated in Fig. 2.22

Equation (2.2.128) has the same form as OQASK with symbol-dependent shaping functions; the shaping function depends on the last two symbols. Because this differs from OQASK as defined in Section 2.2.3.5, we call eq. (2.2.128) modified OQASK.

## 2.3 NONOVERLAPPING SHAPING FUNCTION

### 2.3.1 Baseband signal

In Section 2.2 we have assumed that the shaping functions have the form

$$h_s(t, a_i) = a_i h_s(t)u_T(t) \quad (2.3.1)$$

In this section we relax only one condition. Thus we assume that

$$h_s(t, a_i) = h_s(t, a_i)u_T(t) \quad (2.3.2)$$

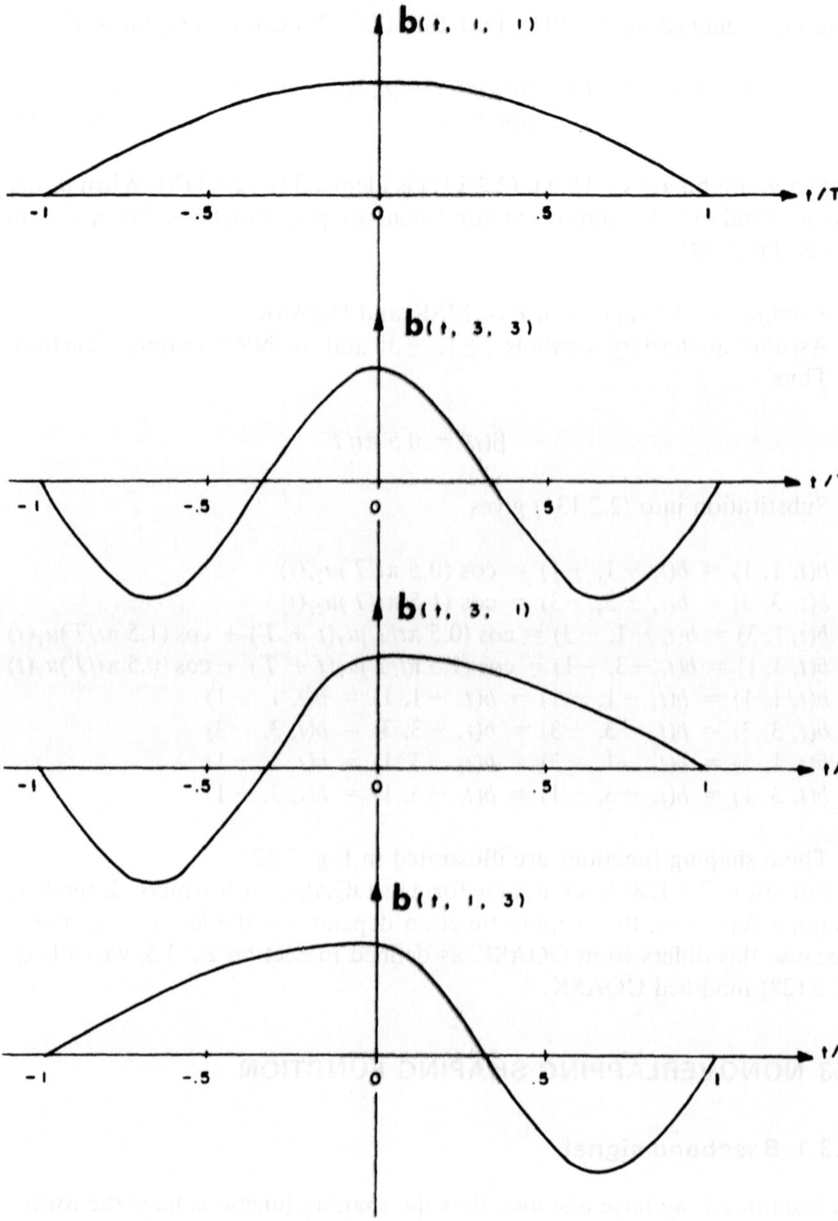


Fig. 2.22. Equivalent modified OQASK shaping functions of quaternary MSK with NRZ shaping function (I. Korn, "Gerneralized Minimum Shift Keying," *IEEE Tr. Inf. Theory*, Vol. IT-26, Mar. 1980. pp. 234–238. Copyright © 1980 IEEE).

which means that the shaping function is symbol-dependent (not via the amplitude only), but still of duration $T$. That this more general form needs to be investigated is already obvious from the FSK or PSK complex envelope in which the equivalent shaping function has this form or from the modified OQASK representation of nonbinary MSK. However, even in baseband there are simple examples for which a symbol-dependent shaping function is the only representation.

*Example* 2.3.1
In binary *pulse position modulation* (PPM), the symbols are represented by the shaping functions

$$h_s(t, 1) = u_{0.5T}(t), \; h_s(t, -1) = u_{0.5T}(t - 0.5\,T) \tag{2.3.3}$$

This is illustrated in Fig. 2.23.

The baseband signal thus has the form

$$s_b(t) = \sum_i h_s(t - iT, a_i) \tag{2.3.4}$$

### 2.3.2 Modulated signal

The modulated signal has here also the general form

$$s(t) = \text{Re}\,\{s(t)\,\exp\,(j(2\,\pi f_c t + \phi_T))\} \tag{2.3.5}$$

where

$$s(t) = A \sum_i b(t - iT, \mathbf{a}_i) \tag{2.3.6}$$

and the form of $b(t, \mathbf{a}_i)$ depends on the form of modulation.

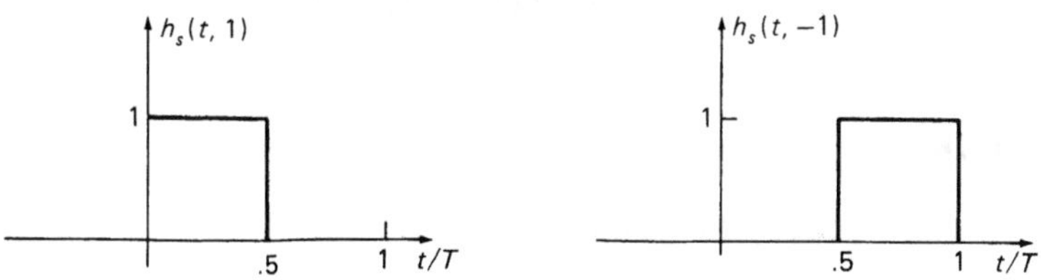


Fig. 2.23. Symbol-dependent shaping functions for binary symbols.

### 2.3.3 LSK

For LSK

$$b(t, \mathbf{a}_i) = \begin{cases} h_s(t, a_i) * \{\delta(t) + jv(t)\} & \text{ASK} \\ h_s(t, a_{Ii}) + jh_s(t, a_{Qi}) & \text{QASK} \\ h_s(t, a_{Ii}) + jh_s(t - 0.5\,T, a_{Qi}) & \text{OQASK} \end{cases} \tag{2.3.7}$$

and $v(t)$ has the form

$$v(t) = \begin{cases} 0 & \text{DSB} \\ h_{\text{SSB}}(t) & \text{SSB} \\ h_{\text{VSB}} & \text{VSB} \end{cases} \tag{2.3.8}$$

where $h_{\text{SSB}}(t)$ and $h_{\text{VSB}}(t)$ are defined in (2.2.19) and (2.2.24), respectively.

### 2.3.4 PSK and FSK

For PSK and FSK, we obtain

$$b(t, a_i) = \begin{cases} \exp\{jK_p h_s(t, a_i)\}u_T(t) & \text{PSK} \\ \exp\{j(\phi_i + \beta(t, a_i)\}u_T(t) & \text{FSK} \end{cases} \tag{2.3.9}$$

where $K_p$ is such that the maximum value of $K_p h_s(t, a_i)$ is $(M - 1)\pi/M$ for $a_i \in \mathring{A}_\pm$

$$\beta(t, a_i) = \begin{cases} 0 & t \leqq 0 \\ K_F \int_0^t h_s(t', a_i)\, dt' & 0 \leqq t \leqq T \\ \beta(T, a_i) & T \leqq t \end{cases} \tag{2.3.10}$$

and

$$\phi_i = \sum_{-\infty}^{i-1} \beta(t, a_k) \qquad \phi_0 = 0 \tag{2.3.11}$$

### 2.3.5 MSK

MSK is defined here by the condition

$$\beta(T, a_i) = 0.5\,\pi a_i \tag{2.3.12}$$

so that, here also, during a $T$ interval the phase changes by $0.5\,\pi$ for $a_i \in \mathring{A}_{\pm}$. In this case also MSK has an OQASK representation. The proof of equivalence is as follows: instead of eq. (2.2.99) and eq. (2.2.100), we have now

$$s(t) = A \sum_i \exp\{j(\phi_{2i-1} + \beta(t - (2i - 1)T, a_{2i-1}))\}u_T(t - (2i - 1)T) + \exp\{j(\phi_{2i} + \beta(t - 2\,iT, a_{2i}))\}u_T(t - 2\,iT) \qquad (2.3.13)$$

and

$$s(t) = A \sum_i \exp\{j(\phi_{2i} + \beta(t - 2\,iT, a_{2i}))\}u_T(t - 2\,iT) + \exp\{j(\phi_{2i+1} + \beta(t - (2i + 1)T, a_{2i+1}))\}u_T(t - (2i + 1)T \qquad (2.3.14)$$

and because of (2.3.12), we still have

$$\phi_k = \phi_{k+1} - 0.5\,\pi a_k \qquad (2.3.15)$$

$$\phi_k = \sum_0^{k-1} 0.5\,\pi a_i \qquad (2.3.16)$$

The definitions of $d_k$, $m_k$, $a_{Ii}$, and $a_{Qi}$ remain as in (2.2.104), (2.2.105), (2.2.129), and (2.2.130).

We substitute

$$\phi_{2i-1} = \phi_{2i} - 0.5\,\pi a_{2i-1} \qquad (2.3.17)$$

into eq. (2.3.13) and

$$\phi_{2i} = \phi_{2i+1} - 0.5\,\pi a_{2i} \qquad (2.3.18)$$

into eq. (2.3.14) and taking the real part of (2.3.13) and the imaginary part of (2.3.14), we obtain

$$s(t) = A \sum_i a_{Ii} b(t - iT, \mathbf{a}_{2i}) + j a_{Qi} b(t - iT - 0.5\,T, \mathbf{a}_{2i+1}) \qquad (2.3.19)$$

where

$$b(t, \mathbf{a}_i) = \sin(0.5\,\pi a_{i-1}) \sin\beta(t + T, a_{i-1})u_T(t + T) + \cos\beta(t, a_i)u_T(t) \qquad (2.3.20)$$

All formulas in this subsection are reduced to the formulas of Subsection 2.2.5.5 when the shaping function is of the form (2.3.1).

## 2.4 OVERLAPPING SHAPING FUNCTIONS[2.13, 2.21, 2.25–2.30]

### 2.4.1 Baseband signal

Here we assume that the shaping function has duration $KT$, where $K$ is a positive integer and hence can be written as

$$h_s(t, a_i) = h_s(t, a_i)u_{KT}(t) \tag{2.4.1}$$

When the shaping functions for all symbols are identical except for the amplitude, then the common shaping function is of duration KT

$$h_s(t) = h_s(t)u_{KT}(t) \tag{2.4.2}$$

The common overlapping shaping function is also called in the literature *Partial response signal* (PRS), because it is generated by a filter whose response is only partially during the $T$ interval and the rest of the signal is beyond that interval. In Fig. 2.24 we show several examples of overlapping shaping functions: duobinary, modified duobinary, a raised cosine, and half-cycle of a sinusoid of duration 2 $T$. Mathematically these shaping functions can be described by

$$h_s(t) = \begin{cases} u_{2T}(t) & \text{duobinary (DB)} \\ u_T(t) - u_T(t - 2\,T) & \text{modified DB} \\ 0.5\,\{1 - \cos(\pi t/T)\}u_{2T}(t) & \text{RC} \\ \sin(0.5\,\pi t/T)u_{2T}(t) & \text{HS} \end{cases} \tag{2.4.3}$$

Overlapping shaping functions are used because they require a narrower bandwidth and hence are more efficient in the frequency sense.

Even if we design the system with a nonoverlapping shaping function due to filtering in the system the original shaping function is distorted and expanded beyond the $T$ interval. There is no analytical difficulty in dealing with overlapping shaping functions in LSK and linear systems; the problem rises only in nonlinear modulation (PSK and FSK) and in nonlinear systems—for example, a system with nonlinear amplifier.

The difficulty is circumvented by defining an equivalent shaping function of duration $T$ only; however, this nonoverlapping shaping function may depend on the last $K$ symbols.

Because

$$u_{KT}(t) = \sum_{0}^{K-1} u_T(t - kT) \tag{2.4.4}$$

we can rewrite (2.4.1) in the form

$$h_s(t, a_i) = \sum_0^{K-1} h_s(t, a_i)u_T(t - kT)$$

$$= \sum_0^{K-1} h_{sk}(t - kT, a_i)u_T(t - kT) \tag{2.4.5}$$

where

$$h_{sk}(t, a_i) = h_s(t + kT, a_i)u_T(t) \tag{2.4.6}$$

is the segment of the original overlapping shaping function of duration $T$, shifted from $kT - (k + 1)T$ to $0 - T$.

*Example* 2.4.1 Segments of triangular shaping function
A triangular shaping function of duration 3 $T$ and its three segments are shown in Fig. 2.25

The baseband signal has the form

$$s_b(t) = \sum_i h_s(t - iT, a_i) \tag{2.4.7}$$

we obtain, after substitution of (2.4.5) into (2.4.7)

$$s_b(t) = \sum_i \left( \sum_{k=0}^{K-1} h_{sk}(t - (i + k)T, a_i)u_T(t - (i + k)T) \right) \tag{2.4.8}$$

Changing the subscript

$$m = i + k \rightarrow i = m - k \tag{2.4.9}$$

we obtain

$$s_b(t) = \sum_{m=-\infty}^{\infty} \sum_{k=0}^{K-1} h_{sk}(t - mT, a_{m-k})u_T(t - mT) \tag{2.4.10}$$

Denoting

$$h_s(t, \mathbf{a}_i) = \sum_{k=0}^{K-1} h_{sk}(t, a_{i-k})u_T(t) \tag{2.4.11}$$

we obtain

$$s_b(t) = \sum_i h_s(t - iT, \mathbf{a}_i) u_T(t - iT) \tag{2.4.12}$$

where the vector (or sequence) $a_i$ is

$$\mathbf{a}_i = \{a_i, a_{i-1}, \ldots, a_{i-K+1}\} \tag{2.4.13}$$

Thus the equivalent shaping function of duration $T$, $h_s(t, \mathbf{a}_i)$ depends on the last $K$ symbols.

*Example* 2.4.2 Equivalent shaping function of 2-HS
Assume a common shaping function HS of duration 2 $T$. Assume also binary symbols $\pm 1$. The equivalent nonoverlapping shaping function is

$$h_s(t, \mathbf{a}_i) = a_i h_{s0}(t) + a_{i-1} h_{s1}(t) \tag{2.4.14}$$

with

$$h_{s0}(t) = \sin(0.5\,\pi t/T) u_T(t)$$

$$h_{s1}(t) = \sin(0.5\,\pi t/T + 0.5\,\pi) u_T(t) = \cos(0.5\,\pi t/T) u_T(t)$$

The four different values of $h_s(t, \mathbf{a}_i)$ are presented in Fig. 2.26.

*Example* 2.4.3 Duobinary signal
Assume binary symbols ($\pm 1$) and the duobinary shaping function. Sketch $s_b(t)$ for the sequence of symbols $(a_{-1}) a_0 a_1 a_2 a_3 a_4 a_5 a_6 = (+1) + 1 - 1 - 1 + 1 + 1 + 1 - 1$.
For duobinary symbols

$$h_{s0}(t) = h_{s1}(t) = u_T(t)$$

hence

$$h_s(t, a_i) = (a_i + a_{i-1}) u_T(t)$$

Because the sum of these two symbols is $0 \pm 2$, the result is as in Fig. 2.27.

Note that because $\mathbf{a}_i$ and $\mathbf{a}_{i+1}$ have $K - 1$ symbols in common, the shaping functions at two neighboring $T$ intervals are correlated. In fact, because $\mathbf{a}_i$ and $\mathbf{a}_{i+K-1}$ have one symbol in common (the symbol $a_i$), there is correlation between shaping functions that are up to $(K - 1)T$ seconds apart. For that reason partial response signals are also called *correlative level signals*.

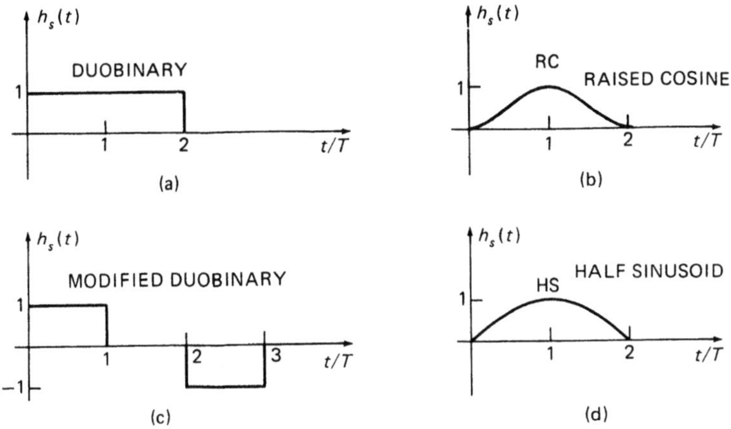


Fig. 2.24. Overlapping (partial response) shaping functions.

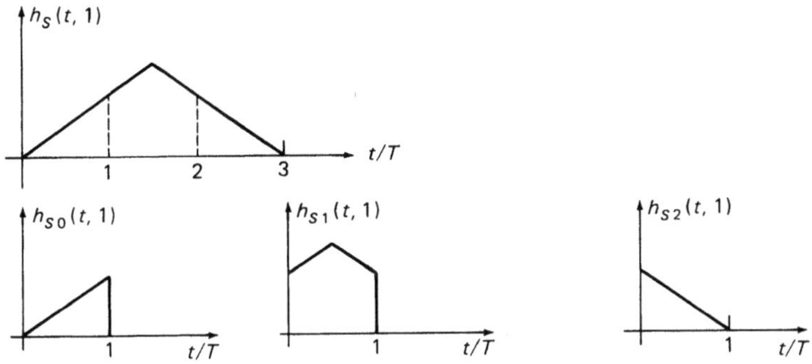


Fig. 2.25. Shaping function of duration 3 $T$ and its three segments.

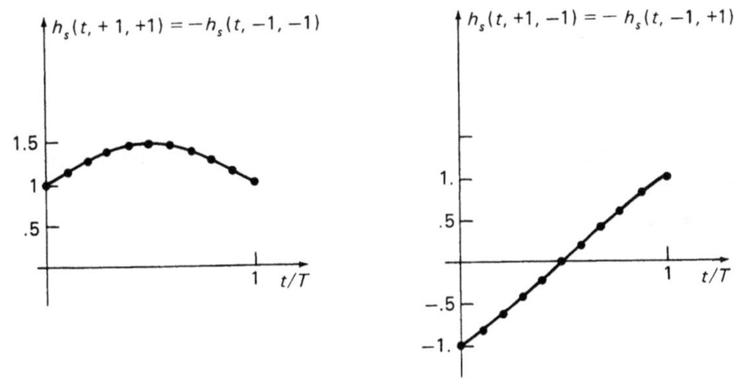


Fig. 2.26. Correlated nonverlapping shaping functions of a HS shaping function of duration 2 $T$.

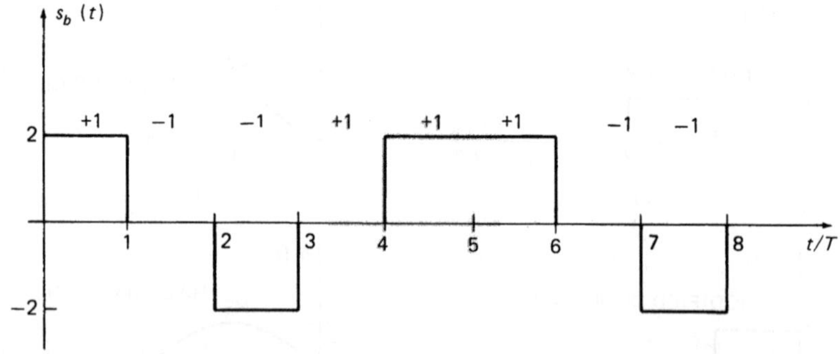


Fig. 2.27 Baseband signal with binary symbols and duobinary shaping function.

### 2.4.2 Modulated signal

The modulated signal has the form (2.1.20) with

$$s(t) = A \sum_i b(t - iT, \mathbf{a}_i) \tag{2.4.15}$$

and the form of $b(t, \mathbf{a}_i)$ depends on the method of modulation and the shaping function $h_s(t, a_i)$.

### 2.4.3 LSK

In LSK there are two representations. In the first $b(t, a_i)$ is overlapping, but depends only on a single symbol, $a_i$ (real for ASK and complex for QASK, OQASK).

$$b(t, a_i) = \begin{cases} h_s(t, a_i) * \{\delta(t) + jv(t)\} & \text{ASK} \\ h_{sI}(t, a_{Ii}) + jh_{sQ}(t, a_{Qi}) & \text{QASK} \\ h_{sI}(t, a_{Ii}) + jh_{sQ}(t - 0.5\,T, a_{Qi}) & \text{OQASK} \end{cases} \tag{2.4.16}$$

Here $h_{sI}(t, a_{Ii})$, $h_{sQ}(t, a_{Qi})$ may be identical or different, and the symbols $a_{Ii}$, $a_{Qi}$ may be from the same or different symbol sets. $v(t)$ is defined for the various ASK modulation methods in (2.3.8).

In the second representation

$$b(t, \mathbf{a}_i) = \begin{cases} h_s(t, \mathbf{a}_i) * \{\delta(t) + jv(t)\} & \text{ASK} \\ h_{sI}(t, \mathbf{a}_{Ii}) + jh_{sQ}(t, \mathbf{a}_{Qi}) & \text{QASK} \\ h_{sI}(t, \mathbf{a}_{Ii}) + jh_{sQ}(t - 0.5\,T, \mathbf{a}_{Qi}) & \text{OQASK} \end{cases} \tag{2.4.17}$$

with $h_s(t, \mathbf{a}_i)$ as defined in (2.4.11) and $h_{sI}(t, \mathbf{a}_{Ii})$, $h_{sQ}(t, \mathbf{a}_{Qi})$ defined similarly.

### 2.4.4 PSK and FSK

For these types of modulation we obtain

$$b(t, \mathbf{a}_i) = \begin{cases} \exp\{jK_p h_s(t, \mathbf{a}_i)\}u_T(t) & \text{PSK} \\ \exp\{j(\phi_i + \beta(t, \mathbf{a}_i)\}u_T(t) & \text{FSK} \end{cases} \tag{2.4.18}$$

where $K_p$ is such that the maximal value of $K_p h_s(t, \mathbf{a}_i)$ is $(M - 1)\pi/M$ when $a_i \in \mathring{A}_{\pm}$

$$\beta(t, \mathbf{a}_i) = \begin{cases} 0 & t \leqq 0 \\ K_F \int_0^t h_s(t', \mathbf{a}_i)\, dt' & 0 \leqq t \leqq T \\ \beta(T, \mathbf{a}_i) & T \leqq t \end{cases} \tag{2.4.19}$$

and

$$\phi_i = \sum_{-\infty}^{i-1} \beta(t, \mathbf{a}_k), \qquad \phi_0 = 0 \tag{2.4.20}$$

### 2.4.5 MSK

It is rather difficult to define here an MSK signal. Let

$$\beta_k(t, a_{i-k}) = \begin{cases} 0 & t \leqq 0 \\ K_F \int_0^t h_{sk}(t', a_{i-k})\, dt' & 0 \leqq t \leqq T \\ \beta_k(T, a_{i-k}) & T \leqq t \end{cases} \tag{2.4.21}$$

Then from (2.4.19)

$$\beta(t, \mathbf{a}_i) = \sum_{0}^{K-1} \beta_k(t, a_{i-k}) \tag{2.4.22}$$

To define an MSK signal we have to assume

$$\beta(KT, a_i) = K_F \int_0^{KT} h_s(t, a_i)\, dt = 0.5\, a_i \pi \tag{2.4.23}$$

Hence the phase difference in a single $T$ interval is bounded by

$$|\phi_{i+1} - \phi_i| = |\beta(T, \mathbf{a}_i)| \leq |0.5\ \pi a_i| \tag{2.4.24}$$

with the bound achieved when all symbols in $\mathbf{a}_i$ are identical. For example, assuming binary symbols ($\pm 1$), the phase increase is $\pm 0.5\ \pi$ only if all $K$ symbols are equal.

*Example* 2.4.4 MSK with duobinary shaping function
Assuming a duobinary shaping function (hence $K = 2$), we obtain

$$\Delta\phi_i = \phi_{i+1} - \phi_i = 0.5\ \pi(a_i + a_{i-1})/2 = 0, \pm 0.5\ \pi \tag{2.4.25}$$

If $\Delta\phi_i = 0.5\ \pi$, then $\Delta\phi_{i+1}$ can be either $0.5\ \pi$ (if $a_{i+1} = 1$) or 0 (if $a_{i+1} = -1$), but can never be $-0.5\ \pi$. Similarly if $\Delta\phi_i = -0.5\ \pi$, $\Delta\phi_{i+1}$ can be either 0 or $-0.5\ \pi$, but never $0.5\ \pi$. If, however, $\Delta\phi_i = 0$, $\Delta\phi_{i+1}$ can have all three values. Figure 2.28 is an illustration of the phase tree for this case. This is not, however, a "true" MSK signal as defined for nonoverlapping shaping function because of the zero phase transition option.

## 2.5 CONCLUSIONS

We have shown in this chapter that the baseband signal has in the most general case the form

$$s_b(t) = \sum_i h_s(t - iT, a_i)u_{KT}(t - iT) \tag{2.5.1}$$

where the shaping functions $\{h_s(t, a_i)\}$ depend only on the single symbol $a_i$, but have duration $KT$ or have duration $T$ only, but depend on $K$ last symbols $\mathbf{a}_i = \{a_i, a_{i+1}, \ldots, a_{i-k+1}\}$. In the latter case

$$s_b(t) = \sum_i h_s(t - iT, \mathbf{a}_i)u_T(t - iT) \tag{2.5.2}$$

with

$$h_s(t, \mathbf{a}_i) = \sum_{k=0}^{K-1} h_s(t + kT, a_{i-k})u_T(t) \tag{2.5.3}$$

We have also shown that the modulated signal always has the form

$$s_M(t) = \text{Re}\,\{s(t) \exp\,(j(2\ \pi f_c t + \phi_T))\} \tag{2.5.4}$$

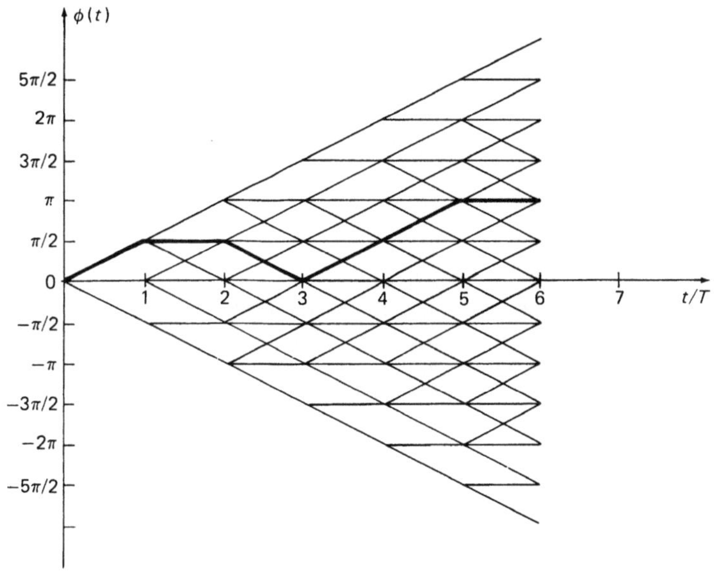


Fig. 2.28. Trellis of duobinary FSK with $\beta_1(t) = \beta_2(t) = 0.25\,\pi$

where the complex envelope is

$$s(t) = A \sum_i b(t - iT, \mathbf{a}_i) u_T(t - iT) \tag{2.5.5}$$

and $b(t, \mathbf{a}_i)$ is presented for the various modulation methods in Table 2.2. For LSK (also MSK and PSK with NRZ shaping function) we can use instead of (2.5.5) the alternative form (as for baseband)

$$s(t) = A \sum_i b(t - iT, a_i) \tag{2.5.6}$$

with

$$b(t, a_i) = \begin{cases} h_s(t, a_i) * \{\delta(t) + jv(t)\} & \text{ASK} \\ h_{sI}(t, a_{Ii}) + jh_{sQ}(t, a_{Qi}) & \text{QASK} \\ h_{sI}(t, a_{Ii}) + jh_{sQ}(t - 0.5\,T, a_{Qi}) & \text{OQASK} \end{cases} \tag{2.5.7}$$

and $h_{sI}(t, a_{Ii})$, $h_{sQ}(t, a_{Qi})$ may be identical or different, and the symbols $a_{Ii}$, $a_{Qi}$ may be from the same or different symbol sets.

In the Table $\beta(t, a_i)$ and $\phi_i$ are as defined in (2.4.19) and (2.4.20). $v(t)$ is defined in (2.3.8). When the shaping functions do not overlap ($K = 1$), the vector $\mathbf{a}_i$ is replaced by $a_i$. When the shaping function is common, we should replace $h_s(t, a_i)$ by $a_i h_s(t)$. In the table only PSK and CPFSK are presented. For DPSK and noncontinuous phase FSK, refer to Sections 2.2.4.1 and 2.2.5.2.

**Table 2.2 Equivalent shaping functions**

| Modulation | | $b(t, \mathbf{a}_i)$ |
|---|---|---|
| Baseband | | $h_s(t, a_i)u_{KT}(t)$ or $h_s(t, \mathbf{a}_i)u_T(t)$ |
| LSK[a] | ASK | $h_s(t, \mathbf{a}_i) * \{\delta(t) + jv(t)\}$ |
| | QASK | $h_{sI}(t, \mathbf{a}_{Ii}) + jh_{sQ}(t, \mathbf{a}_{Qi})$ |
| | OQASK | $h_{sI}(t, \mathbf{a}_{Ii}) + jh_{sQ}(t - 0.5\,T, \mathbf{a}_{Qi})$ |
| PSK | | $\exp\{jK_p h_s(t, \mathbf{a}_i)\}u_T(t)$ |
| FSK | | $\exp(j(\phi_i + \beta(t, \mathbf{a}_i)\}u_T(t)$ |

[a]See eq. (2.5.6), (2.5.7) for alternative forms.

The formulation (2.5.5) and (2.5.6) enables a unified derivation of the *power spectral density* (PSD) for all modulated and baseband signals. In addition it also enables the computation of PSD of the signals distorted by nonlinear amplifiers (soft or hard limiters).

## 2.6 PROBLEMS

2.2.1 Sketch the baseband signal $s_b(t)$ if the shaping function is HS and the symbol sequence is:
 a. $+1 + 1 - 3 + 3 - 1 + 1$
 b. 01100111

2.2.2
 a. Sketch the inphase and quadrature baseband signal components of QASK and OQASK with quaternary symbols generated from a single binary source that produces the sequence $+1 + 1 - 1 - 1 - 1 + 1 - 1 + 1 - 1 + 1 + 1 - 1$. The shaping function is $h_s(t) = \sin(\pi t/T - 0.5 \sin(2\pi t/T))u_T(t)$.
 b. Sketch the envelope in both cases.

2.2.3
 a. Design a symbol constellation with $M = 4$ symbols that maximizes the minimal distance between any two symbols if the sum of the distances between the symbols and the origin is $D$. The distance between the points $(x_I, x_Q)$ and $(y_I, y_Q)$ is $(x_I - y_I)^2 + (x_Q - y_Q)^2$.
 b. Repeat (a) for $M = 16$.

2.2.4

a. Show that a constant envelope OQASK signal is obtained when the shaping function satisfies the condition

$$h_s(t) = \sin \phi(t),\ h_s(t - T_b) = \pm\cos \phi(t), \qquad T_b = 0.5\ T$$

b. Show that condition (a) is satisfied if either

$$\phi(t - T_b) - \phi(t) = \pm 0.5\ \pi + K\ 2\ \pi$$

or

$$\phi(t - T_b) + \phi(t) = \pm 0.5\ \pi + K\ 2\ \pi$$

where $K$ is an integer.

c. Show that the first equation in (b) is satisfied if

$$\phi(t) = (-4\ K \pm 1)(0.5\ \pi t/T) + \alpha(t)$$

and $\alpha(t)$ has the property

$$\alpha(t - T) = \alpha(t)$$

d. Show that the second equation in (b) is satisfied if

$$\phi(t) = \pm 0.25\ \pi + K\pi + \beta(t)$$

and $\beta(t)$ has the property

$$\beta(t - T) = -\beta(t)$$

e. Show that the shaping functions

$$\phi(t) = 0.5\ \pi t/T$$

$$\phi(t) = 0.5\ \pi t/T - C \sin(2\ \pi t/T)$$

$$\phi(t) = 0.5\ \pi t/T - \sum_{1}^{L} A_i \sin^{2i-1}(2\ N\pi t/T)$$

$$\phi(t) = 0.5\ \pi t/T - \sum_{1}^{L} A_i \sin(i\ 2\ \pi t/T)$$

belong to the family defined by (c). $A_i$ is a constant; $L$ and $N$ are integers.

f. Show that the shaping functions with

$$\phi(t) = 0.25\,\pi$$

$$\phi(t) = 0.25\,\pi\{1 - \cos(\pi t/T)\}$$

$$\phi(t) = 0.25\,\pi\{1 - \sum_{1}^{L} A_{2i+1} \cos^{2i+1}(\pi t/T)\}$$

belong to the family defined by (d).

2.2.5

a. Sketch the modulated signal for binary PSK with the SP shaping function and the symbol sequence: $+1 + 1 - 1 - 1 + 1 - 1 + 1$. Assume that the carrier frequency is $f_c = 1/T_b$ and the phase is $\phi_T = -0.5\,\pi$. Here $K_p = 0.5\,\pi$.

b. Repeat (a) for a sequence of quaternary symbols $+1 + 3 - 3 - 1 + 1 - 3$. Here assume $\phi_T = -\pi/4$ and $K_p = \pi/4$.

2.2.6

a. Sketch the modulated signal for binary FSK with the SP shaping function and the symbol sequence: $+1 + 1 - 1 - 1 + 1 - 1 + 1$. Assume that $f_c = 2/T_b$ and $\phi_T = 0$. Assume a frequency deviation of $f_d = 1/T_b$.

b. Repeat (a) for a sequence of symbols: $+1 + 3 - 3 - 1 + 1 - 3$. Assume that $f_c = 2/T_b$ and $\phi_T = 0$. First find the value of $K_F$, so that the frequency corresponding to symbol $-3$ is $0.5/T_b$.

2.2.7 An FSK signal is generated from a baseband signal with HS shaping function.

a. Find the value of $K_F$ so that $\beta(T) = 0.5\,\pi$.

b. Sketch the phase tree and the trellis if the symbol sequence is $+3 - 1 + 1 + 3 - 3 + 1 - 1$.

c. Is this an MSK signal? If yes, what is the shaping function of the equivalent OQASK form for the binary case only.

2.2.8

a. Give at least two examples of shaping functions of duration $T$ and with the property

$$h_s(t + 0.5\,T) = -h_s(0.5\,T - t)$$

b. FSK is generated with the shaping function of (a). Compute $\beta(t)$. What is the value of $\beta(T)$?

c. Assume the FSK of (b). Can you generate the same modulated signal using PSK? What is the shaping function of this PSK?

d. Assume the FSK of (b). Express the FSK signal in the form of inphase and quadrature terms. Show that if the symbols are binary the inphase term is independent of the symbols and only the quadrature term depends on the symbols.

e. Does (d) hold for nonbinary symbols?

2.2.9 Compute and sketch the shaping function of OQASK, which is equivalent to MSK with an RZ shaping function.

2.3.1

a. Sketch the baseband signal if the shaping functions are

$$h_s(t, +1) = u_{0.5T}(t),\ h_s(t, -1) = -u_{0.5T}(t - 0.5\ T)$$

and the sequence of symbols is: $-1 + 1 + 1 - 1 - 1 + 1 + 1 + 1$.

b. The baseband signal of (a) modulates a PSK signal. Determine $K_p$ so that a phase of $0.5\ \pi$ corresponds to symbol $+1$.

c. The baseband signal of (a) modulates an FSK signal. Determine $K_F$ so that the change in phase during a $T$ interval is $0.5\ \pi$.

d. Sketch the phase tree and trellis of (c) for the sequence of (a).

e. Assume we have quaternary symbols. The shaping functions for $\pm 1$ are as in (a) and

$$h_s(t, \pm 3) = 3\ h_s(t, \pm 1)$$

We generate an MSK signal. Compute and sketch the shaping function of the equivalent OQASK.

2.4.1 Generate shaping functions of duration 2 $T$ by convolving pairs of shaping functions each of duration $T$.

a. NRZ and NRZ

b. NRZ and HS

c. NRZ and RC

d. HS and HS

2.4.2

a. Generate a shaping function of duration 3 $T$ by convolving an NRZ of duration $T$ and an NRZ of duration 2 $T$.

b. Define and sketch the three segments of the shaping function, $h_{sk}(t)$, $k = 0, 1, 2$.

c. Sketch the baseband signal if the symbol sequence is $(+1)(+1) + 1 - 1 - 1 + 1 + 1 + 1 - 1 - 1$.

d. The baseband signal is used to modulate a PSK signal. Find the value of $K_p$ so that the maximal phase deviation for any combination of symbols is $\pi/2$.

e. Sketch the phase tree of (d) with the symbols of (c).

## 2.7 REFERENCES

6.1 T. D. Oetting, "A Comparison of Modulation Methods for Digital Radio," *IEEE Tr. Comm.*, Vol. COM-27, Dec. 1979, pp. 1752–1762.

2.2 M. K. Simon and J. G. Smith, "Hexagonal Multiple Phase and Amplitude Shift Keyed Signal Sets," *IEEE Tr. Comm.*, Vol. COM-21, Oct. 1973, pp. 1108–1115.

2.3 G. J. Foschini, R. D. Gitlin, and S. B. Weinstein, "Optimization of Two Dimensional Signal Constellations in the Pressence of Gaussian Noise," *IEEE Tr. Comm.*, Vol. COM-24, Jan. 1974, pp. 28–38.

2.4 C. M. Thomas, M. Y. Weidner, and S. H. Durrani, "Digital Amplitude Phase Shift Keying *M*-ary Alphabets," *IEEE Tr. Comm.*, Vol. COM-22, Feb. 1974, pp. 168–180.

2.5 C. R. Cahn, "Performance of Digital Phase Modulation Communication System," *IRE Tr. Comm. Systems*, Vol. CS-8, Sep. 1960, pp. 150–155.

2.6 T. F. Oberst and D. L. Schilling, "Double Error Probability in Differential PSK," *Proc. IEEE*, Vol. 56, Jun. 1968, pp. 1099–1100.

2.7 A. S. Rosenbaum, "Error Performance of Multiphase DPSK with Noise and Interference," *IEEE Tr. Comm. Techn.*, Vol. COM-18, Dec. 1970, pp. 821–824.

2.8 O. Shimbo, R. J. Fang, and M. Celebiler, "Performance of *M*-ary PSK Systems in Gaussian Noise and Intersymbol Interference," *IEEE Tr. Inf. Theory*, Vol. IT-19, Jan. 1973, pp. 44–58.

2.9 V. K. Prabhu, "PSK Type Modulation with Overlapping Baseband Pulses," *IEEE Tr. Comm.*, Vol. COM-25, Sept. 1977, pp. 980–990.

2.10 R. R. Anderson and J. Salz, "Spectra of Digital FM," *BSTJ*, Vol. 44, Jul–Aug. 1965, pp. 1166–1189.

2.11 T. A. Schonhoff, "Symbol Error Probabilities for *M*-ary CPFSK: Coherent and Noncoherent Detection," *IEEE Tr. Comm.*, Vol. COM-24, Jun. 1976, pp. 644–652.

2.12 T. Aulin and C. E. Sundberg, "Continuous Phase Modulation—(CPM)-Part 1: Full Response Signalling," *IEEE Tr. Comm.*, Vol. COM-29, Mar. 1981, pp. 196–209.

2.13 T. Aulin and C. E. Sundberg, "Continuous Phase Modulation (PM)-Part 2: Partial Response Signalling," *IEEE Tr. Comm.*, Vol. COM-29, Mar. 1981, pp. 210–225.

2.14 T. Aulin and C. E. Sundberg, "On the Minimum Distance for a Class of Signal Space Codes," *IEEE Tr. Inf. Theory*, Vol. IT-28, Jan. 1982, pp. 43–55.

2.15 R. de Buda, "Coherent Demodulation of Frequency Shift Keying with Low Deviation Ratio," *IEEE Tr. Comm.*, Vol. COM-20, Jun. 1972, pp. 429–435.

2.16 F. Amoroso, "Pulse and Spectrum Manipulation in the Minimum (Frequency) Shift Keying (MSK) Format," *IEEE Tr. Comm.*, Vol. COM-24, Mar. 1976, pp. 381–384.

2.17 S. A. Gronomeyer and A. C. McBride, "MSK and Offset QASK Modulation," *IEEE Tr. Comm.*, Vol. COM-24, Aug. 1976, pp. 809–811.

2.18 M. K. Simon, "A Generalization of Minimum Shift Keying (MSK) Type Signalling Based upon Input Data Pulse Shaping," *IEEE Tr. Comm.*, Vol. COM-24, Aug. 1976, pp. 845–856.

2.19 I. Kalet, "A Look at Crosstalk in Quadrature Carrier Modulation Systems," *IEEE Tr. Comm.*, Vol. COM-25, Sep. 1977, pp. 884–892.

2.20 N. Rabsel and S. Pasupathy, "Spectral Shaping in Minimum Shift Keying (MSK)—Type Signalling," *IEEE Tr. Comm.*, Vol. COM-26, Jan. 1978 pp. 189–195.

2.21 F. de Jager and C. B. Dekker, "Tamed Frequency Modulation, a Novel Method to

Achieve Spectrum Economy in Digital Transmission," *IEEE Tr. Comm.*, Vol. COM-26, May 1978, pp. 534–542.

2.22 B. Razin, "A Class of MSK Baseband Pulse Formats with Sharp Spectral Roll-off," *IEEE Tr. Comm.*, Vol. COM-27, May 1979, pp. 826–829.

2.23 I. Korn, "Generalised Minimum Shift Keying," *IEEE Tr. Inf. Theory*, Vol. IT-26, Mar. 1980, pp. 234–238.

2.24 I. Korn, "Shaping Function for Constant Envelope Offset QASK", *Proc. IREE* (Australia), Vol. 41, Sept. 1980, pp. 113–114.

2.25 T. Le-Ngoc, K. Feher, and H. Phan Van, "New Modulation Techniques for Low Cost Power and Bandwidth Efficient Satellite Earth Stations," *IEEE Tr. Comm.*, Vol. COM-30, Jan. 1982, pp. 275–283.

2.26 M. C. Austin and M. U. Chang, "Quadrature Overlapped Raised Cosine Modulation," *IEEE Tr. Comm.*, Vol. COM-29, Mar. 1981, pp. 237–249.

2.27 I. Sasase, V. Harada, and S. Mori, "Bandwidth Efficient Overlapped Modulation," *Proc. IEEE Inter. Conf. on Comm.*, ICC-82, Jun. 1982, pp. 6F.2.1–6F.2.5.

2.28 T. Aulin, C. E. Sundberg, and A. Svenson, "MSK-Type Receivers for Partial Response Continuous Phase Modulation," *Proc. IEEE Inter. Conf. on Comm.*, ICC-82, Jun. 1982, pp. 6F.3.1–6F.3.6.

2.29 P. Gulko and S. Pasupathy, "Linear Receivers for Generalised MSK," *Proc. IEEE Inter. Conf. on Comm.*, ICC-82, Jun. 1982, pp. GF.5.1–6F.5.6.

2.30 P. Kabal and S. Pasupathy, "Partial Response Signalling," *IEEE Tr. Comm.*, Vol. COM-23, Sept. 1975, pp. 921–934.

# 3 POWER SPECTRAL DENSITY (PSD) AND BANDWIDTH

## 3.1 INTRODUCTION

It was shown in Chapter 2 that the modulated signal has the form

$$s_M(t) = \text{Re}\,\{s(t) \exp\,(j(2\,\pi f_c t + \phi_T))\} \qquad (3.1.1)$$

where

$$s(t) = A \sum_i b(t - iT, \mathbf{a}_i) \qquad (3.1.2)$$

It will be shown in this chapter that the power spectral desntiy (PSD) of the modulated signal, $S_{sM}(f)$, is related to the PSD of the complex envelope, $S_s(f)$ by

$$S_{sM}(f) = 0.25\,\{S_s(f - f_c) + S_s(f + f_c)\} \qquad (3.1.3)$$

Thus it is sufficient to compute only $S_s(f)$. It will be shown that

$$S_s(f) = (A^2/T) \sum_n \overline{B(f, \mathbf{a}_n) B^*(f, \mathbf{a}_0)} \exp\,(-j\,2\,\pi f n T) \qquad (3.1.4)$$

where $B(f, \mathbf{a}_n)$ is the Fourier transform (FT) of $b(t, \mathbf{a}_n)$; the asterisk denotes the complex conjugate, and the bar denotes the average operation.

Let $B_x$ be the bandwidth in which $x$% of the signal power is contained. In this chapter we shall find the PSD and $B_x$ for various types of digital modulation with $x = 99\%$ or $x = 99.9\%$. The knowledge of the PSD and bandwidth of the modulated (and baseband) signal is of paramount importance in the design of a digital communications system. The choice of channel bandwidth is determined by the PSD of the signal. Having a choice between two systems that are about equal in all aspects except for the required bandwidth, we shall select the system that needs a smaller bandwidth. There are several reasons for that:

a. Bandwidth costs money.
b. Bandwidth is a limited natural resource that should be used efficiently.
c. There will be less interference with adjacent channels.
d. International regulations specify a mask of bandwidth that may not be

exceeded in various systems. Thus a signal with a smaller bandwidth will require less additional filtering to comply with the mask.

## 3.2 PSD AND BANDWIDTH OF MODULATED SIGNAL[3.1]

Equation (2.1.1) can be rewritten as

$$s_M(t) = 0.5\,\{s(t)\exp(j(2\pi f_c t + \phi_T) + s^*(t)\exp(-j(2\pi f_c t + \phi_T))\} \tag{3.2.1}$$

where $f_c$ is the carrier frequency, and $\phi_T$ is a random phase uniformly distributed in 0—2 $\pi$.

The autocorrelation of a complex random process $x(t)$ is defined by

$$R_x(t+\tau, t) = \overline{x(t+\tau)x^*(t)} = E\{x(t+\tau)x^*(t)\} \tag{3.2.2}$$

where both the bar and the the operator $E$ denote the statistical average. When the process is real, we drop the asterisk in $x^*(t)$. If the process is wide-sense stationary, $R_x(t + \tau, t)$ is only a function of $\tau$. In our case the process happens to be *cyclostationary*, i.e., $R_x(t + \tau, t)$ is periodic in $t$ with period $T$. After averaging with respect to $t$ over one period, we obtain $R_x(\tau)$, which is independent of $t$. Thus the autocorrelation of $s_M(t)$ is from (3.2.2) and (3.2.1)

$$\begin{aligned} R_{sM}(\tau) = {} & 0.25\,\{R_s(\tau)\exp(+j\,2\pi f_c\tau) + R_s^*(\tau)\exp(-j\,2\pi f_c\tau)\} \\ & + 0.25 < \{\overline{s(t+\tau)s(t)}\;\overline{\exp(j\,2\,\phi_T)}\exp(j\,2\pi f_c(2t+\tau)) \\ & + \overline{s^*(t+\tau)s^*(t)}\;\overline{\exp(-j\,2\,\phi_T)}\exp(-j\,2\pi f_c(2t+\tau))\} > \end{aligned} \tag{3.2.3}$$

where $< >$ is the time average operator. In (3.2.3) we have used the property that if $x(t)$ and $y(t)$ are independent processes or variables, then the average of their product is the product of their averages, i.e.,

$$\overline{x(t)y(t)} = \overline{x(t)}\;\overline{y(t)} \tag{3.2.4}$$

Since $s(t)$ and $\phi_T$ are independent, we applied (3.2.4) to (3.2.3) by identifying

$$x(t) = s(t+\tau)s(t),\; y(t) = \exp(j\,2\,\phi_T) \tag{3.2.5}$$

or their complex conjugates. Because $\phi_T$ is uniformly distributed in 0—2 $\pi$, we obtain

$$\overline{\exp(\pm j\,2\,\phi_T)} = (2\pi)^{-1}\int_0^{2\pi}\exp(\pm j\,2\,\phi_T)\,d\phi_T = 0 \tag{3.2.6}$$

Thus (3.2.3) is simplified to

$$R_{sM}(\tau) = 0.25 \{R_s(\tau) \exp(+j 2 \pi f_c \tau) + R_s^*(\tau) \exp(-j 2 \pi f_c \tau)\} \quad (3.2.7)$$

Taking the FT of (3.2.7), we obtain the PSD

$$S_{sM}(f) = 0.25 \{S_s(f - f_c) + S_s^*(-f - f_c)\} \quad (3.2.8)$$

In most cases (the exception is SSB and VSB), $S_s(f)$ is real and symmetric, i.e.

$$S_s^*(f) = S_s(f) = S_s(-f) \quad (3.2.9)$$

Hence (3.2.8) is replaced by

$$S_{sM}(f) = 0.25 \{S_s(f - f_c) + S_s(f + f_c)\} \quad (3.2.10)$$

*Example* 3.2.1 PSD of complex envelope and modulated signal
In Fig. 3.1 we show an example of a triangular PSD of the complex envelope and the resulting $S_M(f)$. In this example we assume that $f_c$ is large enough so that the two terms in (3.2.10) do not overlap.

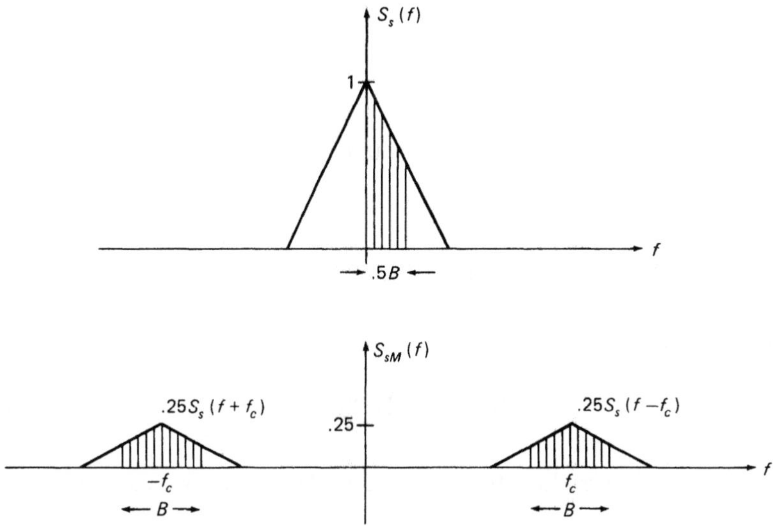


Fig. 3.1. PSD and bandwidth of complex envelope and modulated signal.

The power contained in a bandwidth $B$ is

$$P'_{iB}(B) = \int_{-f_c - B/2}^{-f_c + B/2} S_{sM}(f)\, df + \int_{f_c - B/2}^{f_c + B/2} S_{sM}(f)\, df \quad (3.2.11)$$

which, after substitution of (3.2.10) and (3.2.9), gives

$$P'_{iB}(B) = \int_0^{B/2} S_s(f)\, df \tag{3.2.12}$$

We have illustrated the inband power by the shaded areas in Fig. 3.1. The total power is $P'_{iB}(\infty)$. The normalized power contained in bandwidth $B$ is

$$P_{iB}(B) = P'_{iB}(B)/P'_{iB}(\infty) \tag{3.2.13}$$

If the total power is normalized to 1, there is no need for additional normalization. The power outside bandwidth $B$ is

$$P_{OB}(B) = 1 - P_{iB}(B) \tag{3.2.14}$$

The bandwidth in which $x\%$ of the power is contained is defined by

$$P_{iB}(B_x) = x/100 \tag{3.2.15}$$

or, from (3.2.13) and (3.2.12)

$$\int_0^{0.5B_x} S_s(f)\, df = 0.01\, x \int_0^{\infty} S_s(f)\, df \tag{3.2.16}$$

## 3.3 PSD OF COMPLEX ENVELOPE

The complex envelope is

$$s(t) = A \sum_i b(t - iT, \mathbf{a}_i) \tag{3.3.1}$$

This process is a cyclostationary process; hence first we compute

$$R_s(t + \tau, t) = \overline{s(t + \tau)s^*(t)} \tag{3.3.2}$$

Then we compute

$$R_s(\tau) = \langle R_s(t + \tau, t)\rangle = \int_0^T R_s(t + \tau, t)\, dt/T \tag{3.3.3}$$

and finally the last step is the FT

$$S_s(f) = \int_{-\infty}^{\infty} R_s(\tau) \exp(-j\,2\,\pi f \tau)\, d\tau \tag{3.3.4}$$

*Step 1* We substitute (3.3.1) into (3.3.2) and obtain

$$R_s(t + \tau, t) = A^2 \sum_i \sum_k \overline{b(t + \tau - iT, \mathbf{a}_i) b^*(t - kT, \mathbf{a}_k)} \tag{3.3.5}$$

In writing (3.3.5) we exchanged the order of summation and averaging. To see indeed that (3.3.5) is periodic with repect to $t$ and with period $T$, compute

$$R_s(t + T + \tau, t + T) = A^2 \sum_i \sum_k \overline{b(t + \tau - (i - 1)T, \mathbf{a}_i) b^*(t - (k - 1)T, \mathbf{a}_k)} \tag{3.3.6}$$

Changing indices $i - 1 = i'$, $k - 1 = k'$ and noting that for stationary symbols we can replace the pair $(\mathbf{a}_i, \mathbf{a}_k)$ by the pair $(\mathbf{a}_{i-1}, \mathbf{a}_{k-1})$, we obtain

$$R_s(t + T + \tau, t + T) = A^2 \sum_{i'} \sum_{k'} \overline{b(t + \tau - i'T, \mathbf{a}_{i'}) b^*(t - k'T, \mathbf{a}_{k'})} \tag{3.3.7}$$

which is identical to (3.3.5), because the name of the index does not affect the value of the summation.

*Step 2*

$$R_s(\tau) = (A^2/T) \sum_i \sum_k \int_0^T \overline{b(t + \tau - iT, \mathbf{a}_i) b^*(t - kT, \mathbf{a}_k)\, dt} \tag{3.3.8}$$

Let us denote

$$z = t - kT,\ m = i - k \tag{3.3.9}$$

and change variables in (3.3.8). The result is

$$R_s(\tau) = (A^2/T) \sum_m \sum_k \int_{-kT}^{-kT+T} \overline{b(z + \tau - mT, \mathbf{a}_{m+k}) b^*(z, \mathbf{a}_k)\, dz} \tag{3.3.10}$$

Because of the stationarity of the symbols, we can replace in (3.3.10) the pair $(\mathbf{a}_{m+k}, \mathbf{a}_k)$ by the pair $(\mathbf{a}_m, \mathbf{a}_0)$. Therefore

$$R_s(\tau) = (A^2/T) \sum_m \sum_k \int_{-kT}^{-kT+T} \overline{b(z + \tau - mT, \mathbf{a}_m) b^*(z, \mathbf{a}_0)\, dz} \tag{3.3.11}$$

The summation over $k$ of the segmented integrals is in fact a single integral from $-\infty$ to $\infty$. Replacing in (3.3.10) $z$ by $t$ and $m$ by $i$ (which is of no substance), we obtain thus

$$R_s(\tau) = (A^2/T)\sum_i \int_{-\infty}^{\infty} \overline{b(t + \tau - iT, \mathbf{a}_i)b^*(t, \mathbf{a}_0)\, dt} \tag{3.3.12}$$

*Step 3* We take the FT of (3.3.12) and change again the order of integration, summation, and averaging

$$S_s(f) = A^2 \sum_i \left\{ \int_{-\infty}^{\infty} b^*(t, \mathbf{a}_0) \left( \int_{-\infty}^{\infty} b(t + \tau - iT, \mathbf{a}_i) \right.\right.$$

$$\left. \exp(-j\, 2\, \pi f(\tau + t - iT))d\tau \right)$$

$$\left. \exp(j\, 2\, \pi f t)\, dt \right\} \exp(-j\, 2\, \pi f i T) R \tag{3.3.13}$$

The term in the internal brackets is after changing variables

$$\tau' = t + \tau - iT \tag{3.3.14}$$

simply the FT of $b(t, \mathbf{a}_i)$, i.e., $B(f, \mathbf{a}_i)$. This term can now be removed from the external integral, because it is not a function of $t$, and the resulting external integral is $B^*(f, \mathbf{a}_0)$. Therefore we obtain

$$S_s(f) = (A^2/T) \sum_i S_{b,i}(f) \exp(-j\, 2\, \pi f i T) \tag{3.3.15}$$

where

$$S_{b,i}(f) = \overline{B(f, \mathbf{a}_i) B^*(f, \mathbf{a}_0)} \tag{3.3.16}$$

If the sets of symbols $\mathbf{a}_i$ and $\mathbf{a}_0$ are independent for $|i| \geqq K$, then

$$S_{b,i}(f) = \overline{B(f, \mathbf{a}_i)}\ \overline{B^*(f, \mathbf{a}_0)} \tag{3.3.17}$$

and because of stationarity of the symbols

$$S_{b,i}(f) = \overline{B(f, \mathbf{a}_0)}\ \overline{B^*(f, \mathbf{a}_0)} \qquad |i| \geqq K \tag{3.3.18}$$

Because the average of the complex conjugate is the complex conjugate of the average, i.e., for any complex random variable $x$

$$\overline{x^*} = (\overline{x})^* \tag{3.3.19}$$

we obtain for $|i| \geqq K$

$$S_{b,i}(f) = S_{b,K}(f) = |\overline{B(f, \mathbf{a}_0)}|^2 \tag{3.3.20}$$

which is a real function.

Thus

$$\begin{aligned} S_s(f) = {} & (A^2/T) \sum_{|i|<K} (S_{b,i}(f) - S_{b,K}(f)) \exp(-j\, 2\, \pi\, fiT) \\ & + (A^2/T) S_{b,K}(f) \sum_i \exp(-j\, 2\, \pi fiT) \end{aligned} \tag{3.3.21}$$

Since

$$T \sum_i \exp(-j\, 2\, \pi fiT) = \sum_k \delta(f - kR) \tag{3.3.22}$$

where $R = 1/T$ (this can be simply shown by noting that the right-hand side is a periodic function with period $R$, and the left-hand side is the corresponding Fourier series), we obtain a decomposition of the PSD into a continuous part $S_{sc}(f)$ and discrete part $S_{sd}(f)$.

$$S_s(f) = S_{sc}(f) + S_{sd}(f) \tag{3.3.23}$$

$$S_{sc}(f) = (A^2/T) \sum_{|i|<K} (S_{b,i}(f) - S_{b,K}(f)) \exp(-j\, 2\, \pi fiT) \tag{3.3.24}$$

$$S_{sd}(f) = (A/T)^2 S_{b,K}(f) \sum_k \delta(f - kR) \tag{3.3.25}$$

The continuous part is a continuous function of frequency, though the discrete part has values at frequencies $f = kR$ only.

When we compute eq. (3.3.24), we need only the terms with nonnegative indices because, from (3.3.16) and stationarity of the symbols

$$\begin{aligned} S_{b,-i}(f) &= \overline{B(f, \mathbf{a}_{-i}) B^*(f, \mathbf{a}_0)} = \overline{B(f, \mathbf{a}_0) B^*(f, \mathbf{a}_i)} \\ &= \overline{B^*(f, \mathbf{a}_i) B(f, \mathbf{a}_0)} = \overline{\{B(f, \mathbf{a}_i) B^*(f, \mathbf{a}_0)\}^*} = S^*_{b,i}(f) \end{aligned} \tag{3.3.26}$$

and

$$S_{b,0}(f) = |\overline{B(f, \mathbf{a}_0)}|^2 \tag{3.3.27}$$

$$S_{sc}(f) = (A^2/T)\left\{S_{b,0}(f) - S_{b,K}(f)\right.$$
$$\left. + 2\,\mathrm{Re}\left\{\sum_{i=1}^{K-1}(S_{b,i}(f) - S_{b,K}(f))\exp(-j\,2\,\pi f i T)\right\}\right\} \quad (3.3.28)$$

As formulated in (3.3.16) and (3.3.20) in computing $S_{b,i}(f)$, we first compute the FT of $b(t, \mathbf{a}_i)$ and $b(t, \mathbf{a}_0)$ and then compute their average or the average of their product. In some cases (especially for PSK and FSK) it may be more convenient or computationally more efficient (especially when numerical integration is required) to reverse this order. Thus let

$$m_b(t) = \overline{b(t, \mathbf{a}_0)} \quad (3.3.29)$$

be the average of $b(t, \mathbf{a}_0)$, and let $M_b(f)$ be its FT. Note, that, because of symbol stationarity, the average is independent of the index of the symbol, $\mathbf{a}_i$. Thus

$$S_{b,K}(f) = |M_b(f)|^2 \quad (3.3.30)$$

In many instances $m_b(t)$ is 0; hence $M_b(f)$ is also 0, and the PSD has no discrete part, i.e.

$$S_s(f) = S_{sc}(f) = (A^2/T)\sum_{|i|<K} S_{b,i}(f)\exp(-j\,2\,\pi f i T) \quad (3.3.31)$$

The general term $S_{b,i}(f)$ can also be written as

$$S_{b,i}(f) = \int_{-\infty}^{\infty}\int_{-\infty}^{\infty} \overline{b(t, \mathbf{a}_i)b^*(t', \mathbf{a}_0)}\exp(-j\,2\,\pi(t - t')f)\,dt\,dt' \quad (3.3.32)$$

where we have interchanged the order of FT and statistical average. Let us denote

$$R_{b,i}(t, t') = \overline{b(t, \mathbf{a}_i)b^*(t', \mathbf{a}_0)} \quad (3.3.33)$$

which is the autocorrelation of $b(t, \mathbf{a}_i)$. If the duration of $b(t, \mathbf{a}_i)$ does not exceed $T'$, we can write (3.3.32)

$$S_{b,i}(f) = \int_0^{T'}\int_0^{T'} R_{b,i}(t, t')\exp(-j\,2\,\pi f(t - t'))\,dt\,dt' \quad (3.3.34)$$

After changing variables

$$t - t' = z,\ t' = x \tag{3.3.35}$$

we obtain (see Problem 3.3.3)

$$S_{b,i}(f) = \int_0^{T'} \left\{ \int_0^{T'-z} R_{b,i}(z + x, x)\, dx \right\} \exp(-j\, 2\, \pi\, fz)\, dz$$
$$+ \int_0^{T'} \left\{ \int_0^{T'-z} R_{b,i}(x, z + x)\, dx \right\} \exp(+j\, 2\, \pi fz)\, dz \tag{3.3.36}$$

In many cases

$$R_{b,i}(t, t') = R^*_{b,i}(t', t) \tag{3.3.37}$$

Hence

$$S_{b,i}(f) = 2 \int_0^{T'} \mathrm{Re} \left\{ \left\{ \int_0^{T'-z} R_{b,i}(z + x, x)\, dx \right\} \exp(-j\, 2\, \pi fz) \right\} dz \tag{3.3.38}$$

is real. If in addition $R_{b,i}(t, t')$ is real, then

$$S_{b,i}(f) = 2 \int_0^{T'} \left\{ \int_0^{T'-z} \{R_{b,i}(z + x, x)\, dx\} \cos(2\, \pi\, fz) \right\} dz \tag{3.3.39}$$

It is sufficient to compute the autocorrelation for nonnegative indices because, from (3.3.33) and stationarity of the symbols

$$R_{b,-i}(t, t') = R^*_{b,i}(t', t) \tag{3.3.40}$$

Equation (3.3.34) (hence also eqs. (3.3.36), (3.3.38), and (3.3.39)) defines a transformation from $R_{b,i}(t, t')$ to $S_{b,i}(f)$. We shall call the transformation, for obvious reasons, the *single Fourier transform* (SFT) to distinguish it from the double Fourier transform

$$S_{b,i}(f, f') = \int_0^{T'}\int_0^{T'} R_{b,i}(t, t') \exp(-j\, 2\, \pi ft) \exp(j\, 2\, \pi f't')\, dt\, dt' \tag{3.3.41}$$

Thus from now on $S_{b,i}(f)$ is the SFT of $R_{b,i}(t, t')$.

### 3.3.1 Independent symbols

Here we assume that $b(t, \mathbf{a}_i)$ depends on one symbol only

$$b(t, \mathbf{a}_i) = b(t, a_i) \tag{3.3.42}$$

and that the symbols are independent. Here

$$B(f, \mathbf{a}_i) = B(f, a_i) \tag{3.3.43}$$

$$m_b(t) = \overline{b(t, a_0)} \tag{3.3.44}$$

$$R_{b,i}(t, t') = \overline{b(t, a_i)b^*(t', a_0)} = \begin{cases} \overline{b(t, a_0)b^*(t', a_0)} & i = 0 \\ m_b(t)m_b^*(t') & i \neq 0 \end{cases} \tag{3.3.45}$$

$$S_{b,i}(f) = \begin{cases} \overline{|B(f, a_0|^2} & i = 0 \\ |\overline{B(f, a_0)}|^2 = S_{b,1}(f) & i \neq 0 \end{cases} \tag{3.3.46}$$

Thus from (3.3.24) and (3.3.25) with $K = 1$, we obtain

$$S_{sc}(f) = (A^2/T)\{S_{b,0}(f) - S_{b,1}(f)\} \tag{3.3.47}$$

$$S_{sd}(f) = (A/T)^2 S_{b,1}(f) \sum_k \delta(f - kR) \tag{3.3.48}$$

It is not difficult to show (see Problem 3.3.2) that for equiprobable symbols from the set $\mathring{A} = \{a(1), \ldots, a(M)\}$, we obtain from (3.3.46) and (3.3.47)

$$S_{sc}(f) = (A^2/T) \sum_{i=1}^{M} \sum_{k=1}^{M} |B(f, a(\mathrm{i})) - B(f, a(k))|^2/M \tag{3.3.49}$$

which may be a more convenient form in some instances.

## 3.4 PSD OF BASEBAND SIGNAL

A baseband signal can also be written in the form

$$s(t) = A \sum_i h(t - iT, a_i) \tag{3.4.1}$$

where instead of $s_b(t)$ of Chapter 2, we wrote $s(t)$, instead of $h_s(t, a_i)$ we wrote $h(t, a_i)$, and we have added the amplitude $A$. The baseband signal is a real function. All results of the previous section apply immediately here with $b(t, a_i)$ replaced by $h(t, a_i)$. Thus

$$S_s(f) = (A^2/T) \sum_i S_{h,i}(f) \exp(-j\, 2\, \pi f i T) \tag{3.4.2}$$

$$S_{h,i}(f) = \overline{H(f, a_i) H^*(f, a_0)} \tag{3.4.3}$$

and when the symbols are independent

$$S_s(f) = (A^2/T)\{S_{h,0}(f) - S_{h,1}(f)\} + (A/T)^2 S_{h,1}(f) \sum_k \delta(f - kR) \tag{3.4.4}$$

$$S_{h,1}(f) = |M_h(f)|^2 \tag{3.4.5}$$

where $M_h(f)$ is the FT of

$$m_h(t) = \overline{h(t, a_0)} \tag{3.4.6}$$

### 3.4.1 Common shaping function

Here we assume

$$h(t, a_i) = a_i h(t) \tag{3.4.7}$$

Hence instead of (3.4.2) we have here

$$S_s(f) = (A^2/T)|H(f)|^2 \sum_i \overline{a_i a_0} \exp(-j\, 2\, \pi f i T) \tag{3.4.8}$$

If in addition the symbols are independent (it is sufficient here that the symbols are only uncorrelated), we have, instead of (3.4.4)

$$S_s(f) = (A^2/T)|H(f)|^2\{\overline{a^2}_0 - (\bar{a}_0)^2 + (\bar{a}_0)^2 \sum_k \delta(f - kR)/T\} \tag{3.4.9}$$

When $\overline{a_0} = 0$, we obtain

$$S_s(f) = (A^2/T)|H(f)|^2 \overline{a^2}_0 \tag{3.4.10}$$

For equiprobable symbols this simple formula is obtained when

$$\overline{a_0} = \sum_{k=1}^{M} a(k)/M = 0 \tag{3.4.11}$$

This is true for any symmetric set of symbols and is certainly true for $\mathring{A}_{\pm} = \{\pm 1, \pm 3, \ldots, \pm(M-1)\}$. For this symbol set it is trivial to show that

$$a_0^2 = \sum_{k=1}^{M} a^2(k)/M = (M^2 - 1)/3 \tag{3.4.12}$$

Note from (3.4.8) that in the general case when the symbols are dependent, the PSD is determined by the FT of the shaping function, $H(f)$, and by the correlation between the symbols. From (3.4.9) we conclude that if the symbols are uncorrelated, the PSD is determined solely by the shaping function. The form of the PSD is also independent of the number of symbols $M$. When we substitute (3.4.10) into (3.2.16), we obtain a simple formula for the $x$% bandwidth, which depends only on the shaping function and is the same for all $M$

$$\int_0^{0.5B_x} |H(f)|^2\, df = (x/100) \int_0^{\infty} |H(f)|^2\, df \tag{3.4.13}$$

*Example* 3.4.1 The PSD of baseband signal
In this example we compute the PSD, the power outside bandwidth $B$ and $B_{99}$ for a baseband signal with NRZ, RZ HS, RC, and TR shaping functions defined in Fig. 2.2 and eq. (2.2.3). We substitute (2.2.3) into (3.4.10) and select in each case $A$ so that the total power is 1 watt. The resulting, normalized PSD is presented in Table 3.1. In this table we denoted

$$\text{sinc}(x) = \sin(\pi x)/(\pi x) \tag{3.4.14}$$

**Table 3.1 PSD and $B_{99}$ of baseband and LSK**

| SHAPING FUNCTION | NORMALIZED PSD | $B_{99}T$ |
|---|---|---|
| NRZ | $2\,T\,\text{sinc}^2\,(fT)$ | 19.3 |
| RZ | $T\,\text{sinc}^2\,(0.5\,fT)$ | 38.6 |
| Half-sine | $(4\,T/\pi)\cos^2(\pi fT)\{1-(2\,fT)^2\}^{-2}$ | 2.34 |
| Raised cosine | $(2\,T/3)\,\text{sinc}^2\,(fT)\{1-(fT)^2\}^{-2}$ | 2.86 |
| Triangle | $(3\,T/2)\,\text{sinc}^4\,(0.5\,fT)$ | 2.66 |

Note that the PSD is in each case a function of $fT = f/R$, i.e., the frequency normalized by the symbol rate. The PSD is presented in Fig. 3.2. The 99% bandwidth is the value of $B$ for which $P_{OB}(B) = 0.01$, i.e., log $P_{OB}(B) = -20$. The values of $B_{99}$ are also presented in Table 3.1. There is no curve for the RZ shaping function in Fig. 3.2 and Fig. 3.3, but this

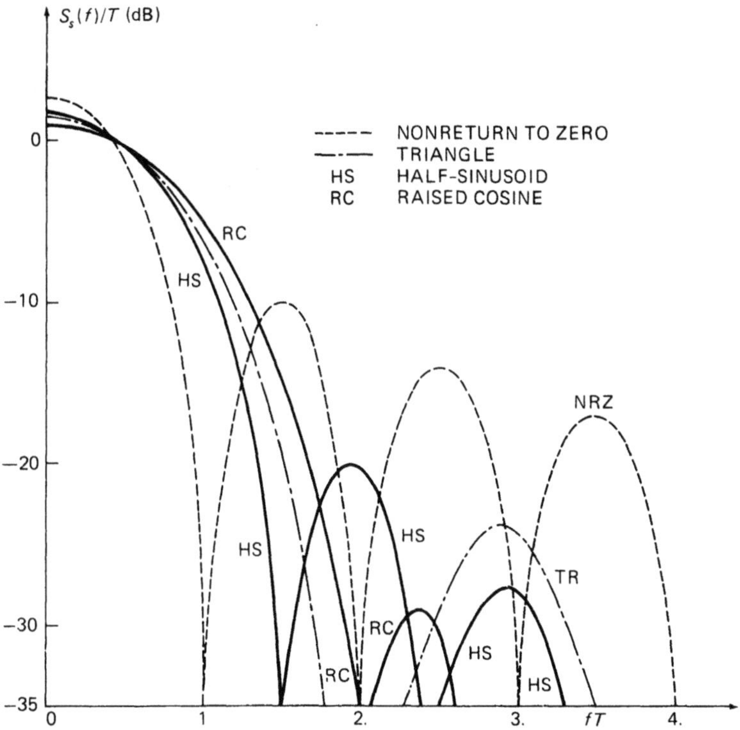


Fig. 3.2. PSD as a function of normalized frequency for baseband and LSK with NRZ, TR, HS, and RC shaping functions.

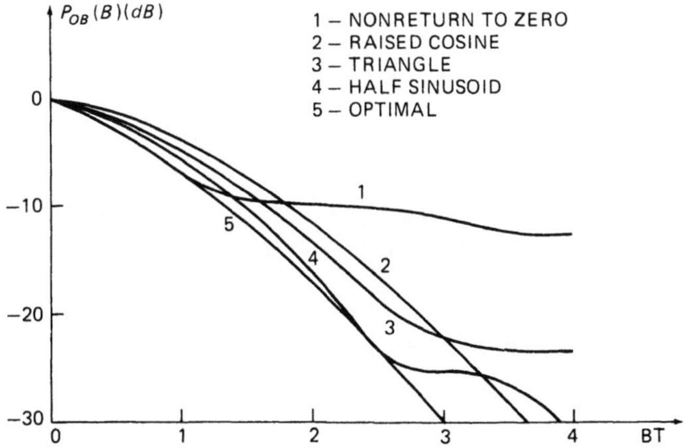


Fig. 3.3. The out-of-band power as a function of normalized bandwidth for baseband and LSK with NRZ, TR, HS, RC, and optimal shaping functions.

curve can be obtained from the NRZ curve by relabeling the horizontal axis from $f/R$ and $B/R$ to $0.5\, f/R$ and $0.5\, B/R$, respectively.

Note from Fig. 3.2 that the main lobe of the NRZ PSD lies within $f/R = 1$, and for the HS the main lobe is within $f/R = 1.43$. This is also shown in Fig. 3.3. Up to $B/R = 1.53$, the best shaping function is NRZ, though after that point the best shaping function is HS. The reason for this behavior is that, although the PSD for HS decreases much faster than the PSD of NRZ for large $f/R$, this does not compensate for the initial difference in the width of the main lobes.

We have in Fig. 3.3 an optimal curve that will be discussed later.

## 3.5 PSD OF LSK

All the results of the previous section apply here also with $B(f, a_i)$ as defined by the FT of the entries in eq. (2.5.7), namely

$$B(f, a_i) = \begin{cases} H(f, a_i)\{1 + jV(f)\} \\ H_I(f, a_{Ii}) + jH_Q(f, a_{Qi}) \\ H_I(f, a_{Ii}) + j \exp(j\, 2\, \pi f T) H_Q(f, a_{Qi}) \end{cases} \tag{3.5.1}$$

where for notational convenience we dropped the subscript $s$ from the shaping function $H_s(f)$

$$V(f) = \begin{cases} 0 & \text{DSB} \\ \pm j \operatorname{sign} f & \text{SSB} \\ H_{\text{VSB}}(f) & \text{VSB} \end{cases} \tag{3.5.2}$$

and $H_{\text{VSB}}(f)$ is defined in (2.2.24). In the case of a common shaping function and identical shaping function in the inphase and quadrature signals, we obtain from (3.5.1)

$$B(f, a_i) = \begin{cases} a_i H(f)\{1 + jV(f)\} & \text{ASK} \\ (a_{Ii} + ja_{Qi})H(f) & \text{QASK} \\ \{a_{Ii} + ja_{Qi} \exp(j\, 2\, \pi T)\}H(f) & \text{OQASK} \end{cases} \tag{3.5.3}$$

If the symbol constellation is symmetric in both directions (and this is in fact the case for all symbol constellations in Fig. 2.8) and the symbols are equiprobable, both conditions normally satisfied in practice, then

$$\overline{a_i} = \overline{a_{Ii}} = \overline{a_{Qi}} = \overline{B(f, a_i)} = 0$$

Hence from (3.5.3) and (3.3.29)

*ASK*

$$S_s(f) = (A^2/T)\overline{a^2_0}|H(f)|^2 W(f)$$

where

$$W(f) = \begin{cases} 1 & & \text{DSB} \\ 4\,u(f) & & \text{SSB} \\ \begin{cases} |1 + H_{od}(f)|^2 & |f| \leqq f_r \\ 4\,u(f) & |f| > f_r \end{cases} & & \text{VSB} \end{cases} \tag{3.5.4}$$

$H_{od}(f)$ is defined in (2.2.23), and $u(f)$ is the unit step function. $S_s(f)$ is not an even function for SSB and VSB, because $|W(f)|^2$ is not symmetric for these cases.

*QASK*

$$S_s(f) = (A^2/T)\overline{|a_i|^2}|H(f)|^2,\ a_i = a_{Ii} + ja_{Qi} \tag{3.5.5}$$

*OQASK*

$$S_s(f) = (A^2/T)\overline{|a_{Ii} + ja_{Qi}\exp(j\,2\,\pi fT)|^2}|H(f)|^2 \tag{3.5.6}$$

The middle term in (3.5.6) is equal to

$$\begin{aligned} &\overline{\{a_{Ii} - a_{Qi}\sin(2\,\pi fT)\}^2 + \{a_{Qi}\cos(2\,\pi fT)\}^2} \\ &= \overline{a^2}_{Ii} - 2\,\overline{a_{Ii}a_{Qi}}\sin(2\,\pi fT) + \overline{a^2}_{Qi} \end{aligned}$$

For symmetrical constellations and equiprobable symbols the middle term is zero; hence here also

$$S_s(f) = (A^2/T)\overline{|a_i|^2}|H(f)|^2,\ a_i = a_{Ii} + ja_{Qi}$$

i.e., the same as for QASK.

We thus have for ASK-DSB, QASK, and OQASK the single formula

$$S_s(f) = (A^2/T)\overline{|a_i|^2}|H(f)|^2 \tag{3.5.7}$$

and this is modified by $W(f)$ for SSB and VSB. Formula (3.5.7) is valid for both overlapping and nonoverlapping shaping functions, because we have not placed any restrictions. Table 3.1 and Figs. 3.2 and 3.3 are thus also valid for ASK-DSB, QASK, and OQASK. In fact (3.5.7) is also valid for binary MSK (because of its equivalence to quaternary OQASK) and for $M$-ary PSK with an NRZ shaping function. In the latter case all symbols are on a circle, hence $\overline{|a_i|^2} = 1$.

Thus the entries of the first line of Table 3.1 represent the PSD and bandwidth of $M$-ary PSK with NRZ shaping function. Similarly, the entries in line 3 of Table 3.1 represent the PSD and bandwidth of binary MSK with NRZ shaping function.

When we apply the results of Table 3.1 it is important to remember that the bandwidth is normalized with respect to the symbol rate, $R$. Because the symbol rate is related to the bit rate by

$$R = R_b/\log_2 M \tag{3.5.8}$$

the actual bandwidth is given by

$$B_{99} = (\text{ent}/\log_2 M)R_b \tag{3.5.9}$$

where ent is the entry in column 3 of Table 3.1. Since binary MSK is equivalent to quaternary OQASK, we should use in (3.5.9) the value $M = 4$ rather than $M = 2$ for MSK.

It is not difficult to show (see Problem 3.5.2) that if the duration of the shaping function is changed from $T$ to $KT$, then the PSD is changed from $S_s(f)$ to $K^2 S_s(Kf)$, and the $x\%$ bandwidth is changed from $B_x$ to $B_x/K$, i.e., the bandwidth is inversely proportional to the duration. This is the main reason for the usage of overlapping or partial response shaping functions.

*Example* 3.5.1 PSD of baseband with shaping functions of duration KT Let us define an NRZ, HS, and RC shaping function of duration KT by

$$h(t) = \begin{cases} u_{KT}(t) & \text{K-NRZ} \\ \sin(\pi t/KT))u_{KT}(t) & \text{K-HS} \\ 0.5\,\{1 - \cos(2\,\pi t/(KT))\}\{u_{KT}(t) & \text{K-RC} \end{cases} \tag{3.5.10}$$

Then the PSD and bandwidth are the same as those presented in Table 3.1 with $T$ replaced by $KT$. Note that 2-NRZ is the duobinary shaping function. Similarly, Figs. 3.2 and Fig. 3.3 are valid by relabeling the horizontal axis (replace $T$ by $KT$ or $R$ by $R/K$).

The 2-RC can be obtained by convolving 1-NRZ and 1-HS. Similarly, many other shaping functions of duration 2 $T$ can be obtained by convolving two shaping functions of duration $T$ each. The PSD of 2-RC is thus the product of the PSD of 1-NRZ and 1-HS. Because 1-NRZ is good for low values of $B/R$, and 1-HS is good for high values of $B/R$, their product PSD, i.e., the PSD of 2-RC should be superior to both. In Fig. 3.4 we show the PSD of 2-RC, 1-HRZ, and 1-HS shaping functions. The figures are reproduced from Ref. 3.12. Other figures can be found in Ref. 3.11.

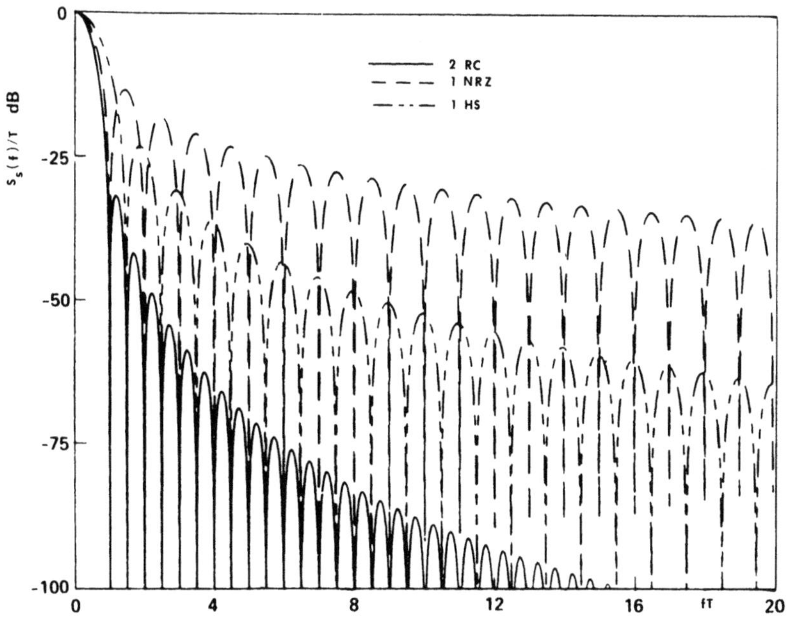


Fig. 3.4. Comparison between PSD of LSK for NRZ and RC of duration $T$ and RC of duration 2 $T$ (M. C. Austin and M. V. Chang, "Quadrature Overlapped Raised Cosine Modulation," *IEEE Tr. Comm.*, Vol. COM-29, March 1981, pp. 237–249. Copyright © 1981 IEEE).

## 3.6 OPTIMIZATION OF SHAPING FUNCTION[3.1–3.5]

In relation to the PSD of baseband and LSK with a common shaping function, the following optimization problem can be formulated. Find the shaping function of duration $T$ so that the out-of-band power $P_{OB}(B)$ is minimized for each $B$, i.e.

$$P_{OB}(B) = \int_{B/2}^{\infty} |H(f)|^2 \, df, \; P_{OB}(0) = 1 \tag{3.6.1}$$

The solution to this problem is presented in Ref. 3.1. The optimal shaping function is the prolate spheroidal wave functions.[3.2, 3.3]

$$h_{op}(t) = C\psi_0(t - 0.5\, T, d)u_T(t), \; d = 0.5\, \pi TB \tag{3.6.2}$$

where $C$ is a normalization constant. The optimal shaping function is shown in Fig. 3.5 for several values of $d$. We conclude that for each value of $B$ we have a different optimal function. In Fig. 3.3 we have also shown the out-of-

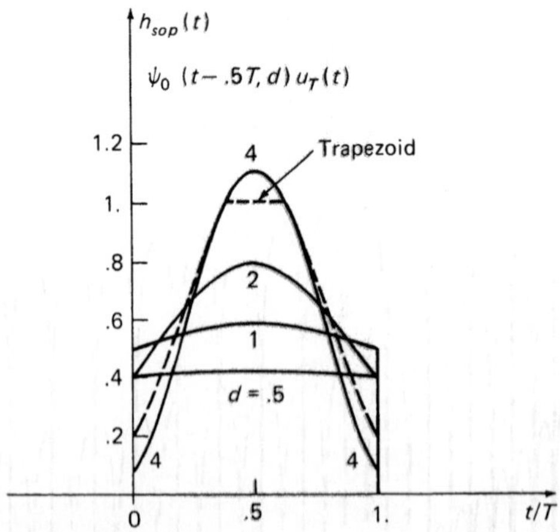


Fig. 3.5. Optimal shaping function.

band power for the optimal shaping function. The value of $B_{99}$ is for the optimal shaping function 2.234 $R$, and this should be compared with the entries in the last column of Table 3.1.

A simple function, a trapezoid described by

$$h(t + 0.5\,T) = \begin{cases} 1 & 0 \leq |t| \leq 0.5\,T\rho \\ \varepsilon + (1 - \varepsilon)\{1 - 2|t|/T\}/(1 - \rho) & 0.5\,T\rho \leq |t| \leq 0.5\,T \\ 0 & 0.5\,T \leq |t| \end{cases} \tag{3.6.3}$$

resembles the function $\psi_0(t, d)$ and in fact for $\varepsilon = \rho = 0.2$ has a 99% bandwidth of 2.24 $R$, which is very close to the optimal. A trapezoid is shown by the dashed line in Fig. 3.5.

It is interesting that if we pose a slightly different optimization problem, namely, find $h_s(t)$ of duration $T$ that minimizes the effective bandwidth

$$f_{cf}^2 = \int_0^\infty f^2 |H(f)|^2\, df \Bigg/ \int_0^\infty |H(f)|^2\, df \tag{3.6.4}$$

the resulting optimal shaping function is[3,4]

$$h_{op}(t) = \sin\,(\pi t/T) u_T(t) \tag{3.6.5}$$

i.e., the half-sinusoidal function.

In many papers it is claimed that shaping functions that are continuous (including the end points $t = 0$ and $t = T$) and have continuous derivatives are preferable from the point of view of bandwidth efficiency. Clearly, this statement is refuted by the optimal shaping functions in (3.6.2), which are discontinuous at the end points. It is true that a function with up to $N$ continuous derivatives has a FT whose asymptotic behavior for large $f$ is[3.5]

$$|H(f)|^2 \propto Cf^{-2(N+2)} \tag{3.6.6}$$

where $C$ is a constant. However, a good asymptotic behavior is not a guarantee that most of the power is concentrated around the origin ($|f| < 1/T$) where the bandwidth is mainly determined.

## 3.7 PSD OF PSK

### 3.7.1 Shaping function of duration $T$

If the shaping function has duration $T$, then from (2.3.9)

$$b(t, a_i) = \exp\{jK_p h(t, a_i)\}u_T(t) \tag{3.7.1}$$

where we have dropped the subscript $s$ from $h_s(t, a_i)$ for notational convenience. Therefore, the PSD is given by (3.3.15) with

$$S_{b,i}(f) = \overline{B(f, a_i)B^*(f, a_0)} \tag{3.7.2}$$

If the symbols are independent, all equations of section (3.3.1) are valid. $S_{b,0}(f)$ can also be computed by taking the SFT of $R_{b,0}(t, t')$ and $S_{b,i}(f)$ by taking the square of the absolute value of the FT of $m_b(t)$ where

$$m_b(t) = \overline{\exp(jK_p h(t, a_0))}u_T(t) \tag{3.7.3}$$

$$R_{b,0}(t, t') = \overline{\exp\{jK_p(h(t, a_0) - h(t', a_0))\}} \tag{3.7.4}$$

### 3.7.2 Common shaping function of duration $T$

Here we assume that

$$h(t, a_i) = a_i h(t) \tag{3.7.5}$$

and the symbols are independent and equiprobable from the set $\mathring{A}_{\pm}$. If we also assume that max $h(t) = 1$ (and this can be assumed without any loss in generality), then $K_p = \pi/M$. Therefore

$$b(t, a_i) = \exp(ja_i K_p h(t)\}u_T(t) \tag{3.7.6}$$

In this case it is easy to show (see Problem 3.7.1) that

$$m_b(t) = M^{-1} \sum_{i=1}^{M} \exp\{j(2\,i - M - 1)K_p h(t)\}$$
$$= \hat{\sin}\{K_p h(t)\} \tag{3.7.7}$$

$$R_{b,0}(t, t') = \hat{\sin}\{K_p(h(t) - h(t'))\} \tag{3.7.8}$$

where we have defined the function

$$\hat{\sin}\, x = \sin(xM)/(M \sin x) = \sum_{i=1}^{M} \exp\{j(2\,i - M - 1)x\}/M \tag{3.7.9}$$

Because $R_{b,0}(t, t')$ satisfies condition (3.3.37) and is real, we can use (3.3.39) to compute $S_{b,0}(f)$ with $T' = T$. $S_{b,1}(f)$ can be computed using (3.3.30), i.e.

$$S_{b,1}(f) = |M_b(f)|^2 \tag{3.7.10}$$

The PSD is computed using eq. (3.3.47) and (3.3.48)

*Example* 3.7.1 PSD of PSK with NRZ shaping function
We assume an NRZ shaping function, $h(t) = u_T(t)$. Thus

$$m_b(t) = \hat{\sin}\{K_p\} = \hat{\sin}\{\pi/M\} = \sin \pi/(M \sin(\pi/M)) = 0$$

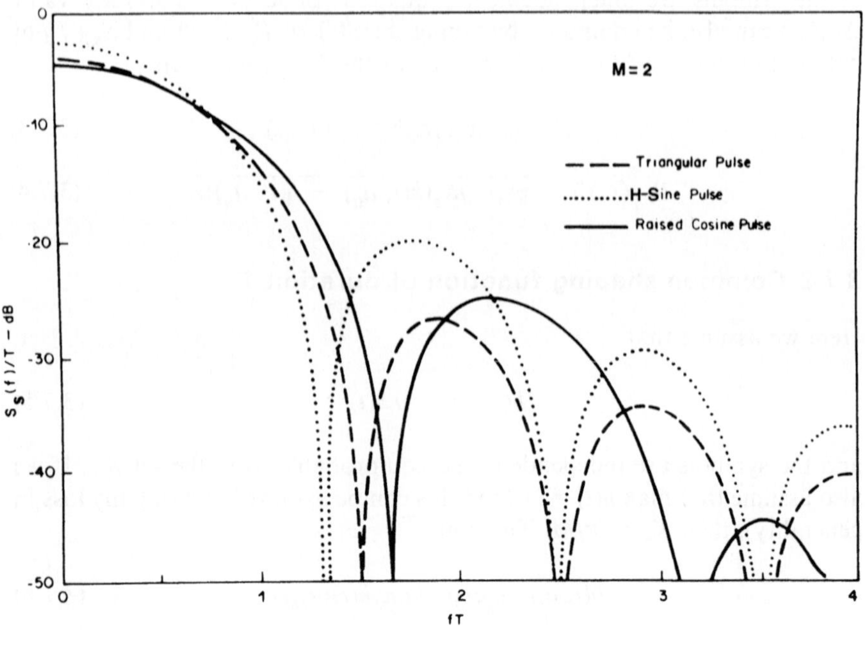

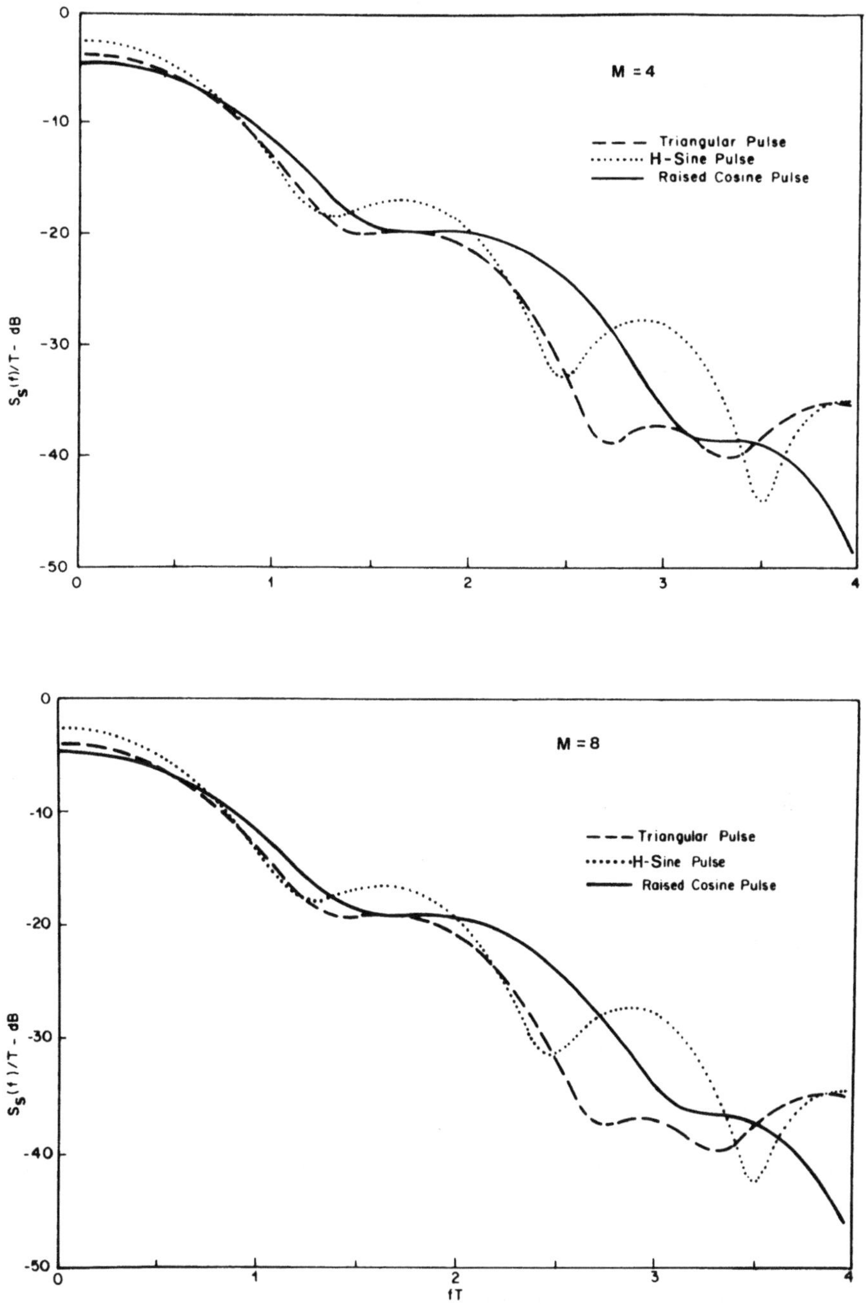


Fig. 3.6. Continuous part of PSD of $M$-ary PSK with HS, RC, and TR shaping functions of duration $T$. (L. J. Greenstein, "Spectra of PSK with Overlapping Baseband Pulses," *IEEE Tr. Comm.*, Vol. COM-25, May 1977, pp. 523–530. Copyright © 1977 IEEE).

Using L'Hopital's rule in (3.7.8), we have

$$R_{b,0}(t, t') = 1$$

and from (3.3.39)

$$S_{b,i}(f) = 2\int_0^T (T - z)\cos(2\pi f z)\,dz = \{T\,\mathrm{sinc}\,(fT)\}^2$$

This is the same as the PSD for LSK with the NRZ shaping function in Table 3.1 as it should be.

The PSD of $M$-ary PSK with HS, RC, and TR shaping functions are presented in Fig. 3.6[3.7] and Fig. 3.7.[3.6] The out-of-band power is presented in Fig. 3.8.[3.1] The trapezoidal shaping function, whose PSD is also shown in Fig. 3.8, is defined in (3.6.3) with $\varepsilon = 0$, $\rho = 0.5$. Table 3.2 presents the bandwidth in which 10, 99, and 99.9% of the power is contained for PSK with various shaping functions and $M = 2, 4$ symbols.[3.1] The fraction of power in the continuous part of the PSD is also included in the table.

**Table 3.2 Bandwidth of PSK with shaping function of duration $T$**

| SHAPING FUNCTION | $M$ | POWER IN $S_{sc}(f)$ | $B_{10}T$ | $B_{99}T$ | $B_{99.9}T$ |
|---|---|---|---|---|---|
| Rectangle | 2 | 1.000 | 1.807 | 19.295 | |
| Rectangle | 4 | 1.000 | 1.807 | 19.295 | |
| Trapezoid | 2 | 0.750 | 2.000 | 4.000 | 8.000 |
| Trapezoid | 4 | 0.769 | 2.000 | 5.389 | 8.672 |
| Triangle | 2 | 0.500 | 2.000 | 3.283 | 6.000 |
| Triangle | 4 | 0.538 | 2.000 | 3.651 | 6.274 |
| Sine | 2 | 0.652 | 2.000 | 3.744 | 6.246 |
| Sine | 4 | 0.682 | 2.000 | 3.839 | 6.270 |
| Raised cosine | 2 | 0.500 | 2.000 | 2.958 | 4.904 |
| Raised cosine | 4 | 0.526 | 2.000 | 4.000 | 5.491 |

It is important to remember that normally for PSK there are no closed form formulas for $M_b(f)$ and $S_{b,0}(f)$, and these are computed using numerical integration.

*Binary optimization problem* In the binary case we have from (3.3.48), (3.3.47), (3.3.49), and (3.7.1)

$$S_{sd}(f) = 0.5\,(A/T)^2|M_b(f)|^2 \sum_k \delta(f - kR) \tag{3.7.11}$$

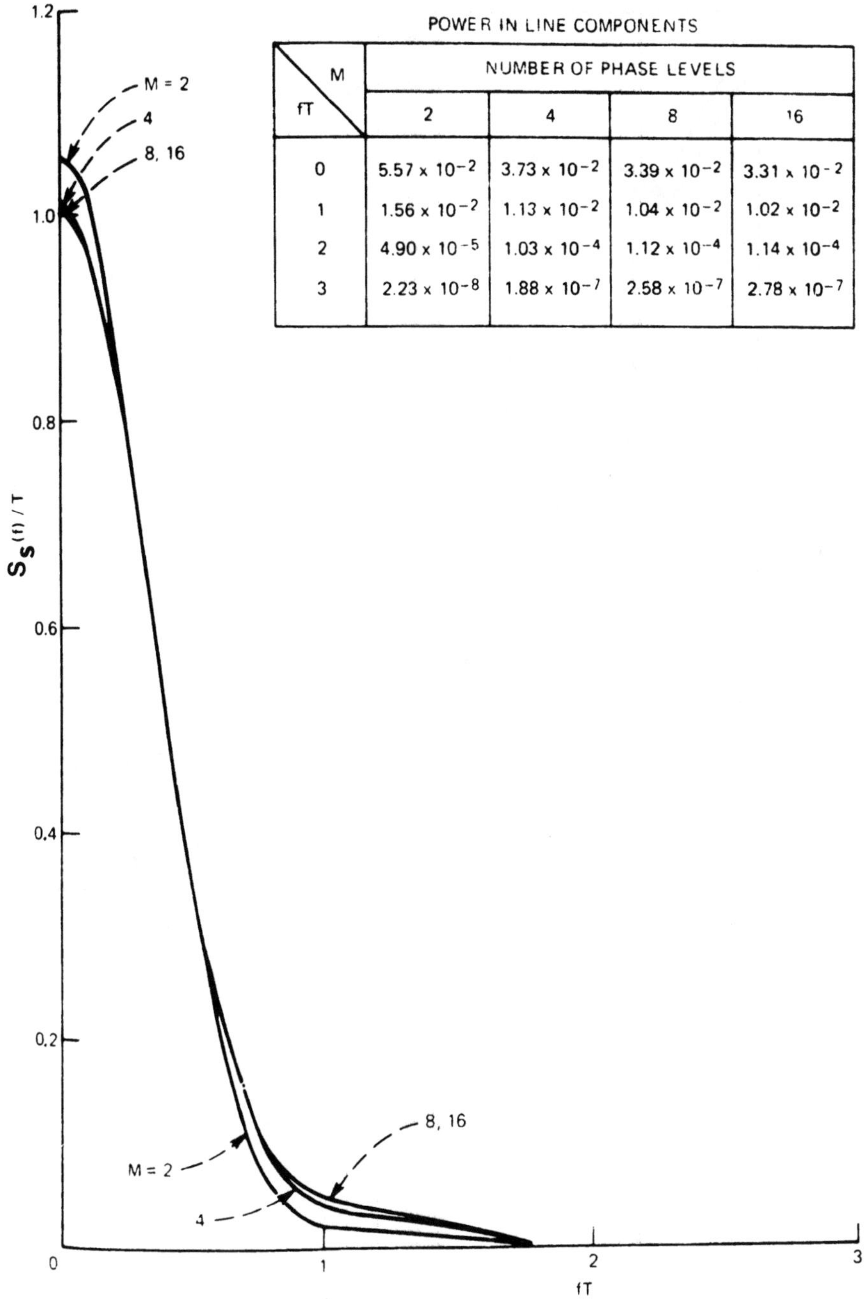


POWER IN LINE COMPONENTS

| fT \ M | NUMBER OF PHASE LEVELS | | | |
|---|---|---|---|---|
| | 2 | 4 | 8 | 16 |
| 0 | $5.57 \times 10^{-2}$ | $3.73 \times 10^{-2}$ | $3.39 \times 10^{-2}$ | $3.31 \times 10^{-2}$ |
| 1 | $1.56 \times 10^{-2}$ | $1.13 \times 10^{-2}$ | $1.04 \times 10^{-2}$ | $1.02 \times 10^{-2}$ |
| 2 | $4.90 \times 10^{-5}$ | $1.03 \times 10^{-4}$ | $1.12 \times 10^{-4}$ | $1.14 \times 10^{-4}$ |
| 3 | $2.23 \times 10^{-8}$ | $1.88 \times 10^{-7}$ | $2.58 \times 10^{-7}$ | $2.78 \times 10^{-7}$ |

Fig. 3.7. The PSD of $M$-ary PSK with RC shaping function of duration $T$, (reprinted with permission from *The Bell System Technical Journal*. Copyright © 1974, AT&T).

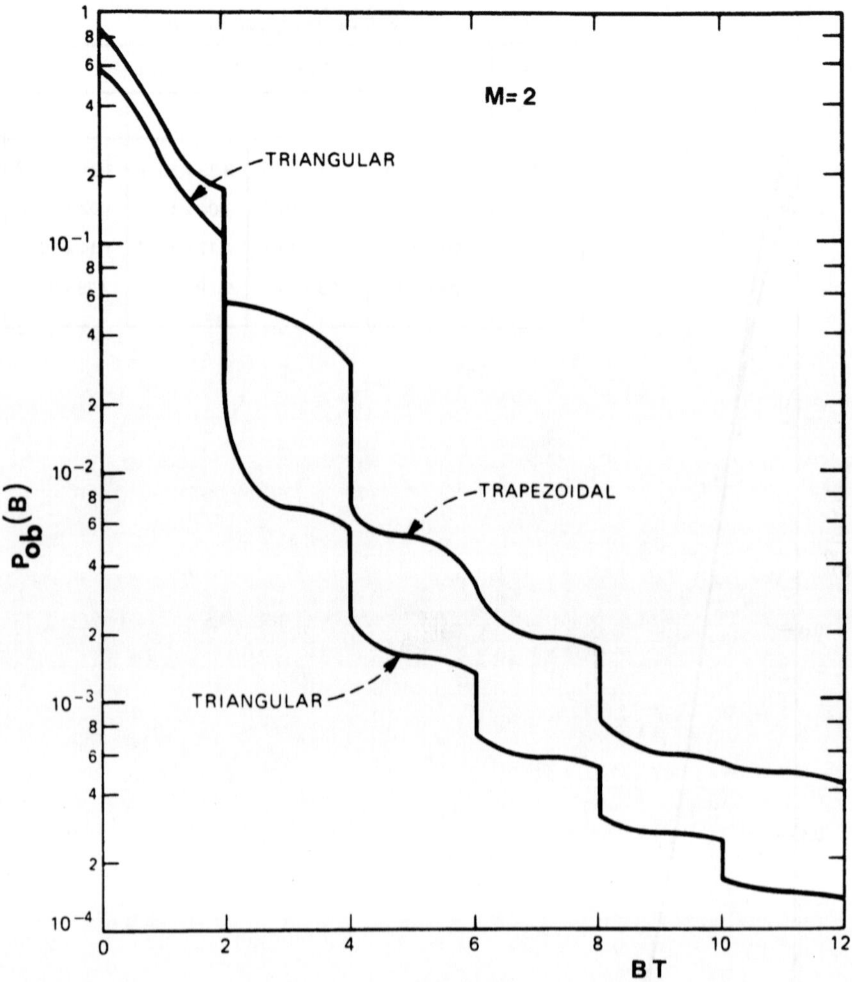
M= 2
TRIANGULAR
TRAPEZOIDAL
TRIANGULAR
$P_{ob}(B)$
1
8
6
4
2
$10^{-1}$
8
6
4
2
$10^{-2}$
8
6
4
2
$10^{-3}$
8
6
4
2
$10^{-4}$
0
2
4
6
8
10
12
BT

Fig. 3.7. (*con't.*)

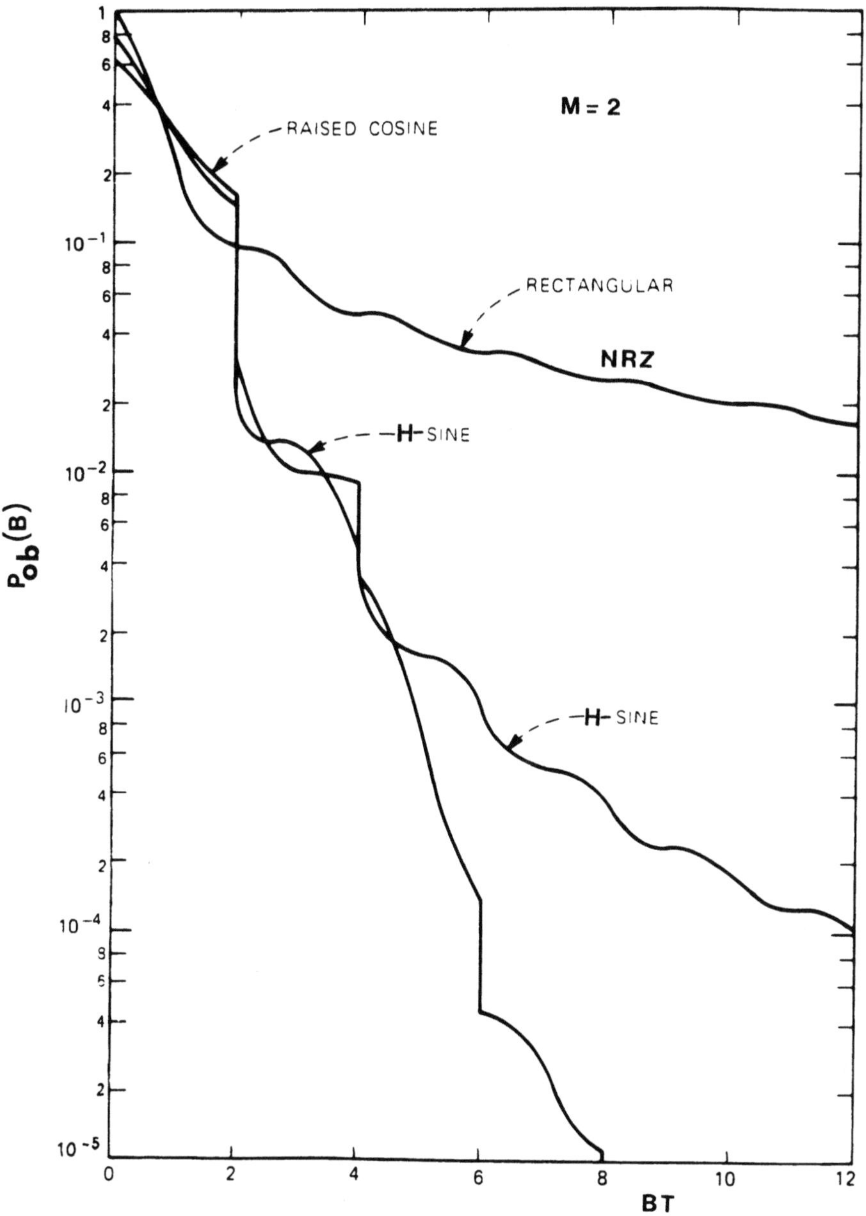
M = 2
RAISED COSINE
RECTANGULAR
NRZ
H-SINE
H-SINE
$P_{ob}(B)$
BT
1
8
6
4
2
$10^{-1}$
$10^{-2}$
$10^{-3}$
$10^{-4}$
$10^{-5}$
0
2
4
6
8
10
12

Fig. 3.7. (*con't.*)

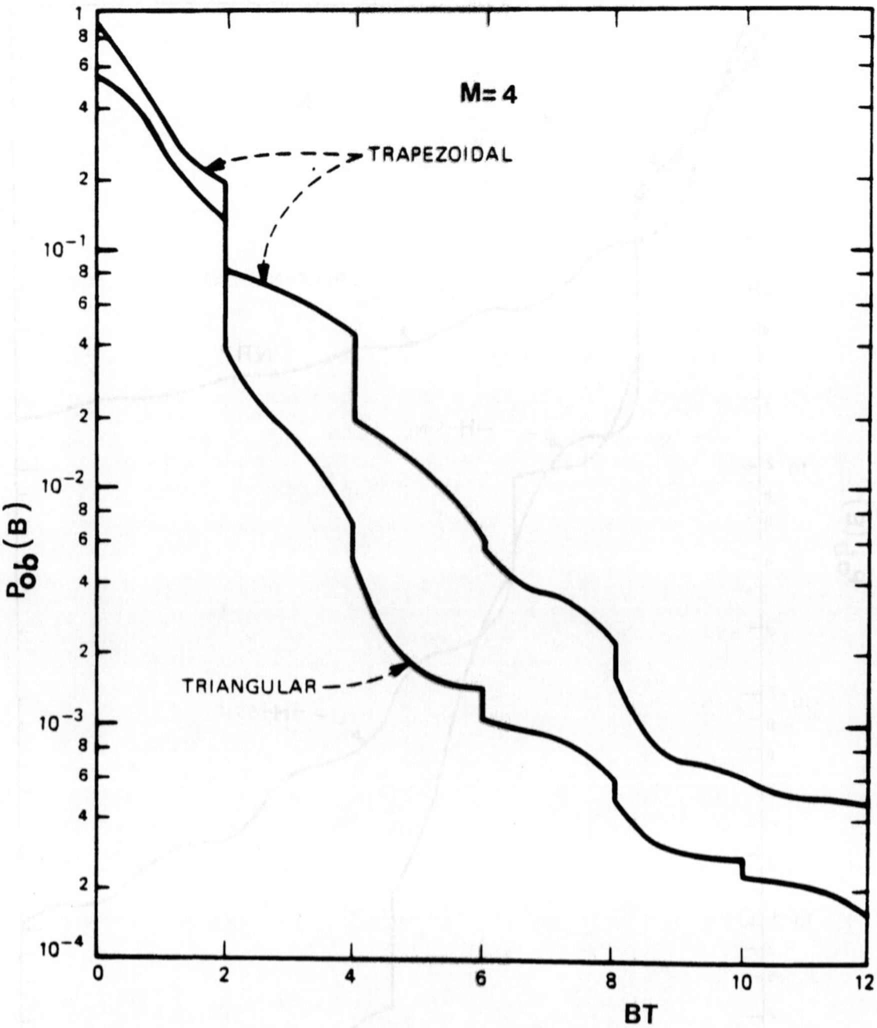
M= 4
TRAPEZOIDAL
TRIANGULAR
$P_{ob}(B)$
BT
1
8
6
4
2
$10^{-1}$
$10^{-2}$
$10^{-3}$
$10^{-4}$
0
2
4
6
8
10
12

Fig. 3.7. (*con't.*)

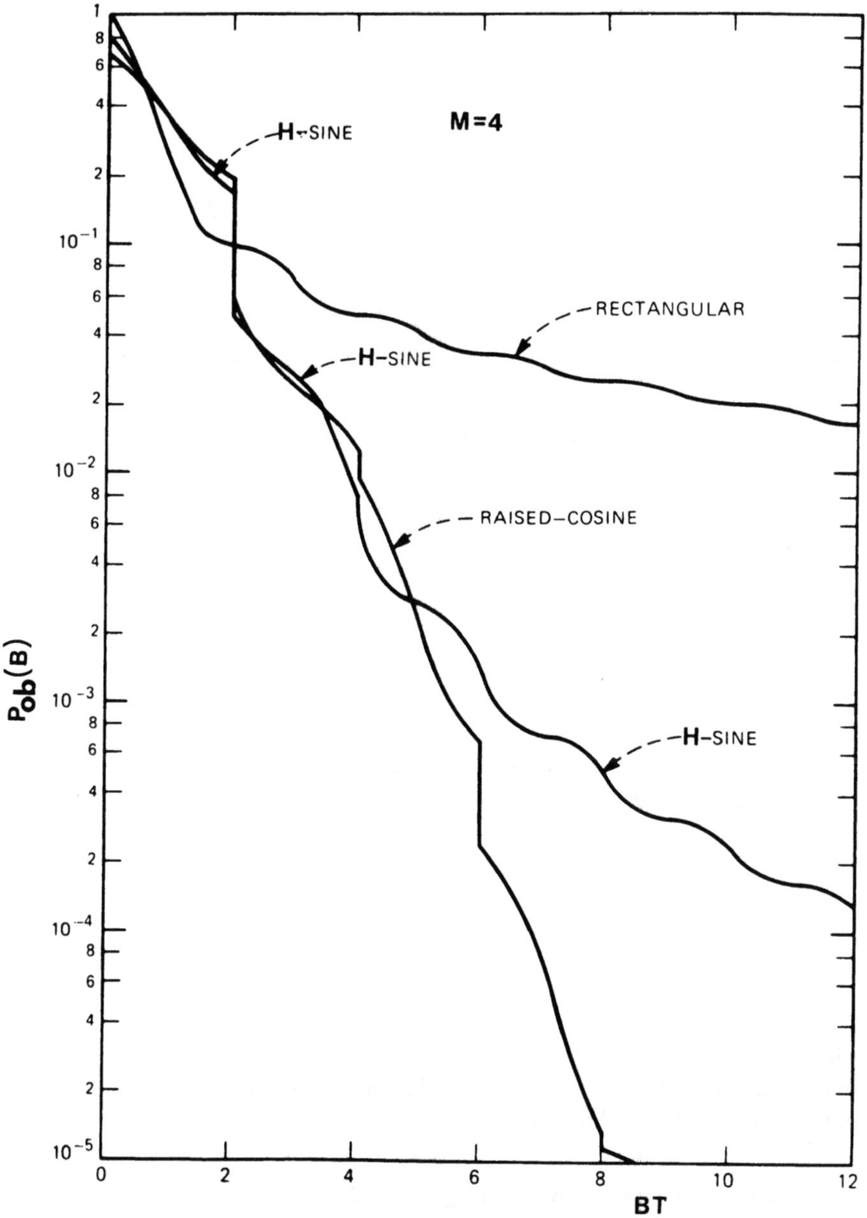


Fig. 3.8. The out-of-band power of PSK ($M$ = 2,4) with NRZ, HS, RC, TR, and trapezoidal shaping functions of duration $T$ (reprinted with permission from *The Bell System Technical Journal.* Copyright © 1976, AT&T).

where $M_b(f)$ is the FT of

$$m_b(t) = \cos(0.5\,\pi h(t)) \tag{3.7.12}$$

and

$$S_{sc}(f) = 0.5\,(A^2/T)|B(f, 1) - B(f, -1)|^2 \tag{3.7.13}$$

Now

$$B(f, 1) - B(f, -1) = \int_0^T \{\exp(j\,0.5\,\pi h(t)) - \exp(-j\,0.5\,\pi h(t)\} \exp(-j\,2\,\pi f t)\,dt \tag{3.7.14}$$

which is the FT of $2\,j\sin(0.5\,\pi h(t))u_T(t)$. Denoting

$$d(t) = \sin(0.5\,\pi h(t))u_T(t) \tag{3.7.15}$$

we obtain

$$S_{sc}(f) = 2\,(A^2/T)|D(f)|^2 \tag{3.7.16}$$

Here we can again pose the optimization problem of Section 3.6. The optimal shaping function is

$$d_{op}(t) = C\psi_0(t - 0.5\,T, d),\ d = 0.5\,\pi TB \tag{3.7.17}$$

i.e.

$$h_{op}(t) = (2/\pi)\sin^{-1}(d_{op}(t)) \tag{3.7.18}$$

This optimal shaping function minimizes the out-of-band power of $S_{sc}(f)$ only. The optimal shaping function that minimizes the total out-of-band power for PSK is not known yet.[3.1]

### 3.7.3 Shaping function of duration 2*T*[3.6, 3.7]

In this section we assume that

$$h(t, a_i) = h_0(t, a_i)u_T(t) + h_1(t - T, a_i)u_T(t - T) \tag{3.7.19}$$

$$h_k(t, a_i) = h(t + kT, a_i)u_T(t) \tag{3.7.20}$$

Hence

$$b(t, \mathbf{a}_i) = b(t, a_i, a_{i-1}) = b_0(t, a_i)b_i(t, a_{i-1}) \tag{3.7.21}$$

where we denoted

$$b_k(t, a_i) = \exp\{jK_p h_k(t, a_i)\}u_T(t) \tag{3.7.22}$$

Note that although the duration of $h(t, a_i)$ is $2T$, the duration of $b(t, \mathbf{a}_i)$ is only $T$. We shall assume from now on that the symbols are independent. In the computation of $S_{b,i}(f)$ we shall need the following notation

$$m_{bk}(t) = \overline{b_k(t, a_0)} \tag{3.7.23}$$

$$\phi_{k,n}(t, t') = \overline{b_k(t, a_0)b_n^*(t', a_0)} \tag{3.7.24}$$

Thus

$$R_{b,i}(t, t') = \overline{b_0(t, a_i)b_1(t, a_{i-1})b_0^*(t', a_0)b_1^*(t', a_{-1})} \tag{3.7.25}$$

We shall compute separately the term $S_{b,0}(f)$, $S_{b,1}(f)$, and $S_{b,i}(f)$ $i > 1$. In each case $S_{b,i}(f)$ is the SFT of $R_{b,i}(t, t')$.

*$i = 0$* From (3.7.25) and independence of symbols

$$R_{b,0}(t, t') = \phi_{0,0}(t, t')\phi_{1,1}(t, t') \tag{3.7.26}$$

*$i = 1$*

$$R_{b,1}(t, t') = m_{b0}(t)\phi_{1,0}(t, t')m_{b1}^*(t) \tag{3.7.27}$$

*$i \geqq 2$*

$$R_{b,i}(t, t') = R_{b,2}(t, t') = m_b(t)m_b^*(t') \tag{3.7.28}$$

where

$$m_b(t) = \overline{b(t, \mathbf{a}_i)} = m_{b0}(t)m_{b1}(t) \tag{3.7.29}$$

In the derivation of the PSD we can use eq. (3.3.28) with $K = 2$ and eq. (3.3.25). In computing the SFT the time limit is $T$ instead of $T'$.

*Common shaping function* Here we assume that

$$h(t, a_i) = a_i h(t)u_{2T}(t) \tag{3.7.30}$$

and the symbols are equiprobable from the set $\mathring{A}_{\pm}$. Assuming also that max $h(t) = 1$ (this is no restriction) we have $K_p = 0.5\ \pi/M$. With these assumptions we obtain from (3.7.23) and (3.7.24)

$$m_{bk}(t) = \hat{\sin}\ \{K_p h_k(t)\} \tag{3.7.31}$$

$$\phi_{k,n}(t, t') = \hat{\sin}\ \{K_p(h_k(t) - h_n(t'))\} \tag{3.7.32}$$

where

$$h_k(t) = h(t + kT)u_T(t) \tag{3.7.33}$$

Since

$$\phi_{k,k}(t, t') = \phi_{k,k}(t', t) \tag{3.7.34}$$

also

$$R_{b,0}(t, t') = R_{b,0}(t', t) \tag{3.7.35}$$

and we can use eq. (3.3.39) with $T = T'$ to obtain $S_{b,0}(f)$. To compute $S_{b,1}(f)$ we still have to use eq. (3.3.36) with $T' = T$.

*Example* 3.72 PSD of PSK with duobinary shaping function
We compute the PSD of $M$-ary PSK with the duobinary shaping function, $h(t) = u_{2T}(t)$. Thus

$$h_0(t) = h_1(t) = u_T(t) \tag{3.7.36}$$

Here we obtain from (3.7.31) and using L'Hopital's rule from (3.7.32)

$$m_{bk}(t) = \{M \sin\ (0.5\ \pi/M)\}^{-1} \tag{3.7.37}$$

$$\phi_{k,n}(t, t') = 1 \tag{3.7.38}$$

Thus

$$S_{b,0}(f) = 2\int_0^T (T - z)\cos\ (2\ \pi f z)\ dz = \{T \operatorname{sinc}\ (fT)\}^2 \tag{3.7.39}$$

$$S_{b,1}(f) = \{M \sin\ (0.5\ \pi/M)\}^{-2} S_{b,0}(f) \tag{3.7.40}$$

$$S_{b,2}(f) = \{M \sin\ (0.5\ \pi/M)\}^{-4} S_{b,0}(f) \tag{3.7.41}$$

Substitution into eq. (3.3.28) and (3.3.25) gives

$$S_s(f) = T\{A \text{ sinc } (fT)\}^2\{1 + 2\, V^2(M) \cos (2\, \pi f T) - V^4(M)(1 + 2 \cos (2\, \pi f T)) + RV^4(M) \sum_k \delta(f - kR)\} \quad (3.7.42)$$

where

$$V(M) = \{M \sin (0.5\, \pi/M)\}^{-1} \quad (3.7.43)$$

In the binary case this is simplified to

$$S_s(f) = 0.5\, T\,\{A \text{ sinc } (fT)\}^2\{1.5 + \cos (2\pi f T) + R \sum_k \delta(f - kR)\} \quad (3.7.44)$$

The continuous part of the PSD for several shaping functions of duration 2 $T$ and various $M$ is given in Fig. 3.9.[3.6] The PSD of PSK with the 2-RC shaping function and $M$ = 2, 4, 6, and 8 is shown in Fig. 3.10.[3.7] The PSD of quaternary PSK with the RC shaping function of duration 2 $\beta T$, $0.5 \leqq \beta \leqq 1$ is shown in Fig. 3.11.[3.7] The methods for the computation of the PSD in Refs. 3.1, 3.6, and 3.7 are different from the method presented here. Refs. 3.1 and

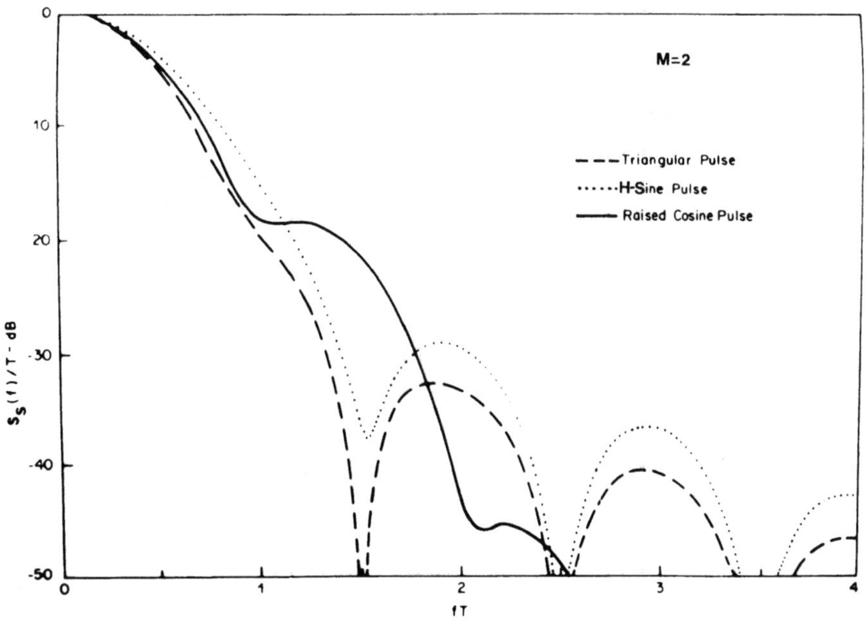


Fig. 3.9. Continuous part of PSD of $M$-ary PSK with TR, HS, and RC shaping functions of duration 2 $T$ (L. J. Greenstein, "Spectra of PSK with Overlapping Baseband Pulses," *IEEE Tr. Comm.*, Vol. COM-25, May 1977, pp. 523–530. Copyright © 1977 IEEE).

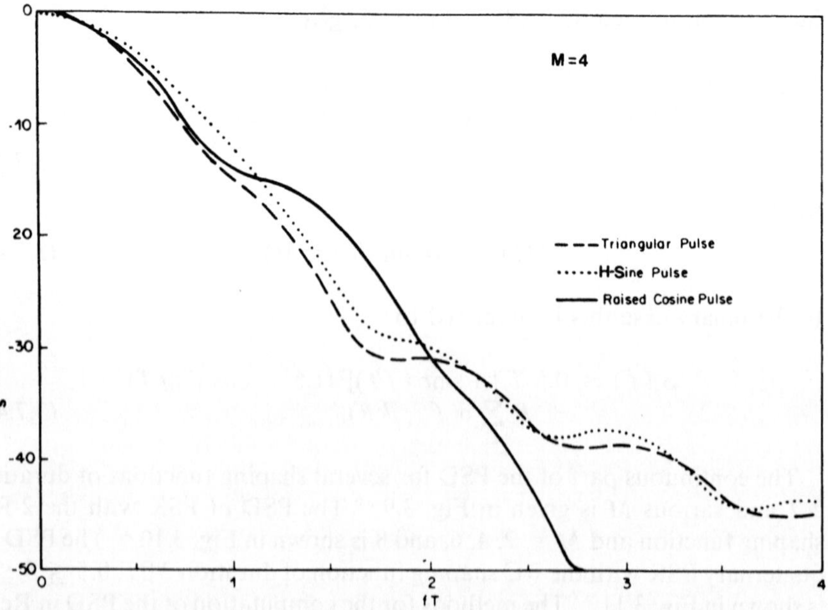

M=4
Triangular Pulse
H-Sine Pulse
Raised Cosine Pulse
$S_s(f)/T$ - dB
fT


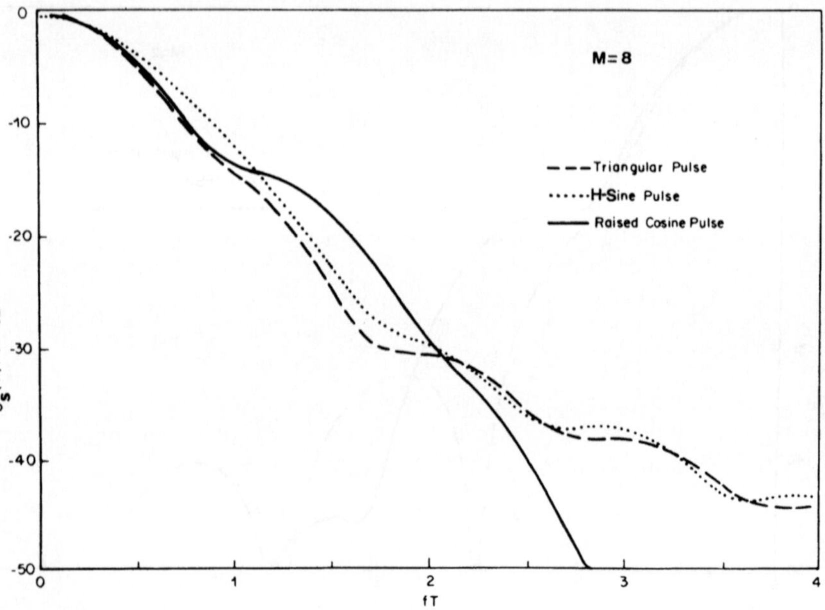

M=8
Triangular Pulse
H-Sine Pulse
Raised Cosine Pulse
$S_s(f)/T$ - dB
fT


Fig. 3.9. (*con't.*)

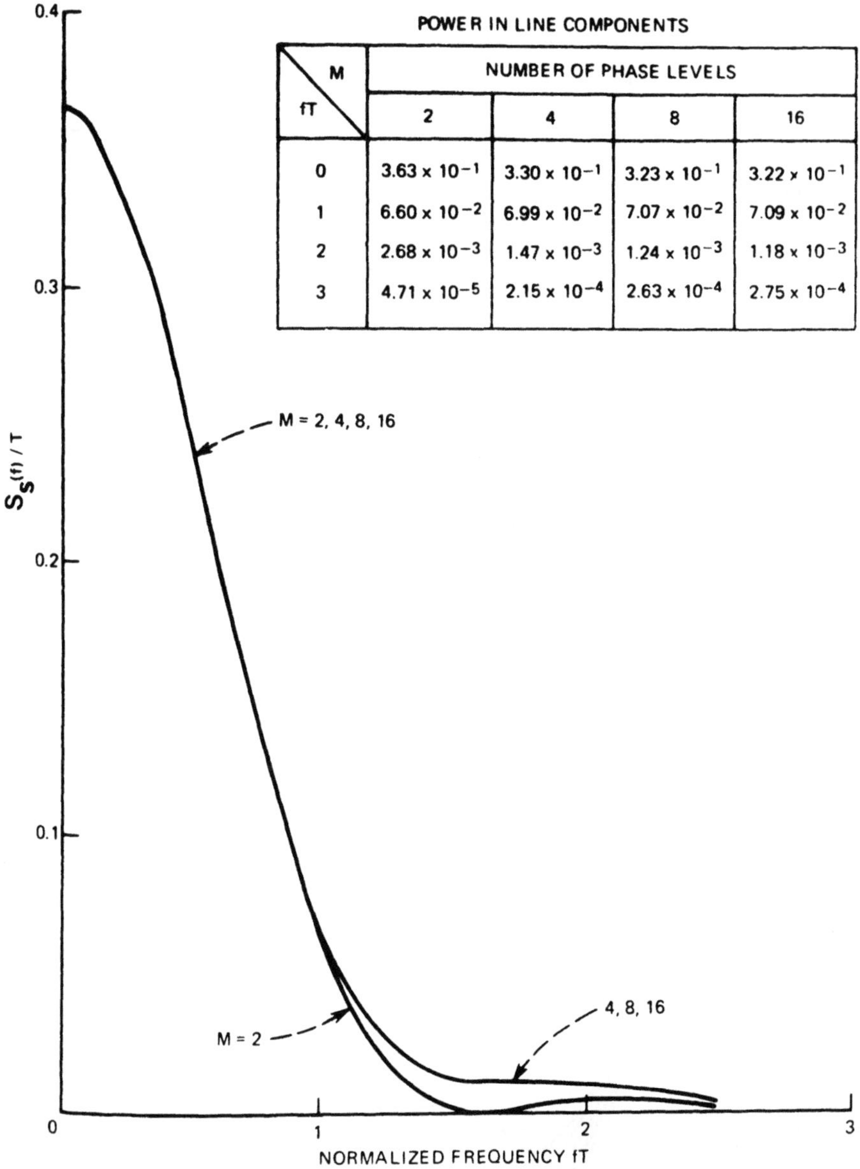


POWER IN LINE COMPONENTS

| fT \ M | NUMBER OF PHASE LEVELS 2 | 4 | 8 | 16 |
|---|---|---|---|---|
| 0 | $3.63 \times 10^{-1}$ | $3.30 \times 10^{-1}$ | $3.23 \times 10^{-1}$ | $3.22 \times 10^{-1}$ |
| 1 | $6.60 \times 10^{-2}$ | $6.99 \times 10^{-2}$ | $7.07 \times 10^{-2}$ | $7.09 \times 10^{-2}$ |
| 2 | $2.68 \times 10^{-3}$ | $1.47 \times 10^{-3}$ | $1.24 \times 10^{-3}$ | $1.18 \times 10^{-3}$ |
| 3 | $4.71 \times 10^{-5}$ | $2.15 \times 10^{-4}$ | $2.63 \times 10^{-4}$ | $2.75 \times 10^{-4}$ |

Fig. 3.10. The PSD of *M*-ary PSK with RC shaping function of duration $2T$ (reprinted with permission from *The Bell System Technical Journal*. Copyright © 1974, AT&T).

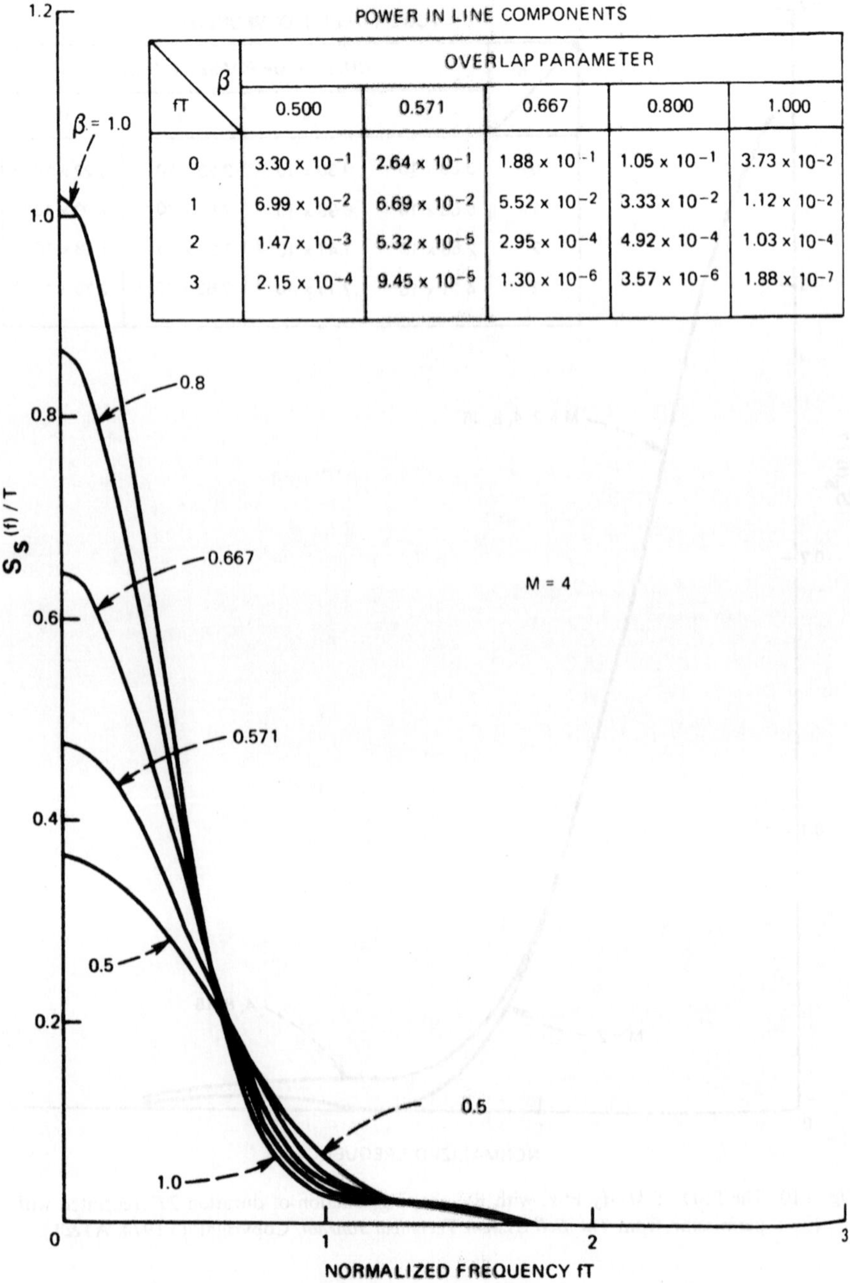


POWER IN LINE COMPONENTS

| fT \ β | OVERLAP PARAMETER 0.500 | 0.571 | 0.667 | 0.800 | 1.000 |
|---|---|---|---|---|---|
| 0 | $3.30 \times 10^{-1}$ | $2.64 \times 10^{-1}$ | $1.88 \times 10^{-1}$ | $1.05 \times 10^{-1}$ | $3.73 \times 10^{-2}$ |
| 1 | $6.99 \times 10^{-2}$ | $6.69 \times 10^{-2}$ | $5.52 \times 10^{-2}$ | $3.33 \times 10^{-2}$ | $1.12 \times 10^{-2}$ |
| 2 | $1.47 \times 10^{-3}$ | $5.32 \times 10^{-5}$ | $2.95 \times 10^{-4}$ | $4.92 \times 10^{-4}$ | $1.03 \times 10^{-4}$ |
| 3 | $2.15 \times 10^{-4}$ | $9.45 \times 10^{-5}$ | $1.30 \times 10^{-6}$ | $3.57 \times 10^{-6}$ | $1.88 \times 10^{-7}$ |

Fig. 3.11. The PSD of quaternary PSK with RC shaping function of duration $2\beta T$, $0.5 \leqq \beta \leqq 1.0$ (reprinted with permission from *The Bell System Technical Journal*. Copyright © 1974, AT&T).

3.6 describe a matrix method, and in Ref. 3.7 the function $b(t, \mathbf{a}_i)$ is not restricted to a $T$ interval.

### 3.7.4 Shaping function of duration *KT*

Here we assume

$$h(t, a_i) = \sum_{k=0}^{K-1} h_k(t - kT, a_i)u_T(t - kT) \tag{3.7.45}$$

Hence

$$h(t, \mathbf{a}_i) = h(t, a_i, a_{i-1} \ldots a_{i-k}) = \sum_{k=0}^{K-1} h_k(t, a_{i-k})u_T(t) \tag{3.7.46}$$

Thus the difference is

$$\begin{aligned} h(t, \mathbf{a}_i) - h(t', \mathbf{a}_0) = \Bigg\{ &\sum_{k=0}^{i-1} h_k(t, a_{i-k}) + \sum_{k=i}^{K-1} \{h_k(t, a_{i-k}) \\ &- h_{k-i}(t', a_{i-k})\} - \sum_{k=K-i}^{K-1} h_k(t', a_{-k}) \Bigg\} u_T(t) \end{aligned} \tag{3.7.47}$$

The second term is nonzero only if $K > i$. Thus for $i \geqq K$, $h(t, \mathbf{a}_i)$ and $h(t', \mathbf{a}_0)$ are independent if the symbols are independent. This implies that

$$b(t, \mathbf{a}_i) = \exp\{K_p h(t, \mathbf{a}_i)\} = \prod_{k=0}^{K-1} b_k(t, a_{i-k}) \tag{3.7.48}$$

is independent from $b(t', \mathbf{a}_0)$ for $i \geqq K$. We can use eqs. (3.3.24) and (3.3.25) for the computation of the PSD. Now we compute the various $S_{bi}(f)$.

<u>$S_{b,i}(f)\ 0 \leqq i \leqq K$</u>

$$\begin{aligned} R_{b,i}(t, t') &= \overline{b(t, \mathbf{a}_i)b^*(t', \mathbf{a}_0)} \\ &= \prod_{k=0}^{i-1} m_{bk}(t) \prod_{k=i}^{K-1} \phi_{k,k-i}(t, t') \prod_{k=i}^{K-1} m_{bk}{}^*(t') \end{aligned} \tag{3.7.49}$$

Generally we have to use eq. (3.3.36) with $T' = T$ to obtain the SFT; however, for $i = 0$

$$R_{b,0}(t, t') = R_{b,0}(t', t) \tag{3.7.50}$$

and eq. (3.3.39) is more convenient.

$S_{b,i}(f)\ i \geqq K$

In this case

$$R_{b,i}(t, t') = \prod_{k=0}^{K-1} m_{bk}(t)m_{bk}{}^*(t') = m_b(t)m_b{}^*(t') \tag{3.7.51}$$

where

$$m_b(t) = \overline{b(t, \mathbf{a}_0)} = \sum_{k=0}^{K-1} m_{bk}(t) \tag{3.7.52}$$

To obtain $S_{b,i}(f)$ here we can use either (3.3.30) or (3.3.38), because condition (3.3.37) is satisfied. In each case we substitute $T$ for $T'$.

*Common shaping function* If we assume that

$$h(t, a_i) = a_i h(t) u_{KT}(t) \tag{3.7.53}$$

that the symbols are equiprobable from the set $\mathring{A}_{\pm}$ and max $h(t) = 1$ (hence $K_p = \pi/(KM)$), we obtain $m_{bk}(t)$ and $\phi_{k,n}(t)$ as in (3.7.31) and (3.7.32). Because $m_{bk}(t)$ and $\phi_{k,n}(t)$ are now real, $R_{b,i}(t, t')$ is also real, and we can use (3.3.39) or (3.3.30) to compute $S_{b,i}(f)$ for $i \geqq K$.

The PSD of PSK with shaping function from the partial response family with various durations and symbol levels is presented in Ref. 3.18.

## 3.8 PSD OF FSK[3.1, 3.8, 3.9, 3.10, 3.13, 3.15, 3.19, 3.20]

### 3.8.1 Shaping function of duration T

If the shaping function has duration $T$, then from (2.3.9)

$$b(t, a_i) = \exp\{j(\phi_i + \beta(t, a_i))\}u_T(t) \tag{3.8.1}$$

where

$$\beta(t, a_i) = \begin{cases} 0 & t \leqq 0 \\ k_F \displaystyle\int_0^t h(t', a_i)\, dt' & 0 \leqq t \leqq T \\ \beta(T, a_i) & T \leqq t \end{cases} \tag{3.8.2}$$

and

$$\phi_i = \sum_{k=-\infty}^{i-1} \beta(T, a_k) \tag{3.8.3}$$

We define here

$$r(t, a_i) = \exp\{j\beta(t, a_i)\}u_T(t) \tag{3.8.4}$$

with average value

$$m_r(t) = \overline{r(t, a_0)} \tag{3.8.5}$$

and

$$R_{r,0}(t, t') = \overline{r(t, a_0)r^*(t', a_0)}$$

Hence

$$\begin{aligned} R_{b,i}(t, t') &= \overline{\exp\{j(\phi_i - \phi_0)\}r(t, a_i)r^*(t', a_0)} \\ &= \overline{\prod_{k=0}^{i-1} r(T, a_k)r(t, a_i)r^*(t', a_0)} \\ &= \overline{\prod_{k=1}^{i-1} r(T, a_k)r(t, a_i)r(T, a_0)r^*(t', a_0)} \end{aligned} \tag{3.8.6}$$

Assuming independent symbols, we obtain for $i > 0$

$$R_{b,i}(t, t') = m_r^{i-1}(T)m_r(t)R_{r,0}(T, t') \tag{3.8.7}$$

and for $i = 0$

$$R_{b,0}(t, t') = R_{r,0}(t, t') = \overline{\exp\{j(\beta(t, a_0) - \beta(t', a_0))} \tag{3.8.8}$$

Taking the SFT of (3.8.7) and (3.8.8), we obtain $S_{b,i}(f)$. We can also write

$$S_{b,i}(f) = \begin{cases} \overline{|R(f, a_0)|^2} = S_{r,0}(f) & i = 0 \\ m_r^{i-1}(T)M_r(f)\overline{r(T, a_0)R^*(f, a_0)} & i > 0 \end{cases} \tag{3.8.9}$$

Since

$$S_{b,-i}(f) = S_{b,i}^*(f) \tag{3.8.10}$$

we have from (3.3.15)

$$S_s(f)T/A^2 = S_{r,0}(f) + 2\,\mathrm{Re}\,\{M_r(f)\hat{M}_r^*(f) \sum_{n=1}^{\infty}(m_r(T)\exp(-j\,2\,\pi fT))^n \exp(-j\,2\,\pi fT)\} \quad (3.8.11)$$

where

$$\hat{M}_r^*(f) = \overline{r(T, a_0)R^*(f, a_0)} \quad (3.8.12)$$

We have from (3.8.2) that $|r(t, a_i)|$ can not exceed 1; therefore the term in the summation

$$|m_r(T)\exp(-j\,2\,\pi fT)| = |m_r(T)| \leq 1 \quad (3.8.13)$$

We shall analyze the case of inequality first.

$\underline{|m_r(T)| < 1}$

In this case the summation in (3.8.11) converges. The result is a PSD that is a continuous function of frequency only

$$S_s(f)T/A^2 = S_{r,0}(f) + 2\,\mathrm{Re}\,\{M_r(f)\hat{M}_r^*(f)/(\exp(j\,2\,\pi fT) - m_r(T))\} \quad (3.8.14)$$

$\underline{|m_r(T)| = 1}$

This is possible only if

$$|m_r(T)| = \left|\sum_{i=1}^{M}\exp(j\beta(T, a(i)))P_i\right| = 1 \quad (3.8.15)$$

where we assumed that the symbols belong to the general set $\mathring{A} = \{a(1), a(2), \ldots, a(M)\}$ and $P_i$ is the probability of the symbol $a(i)$ $i = 1, \ldots, M$. To satisfy (3.8.15), each term must be equal

$$\exp(j\beta(T, a(\mathrm{i})) = \exp(jc) \quad (3.8.16)$$

where $c$ is the same constant for all $i = 1, \ldots, M$. This is possible only if

$$\beta(T, a(i)) = c\ (\text{modulo } 2\,\pi) \quad (3.8.17)$$

Let us write the constant in a more convenient form

$$c = 2\,\pi f_d T \quad (3.8.18)$$

where $f_d$ is a constant (frequency). This means that

$$r(T, a_0) = \exp(j\, 2\, \pi f_d T) \tag{3.8.19}$$

is a constant and not a random variable. This implies, from (3.8.5) and (3.8.12)

$$m_r(T) = \exp(j\, 2\, \pi f_d T) \tag{3.8.20}$$

$$\hat{M}_r^*(f) = \exp(j\, 2\, \pi f_d T) M_r^*(f) \tag{3.8.21}$$

We substitute (3.8.20) and (3.8.21) with (3.8.11) and obtain

$$\begin{aligned} S_s(f)T/A^2 &= S_{b,0}(f) + 2\,\mathrm{Re}\,\{|M_r(f)|^2 \sum_{n=1}^{\infty} \exp(-j\, 2\, \pi(f - f_d)nT\} \\ &= S_{b,0}(f) - |M_r(f)|^2 + R|M_r(f)|^2 \sum_k \delta(f - f_d - kR) \end{aligned} \tag{3.8.22}$$

This is very similar to expression (3.4.4) for baseband and LSK, provided we replaced $h(t, a_0)$ by $r(t, a_0)$, and the discrete components are shifted in frequency by $f_d$.

*Common shaping function* Here we assume that $h(t, a_i) = a_i h(t)$; hence

$$\beta(t, a_i) = a_i \beta(t) \tag{3.8.23}$$

and

$$r(t, a_i) = \exp\{j a_i \beta(t)\} u_T(t) \tag{3.8.24}$$

Assuming equiprobable symbols from the set $\mathring{A}_{\pm}$, we obtain

$$m_r(t) = \hat{\sin}\,\beta(t) \tag{3.8.25}$$

$$R_{r,0}(t, t') = \hat{\sin}\,\{\beta(t) - \beta(t')\} \tag{3.8.26}$$

and the function $\hat{\sin}$ (.) is defined in (3.7.9). The PSD has a discrete component if for all symbols in $\mathring{A}_{\pm}$

$$a_0 \beta(T) = 2\, \pi f_d T \qquad (\text{modulo } 2\, \pi) \tag{3.8.27}$$

which means that

$$\beta(T) = 2\, \pi f_d T \tag{3.8.28}$$

must be an integer multiple of 2 π, i.e., $f_d T$ is an integer. The normalized frequency deviation (already defined in Section 2) is

$$h = \beta(T)/\pi = 2 f_d T \tag{3.8.29}$$

Thus $h$ must be an integer if the PSD contains discrete components.

*Example* 3.8.1 PSD of FSK with NRZ shaping function
We compute the PSD of FSK with the NRZ shaping function. The symbols are equiprobable from the Set $\mathring{A}_{\pm}$. Thus from (2.3.10)

$$\beta(t) = K_F t = 2 \pi f_d t \tag{3.8.30}$$

where here $f_d$ is also the frequency deviation from the carrier.

*$f_d T \neq$ integer*

*Method 1*

$$R(f, a_0) = \int_0^T \exp(j 2 \pi f_d t a_0) \exp(-j 2 \pi f t)\, dt$$

$$= T \exp(-j \pi (f - a_0 f_d) T \operatorname{sinc} \{(f - a_0 f_d) T\} \tag{3.8.31}$$

$$M_r(f) = \overline{R(f, a_0)} = M^{-1} T \sum_{i=1}^{M} \exp\{-j\pi(f - (2i - 1 - M) f_d) T\}$$
$$\operatorname{sinc}\{(f - (2i - 1 - M) f_d T\} \tag{3.8.32}$$

$$S_{r,0}(f) = \overline{|R(f, a_0)|^2} = T^2 \sum_{i=1}^{M} \operatorname{sinc}^2 \{(f - (2i - 1 - M) f_d) T\}/M \tag{3.8.33}$$

$$\hat{M}_r^*(f) = M^{-1} T \sum_{i=1}^{M} \exp\{j\pi(f + (2i - 1 - M) f_d) T\}$$
$$\operatorname{sinc}\{(f - (2i - 1 - M) f_d) T\} \tag{3.8.34}$$

$$m_r(T) = \hat{\sin}(2 \pi f_d T)$$

These equations are substituted into (3.8.14) to obtain the PSD.

*Method 2*

$$m_r(t) = \hat{\sin}(2 \pi f_d t) u_T(t) \tag{3.8.36}$$

$$R_{r,0}(t, t') = \hat{\sin}\,\{2\,\pi f_d(t - t')\}u_T(t)u_T(t') \tag{3.8.37}$$

$$S_{r,0}(f) = \int_0^T \left\{ \int_0^{T-z} \hat{\sin}\,\{2\,\pi f_d z\}\,dx \right\} \cos\,(2\,\pi f z)\,dz$$

$$= \int_0^T (T - z)\,\hat{\sin}\,(2\,\pi f_d z)\cos\,(2\,\pi f z)\,dz \tag{3.8.38}$$

We substitute (3.7.9) into (3.8.38) and obtain again eq. (3.8.33). To compute the other terms of (3.8.14), $S_{b,i}(f)$, we need also the FT of $m_r(t)$ and $R_{r,0}(T, t')$.

$f_dT$ = *integer*

We use eq. (3.8.22) with

$$M_r(f) = T\exp\,(-j\,2\,\pi f T)\sin\,(\pi f T)\sum_{i=1}^{M}\{M\pi(f - (2\,i - 1 - M)f_d)T\} \tag{3.8.39}$$

$$S_{b,0}(f) = T^2\sin^2\,(\pi f T)\sum_{i=1}^{M}\{\pi(f - (2\,i - 1 - M)f_d)T\}^{-2}/M \tag{3.8.40}$$

In Fig. 3.12 we show the PSD for $M = 2, 4, 8$ and various values of $h = 2\,f_dT$. In Fig. 3.13 is shown the PSD for the same case, but here $h = 1/M$. The inband power for the binary case, but various $h$ is shown in Fig. 3.14.

Figures 3.12 and 3.13 are reproduced from Ref. 3.8 and Fig. 3.14 from Ref. 3.9.

This seems to be the only example where it is easier to compute first the FT and then the average value, rather than the other way around. The reason for that is that here the FT has a closed form solution, and no numerical intergration is required.

In Fig. 3.15 we show the PSD of FSK with the RC shaping function of duration $T$. This figure is reproduced from Ref. 3.10.

In Table 3.3 is presented the 99% bandwidth for binary FSK with rectangular shaping function and various normalized frequency deviations.

In Table 3.4 is presented the 99% bandwidth for binary FSK and raised cosine, triangular, and half-sinusoidal shaping functions.

The PSD of multi-$h$ FSK is presented in Ref. 3.19. In this reference the PSD was obtained by simulation.

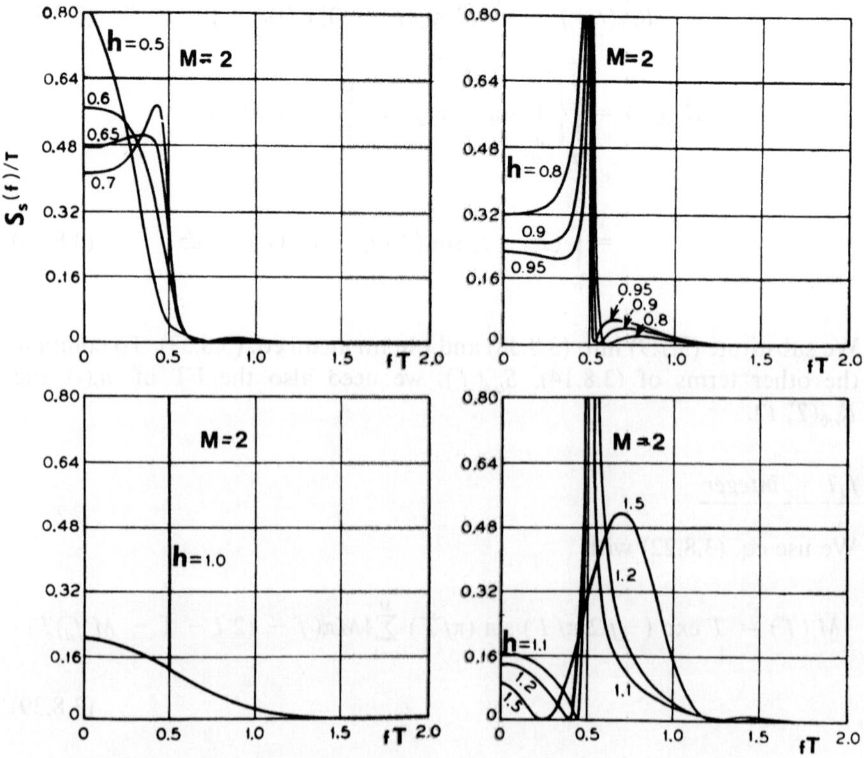


Fig. 3.12. The PSD of $M$-ary FSK with NRZ shaping function of duration $T$ and various values of normalized frequency deviation, $h = 2f_dT$ (reprinted with permission from *The Bell System Technical Journal*. Copyright 1965, AT&T).

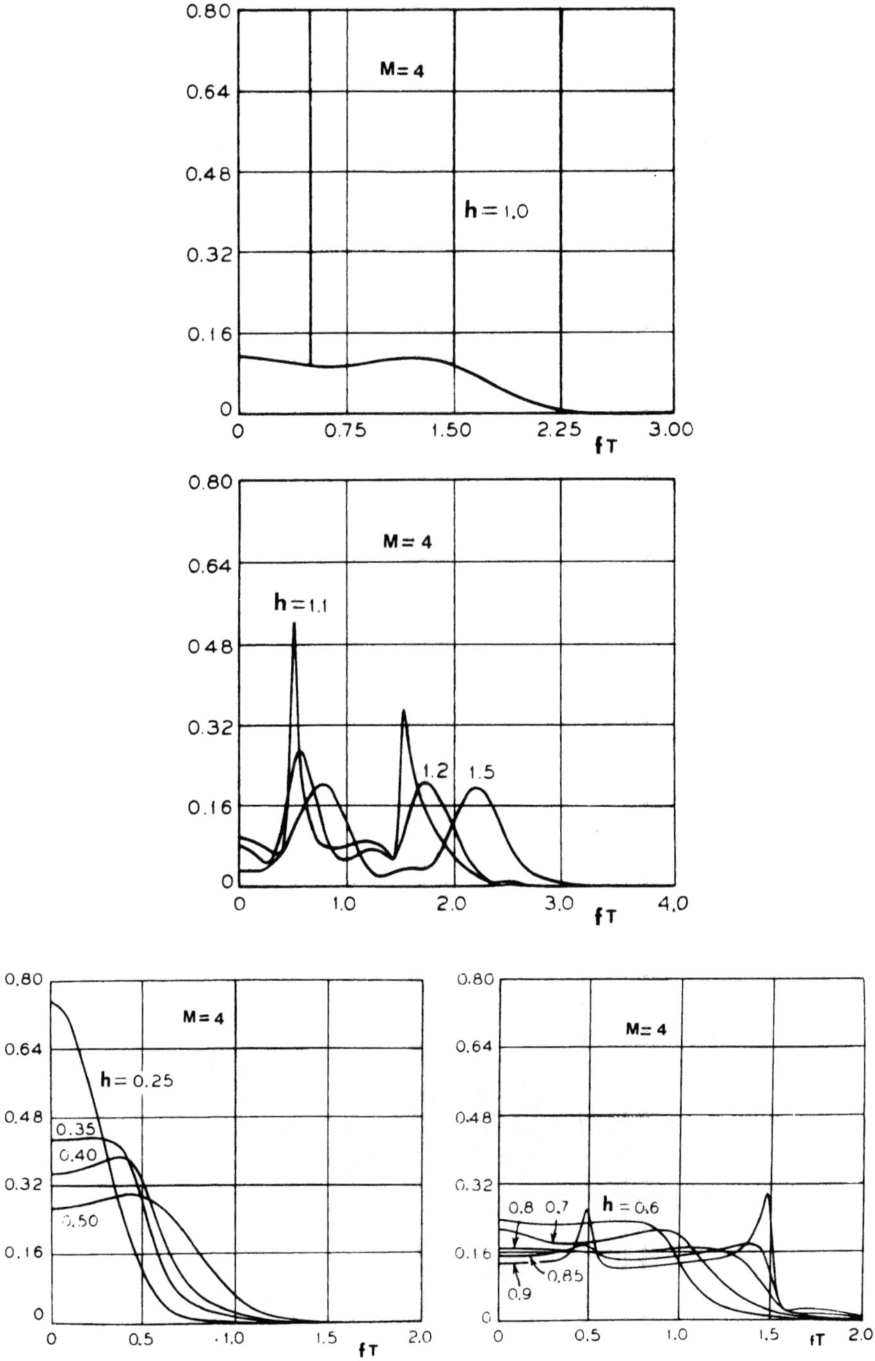
0.80
0.64
0.48
0.32
0.16
0
M= 4
h = 1.0
0
0.75
1.50
2.25
3.00
fT
M= 4
h = 1.1
1.2
1.5
0
1.0
2.0
3.0
4.0
fT
M = 4
h = 0.25
0.35
0.40
0.50
0
0.5
1.0
1.5
2.0
fT
M= 4
0.8
0.7
h = 0.6
0.85
0.9
0
0.5
1.0
1.5
fT
2.0

Fig. 3.12. (*con't.*)

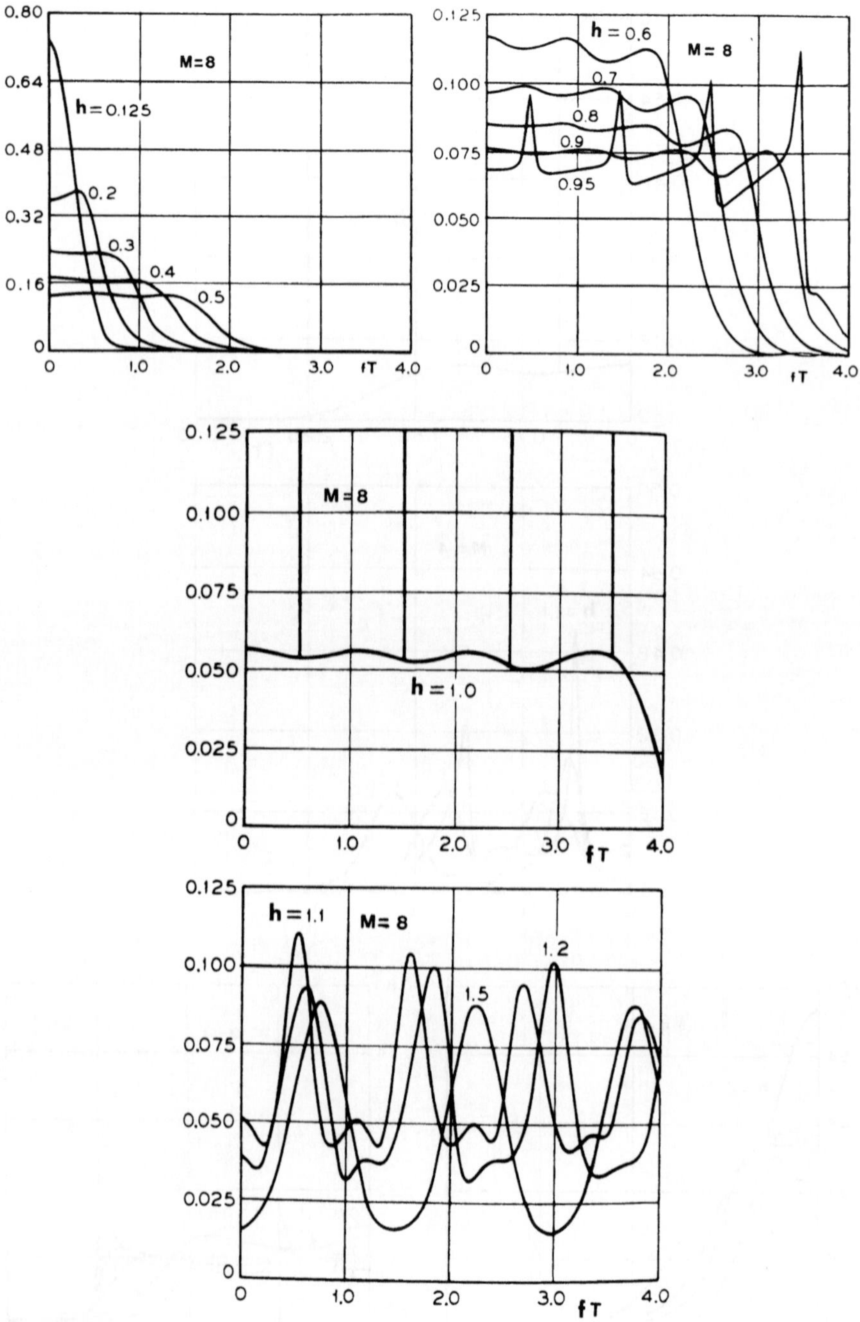

0.80
0.64
0.48
0.32
0.16
0
M=8
h=0.125
0.2
0.3
0.4
0.5
0
1.0
2.0
3.0
fT
4.0
0.125
0.100
0.075
0.050
0.025
0
h = 0.6
M = 8
0.7
0.8
0.9
0.95
0
1.0
2.0
3.0
fT
4.0
0.125
0.100
0.075
0.050
0.025
0
M = 8
h = 1.0
0
1.0
2.0
3.0
fT
4.0
0.125
0.100
0.075
0.050
0.025
0
h = 1.1
M = 8
1.2
1.5
0
1.0
2.0
3.0
fT
4.0


Fig. 3.12. (*con't.*)

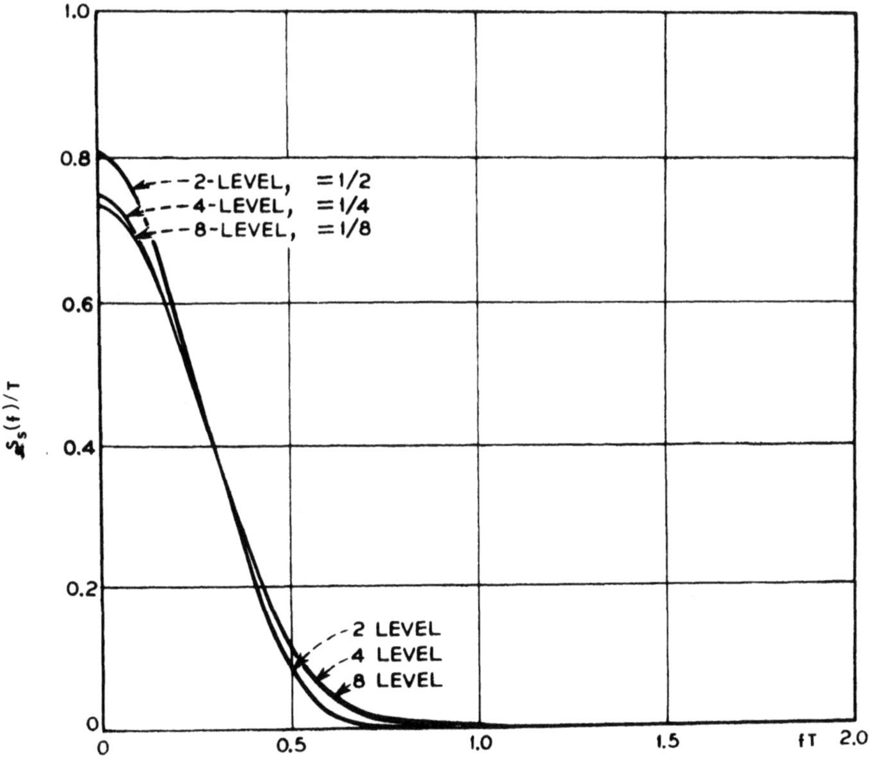


Fig. 3.13. The PSD of $M$-ary FSK with NRZ shaping function of duration $T$ and $h = 1/M$ (reprinted with permission from *The Bell System Technical Journal*. Copyright © 1965, AT&T).

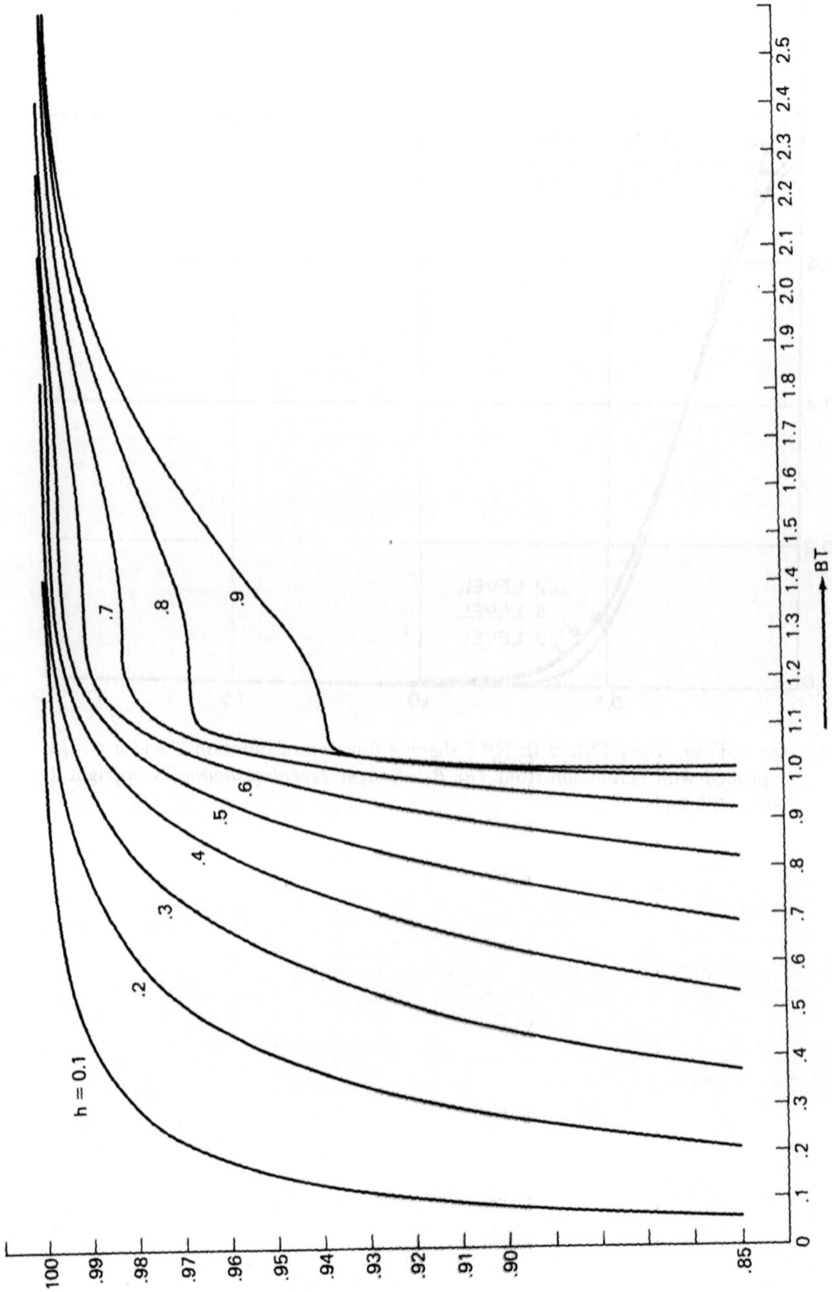


Fig. 3.14 The inband power for binary FSK with NRZ shaping function of duration $T$ and various $h$ (T. Tjhung, "Band Occupancy of Digital FM Signals," *IEEE Tr. Comm. Techn.*, Vol. COM-12, Dec. 1964, pp. 211–216. Copyright © 1964 IEEE).

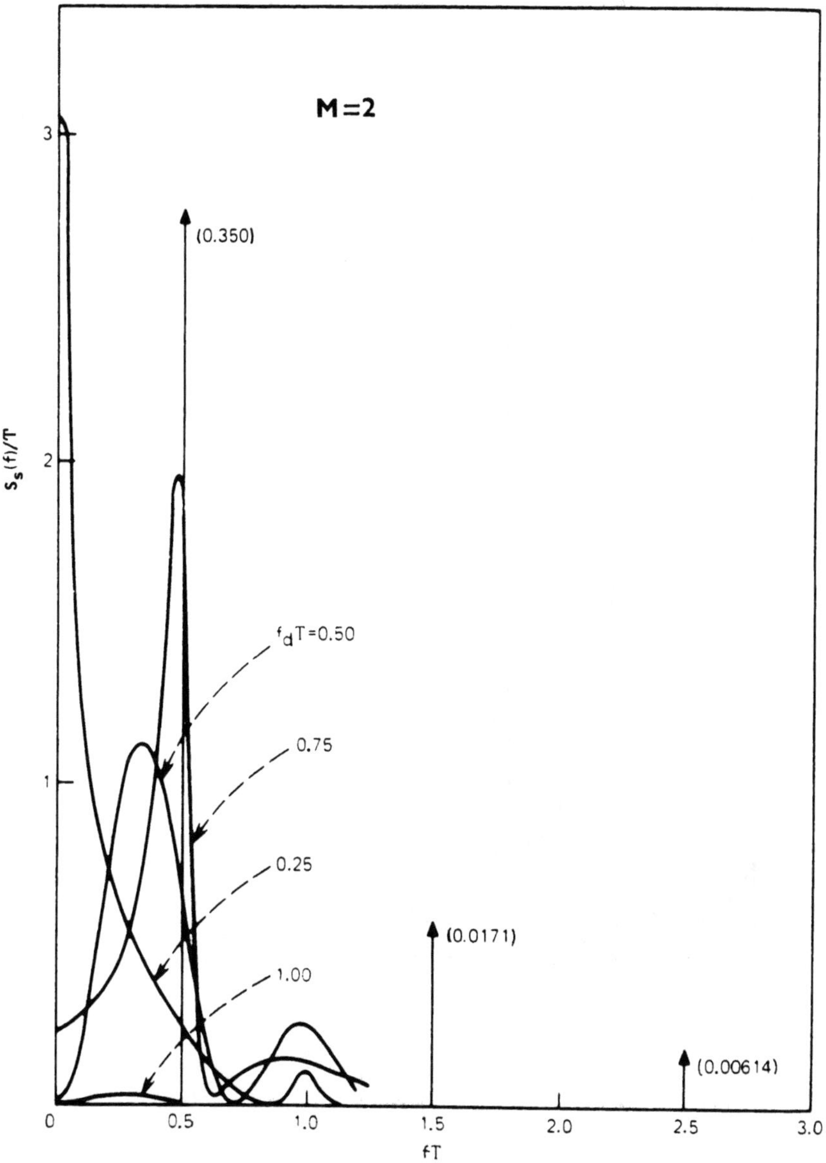


Fig. 3.15. The PSD of $M$-ary FSK with RC shaping function of duration $T$ (reprinted with permission from *The Bell System Technical Journal*. Copyright © 1975, AT&T).

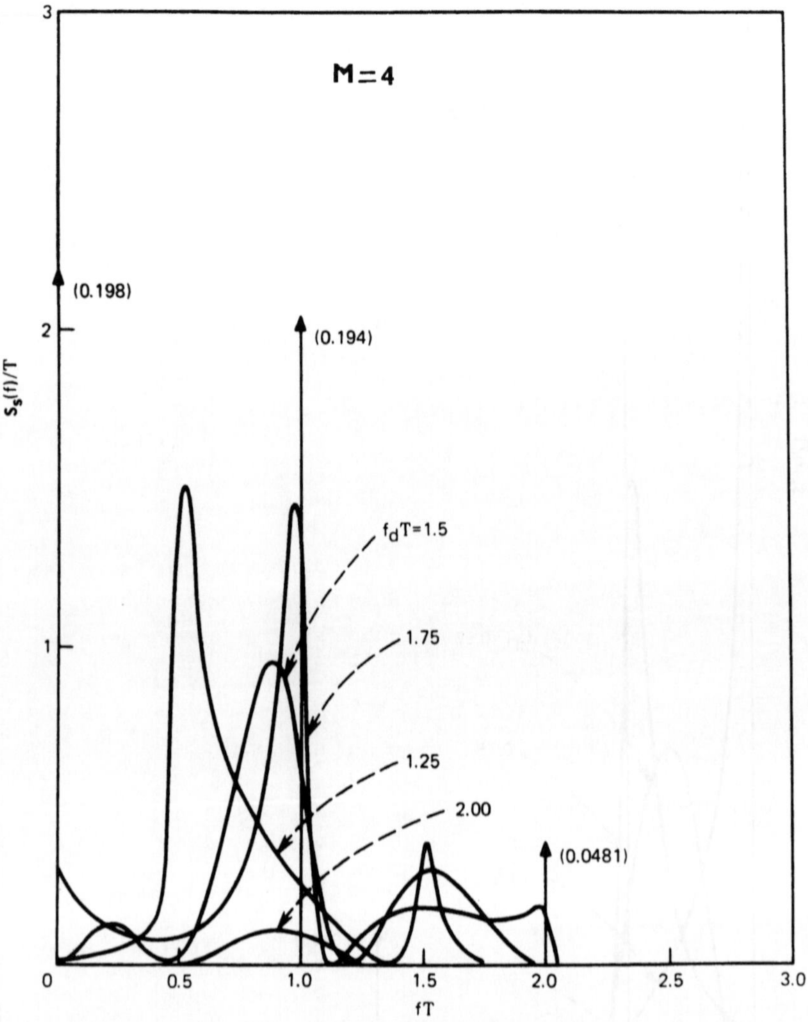

M=4
$S_s(f)/T$
fT
(0.198)
(0.194)
(0.0481)
$f_dT$=1.5
1.75
1.25
2.00
0
0.5
1.0
1.5
2.0
2.5
3.0
1
2
3


Fig. 3.15. (*con't.*)

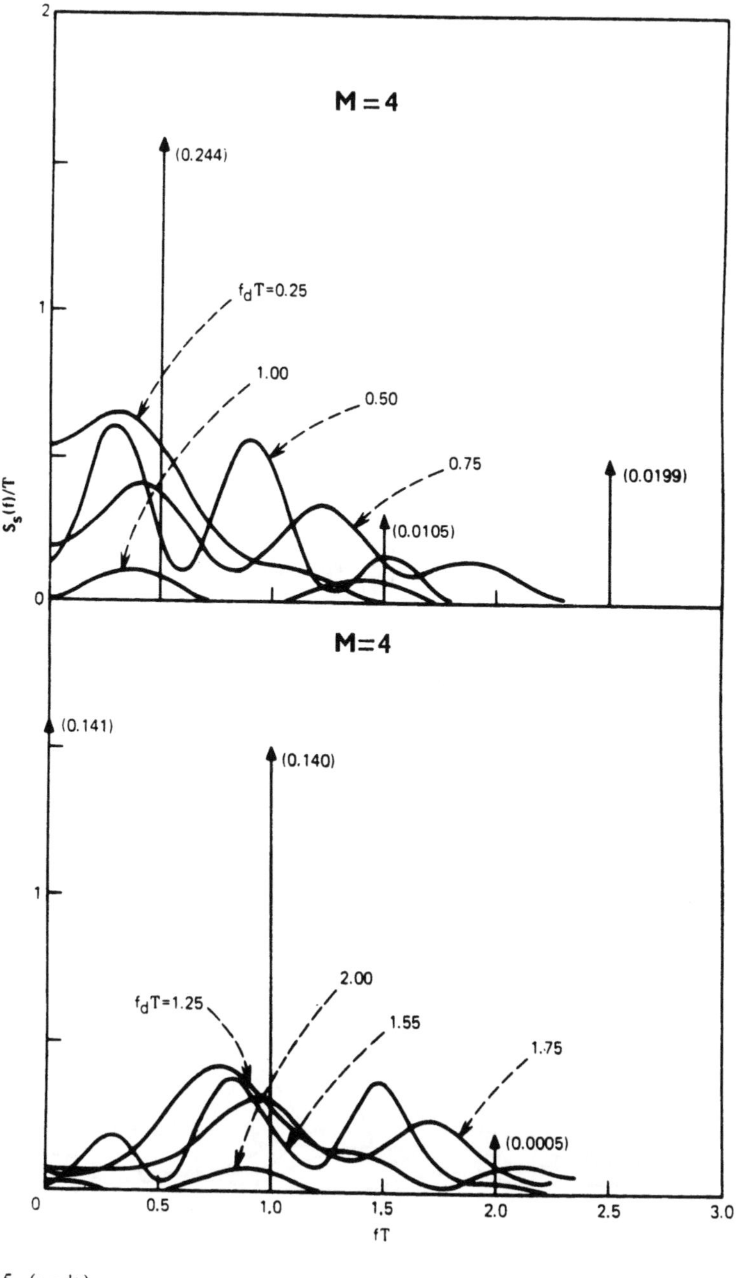

M=4
(0.244)
$f_dT$=0.25
1.00
0.50
0.75
(0.0199)
(0.0105)
M=4
(0.141)
(0.140)
2.00
$f_dT$=1.25
1.55
1.75
(0.0005)
$S_s(f)/T$
2
1
0
0.5
1.0
1.5
2.0
2.5
3.0
fT


Fig. 3.15. (*con't.*)

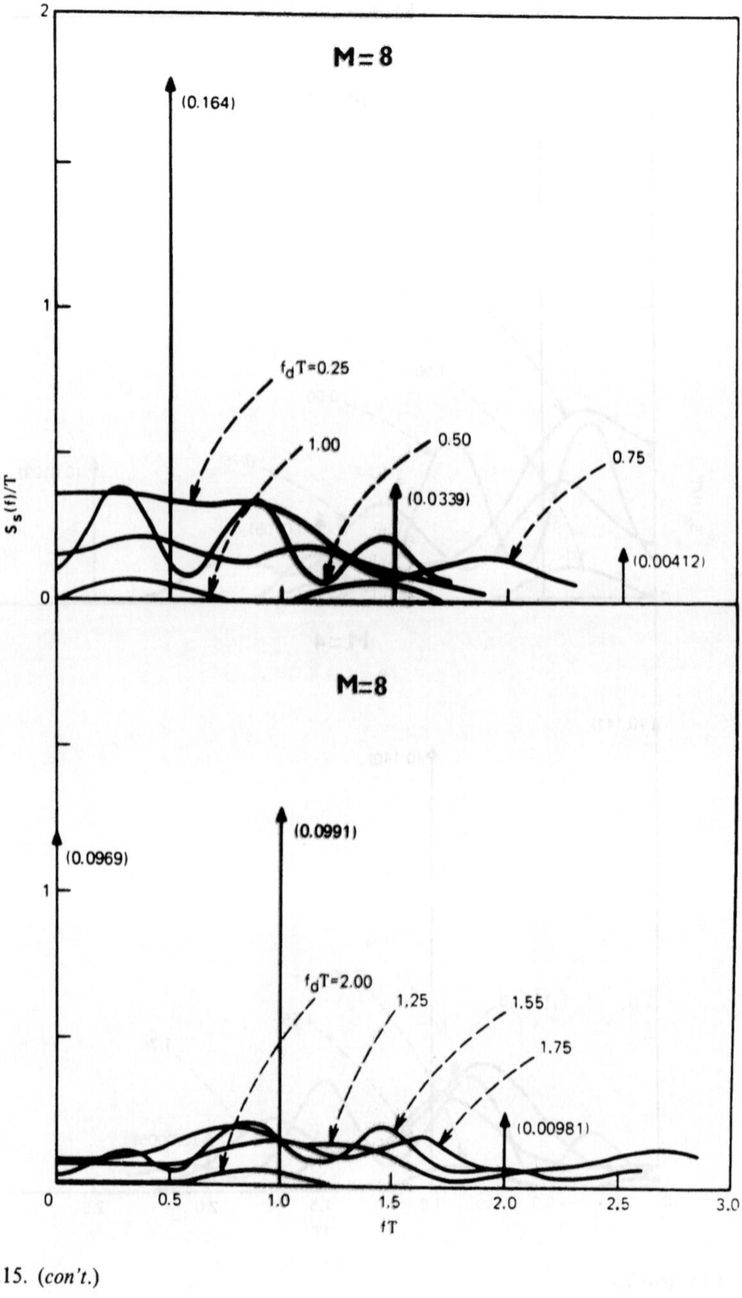
M=8
(0.164)
$f_dT$=0.25
1.00
0.50
0.75
(0.0339)
(0.00412)
$S_s(f)/T$
2
1
0
M=8
(0.0969)
(0.0991)
$f_dT$=2.00
1.25
1.55
1.75
(0.00981)
0
0.5
1.0
1.5
2.0
2.5
3.0
fT

Fig. 3.15. *(con't.)*

**Table 3.3 Bandwidth for binary FSK with NRZ shaping function of duration $T$**

| | | | | | | | | | |
|---|---|---|---|---|---|---|---|---|---|
| $h = 2f_dT$ | 0.1 | 0.2 | 0.3 | 0.4 | 0.5 | 0.6 | 0.7 | 0.8 | 0.9 |
| $B_{99}T$ | 0.45 | 0.78 | 1.00 | 1.10 | 1.17 | 1.25 | 1.78 | 1.93 | 2.05 |

**Table 3.4 Bandwidth of binary FSK with RC, TR, and HS shaping functions of duration $T$**

| SHAPING FUNCTION | RAISED COSINE | | TRIANGLE | | HALF-SINE |
|---|---|---|---|---|---|
| $h$ | 0.4 | 0.5 | 0.4 | 0.5 | 0.5 |
| $2f_dT$ | 0.8 | 1.0 | 0.8 | 1.0 | 0.785 |
| $B_{99}T$ | 1.42 | 2.20 | 1.08 | 1.92 | 1.5 |

### 3.8.2 Shaping function of duration 2 $T$

Here $h(t, a_i)$ is as in (3.7.19) and (3.7.20); hence

$$b(t, \mathbf{a}_i) = \exp\{j(\phi_i + \beta(t, \mathbf{a}_i)\}u_T(t) \tag{3.8.41}$$

where

$$\beta(t, \mathbf{a}_i) = \beta(t, a_i, a_{i-1}) = \beta_0(t, a_i) + \beta_1(t, a_{i-1}) \tag{3.8.42}$$

$$\begin{aligned}\phi_i &= \sum_{-\infty}^{i-1} \beta(T, \mathbf{a}_k) = \sum_{-\infty}^{i-1} \{\beta_0(T, a_k) + \beta_1(T, a_{k-1})\} \\ &= \sum_{-\infty}^{i-1} \beta(2\,T, a_{k-1}) + \beta_0(T, a_{i-1})\end{aligned} \tag{3.8.43}$$

and

$$\beta_k(t, a_i) = K_F \int_0^t h_k(t', a_i)u_T(t')\,dt' \tag{3.8.44}$$

$$\beta(t, a_i) = K_F \int_0^t h(t', a_i)u_{2T}(t')\,dt' \tag{3.8.45}$$

Note that although the duration of the shaping function $h(t, a_i)$ is 2 $T$, the duration of $b(t, \mathbf{a}_i)$ is only $T$; hence when we compute the SFT we use $T' = T$.

We shall denote here also

$$r_k(t, \mathbf{a}_i) = \exp(j\beta_k(t, \mathbf{a}_i))u_T(t) \tag{3.8.46}$$

$$r(t, \mathbf{a}_i) = \exp(j\beta(t, \mathbf{a}_i)) = r_0(t, a_i)r_1(t, a_{i-1}) \tag{3.8.47}$$

$$R_{r,0}(t, t') = \overline{r(t, \mathbf{a}_i)r^*(t', \mathbf{a}_i)} \tag{3.8.48}$$

In the last equation we have assumed that the symbols are independent. We shall compute each of the PSD terms separately.

$\underline{S_{b,0}(f)}$

$$S_{b,0}(f) = \overline{|B(f, \mathbf{a}_i)|^2} = \overline{|R(f, \mathbf{a}_i)|^2} \tag{3.8.49}$$

This can also be computed using the alternative method

$$S_{b,0}(f) = \int_0^T \left\{ \int_0^{T-z} R_{r,0}(x + z, x)\, dx \right\} \cos(2\,\pi f z)\, dz \tag{3.8.50}$$

$\underline{S_{b,1}(f)}$

$$S_{b,1}(f) = \overline{\exp\{j(\phi_1 - \phi_0)\}R(f, \mathbf{a}_1)R^*(f, \mathbf{a}_0)} \tag{3.8.51}$$

The phase difference is from (3.8.43)

$$\phi_1 - \phi_0 = \beta_0(T, a_0) + \beta_1(T, a_{-1}) \tag{3.8.52}$$

Thus

$$S_{b,1}(f) = \int_0^T\int_0^T \overline{r_0(t, a_1)r_l(t, a_0)r_0^*(t', a_0)r_0(T, a_0)r_l(T, a_{-1})r_1^*(t, a_{-1})}$$
$$\exp(-j\,2\,\pi f(t - t'))\, dt\, dt' \tag{3.8.53}$$

Assuming independent symbols (we have already assumed in the beginning that they are stationary), the integrand is

$$R_{b,1}(t, t') = \overline{m_{r0}(t)r_1(t, a_0)r_0(T, a_0)r_0^*(t', a_0)}\ \overline{r_1(T, a_0)r_1^*(t, a_0)} \tag{3.8.54}$$

where

$$m_{rk}(t) = \overline{r_k(t, a_0)} \tag{3.8.55}$$

$\underline{S_{b,i}(f) \quad i \geqq 2}$

$$S_{b,i}(f) = \overline{\exp\{j(\phi_i - \phi_0)R(f, a_i)R^*(f, a_0)} \tag{3.8.56}$$

Here, from (3.8.43)

$$\phi_i - \phi_0 = \sum_{k=1}^{i-2} \beta(2\,T, a_k) + \beta_1(T, a_{-1}) + \beta_0(T, a_{i-1}) + \beta(2\,T, a_0) \tag{3.8.57}$$

When we substitute (3.8.57) and (3.8.47) into (3.8.56), we see that $S_{b,i}(f)$ is the SFT of

$$\begin{aligned} R_{b,i}(t, t') &= m_r^{i-2}(2\,T)m_{r0}(t)\overline{r_1(t, a_{i-1})r_0(T, a_{i-1})} \\ &\quad \overline{r_1(T, a_l)r_1^*(t, a_l)}\ \overline{r(2\,T, a_0)r_0^*(t', a_0)} \\ &= m_r^{i-2}(2\,T)w(t, t') \end{aligned} \tag{3.8.58}$$

where

$$m_r(t) = \overline{r(t, a_i)} \tag{3.8.59}$$

$$r(t, a_i) = \exp(j\beta(t, a_i)u_{2T}(t) \tag{3.8.60}$$

and

$$w(t, t') = m_{r0}(t)\overline{r_1(t, a_0)r_0(t, a_0)}\ \overline{r_1(T, a_0)r_1^*(t, a_0)}\ \overline{r(2\,T, a_0)\ r_0^*(t', a_0)} \tag{3.8.61}$$

Since

$$S_{b,-1}(f) = S^*_{b,i}(-f) \tag{3.8.62}$$

We have all the necessary information to compute the PSD. Thus

$$S_{b,i}(f) = m_r^{i-2}(2\,T)W(f) \tag{3.8.63}$$

where $W(f)$ is the SFT of $w(t, t')$, and using eq. (3.3.15) we obtain

$$\begin{aligned} S_s(f)T/A^2 &= S_{b,0}(f) + 2\,\mathrm{Re}\{S_{b,i}(f)\exp(j\,2\,\pi f T)\} + 2\,\mathrm{Re}\{W(f)m_r(2\,T) \\ &\quad \exp(-j\,4\,\pi f T)\sum_{n=0}^{\infty}\{m_r(2\,T)\exp(-j\,2\,\pi f T)\}^n \end{aligned} \tag{3.8.64}$$

We have here again two cases:

$|m_r(2\,T)| < 1$

In this case the summation converges, and the PSD is a continuous function of frequency

$$S_s(f)T/A^2 = S_{b,0}(f) + 2\,\mathrm{Re}\left\{\left(S_{b,1}(f) + \frac{W(f)m_r(2\,T)}{\exp(j\,2\,\pi fT) - m_r(2\,T)}\right)\exp(-j\,2\,\pi fT)\right\} \tag{3.8.65}$$

$|m_r(2\,T)| = 1$

In this case the summation does not converge, and the PSD has both a continuous and a discrete part. The condition $|m_r(2\,T)| = 1$ is possible only if

$$\beta(2\,T, a_0) = 2\,\pi f_d T \quad (\text{modulo } 2\,\pi) \tag{3.8.66}$$

is a constant for all $a_0 \in \mathring{A}$, which means that $r(2\,T, a_0)$ is the constant $\exp(j\,2\,\pi f_d t)$ and not a random variable. Thus in this case we have

$$m_r(2\,T) = \exp(j\,2\,\pi f_d \mathrm{T}) \tag{3.8.67}$$

and

$$\overline{r(2\,T, a_0)r_0^*(t', a_0)} = r(2\,T, a_0)\overline{r_0^*(t', a_0)} = \exp(j\,2\,\pi f_d T)m_{r0}^*(t') \tag{3.8.68}$$

Since

$$\beta_1(T, a_i) = \beta(2\,T, a_i) - \beta_0(T, a_i) \tag{3.8.69}$$

we can also rewrite

$$\begin{aligned}\overline{r_1(T, a_0)r_1^*(t', a_0)} &= \overline{r(2\,T, a_0)r_1^*(t', a_0)r_0^*(T, a_0)} \\ &= \exp(j\,2\,\pi f_d T)\overline{r_1^*(t', a_0)r_0^*(T, a_0)}\end{aligned} \tag{3.8.70}$$

When we substitute (3.8.67), (3.8.68), and (3.8.70) into (3.8.58), we obtain

$$R_{b,i}(t, t') = \exp(j\,2\,\pi f_d iT)\hat{w}(t, t') \tag{3.8.71}$$

with

$$\hat{w}(t, t') = m_{r0}(t)\overline{r_1(t', a_0)r_0(T, a_0)}m_{r0}^*(t')\overline{r_1^*(t', a_0)r_0^*(T, a_0)} \tag{3.8.72}$$

The SFT of $\hat{w}(t, t')$, $\hat{W}(f)$ is a real function of $f$; hence

$$
\begin{aligned}
S_s(f)T/A^2 &= S_{b,0}(f) + 2\,\mathrm{Re}\,\{S_{b,1}(f)\exp(-j\,2\,\pi f T)\} \\
&\quad + 2\,\hat{W}(f)\,\mathrm{Re}\left\{\sum_{i=2}^{\infty}\exp(-j\,2\,\pi(f - f_d)iT)\right\} \\
&= S_{b,0}(f) - \hat{W}(f) + 2\,\mathrm{Re}\,\{(S_{b,1}(f) - \hat{W}(f)\exp(-j\,2\,\pi f T)\} \\
&\quad + R\hat{W}(f)\sum_k \delta(f_d - kR)
\end{aligned}
\tag{3.8.73}
$$

<u>*Common shaping function*</u> Here we assume

$$h(t, a_i) = a_i\{h_0(t)u_T(t) + h_1(t - T)u_T(t - T))\} = a_i h(t) \tag{3.8.74}$$

hence

$$\beta(t, a_i) = a_i\beta_0(t) + a_{i-1}\beta_1(t) \tag{3.8.75}$$

$$\beta(t) = K_F \int_0^t h(t')u_{2T}(t')\,dt' \tag{3.8.76}$$

$$\beta_k(t) = K_F \int_0^t h_k(t')u_T(t')\,dt' \tag{3.8.77}$$

We also assume that the symbols are independent and from the set $\mathring{A}_{\pm}$, thus

$$\overline{r_k(t, a_0)r_n^*(t', a_0)} = \hat{\sin}\,\{(\beta_k(t) - \beta_n(t')\} \tag{3.8.78}$$

$$m_{rk}(t) = \hat{\sin}\,\{\beta_k(t)\} \tag{3.8.79}$$

$$\overline{r_1(t, a_0)r_0(T, a_0)r_0^*(t', a_0)} = \hat{\sin}\,\{\beta_1(t) + \beta_0(T) - \beta_0(t')\} \tag{3.8.80}$$

$$\overline{r(2\,T, a_0)r_0^*(t', a_0)} = \hat{\sin}\,\{\beta(2\,T) - \beta_0(t'))\} \tag{3.8.81}$$

$$\overline{r_k(t, a_0)r_n(t', a_0)} = \hat{\sin}\,\{\beta_k(t) + \beta_n(t')\} \tag{3.8.82}$$

$$m_r(t) = \hat{\sin}\,\{\beta(t)\} \tag{3.8.83}$$

*Example* 3.8.2 PSD of FSK with duobinary shaping function.
We compute the PSD of FSK with a duobinary shaping function

$$h(t) = u_{2T}(t) \tag{3.8.84}$$

Hence

$$h_0(t) = h_1(t) = u_T(t) \tag{3.8.85}$$

$$\beta_1(t) = \beta_0(t) = \beta(t) = 2\,\pi f_d t \tag{3.8.86}$$

In this case we obtain

$$m_r(t) = \hat{\sin}\,(2\,\pi f_d t) \tag{3.8.87}$$

$$R_{b,0}(t, t') = \hat{\sin}^2\,(2\,\pi f_d(t - t')) \tag{3.8.88}$$

$$R_{b,1}(t, t') = \hat{\sin}\,(2\,\pi f_d T)\,\hat{\sin}\,\{2\,\pi f_d(t + T - t')\}\,\hat{\sin}\,\{2\,\pi f_d(T - t')\} \tag{2.8.89}$$

$$w(t, t') = \hat{\sin}\,(2\,\pi f_d t)\,\hat{\sin}\,\{2\,\pi f_d(t + T)\}\,\hat{\sin}\,\{2\,\pi f_d(2\,T - t')\}\,\hat{\sin}\,\{2\,\pi f_d(t - t')\} \tag{3.8.90}$$

$$\hat{w}(t, t') = \hat{\sin}\,(2\,\pi f_d t)\,\hat{\sin}\,\{2\,\pi f_d(t + T)\}\,\hat{\sin}\,(2\pi\,f_d t')\,\hat{\sin}\,(2\,\pi f_d(t' + T)) \tag{3.8.91}$$

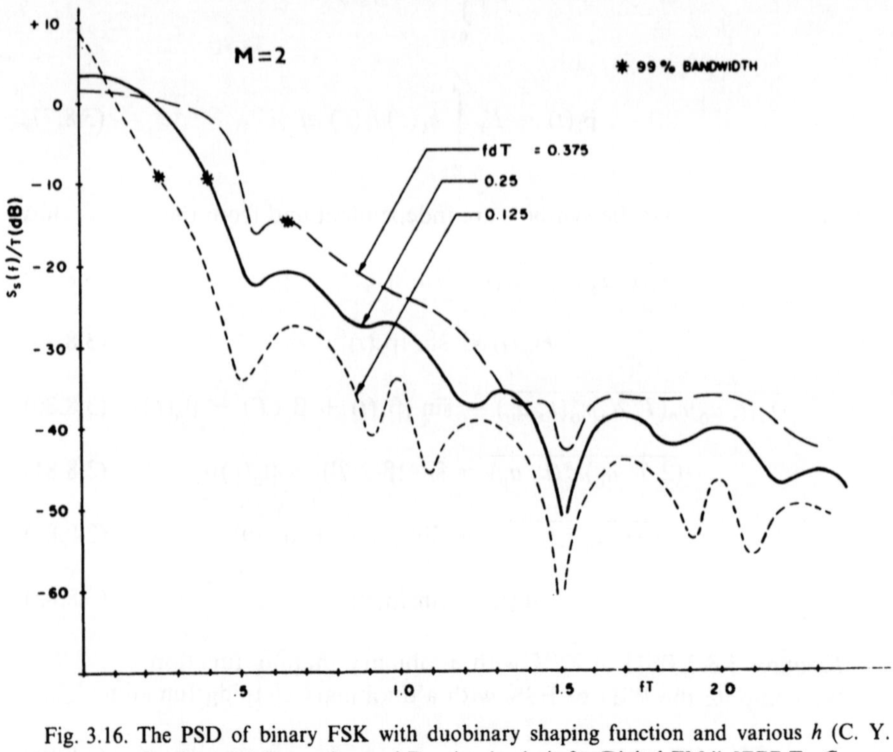


Fig. 3.16. The PSD of binary FSK with duobinary shaping function and various $h$ (C. Y. Garrison, "A Power Spectral Density Analysis for Digital FM," *IEEE Tr. Comm.*, Vol. COM-23, Nov. 1975, pp. 1228–1243. Copyright © 1975 IEEE).

We take the SFT of these four functions and obtain the PSD. The PSD of binary FSK with duobinary shaping function is shown in Fig. 3.16. Figure 3.17 is the same as Fig. 3.16, but the symbols are quaternary. These figures are reproduced from Refs. 3.13.

In Fig. 3.18 we present the PSD of binary FSK with raised cosine and triangular shaping functions of duration 2 $T$. This figure is reprinted from Ref. 3.17. The PSD of FSK with these and other functions can be found in Refs. 3.10, 3.13, 3.14, and 3.15.

In Table 3.5 we present the 99% bandwidth for FSK with triangular, raised cosine, and duobinary shaping functions, all of duration 2 $T$.

**Table 3.5 Bandwidth of FSK with various shaping functions of duration 2 *T***

| SHAPING FUNCTION | TRIANGLE | | | RAISED COSINE | | | DUOBINARY | | | MODIFIED DUOBINARY | | |
|---|---|---|---|---|---|---|---|---|---|---|---|---|
| $2f_dT$ | 0.7 | 0.8 | 1.25 | 0.5 | 0.8 | 1.25 | 0.25 | 0.5 | 0.75 | 0.25 | 0.5 | 0.75 |
| $B_{99}T$ | 1.08 | 1.12 | 1.86 | 1.06 | 1.45 | 1.94 | 0.54 | 0.5 | 1.34 | 0.7 | 1.1 | 1.5 |

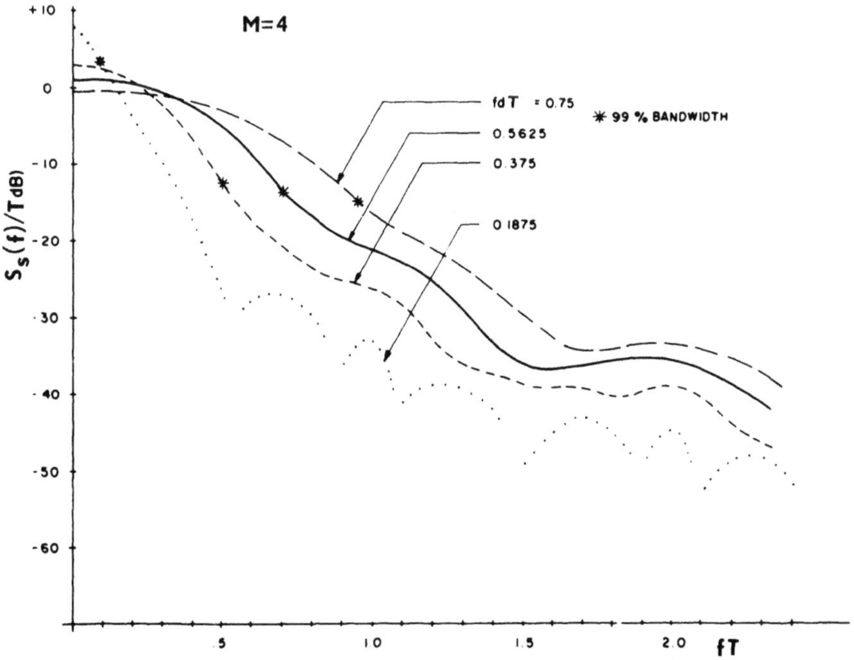


Fig. 3.17. The PSD of quaternary FSK with duobinary shaping function and various $h$ (C. Y. Garrison, "A Power Spectral Density Analysis for Digital FM," *IEEE Tr. Comm.*, Vol. COM-23, Nov. 1975, pp. 1228–1243. Copyright © 1975 IEEE).

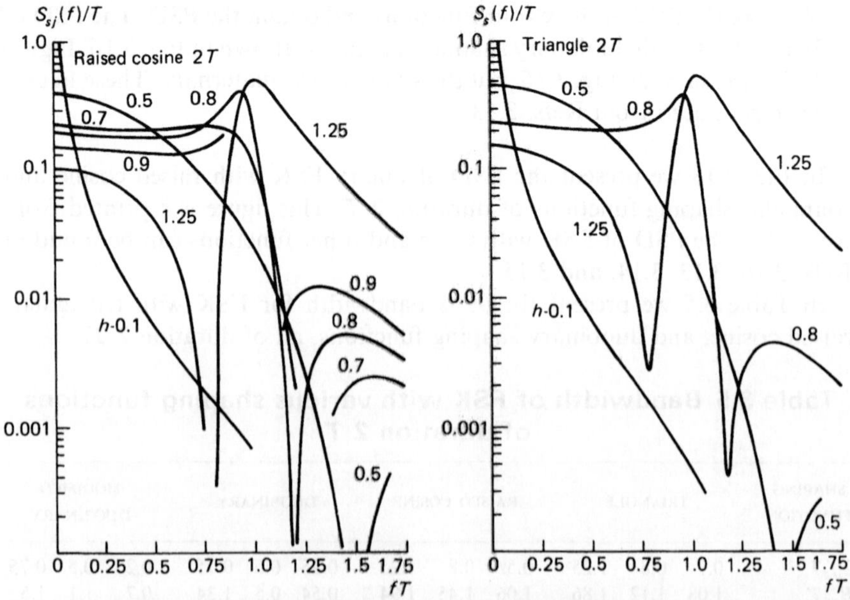


Fig. 3.18. The PSD of binary FSK with RC and TR shaping functions of duration 2 $T$ (reprinted from T. Tjeng and T. Tjhung, "Power Spectra and Power Distribution of Random Binary FM Signals with Premodulation Shaping," *Electronic Letters*, Vol. 1, Aug. 1965, pp. 176–178).

### 3.8.3 Shaping function of duration *KT*

Here $h(t, a_i)$ is as in (3.7.45); hence

$$b(t, \mathbf{a}_i) = \exp\{j(\phi_i + \beta(t, \mathbf{a}_i)\}u_T(t) \tag{3.8.92}$$

where

$$\begin{aligned}\beta(t, \mathbf{a}_i) &= \beta(t, a_i, a_{i-1}, \ldots, a_{i-k}) \\ &= \sum_{k=0}^{K-1} \beta_k(t, a_{i-k})\end{aligned} \tag{3.8.93}$$

and

$$\phi_i = \sum_{-\infty}^{i-1} \beta(T, a_n) = \sum_{-\infty}^{i-1} \sum_{k=0}^{K-1} \beta_k(T, a_{n-k}) \tag{3.8.94}$$

We denote as before

$$r_k(t, a_i) = \exp(j\beta_k(t, a_i)u_T(t)) \tag{3.8.95}$$

$$r(t, \mathbf{a}_i) = \exp\{j\beta(t, \mathbf{a}_i)\} = \prod_{k=0}^{K-1} r_k(t, a_{i-k})u_T(t) \tag{3.8.96}$$

$$r(t, a_i) = \exp\{j\beta(t, a_i)\}u_{KT}(t) \tag{3.8.97}$$

The general term in the PSD formula is

$$S_{b,i}(f) = \overline{\exp\{j(\phi_i - \phi_0)\}R(f, \mathbf{a}_i)R^*(f, \mathbf{a}_0)} \tag{3.8.98}$$

The phase difference is from (3.8.94)

$$\Delta\phi_i = \phi_i - \phi_0 = \sum_{n=0}^{i-1}\sum_{k=0}^{K-1} \beta_k(T, a_{n-k}) \tag{3.8.99}$$

Changing indices

$$n - k = z \tag{3.8.100}$$

It is not difficult to see (Problem 3.8.3) that we have two expressions depending whether $i < K$ or $i \geqq K$.

$\underline{i < K}$

$$\Delta\phi_i = \sum_{z=-K+1}^{-K+i}\sum_{k=-z}^{K-1} \beta_k(T, a_z) + \sum_{z=-K+i+1}^{0}\sum_{k=-z}^{i-1-z} \beta_k(T, a_z) + \sum_{z=1}^{i-1}\sum_{k=0}^{i-1-z} \beta_k(T, a_z) \tag{3.8.101}$$

$\underline{i \geqq K}$

$$\Delta\phi_i = \sum_{z=-K+1}^{0}\sum_{k=-z}^{K-1} \beta_k(T, a_z) + \sum_{z=1}^{i-K}\sum_{k=0}^{K-1} \beta_k(T, a_z) + \sum_{z=i-K+1}^{i-1}\sum_{k=0}^{i-1-z} \beta_k(T, a_z) \tag{3.8.102}$$

and we use the conventional notation that $\sum_{k}^{n} = 0$ for $n < k$.

We can also write

$$r(t, \mathbf{a}_i) = r_0(t, a_i) \prod_{z=i-K+1}^{i-1} r_{i-z}(t, a_z) \tag{3.8.103}$$

$$r^*(t', \mathbf{a}_0) = \prod_{z=-K+1}^{0} r^*_{-z}(t', a_z) \tag{3.8.104}$$

Thus for $i < K$, we obtain, assuming independent symbols

$$R_{b,i}(t, t') = \overline{\exp\{j\Delta\phi_i\}r(t, \mathbf{a}_i)r^*(t, \mathbf{a}_0)}$$

$$= \prod_{z=-K+1}^{-K+i} E\{r^*_{-z}(t', a_z) \prod_{k=-z}^{K-1} r_k(T, a_z)\}$$

$$\prod_{z=-K+i-1}^{0} E\{r_{i-z}(t, a_z)r^*_{-z}(t', a_z) \prod_{k=-z}^{i-1-z} r_k(T, a_z)\}$$

$$\prod_{z=1}^{i-1} E\{r_{i-z}(t, a_z) \prod_{k=0}^{i-1-z} r_k(T, a_z)\}\overline{r_0(t, a_i)} \tag{3.8.105}$$

where we have used for convenience the $E$ notation for the average instead of the bar. We also use here the convention for $\prod_k^n = 1$ $n < k$. Because of stationarity we can replace in (3.8.105) $a_z$ by $a_0$. Again changing indices we obtain

$$R_{b,i}(t, t') = \prod_{n=K-i}^{K-1} E\{r^*_n(t', a_0) \prod_{k=n}^{K-1} r_k(T, a_0)\} \prod_{n=0}^{K+1-i} E\{r_{i+n}(t, a_0)r^*_n(t', a_0)$$

$$\prod_{k=n}^{n+i-1} r_k(T, a_0)\} \prod_{n=1}^{i-1} E\{r_n(t, a_0) \prod_{k=0}^{n-1} r_k(T, a_0)\}\overline{r_0(t, a_0)} \tag{3.8.106}$$

Similarly for $i \geqq K$

$$R_{b,i}(t, t') = \prod_{z=-K+1}^{0} E\{r^*_{-z}(t', a_z) \prod_{k=-z}^{K-1} r_k(T, a_z)\} \prod_{z=1}^{i-K} E\left\{\sum_{k=0}^{K-1} r_k(T, a_z)\right\}$$

$$\prod_{z=i-K+1}^{i-1} E\{r_{i-z}(t, a_z) \prod_{k=0}^{i-1-z} r_k(T, a_z)\}\overline{r_0(t, a_i)} \tag{3.8.107}$$

Here also we can replace, because of stationarity, $a_z$ by $a_0$. Because

$$\sum_{k=0}^{K-1} \beta_k(T, a_z) = \beta(KT, a_z) \tag{3.8.108}$$

the second average in (3.8.107) is

$$E\left\{\prod_{k=0}^{K-1} r_k(T, a_z)\right\} = E\{r(KT, a_z)\} = m_r(kT) \tag{3.8.109}$$

and the product of these averages is simply

$$\prod_{z=1}^{i-K} m_r(KT) = m_r^{i-K}(KT) \tag{3.8.110}$$

In the third product of averages we first change variables $i - z = n$ and then replace $n$ by $-z$. The result is

$$\prod_{z=-K+1}^{-1} E\{r_{-z}(t, a_0) \prod_{k=0}^{-z-1} r_k(T, a_0)\} \tag{3.8.111}$$

which is independent of $i$. Thus for $i \geqq K$, only one term in (3.8.107), namely, (3.8.110), depends on $i$. Thus we can write

$$R_{b,i}(t, t') = m_r^{i-K}(KT)w(t, t') \tag{3.8.112}$$

where

$$\begin{aligned} w(t, t') &= \prod_{z=-K+1}^{0} E\{r^*_{-z}(t', a_0) \prod_{k=-z}^{K-1} r_k(T, a_0)\} \prod_{z=-K+1}^{-1} E\{r_{-z}(t, a_0) \\ &\quad \prod_{k=0}^{-z-1} r_k(T, a_0)\} m_{r0}(t) \\ &= \prod_{n=0}^{K-1} E\{r^*_n(t', a_0) \prod_{k=n}^{K-1} r_k(T, a_0)\} \\ &\quad \prod_{n=1}^{K-1} E\{r_n(t, a_0) \prod_{k=0}^{n-1} r_k(T, a_0) m_{r0}(t)\} \end{aligned} \tag{3.8.113}$$

Let $W(f)$ be the SFT of $w(t, t')$. Then for $i \geqq K$ we obtain

$$S_{b,i}(f) = m_r^{i-K}(KT)W(f) \tag{3.8.114}$$

Since

$$S_{b,i}(f) = S^*_{b,i}(f) \tag{3.8.115}$$

we obtain from (3.3.15)

$$\begin{aligned} S_s(f)T/A^2 &= S_{b,0}(f) + 2\,\mathrm{Re}\left\{\sum_{i=1}^{K-1} S_{b,i}(f) \exp(-j\,2\,\pi f i T)\right\} \\ &\quad + 2\,\mathrm{Re}\,\{W(f) \sum_{i=K}^{\infty} m_r^{i-K}(KT) \exp(-j\,2\,\pi f i T)\} \\ &= S_{b,0}(f) + 2\,\mathrm{Re}\left\{\sum_{i=1}^{K-1} S_{b,i}(f) \exp(-j\,2\,\pi f i T)\right\} \\ &\quad + 2\,\mathrm{Re}\,\{W(f) \exp(-j\,2\,\pi f K T) \sum_{n=0}^{\infty} (m_r(KT) \exp(-j\,2\,\pi f T))^n\} \end{aligned} \tag{3.8.116}$$

We have again the two cases

$|m_r(KT)| < 1$

In this case the summation in (3.8.116) converges, and the PSD is a continuous function of $f$.

$$S_s(f)T/A^2 = S_{b,0}(f) + 2\,\mathrm{Re}\left\{\sum_{i=1}^{K-1} S_{b,i}(f)\exp(-j\,2\,\pi f iT)\right\} + 2\,\mathrm{Re}\left\{\frac{W(f)\exp(-j\,2\,\pi fKT)}{1 - m_r(KT)\exp(-j\,2\,\pi fT)}\right\} \tag{3.8.117}$$

$|m_r(KT)| = 1$

In this case the summation does not converge, and the PSD has a discrete part. This can happen only if

$$\beta(KT, a_0) = 2\,\pi f_d T \qquad (\text{modulo } 2\,\pi) \tag{3.8.118}$$

is a constant for all $a_0 \in \mathring{A}$, which means that $r(KT, a_0)$ is the constant exp $(j\,2\,\pi f_d T)$ and not a random variable. With this in mind we can write

$$\begin{aligned}\sum_{k=-z}^{K-1} \beta_k(T, a_0) &= \sum_{k=0}^{K-1} \beta_k(T, a_0) - \sum_{k=0}^{-z-1} \beta_k(T, a_0)\\ &= \beta(KT, a_0) - \sum_{k=0}^{-z-1} \beta_k(T, a_0)\\ &= 2\,\pi f_d T - \sum_{k=0}^{-z-1} \beta_k(T, a_0) \quad (\text{modulo } 2\,\pi)\end{aligned} \tag{3.8.119}$$

This enable us to change (3.8.113) to

$$w(t, t') = \{\exp(j\,2\,\pi f_d \mathrm{T})\}^K \hat{w}(t, t') \tag{3.8.120}$$

with

$$\begin{aligned}\hat{w}(t, t') = &\prod_{n=1}^{K-1} E\{r_n^*(t', a_0)\prod_{k=n}^{K-1} r_k^*(T, a_0)\}\\ &\prod_{n=1}^{K-1} E\{r_n(t, a_0)\prod_{k=n}^{K-1} r_k(T, a_0)\} m_{r0}^*(t') m_{r0}(t)\end{aligned} \tag{3.8.121}$$

The SFT of $\hat{w}(t, t')$ is the real function $\hat{W}(f)$. Since

$$m_r(KT) = \overline{r(KT, a_0)} = \exp(j\,2\,\pi f_d T) \tag{3.8.122}$$

we have, instead of (3.8.116)

$$
\begin{aligned}
S_s(f)T/A^2 &= S_{b,0}(f) + 2\,\mathrm{Re}\left\{\sum_{i=1}^{K-1} S_{b,i}(f) \exp(-j\,2\,\pi f i T)\right\} \\
&\quad + \hat{W}(f) \sum_{|i| \geq K}^{\infty} \exp(-j\,2\,\pi(f - f_d)iT) \\
&= S_{b,0}(f) + 2\,\mathrm{Re}\left\{\sum_{i=1}^{K-1} S_{b,i}(f) \exp(-j\,2\,\pi f i T)\right\} \\
&\quad - \hat{W}(f) \sum_{|i| < K} \exp(-j\,2\,\pi(f - f_d)iT) \\
&\quad + R\hat{W}(f) \sum_{k} \delta(f - f_d - kR)
\end{aligned} \tag{3.8.123}
$$

<u>*Common shaping function*</u> Here we assume that

$$h(t, a_i) = a_i h(t) \tag{3.8.124}$$

Hence

$$\beta(t, a_i) = a_i \beta(t) \tag{3.8.125}$$

$$\beta_k(t, a_i) = a_i \beta_k(t) \tag{3.8.126}$$

We also assume that the symbols are equiprobable from the set $\mathring{A}_{\pm}$. From these assumptions we obtain instead of (3.8.106), (3.8.113), and (3.8.121)

$$
\begin{aligned}
R_{b,i}(t, t') = &\prod_{n=K-i}^{K-1} \left\{ \hat{\sin}\left( \prod_{k=n}^{K-1} \beta_k(T) - \beta_n(t') \right) \right\} \\
&\prod_{n=0}^{K+1-i} \{\hat{\sin}\,(\beta_{i+n}(t) + \sum_{k=n}^{n+i-1} \beta_k(T) - \beta_n(t'))\} \\
&\prod_{n=1}^{i-1} \{\hat{\sin}\,(\beta_n(t) + \sum_{k=0}^{n-1} \beta_k(T))\}\hat{\sin}\,\{\beta_0(t)\}
\end{aligned} \tag{3.8.127}
$$

$$
\begin{aligned}
w(t, t') = &\prod_{n=0}^{K-1} \hat{\sin} \left\{ \prod_{k=b}^{K-1} \beta_k(T) - \beta_n(t') \right\} \\
&\prod_{n=1}^{k-1} \hat{\sin}\,\{\beta_n(t, a_0) + \sum_{k=0}^{n-1} \beta_k(T))\}\ \hat{\sin}\,\{\beta_0(t)\}
\end{aligned} \tag{3.8.128}
$$

$$
\begin{aligned}
\hat{w}(t, t') = &\prod_{n=1}^{K-1} \hat{\sin} \left\{ \sum_{k=n}^{K-1} \beta_k(T) + \beta_n(t') \right\} \\
&\prod_{n=1}^{K-1} \hat{\sin} \left\{ \sum_{k=n}^{K-1} \beta_k(T) + \beta_n(t) \right\} \hat{\sin}\,\beta_0(t)\ \hat{\sin}\,\beta_0(t')
\end{aligned} \tag{3.8.129}
$$

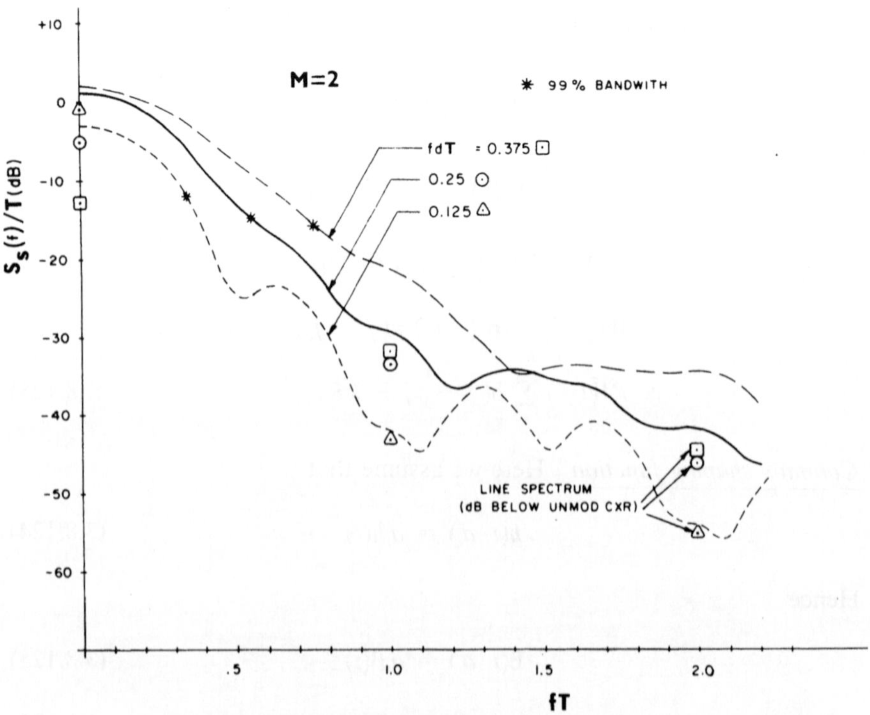


Fig. 3.19. The PSD of binary FSK with modified duobinary shaping function. (C. Y. Garrison, "A Power Spectral Density Analysis for Digital FM," *IEEE Tr. Comm.*, Vol. COM-23, Nov. 1975, pp. 1228–1243. Copyright © 1975 IEEE).

In Fig. 3.19 we show the PSD of binary FSK with modified duobinary shaping function (the duration is 3 $T$). This figure is also taken from Ref. 3.13. Table 3.5 contains a column for the 99% bandwidth of binary FSK with this shaping function.

In Fig. 3.20 we show the PSD of binary FSK with raised cosine function of duration 4 $T$ and $\beta(4\,T) = \pi h$ ($h$ = 0.5, 0.8, 1.2). Similarly in Fig. 3.21 we present the PSD of quaternary FSK with raised cosine shaping function of duration 3 $T$ and $\beta(3\,T) = \pi h$ ($h$ = 0.25, 0.4, 0.5, 0.6). These two figures are reprinted from Ref. 3.20.

It is important to recognize that if $\beta(KT, a_i) = 0$ for shaping functions of duration $KT$, then FSK is reduced to PSK if we replace $\beta(t, a_i)$ by $K_p h(t, a_i)$. Thus the results obtained for PSK (which are much simpler then those for FSK) can be used in this case.

Recently several papers (Ref. 3.26–3.29) have been published on this subject which may be useful to the reader.

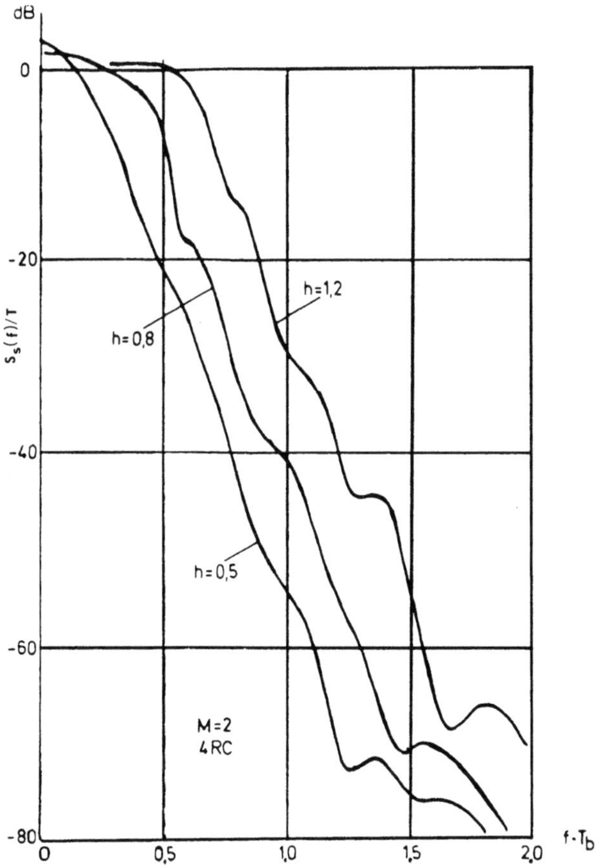


Fig. 3.20. PSD of binary FSK with RC shaping function of duration 4 $T$ and $\beta(4\ T) = \pi h$ ($h$ = 0.5, 0.8, 1.2). T. Aulin, N. Rydbeck, and C. E. W. Sundberg, "Continuous Phase Modulation—Part 2: Partial Response Signalling," *IEEE Tr. Comm.*, Vol. COM-29, Mar. 1981, pp. 210–225. Copyright © 1981 IEEE).

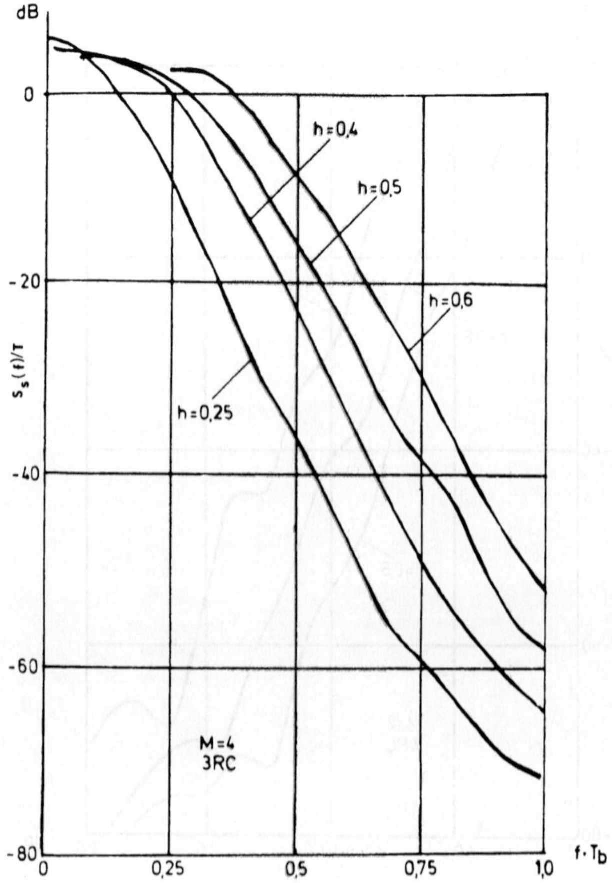


Fig. 3.21. PSD of quaternary FSK with RC shaping function of duration 3 $T$ and $\beta(3\,T) = \pi h$ ($h$ = 0.25, 0.4, 0.5, 0.6) (T. Aulin, N. Rydbeck, and C. E. W. Sundberg, "Continuous Phase Modulation—Part 2: Partial Response Signalling," *IEEE Tr. Comm.*, Vol. COM-29, Mar. 1981, pp. 210–225. Copyright © 1981 IEEE).

## 3.9 THE PSD OF MSK[3.10, 3.16, 3.17]

### 3.9.1 Binary MSK and common shaping function

In this section we assume that $h(t, a_i) = a_i h(t)$ and $a_i = \pm 1$. The PSD can be computed from (3.8.14), because MSK is a special case of FSK with $h = 0.5$ ($\beta(T) = 0.5\,\pi$). It can also be computed using eq. (3.5.7), because MSK is a special case of OQASK, but with $H(f)$ in (3.5.7) replaced by the FT of

$$b(t) = \sin\beta(t + T_b)u_{Tb}(t + T_b) + \cos\beta(t)u_{Tb}(t) \qquad (3.9.1)$$

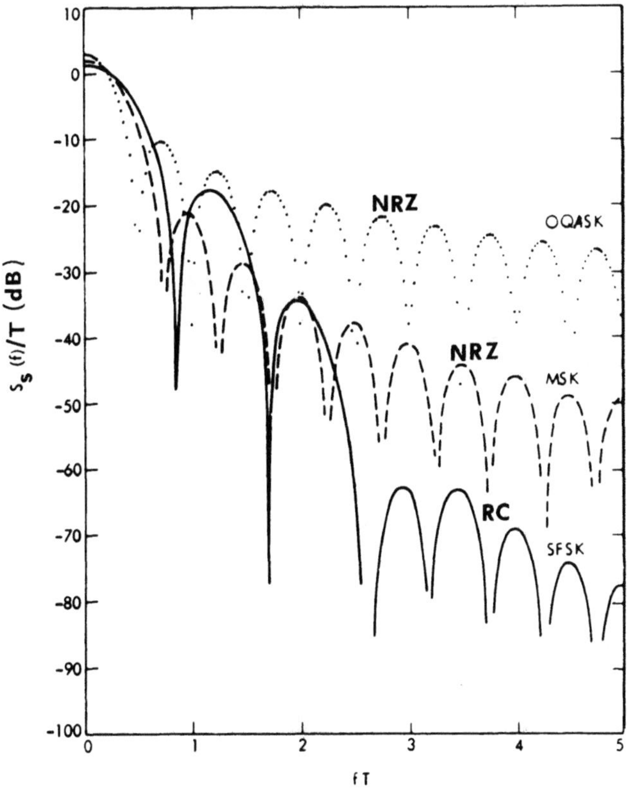


Fig. 3.22. PSD of binary MSK with NRZ and RC shaping functions of duration $T$ (M. K. Simon, "A Generalisation of Minimum Shift Keying (MSK)—Type Signalling Based upon Input Data Symbol Pulse Shaping," *IEEE Tr. Comm.*, Vol. COM-24, Aug. 1976, pp. 845–856. Copyright © 1976 IEEE).

which has duration $2\,T_b$. The PSD is simply given by

$$S_s(f) = (A^2/T)|B(f)|^2 \tag{3.9.2}$$

In Fig. 3.22 is presented the PSD of binary MSK with the NRZ and RC shaping functions. In this figure OQASK represents the PSD of OQASK with the NRZ shaping function. The out-of-band fractional power for these shaping functions is shown in Fig. 3.23. The out-of-band fractional power of binary MSK with HS, TR, and modified TR shaping function defined by

$$K_F h(t + 0.5\,T_b) = \frac{(n+1)\pi}{2\,T_b}(1 - 2|t|/T_b)^n u_{Tb}(t + 0.5\,T_b) \tag{3.9.3}$$

are presented in Fig. 3.24. These three figures are reproduced from Ref. 3.16. The modified TR is a TR shaping function for $n = 1$.

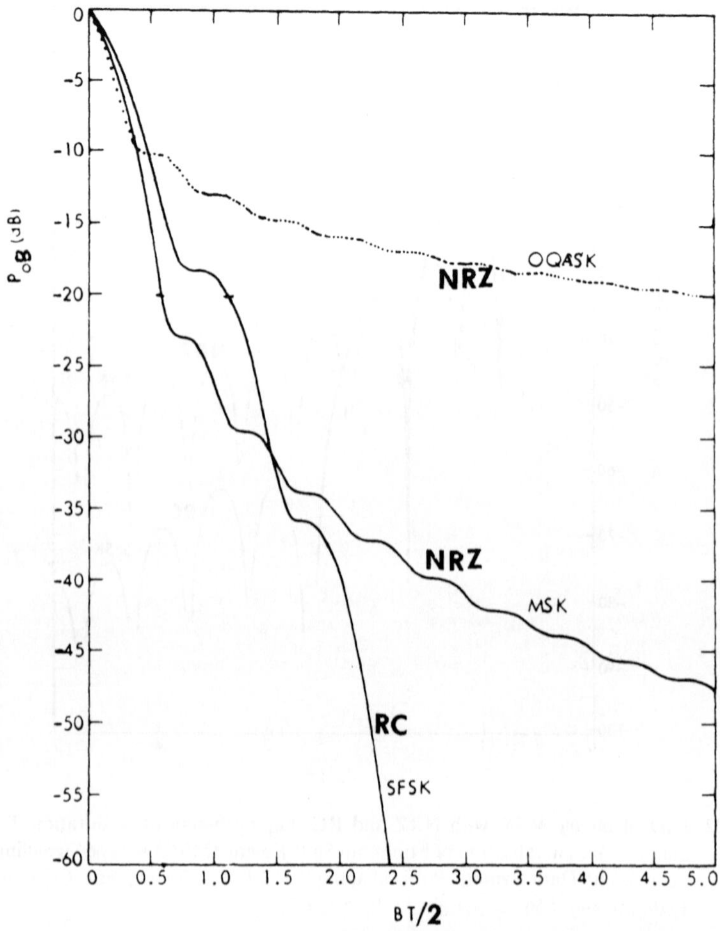


Fig. 3.23 The out-of-band power of binary MSK with NRZ and RC shaping functions of duration $T$ (M. K. Simon, "A Generalization of Minimum Shift Keying (MSK)—Type Signalling Based upon Input Data Symbol Pulse Shaping," *IEEE Tr. Comm.*, Vol. COM-24, Aug. 1976, pp. 845–856. Copyright © 1976 IEEE).

Note from these figures that, although for large $f$ SFSK (MSK with RC) is better than MSK (MSK with NRZ) and this is better than OQPSK (with NRZ), this is not true for small values of $f$. In fact the main lobe of OQPSK is narrower than MSK, and this in turn is narrower than SFSK. This means that in systems with narrowband channels OQPSK is not worse than MSK, and both are better than SFSK.

In Fig. 3.25 is shown the PSD of binary MSK with raised cosine shaping function of duration $KT_b$ ($K$ = 2, 3, 4). This figure is taken from Ref. 3.20.

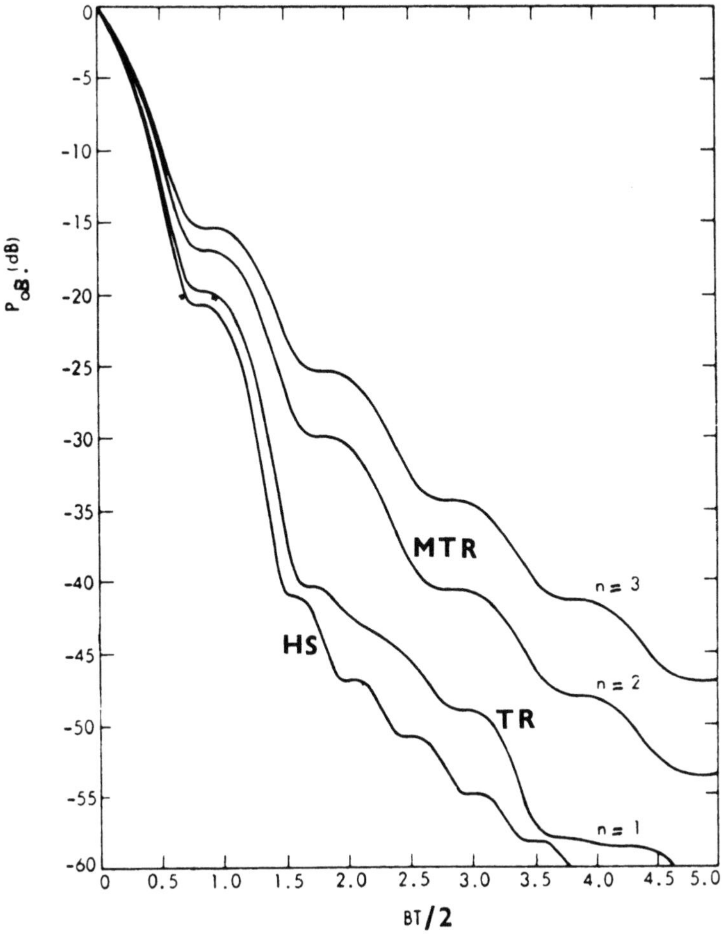


Fig. 3.24 The out-of-band power of binary MSK with HS, TR and modified TR shaping functions of duration $T$ (M. K. Simon, "A Generalization of Minimum Shift Keying (MSK)-type Signalling Based upon Input Data Symbol Pulse Shaping," *IEEE Tr. Comm.*, Vol. COM-24, Aug. 1976, pp. 845–856. Copyright © 1976 IEEE).

### 3.9.2 Optimization problem

We know that $\beta(t)$ is a continuous function of time with $\beta(0) = 0$ and $\beta(T) = 0.5\ \pi$. Because both sin (.) and cos (.) are continuous functions of the argument, we see from (3.9.1) that $b(t)$ is a continuous function of $t$ with

$$b(-T_b) = b(T_b) = 0,\ b(0) = 1$$

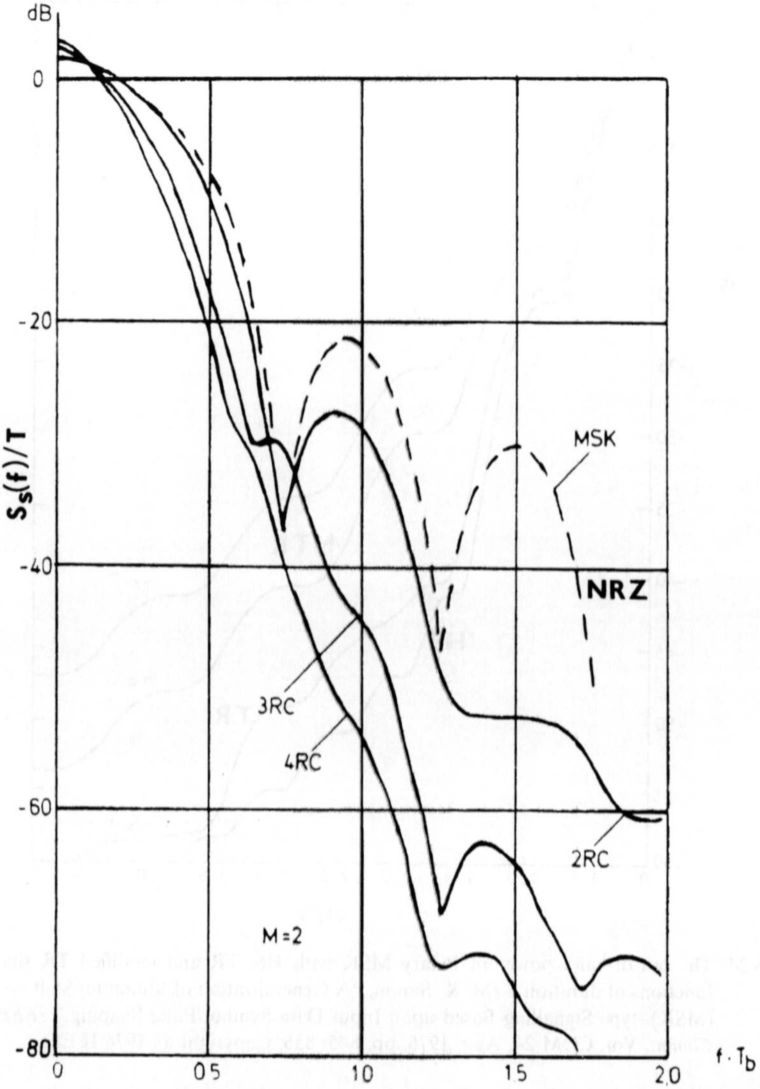


Fig. 3.25 The PSD of binary MSK with RC shaping function of duration KT ($K$ = 2, 3, 4) (T. Aulin, N. Rydbeck, and C. E. W. Sundberg, "Continuous Phase Modulation—Part 2: Partial Response Signalling," *IEEE Tr. Comm.*, Vol. COM-29, Mar. 1981, pp. 210–225. Copyright © 1981 IEEE).

We can formulate now the following optimization problem. Find a continuous function $b(t)$ of duration $2\ T_b$, so that the out-of-band power is minimized.

The solution to this problem with no continuity constraint at the endpoints $(t = \pm T_b)$ is the prolate spheroidal wave function mentioned in Section 3.6. The optimal solution to the constrained problem is not yet known.

### 3.9.3 General MSK

We assume without loss of generality that $a_i \in \mathring{A}_{\pm}$.

In this case also we can use eq. (3.8.14) with the condition

$$\begin{aligned} \beta(T, a_i) &= a_i\ 0.5\ \pi \rightarrow m_r(T) = \overline{\exp\{j\beta(T, a_i)\}} \\ &= \hat{\sin}\ (0.5\ \pi) = 0 \end{aligned} \tag{3.9.4}$$

Here

$$\hat{M}_r^*(f) = \overline{\exp\ (j\ 0.5\ \pi a_0) R^*(f, a_0)} \tag{3.9.5}$$

Thus

$$\begin{aligned} S_s(f)T/A^2 = &\ \overline{|R(f, a_0|^2} + 2\ \mathrm{Re}\ \{\overline{R(f, a_0)} \\ &\ \overline{\exp\ (j\ 0.5\ \pi a_0) R^*(f, a_0)} \exp\ (-j\ 2\ \pi f T)\} \end{aligned} \tag{3.9.6}$$

However, using the modified OQASK representation of general MSK, a different formula was obtained in Ref. 3.17. It is shown there that

$$\begin{aligned} S_s(f)T/A^2 = &\ \overline{|B(f, a_0, a_1)|^2} - 2\ \mathrm{Re}\ \{\overline{m_0 B(f, a_0, a_1)} \\ &\ \overline{m_1 B^*(f, a_0, a_1)} \exp\ (-j\ 4\ \pi f T)\} \\ &+ 2\ Im\ \{\overline{m_1 B(f, a_0, a_1) B^*(f, a_1, a_2)} \exp\ (j\ 2\ \pi f T)\} \end{aligned} \tag{3.9.7}$$

where

$$m_i = \sin\ (0.5\ a_i \pi) \tag{3.9.8}$$

and

$$\begin{aligned} b(t, a_0, a_1) = &\ m_0 \sin\ (\beta(t + T, a_0) u_T(t + T) \\ &+ \cos\ \beta(t, a_1) u_T(t) \end{aligned} \tag{3.9.9}$$

If the shaping functions are pairwise antipodal, i.e.

$$h\ (t, a_i) = -h(t, -a_i) \tag{3.9.10}$$

then in the same reference it is shown that

$$S_s(f) = (A^2/T)\overline{|B(f, a_0, a_1)|^2}$$
$$= 4\,A^2/T \sum_{a_0, a_1 \in I_+}\sum |B(f, a_0, a_1)|^2/M^2 \quad (3.9.11)$$

where

$$I_+ = \{1, 3, \ldots, M - 1)\} \quad (3.9.12)$$

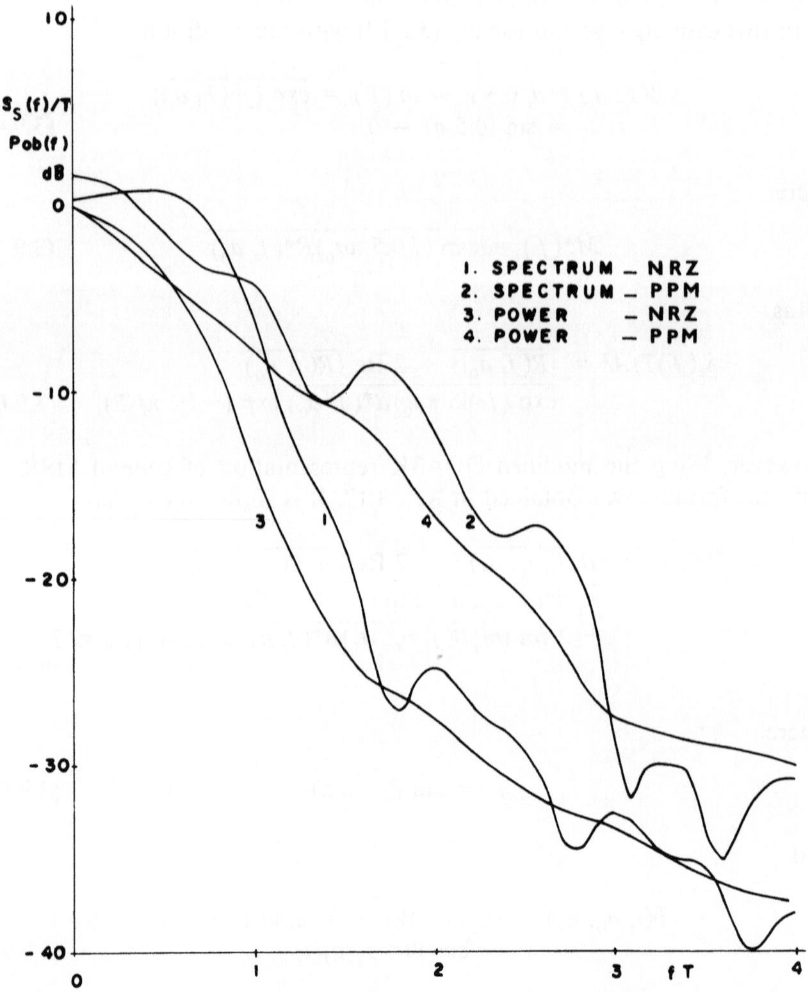


Fig. 3.26. The PSD and out-of-band power of quaternary MSK with NRZ and PPM shaping functions (I. Korn "Generalised Minimum Shift Keying," *IEEE Tr. Inf. Theory*), Vol. IT-26, Mar. 1980, pp. 234–238. Copyright © 1980 IEEE).

For binary symbols this is reduced to

$$S_s(f) = (A^2/T)|B(f, 1, 1)|^2 \tag{3.9.13}$$

*Example* 3.9.1 PSD of quaternary MSK with common shaping function
We compute the PSD of quaternary MSK with common shaping function

$$h(t, a_i) = a_i(2\, T_b)^{-1}\pi u_{Tb}(t),\ a_i = \pm 1, \pm 3 \tag{3.9.14}$$

The equivalent OQASK shaping functions are shown in the previous chapter in Fig. 2.22. The PSD and the out-of-band power are shown in Fig. 3.26. The figure is taken from Ref. 3.17.

*Example* 3.9.2 PSD of quaternary MSK and noncommon shaping functions
We compute the PSD of quaternary MSK with shaping functions

$$h(t, \pm 1) = \pm \pi/T_b u_{0.5Tb}(t)$$

$$h(t, \pm 3) = \pm 3\, \pi/T_b u_{0.5Tb}(t - 0.5\, T_b) \tag{3.9.15}$$

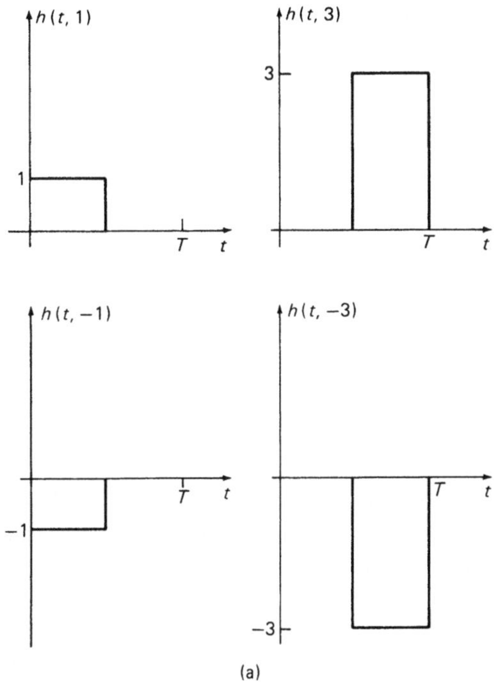


Fig. 3.27 (a) The PPM shaping functions of quaternary MSK and (b) equivalent OQASK shaping functions (I. Korn, "Generalised Minimum Shift Keying," *IEEE Tr. Inf. Theory*, Vol. IT-26, Mar. 1980, pp. 234–238. Copyright © 1980 IEEE).

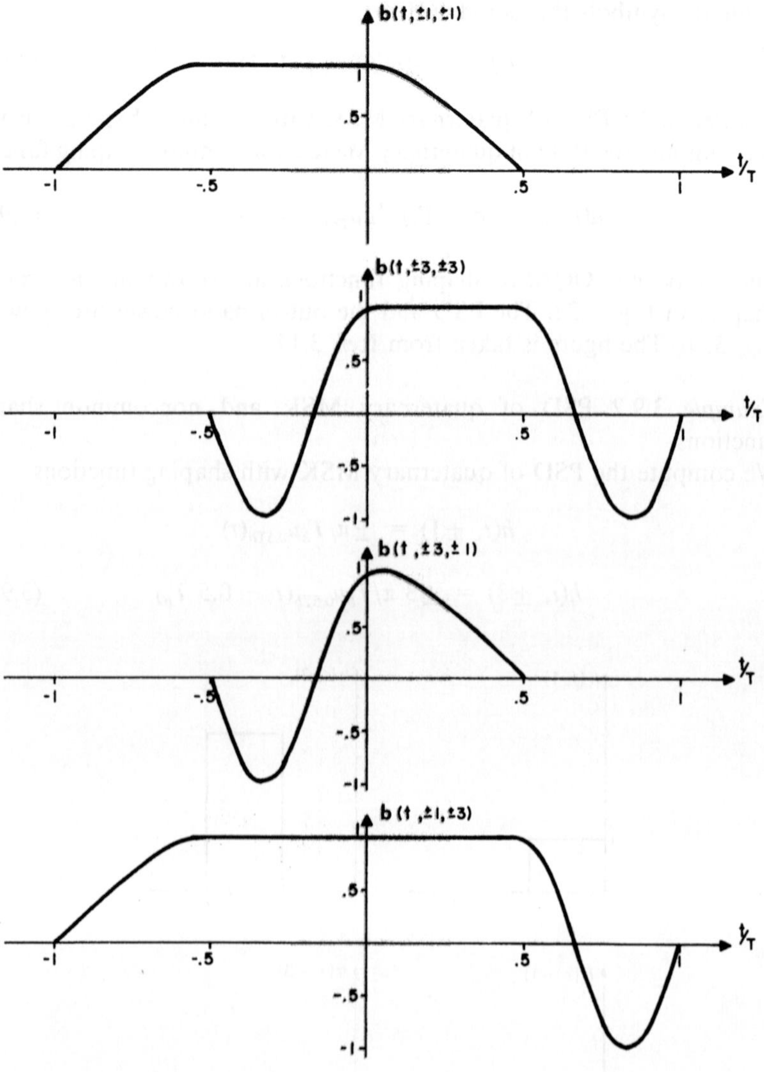


Fig. 3.27. (*con't.*)

These shaping functions and the equivalent OQASK shaping functions are shown in Fig. 3.27. The PSD and the out-of-band power are shown in Fig. 3.26. This is also reproduced from Ref. 3.17.

The PSD and out-of-band power for $M$-ary MSK with NRZ shaping function is shown in Fig. 3.28, which is reproduced from Ref. 3.16. In Tables 2.3–2.5 we can find the 99% bandwidth for binary MSK under the heading $h = 0.5$.

## 3.10 THE PSD OF QASK AND OQASK WITH NONLINEAR BANDPASS FILTERING[3.22]

### 3.10.1 Bandpass, memoryless nonlinearity

If the modulated signal $s_M(t)$ with PSD $S_{sM}(f)$ is passed through a linear bandpass filter with transfer function $H_{TM}(f)$, the PSD of the output $y(t)$ is

$$S_{yM}(f) = S_{sM}(f)|H_{TM}(f)|^2 \tag{3.10.1}$$

and this is indeed one method used to achieve compliance with international regulations on frequency allocations. For LSK signals this can also be

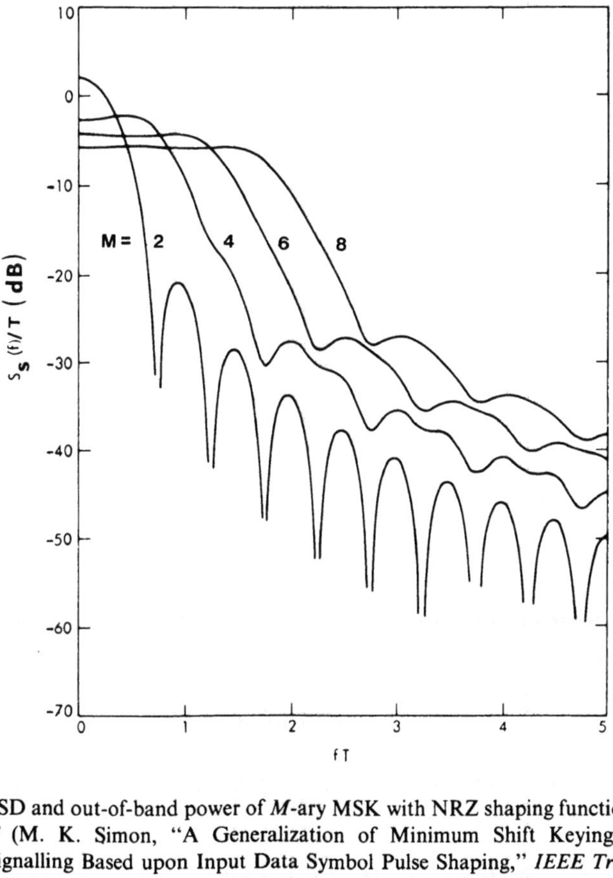


Fig. 3.28. PSD and out-of-band power of $M$-ary MSK with NRZ shaping function of duration $T$ (M. K. Simon, "A Generalization of Minimum Shift Keying (MSK)–type Signalling Based upon Input Data Symbol Pulse Shaping," *IEEE Tr. Comm.*, Vol. COM-24, Aug. 1976, pp. 845–856. Copyright © 1976 IEEE).

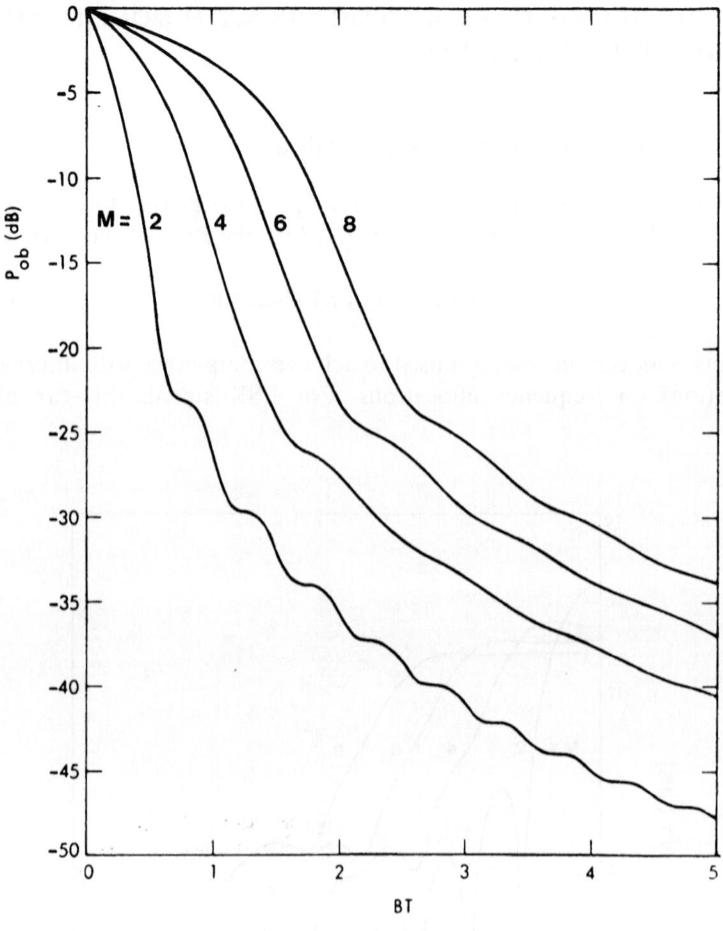


Fig. 3.28. (*con't.*)

achieved by filtering the baseband signals, so that the PSD of the complex envelope is modified from $S_s(f)$ to

$$S_y(f) = S_s(f)|H_T(f)|^2 \tag{3.10.2}$$

where $H_T(f)$ is the low-pass equivalent transfer function of the bandpass filter $H_{TM}(f)$, i.e.

$$H_T(f) = H_{TM}(f + f_c)u(f + f_c) \tag{3.10.3}$$

and $f_c$ is the carrier frequency ($u(.)$ is the step function).

When the filter is nonlinear, the equations are not valid. We shall assume that the nonlinear filter is memoryless, i.e., the output depends only on the instantaneous value of the input. Thus let

$$x = A \cos \theta \tag{3.10.4}$$

and let $f(x)$ be a nonlinear function of $x$. Denote

$$z(A, \theta) = f(x) = f(A \cos \theta) \tag{3.10.5}$$

Because $\cos \theta$ is a periodic, even function of $\theta$ with period $2\pi$, this is also true for $z(A, \theta)$. Hence $z(A, \theta)$ can be represented by a Fourier series in $\theta$

$$z(A, \theta) = \sum_{k=0}^{\infty} z_k(A) \cos (k\theta) \tag{3.10.6}$$

The first (fundamental) coefficient is

$$z_1(A) = 0.5 \int_{-\pi}^{\pi} f(A \cos \theta) \cos \theta \, d\theta/\pi \tag{3.10.7}$$

We shall denote this function by $g(A)$, i.e.

$$g(A) = z_1(A) \tag{3.10.8}$$

A model of such a nonlinearity in which $\theta = \omega_c t + \phi$ ($\omega_c = 2\pi f_c$) is presented in Fig. 3.29.

A bandpass nonlinearity is a nonlinear device followed by a bandpass filter that retains only the fundamental frequency term. Thus let the input be

$$x_M(t) = A_x(t) \cos (w_c t + \phi_x(t)) \tag{3.10.9}$$

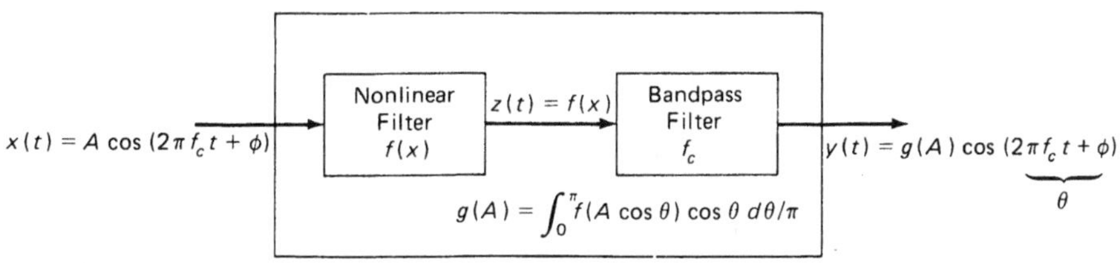


Fig. 3.29. A model of memoryless, bandpass nonlinear filter.

Then the output is

$$y_M(t) = A_y(t) \cos (w_c t + \phi_y(t)) \tag{3.10.10}$$

and the relations are

$$A_y(t) = g_A(A_x(t)) \tag{3.10.11}$$

$$\phi_y(t) = g_\phi(A_x(t)) + \phi_x(t) \tag{3.10.12}$$

where $A_x(t)$ denoted the envelope and $\phi_x(t)$ the phase of the bandpass signal $x_M(t)$ (the same notation for $y_M(t)$ and other bandpass signals). $g_A(.)$ represents the change in the amplitude of the signal and is thus the AM-to-AM conversion, while $g_\phi(.)$ represents the change in phase and is the AM-to-PM conversion, where AM means amplitude modulation and PM means phase modulation. Both are functions of the envelope only. Note that (3.10.11) is obtained from (3.10.4)–(3.10.8) if we identify $A = A_x(t)$, $\theta = w_c t + \phi_x(t)$ and $g(.) = g_A(.)$.

A hard limiter is a nonlinearity for which

$$f(x) = A \operatorname{sign} x \tag{3.10.13}$$

$$g_A(A_x) = \gamma,\ g_\phi(A_x) = 0 \tag{3.10.14}$$

where $\gamma$ is a constant. A TWT (traveling wave tube), which is used as an amplifier in satellite communication and other applications, is a nonlinearity that can be modeled by[3.21]

$$g_A(A_x) = \alpha_A A_x/(1 + \beta_A A_x^2)$$

$$g_\phi(A_x) = \alpha_\phi A_x^2/(1 + \beta_\phi A_x^2) \tag{3.10.15}$$

where $\alpha_A$, $\beta_A$, $\alpha_\phi$, and $\beta_\phi$ are constants selected to fit the experimentally obtained characteristic.

Instead of using (3.10.9), (3.10.10), we can also use their complex envelope form

$$x(t) = A_x(t) \exp \{j\phi_x(t)\} \tag{3.10.16}$$

$$\begin{aligned} y(t) &= A_y(t) \exp \{j\phi_y(t)\} \\ &= g_A(A_x) \exp \{jg_\phi(A_x)\} \exp (j\phi_x(t)) \end{aligned} \tag{3.10.17}$$

Three different but equivalent models of the complex nonlinearity are shown in Fig. 3.30. The relations between the different representations are

$$A_x = (x_I^2 + x_Q^2)^{1/2}, \ \phi_x = \tan^{-1}(x_Q/x_I) \tag{3.10.18}$$

$$g_I = g_A \cos g_\phi, \ g_Q = g_A \sin g_\phi \tag{3.10.19}$$

$$g_c = g_I/A_x, \ g_s = g_Q/A_x \tag{3.10.20}$$

For example a hard limiter and TWT[3.21] can be represented by

$$g_I(A_x) = \gamma \qquad g_Q(A_x) = 0 \tag{3.10.21}$$

$$g_I(A_x) = \alpha_I/(1 + \beta_I A_x^2)$$

$$g_Q(A_x) = \alpha_Q A_x^3/(1 + \beta_Q A_x^2) \tag{3.10.22}$$

where again $\alpha_I$, $\beta_I$, $\alpha_Q$, and $\beta_Q$ are proper constants. To simplify the notation we have omitted the explicit time dependence in all these equations. A real-time representation of the first model of Fig. 3.30 is shown in Fig. 3.31. Similar real-time models can be given for the other complex models. Several memoryless, bandpass nonlinearities in cascade can be combined into a single nonlinear, memoryless filter. Thus let $x(t)$, $y(t)$, and $s(t)$ be the input to the first nonlinearity, second nonlinearity, and output, as shown in Fig. 3.32. We obtain

$$A_s = g_{A2}(A_y) = g_{A2}\{g_{A1}(A_x)\} = g_A(A_x) \tag{3.10.23}$$

$$\phi_s = \phi_y + g_{\phi 2}(A_y) = \phi_x + g_{\phi 1}(A_x) + g_{\phi 2}\{g_{A1}(A_x)\} = \phi_x + g_\phi(A_x) \tag{3.10.24}$$

where we again suppressed the time dependence.

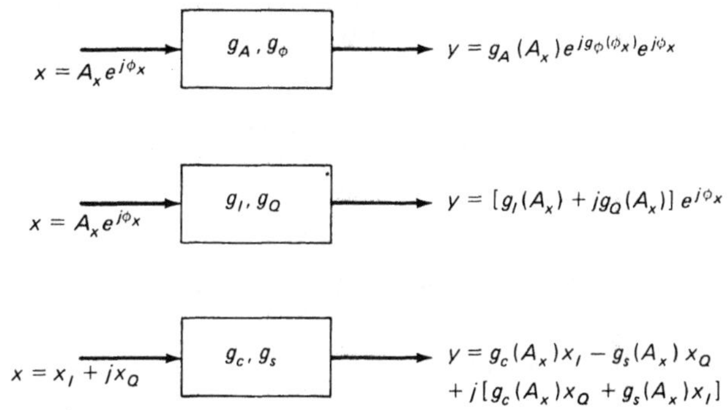


Fig. 3.30. Three equivalent models of a bandpass nonlinearity with both AM-to-AM and AM-to-PM conversion.

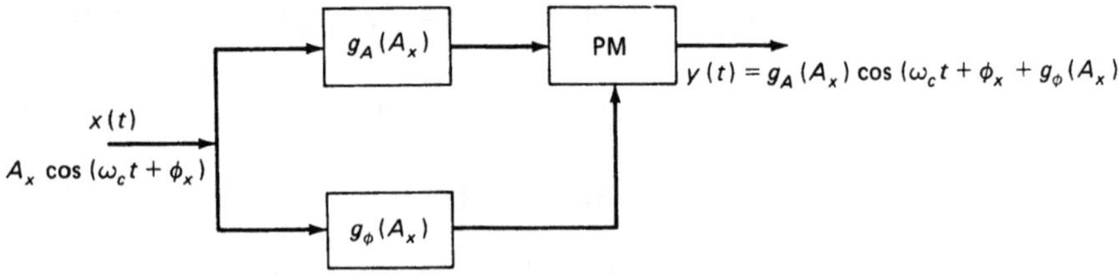


Fig. 3.31. Real-time model of memoryless, bandpass nonlinearity.

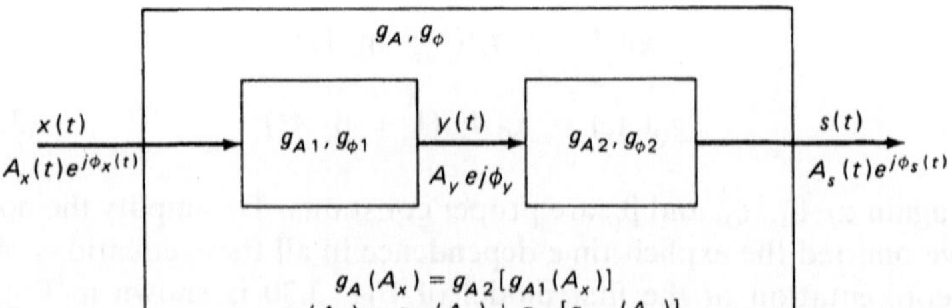


Fig. 3.32. Two bandpass nonlinearities in cascade.

## 3.10.2 THE PSD

Now we assume that $x_M(t)$ is a QASK or OQASK signal with quaternary symbols and common shaping function of duration $KT$. The complex envelope of the signal is

$$x(t) = A\left\{\sum_i a_{I,i}h(t - iT) + ja_{Q,i}h(t - iT - \varepsilon T_b)\right\} \tag{3.10.25}$$

where $\{a_{I,i}\}$, $\{a_{Q,i}\}$ are independent sequences of binary ($\pm 1$), equiprobable symbols, $T = 2\,T_b$ and $\varepsilon = 0$ for QASK and $\varepsilon = 1$ for OQASK. Since $h(t)$ is limited in duration to $KT$, we can write

$$h(t) = \sum_{k=0}^{K-1} h_k(t - kT)u_T(t - KT) \tag{3.10.26}$$

and

$$h_k(t, \varepsilon) = h(t + kT - \varepsilon T)u_T(t) \tag{3.10.27}$$

When $\varepsilon = 0$ we shall also write

$$h_k(t, 0) = h_k(t) \tag{3.10.28}$$

Using these equations, (3.10.25) can be written as

$$x(t) = \sum_i h_I(t - iT, \mathbf{a}_{I,i}) + j \sum_i h_Q(t - iT, \mathbf{a}_{Q,i}) \qquad (3.10.29)$$

where

$$h_I(t, \mathbf{a}_{I,i}) = A \sum_{k=0}^{K-1} a_{I,i-k} h_k(t, 0) u_T(t) \qquad (3.10.30)$$

and

$$h_Q(t, \mathbf{a}_{Q,i}) = A \sum_{k=0}^{K-1+\varepsilon} a_{Q,i-k} h_k(t, \varepsilon) u_T(t) \qquad (3.10.31)$$

Note that $h_I(.\,,.)$ and $h_Q(.\,,.)$ are confined to the interval $0$–$T$ only. Note also that $h_I(.\,,.)$ depends only on $K$ symbols $\mathbf{a}_{I,i} = \{a_{I,i}, a_{I,i-1}, \ldots, a_{I,i-K+1}\}$, though $h_Q(.\,,.)$ depends either on $K$ symbols ($\varepsilon = 0$) or $K + 1$ symbols ($\varepsilon = 1$), $\mathbf{a}_{Q,i} = \{a_{Q,i}, a_{Q,i-1}, \ldots\, a_{Q,i-K+1}\}$. Note also that for $\varepsilon = 1$ $h_0(t, 1)$ is confined to the interval $T_b$–$T$ only and $h_K(t, 1)$ to the interval $0$–$T_b$ only.

It follows from (3.10.29)–(3.10.31) that the amplitude and phase functions are

$$A_x(t, \mathbf{a}_i) = \{h_I^2(t, \mathbf{a}_{I,i}) + h_Q^2(t, \mathbf{a}_{Q,i})\}^{1/2} \qquad (3.10.32)$$

$$\tan \phi_x(t, \mathbf{a}_i) = h_Q(t, \mathbf{a}_{Q,i})/h_I(t, \mathbf{a}_{I,i}) \qquad (3.10.33)$$

where

$$\mathbf{a}_i = \{\mathbf{a}_{I,i}, \mathbf{a}_{Q,i}\} \qquad (3.10.34)$$

The output of the bandpass nonlinearity has, from (3.10.18)–(3.10.20), the complex envelope

$$y(t) = \sum_i b(t - iT, \mathbf{a}_i) \qquad (3.10.35)$$

$$b(t, \mathbf{a}_i) = b_I(t, \mathbf{a}_i) + j b_Q(t, \mathbf{a}_i) \qquad (3.10.36)$$

$$b_I(t, \mathbf{a}_i) = g_c(A_x) h_I(t, \mathbf{a}_{I,i}) - g_s(A_x) h_Q(t, \mathbf{a}_{Q,i}) \qquad (3.10.37)$$

$$b_Q(t, \mathbf{a}_i) = g_c(A_x) h_Q(t, \mathbf{a}_{Q,i}) + g_s(A_x) h_I(t, \mathbf{a}_{I,i}) \qquad (3.10.38)$$

where $A_x$ stands for $A_x(t, \mathbf{a}_i)$.

Note from (3.10.30) and (3.10.31) that if we replace each symbol in $\mathbf{a}_i$ by its complementary value (i.e., $1 \to -1$, $-1 \to 1$), then

$$h_I(t, -\mathbf{a}_{I,i}) = -h_I(t, \mathbf{a}_{I,i}) \tag{3.10.39}$$

$$h_Q(t, -\mathbf{a}_{Q,i}) = -h_Q(t, \mathbf{a}_{Q,i}) \tag{3.10.40}$$

However, $A_x$ in (3.10.32) remains unchanged. Therefore both $g_c(A_x)$ and $g_s(A_x)$ are not affected, and from (3.10.36)–3.10.38)

$$b(t, -\mathbf{a}_i) = -b(t, \mathbf{a}_i) \tag{3.10.41}$$

This implies that the average value is 0

$$m_b(t) = \overline{b(t, a_i)} = 0 \tag{3.10.42}$$

and hence the FT

$$\overline{B(f, \mathbf{a}_i)} = M_b(f) = 0 \tag{3.10.43}$$

In computing the PSD we need the terms

$$S_{b,i}(f) = \overline{B(f, \mathbf{a}_i)B^*(f, \mathbf{a}_0)} \tag{3.10.44}$$

However, since the sets $\mathbf{a}_i$ and $\mathbf{a}_0$ are independent for $|i| \geq K + \varepsilon$, for such $i$

$$S_{b,i}(f) = 0 \tag{3.10.45}$$

We thus obtain from (3.3.21) the PSD

$$TS_y(f) = S_{b,0}(f) + 2 \operatorname{Re} \sum_{i=1}^{K+\varepsilon-1} S_{b,i}(f) \exp(-j\, 2\pi f i T) \tag{3.10.46}$$

In the case of shaping functions of duration 2 $T$ ($K = 2$), we obtain

$$TS_y(f) = S_{b,0}(f) + \begin{cases} 2 \operatorname{Re}\{S_{b,1}(f) \exp(-j\, 2\,\pi f T)\} & \text{QASK} \\ 2 \operatorname{Re}\{S_{b,1}(f) \exp(-j\, 2\,\pi f T) + S_{b,2}(f) \exp(-j\, 4\,\pi f T)\} & \text{OQASK} \end{cases} \tag{3.10.47}$$

### 3.10.3 PSD of hard-limited QASK

In this section we assume that the signal is QASK (hence $\varepsilon = 0$), the nonlinearity is a hard limiter, and the shaping function has duration 2 $T$. We thus obtain from (3.10.20), (3.10.21), (3.10.37), and (3.10.38)

$$b_I(t, \mathbf{a}_i) = \gamma h_I(t, \mathbf{a}_{I,i})/A_x(t, \mathbf{a}_i) \tag{3.10.48}$$

$$b_Q(t, \mathbf{a}_i) = \gamma h_Q(t, \mathbf{a}_{Q,i})/A_x(t, \mathbf{a}_i) \tag{3.10.49}$$

where from (3.10.30)–(3.10.32) and (3.10.28) and $K = 2$, $\varepsilon = 0$

$$h_I(t, \mathbf{a}_{I,i}) = A\{a_{I,i}h_0(t) + a_{I,i-1}h_1(t)\}u_T(t) \tag{3.10.50}$$

$$h_Q(t, \mathbf{a}_{Q,i}) = A\{a_{Q,i}h_0(t) + a_{Q,i-1}h_1(t)\}u_T(t) \tag{3.10.51}$$

$$A_x(t, \mathbf{a}_i) = 2^{1/2}A\{h_0^2(t) + h_1^2(t) + (v_i + w_i)h_0(t)h_I(t)\}^{1/2} \tag{3.10.52}$$

and

$$v_i = a_{I,i}a_{I,i-1} \qquad w_i = a_{Q,i}a_{Q,i-1} \tag{3.10.53}$$

Note that $\{v_i\}$ and $\{w_i\}$ are sequences of independent, equiprobable, binary ($\pm 1$) random variables. $v_i$ and $w_i$ are independent. $v_i$ is also independent of $a_{I,i}$ and $a_{I,i-1}$ when each of them is taken separately, and $w_i$ is independent separately of $a_{Q,i}$ and $a_{Q,i-1}$. These facts have important implications in the computation of the PSD.

When we substitute (3.10.50)–(3.10.52) into (3.10.48) and (3.10.49), we obtain

$$b_I(t, \mathbf{a}_i) = \gamma\, 2^{-1/2}a_{I,i}g(t, v_i, w_i) \tag{3.10.54}$$

$$b_Q(t, \mathbf{a}_i) = \gamma\, 2^{-1/2}a_{Q,i}g(t, w_i, v_i) \tag{3.10.55}$$

where

$$g(t, v_i, w_i) = \frac{h_0(t) + v_ih_1(t)}{\{h_0^2(t) + h_1^2(t) + (v_i + w_i)h_0(t)h_1(t)\}^{1/2}}u_T(t) \tag{3.10.56}$$

Thus

$$g(t, 1, 1) = g(t, -1, -1) = u_T(t) \tag{3.10.57}$$

$$g(t, 1, -1) = (h_0(t) + h_1(t))/\{h_0^2(t) + h_1^2(t)\}^{1/2} \tag{3.10.58}$$

$$g(t, -1, 1) = (h_0(t) - h_1(t))/\{h_0^2(t) + h_1^2(t)\}^{1/2} \tag{3.10.59}$$

with an average value of

$$m_g(t) = 0.5\,\{1 + h_0(t)/(h_0^2(t) + h_1^2(t))^{1/2}\}u_T(t) \tag{3.10.60}$$

The first term in (3.10.47) is from (3.10.36), (3.10.54), and (3.10.55)

$$S_{b,0}(f) = \overline{|B(f, \mathbf{a}_0)|^2} = \overline{\gamma^2/2|a_{I,0}G(f, v_0, w_0) + ja_{Q,0}G(f, w_0, v_0)|^2}$$
$$= \gamma^2\overline{|G(f, v_0, w_0)|^2} \tag{3.10.61}$$

The last equality follows from the fact that the crossterms are zero and the mean square values of $G(f, v_0, w_0)$ and $G(f, w_0, v_0)$ are identical. The crossterms are zero because $a_{I,0}a_{Q,0}$ is independent of $v_0$, $w_0$ and $\overline{a_{I,0}a_{Q,0}} = 0$. The second term in (3.10.47) is

$$S_{b,1}(f) = \overline{B(f, \mathbf{a}_1)B(f, \mathbf{a}_0)} = \overline{\gamma^2 v_1 G(f, v_1, w_1)G^*(f, v_0, w_0)}$$
$$= \gamma^2 \overline{v_0 G(f, v_0, w_0)}\ \overline{G^*(f, v_0, w_0)} \tag{3.10.62}$$

The last equality follows from the independence of $(v_1, w_1)$ and $(v_0, w_0)$ and symbol stationarity. The second equality follows from the fact that the crossterms are zero and the averages of $v_1 g(t, v_1, w_1)$ and $w_1 g(t, w_1, v_1)$ are identical. The crossterms are zero because $a_{I,1}a_{Q,0}$ is independent of $(v_1, w_1, v_0, w_0)$ and $\overline{a_{I,1}a_{Q,0}} = 0$. Let us denote

$$\hat{m}_g(t) = \overline{v_0 g(t, v_0, w_0)} = 0.5\,\{1 + h_1(t)/(h_0^2(t) + h_1^2(t))^{1/2}\}u_T(t) \tag{3.10.63}$$

where the last equality follows from (3.10.56)–(3.10.59). We thus obtain

$$S_{b,1}(f) = \gamma^2 \hat{M}_g(f) M_g^*(f) \tag{3.10.64}$$

When we substitute (3.10.61) and (3.10.64) into (3.10.47), we obtain the PSD

$$S_y(f) = (\gamma^2/T)\{\overline{|G(f, v_0, w_0|^2} + \mathrm{Re}\,\{\hat{M}_g(f)M_g^*(f)\exp(-j\,2\,\pi f T)\}\} \tag{3.10.65}$$

*Example* 3.10.1 PSD of hardlimited QASK with 2-RC shaping function
We assume that the shaping function is the RC of duration 2 $T$, i.e.

$$h(t) = \sin^2(0.5\,\pi t/T)u_{2T}(t) \tag{3.10.66}$$

Hence

$$h_0(t) = \sin^2(0.5\,\pi t/T)u_T(t) \tag{3.10.67}$$

$$h_1(t) = \sin^2(0.5\,\pi(t + T)/T) = \cos^2(0.5\,\pi t/T)u_T(t) \tag{3.10.68}$$

Therefore noting that

$$\sin^4\alpha + \cos^4\alpha = 0.25(3 + \cos^4\alpha) \tag{3.10.69}$$

we obtain

$$g(t, 1, 1) = g(t, -1, -1) = u_T(t) \tag{3.10.70}$$

$$g(t, 1, -1) = 2(3 + \cos(2\pi t/T))^{-1/2} u_T(t) \tag{3.10.71}$$

$$g(t, -1, 1) = -2\cos(\pi t/T)(3 + \cos(2\pi t/T))^{-1/2} u_T(t) \tag{3.10.72}$$

$$m_g(t) = 0.5\{1 + 2\sin^2(0.5\pi t/T)/(3 + \cos(2\pi t/T))^{1/2}\} u_T(t) \tag{3.10.73}$$

$$\hat{m}_g(t) = 0.5\{1 + 2\cos^2(0.5\pi t/T)/(3 + \cos(2\pi t/T))^{1/2}\} u_T(t) \tag{3.10.74}$$

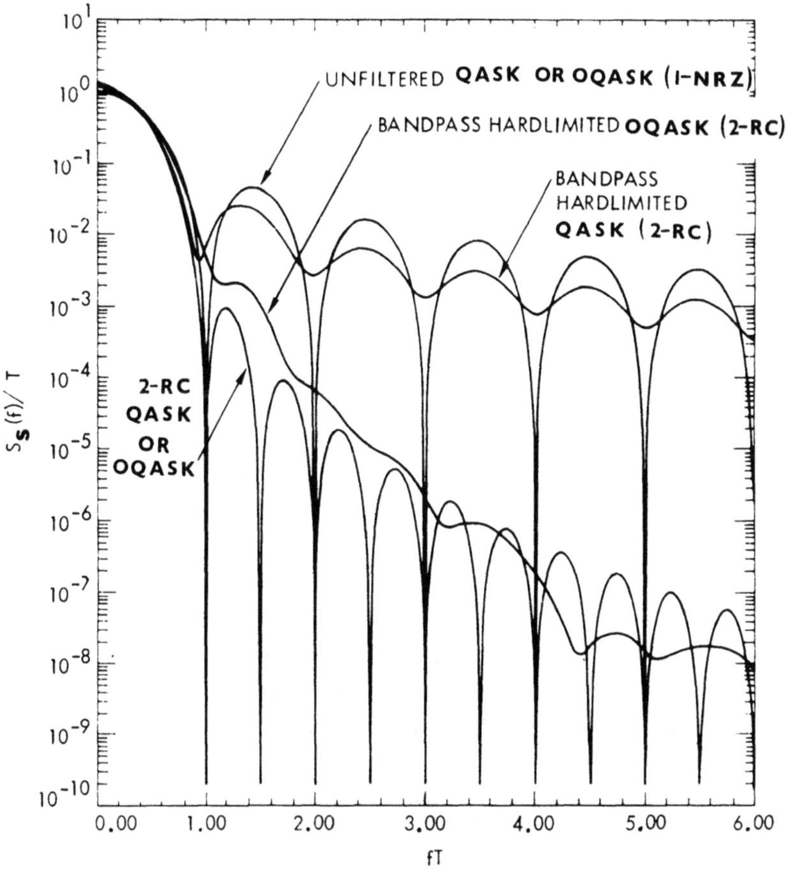


Fig. 3.33. The PSD of QASK and OQASK with NRZ shaping function of duration $T$, with RC shaping function of duration $2T$, and after a bandpass hard limiter operation on the 2-RC signals (D. Divasalar and M. K. Simon, "The Power Spectral Density of Digital Modulation Transmitted over Nonlinear Channels," *IEEE Tr. Comm.*, Vol. COM-30, Jan. 1982, pp. 142–151. Copyright © 1982 IEEE).

It is a curiosity here that

$$M_g^*(f) \exp(-j\,2\,\pi f T) = \int_0^T m_g(t) \exp(j\,2\,\pi f)(t - T)\, dt \qquad (3.10.75)$$

after changing variables $t - T = z$, is equal to

$$\int_0^T m_g(T - z) \exp(-j\,2\,\pi f z)\, dz = \int_0^T \hat{m}_g(z) \exp(-j\,2\,\pi f z)\, dz = \hat{M}_g(f) \qquad (3.10.76)$$

Therefore here, instead of (3.10.65), we have

$$S_y(f) = (\gamma^2/T)\{\overline{|G(f, v_0, w_0)|^2} + \mathrm{Re}\,(\hat{M}_g{}^2(f))\} \qquad (3.10.77)$$

Both $G(f, v_0, w_0)$ and $\hat{M}_g(f)$ are computed here using numerical integeration. In Fig. 3.33 is shown the PSD of QASK with the RC shaping function of duration 2 $T$ with and without a hard limiter. In the same figure is shown QASK with an NRZ shaping function of duration $T$. We may consider the 2-RC QASK as a linearly filtered version of 1-NRZ QASK. Note that the linearly filtered QASK has reduced sidelobes that are almost restored to their original value after the bandpass hard limiter. This implies that there is no sense in filtering a QASK signal to reduce its bandwidth if the signal is applied at a later stage to a hard limiter. This figure is taken from Ref. 3.22, where for the first time the PSD of a signal filtered by a bandpass nonlinearity was obtained analytically.

### 3.10.4 PSD of hard-limited OQASK

In this section we assume that the signal is OQASK (hence $\varepsilon = 1$), the nonlinearity is a hard limter, and the shaping function has duration 2 $T$. We thus obtain $b_I(t, \mathbf{a}_i)$ and $b_Q(t, \mathbf{a}_i)$ as in (3.10.48), (3.10.49), however here from (3.10.30)–(3.10.32) and (3.10.28) with $K = 2$, $\varepsilon = 1$

$$h_I(t, \mathbf{a}_{I,i}) = A\{a_{I,i} h_0(t) + a_{I,i-1} h_1(t)\} u_T(t) \qquad (3.10.78)$$

$$h_Q(t, \mathbf{a}_{Q,i}) = A\{a_{Q,i} h_0(t, 1) + a_{Q,i-1} h_1(t, 1) + a_{Q,i-2} h_2(t, 1)\} \qquad (3.10.79)$$

$$A_x(t, \mathbf{a}_i) = A\{(h_0(t) + v_i h(t))^2 + (h_0(t, 1) + w_i h_1(t, 1) + w_i w_{i-1} h_2(t, 1))^2\}^{1/2} \qquad (3.10.80)$$

where here $\mathbf{a}_i$ denotes the triple

$$\mathbf{a}_i = (v_i, w_i, w_{i-1}) \tag{3.10.81}$$

Denote

$$g_I(t, \mathbf{a}_i) = A\{h_0(t) + v_i h_1(t)\}/A_x(t, \mathbf{a}_i) \tag{3.10.82}$$

$$g_Q(t, \mathbf{a}_i) = A\{h_0(t, 1) + w_i h_1(t, 1) + w_i w_{i-1} h_2(t, 1)\}/A_x(t, \mathbf{a}_i) \tag{3.10.83}$$

then

$$b_I(t, \mathbf{a}_i) = \gamma a_{I,i} g_I(t, \mathbf{a}_i) \tag{3.10.84}$$

$$b_Q(t, \mathbf{a}_i) = \gamma a_{Q,i} g_Q(t, \mathbf{a}_i) \tag{3.10.85}$$

Note that $(a_{I,i}, a_{Q,i})$ is independent of $(v_i, w_i, w_{i-1})$ and $\overline{a_{I,i} a_{Q,i}} = 0$; therefore all crossterms in products

$$S_{b,i}(f) = \overline{\{B_I(f, \mathbf{a}_i) + jB_Q(f, \mathbf{a}_0)\}\{B_I^*(f, \mathbf{a}_0) - jB_q^*(f, \mathbf{a}_0)\}} \tag{3.10.86}$$

are zero. Thus

$$S_{b,0}(f) = \gamma^2\{\overline{|G_I(f, \mathbf{a}_0)|^2} + \overline{|G_Q(f, \mathbf{a}_0)|^2}\} \tag{3.10.87}$$

$$S_{b,1}(f) = \gamma^2\{\overline{v_1 G_I(f, \mathbf{a}_i) G_I^*(f, \mathbf{a}_0)} + \overline{w_1 G_Q(f, \mathbf{a}_1) G_Q^*(f, \mathbf{a}_0)}\} \tag{3.10.88}$$

$$S_{b,2}(f) = \gamma^2\{\overline{v_2 v_1 G_I(f, \mathbf{a}_2) G_I^*(f, \mathbf{a}_0)} + \overline{w_2 w_1 G_Q(f, \mathbf{a}_2) G_Q^*(f, \mathbf{a}_0)}\} \tag{3.10.89}$$

Since $\mathbf{a}_1 = (v_1, w_1, w_0)$ and $\mathbf{a}_0 = (v_0, w_0, w_{-1})$, we cannot separate the terms in (3.10.88) as we have done in (3.10.62). The reason is that $v_1$ is common to $v_I$ and $G_I(f, \mathbf{a}_1)$ and $w_0$ is common to $G_I(f, \mathbf{a}_1)$ and $G_I^*(f, \mathbf{a}_0)$. Similarly $w_1$ is common to $w_1$ and $G_Q(f, \mathbf{a}_1)$ and $w_0$ is common to $G_Q(f, \mathbf{a}_2)$ and $G_Q^*(f, \mathbf{a}_0)$. Since $\mathbf{a}_2 = (v_2, w_2, w_1)$ and $\mathbf{a}_0 = (v_0, w_0, w_{-1})$, $v_1$ can be separated from the other terms in (3.10.89), and since $\overline{v_1} = 0$, the first term in the summation of (3.10.89) is 0. The second term in this summation can be separated into two parts. Hence

$$S_{b,2}(f) = \gamma^2 \, \overline{w_2 w_1 G_Q(f, \mathbf{a}_2)} \; \overline{G_Q(f, \mathbf{a}_0)} \tag{3.10.90}$$

The PSD is found by substitution of (3.10.87), (3.10.88), and (3.10.90) into (3.10.47).

*Example* 3.10.2 PSD of hard-limited OQASK with 2-RC shaping function We assume that the shaping function is the RC of duration 2 $T$ as in the previous example. $h_0(t)$ and $h_1(t)$ are presented in (3.10.67) and (3.10.68), while

$$\begin{aligned} h_0(t, 1) &= \sin^2(0.5\,\pi t/T - \pi/4)u_{Tb}(t - T_b) \\ &= \cos^2(0.5\,\pi t/T + \pi/4)u_{Tb}(t - T_b) \end{aligned} \tag{3.10.91}$$

$$h_1(t, 1) = \sin^2(0.5\,\pi t/T + \pi/4)u_T(t) \tag{3.10.92}$$

$$\begin{aligned} h_2(t, 1) &= \sin^2(0.5\,\pi t/T + \pi + \pi/4)u_T(t) \\ &= \cos^2(0.5\,\pi t/T + \pi/4)u_{Tb}(t) \end{aligned} \tag{3.10.93}$$

where $T = 2\,T_b$.

The PSD for this case has not yet been computed. However, if we consider only the real part of $y(t)$, i.e.

$$y_I(t) = \sum_i b_I(t - iT, \mathbf{a}_i) \tag{3.10.94}$$

then the PSD can be computed if we ignore the terms with the quadrature subscript. The result is

$$S_{yI}(f) = (\gamma^2/T)\{\overline{|G_I(f, \mathbf{a}_0)|^2} + \mathrm{Re}\,\overline{(v_1 G_I(f, \mathbf{a}_1)G_I^*(f, \mathbf{a}_0)}\exp(-j\,2\,\pi f\,T))\} \tag{3.10.95}$$

Using this equation, the PSD of $S_{yI}(f)$ was computed in Ref. 3.22, and the result is presented under the heading OQASK in Fig. 3.33. As can be seen the sidelobes are not restored by the nonlinear operation as in the QASK case. Thus baseband, linear filtering of OQASK signal is an effective means of bandlimiting the PSD, because the bandwidth is not restored subsequently by the nonlinear operation.

## 3.11 FILTER BANDWIDTH FOR DIGITAL RADIO[3.24]

The bandwidth of LSK signals was derived in Section 3.5, and the result was (see eq. (3.5.7))

$$S_s(f) = (A^2\overline{|a_i|^2}/T)|H(f)|^2 = C|H(f)|^2 \tag{3.11.1}$$

where $C$ is a constant. According to FCC regulations,[3.23] the PSD of the transmitted signal must not exceed an emmission mask that depends on the bandwidth and carrier frequencies. The FCC states that outside the authorized channel bandwidth $B_c$, the signal power in an interval $\Delta f$ centered on frequency $f$ must be at least $D(f)$ dB below the total transmitted power. The values of $\Delta f$ and $D(f)$ are

$$\Delta f = \begin{cases} 4 \text{ kHz} & f < 15\text{-GHz bands} \\ 1 \text{ MHz} & f > 15\text{-GHz hand} \end{cases} \tag{3.11.2}$$

$$D(f) = \begin{cases} \text{Max}\,\{-80, \text{Min}\,(-50, (5-10 \log B_c \; - \; 80\,(f/B_c)))\} \\ \qquad\qquad\qquad\qquad\qquad\qquad f < 15\text{-GHz band} \\ \text{Max}\,\{-56, \text{Min}\,(-11, (9-10 \log B_c \; - \; 40\,(f/B_c)))\} \\ \qquad\qquad\qquad\qquad\qquad\qquad f > 15\text{-GHz band} \end{cases} \tag{3.11.3}$$

The function $D(f)$ (called *emission mask*) is shown in Fig. 3.34[3.24] for channel bandwidths of $B_c = 20$, 30, and 40 MHz, which are allocated in the 4, 6, and 11 GHz bands, respectively.

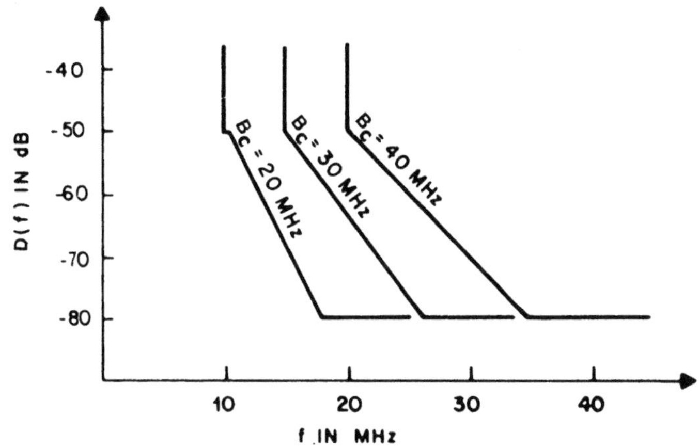


Fig. 3.34. Emission masks of digital radio (L. J. Greenstein and D. Vitello, "Required Transmit Filter Bandwidths in Digital Radio Systems," *IEEE Tr. Comm.*, Vol. COM-29, Sept. 1981, pp. 1405–1408. Copyright © 1981 IEEE).

We assume that the shaping functions are the NRZ, HS, and SFSK, which although mentioned before, are specified again by

$$h(t) = \begin{cases} u_T(t) & \text{NRZ} \\ \sin\,(\pi t/T) u_T(t) & \text{HS} \\ \sin\,\{\pi t/T \; - \; 0.25 \sin\,(4\,\pi t/T)\} & \text{SFSK} \end{cases} \tag{3.11.4}$$

The normalized power of the signal in a bandwidth $\Delta f$ around $f$ is

$$P_s(f, \Delta f) = \int_{f-0.5\Delta f}^{f+0.5\Delta f} |H(f)|^2 \, df/E_H \simeq \Delta f\,|H(f)|^2/E_H \tag{3.11.5}$$

where

$$E_H = \int_{-\infty}^{\infty} |H(f)|^2 \, df \tag{3.11.6}$$

The normalized power will exceed the emission mask, $D(f)$, and hence must be modified before transmission by a filter, which we shall assume to be either a Butterworth or a Chebyshev filter

$$|H_T(f)|^2 = \begin{cases} \{1 + (f/f_0)^{2n}\}^{-1} & \text{Butterworth} \\ \{1 + \varepsilon C_n^2(f/f_0)\}^{-2} & \text{Chebyshev} \end{cases} \tag{3.11.7}$$

Here $C_n(.)$ is an $n$th order Chebyshev polynomial, $f_0$ is the 3-dB bandwidth (one sided) of the Butterworth filter and the ripple bandwidth of the Chebyshev filter (i.e., $f_0$ is the least value of frequency such that for all $f > f_0$ $|H_T(f)|^2 < (1 + \varepsilon^2)^{-1}$). It will be assumed that $n = 4, 6, 8$ for Butterworth filters and $n = 4, 6$ for Chebyshev filters. The ripple factor is assumed to be

$$r = 10 \log (1 + \varepsilon^2) = 0.1, 0.5 \text{ dB}$$

Let $y(t)$ be the modified signal, with normalized power in the bandwidth $\Delta f$

$$P_y(f, \Delta f) \simeq \Delta f \, |H(f)H_T(f)|^2 / E_y(f) \tag{3.11.8}$$

$$E_y(f) = \int_{-\infty}^{\infty} |H(f)H_T(f)|^2 \, df \tag{3.11.9}$$

For each value of $f$ we can find the largest value of $f_0$ such that $P_y(f_0, \Delta f) \leq D(f)$. Such a $f_0$ is called optimal. An emission mask and filtered and unfiltered fractional powers are shown in Fig. 3.35. The values of $f_0 T$ for values of $B_c T$ between 0.8–2.0 and $B_c = 30$ MHz are shown in Table 3.6. For $B_c = 20, 40$ MHz, the values will differ from those in the table by less than 3%. This table is reproduced from Ref. 3.24.

## 3.12 SUMMARY

In this chapter we have presented the PSD of LSK, PSK, FSK, and MSK modulated signals. The PSD and the bandwidth are affected by the duration of the shaping functions, and generally speaking the bandwidth is reduced when the duration is increased. International regulations require efficient use of the available frequency spectrum; hence in designing a digital communic-

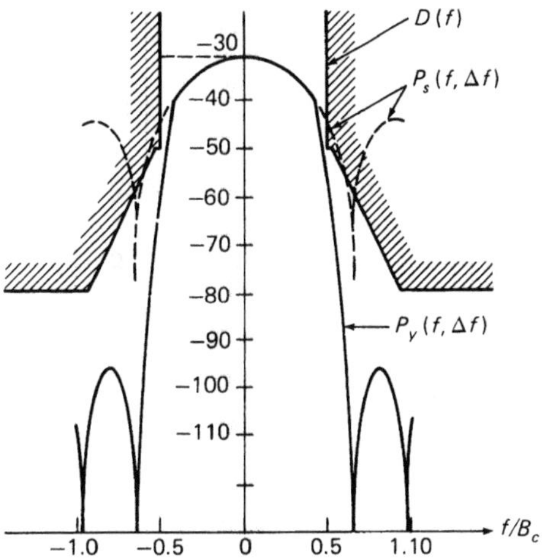


Fig. 3.35. Emission mask, filtered and unfiltered signals.

ation system signals with narrow bandwidth are preferred. A brute force approach in achieving this goal is filtering the signal in order to comply with specified emission masks. The result is a distorted signal that will cause intersymbol interference that degrades the error probability of the system. In addition, the bandwidth may almost be restored to its original value if nonlinear amplifiers are present at later stages of the system. A narrow bandwidth by itself is not the main goal in a system design, rather it is associated with the resulting error probability. We can always achieve a negligible bandwidth if we allow the error probability to be close to 1/M; in fact in this case no communications system is required. The aim is; given an error probability, find a signal with the minimum bandwidth. Constant envelope signals, especially PSK and FSK signals with continuous phase and overlapping shaping functions, show promising results in both these respects. Several papers in the special issue of the IEEE *Transactions on Communication*, vol. COM-29, March 1981, prove this point.

In digital radio and other systems with linear amplifiers, $M$-ary LSK systems ($M$ up to 64 at present) are also both frequency and performance efficient.

In Table 3.7[3.25] we present the bandwidth for various modulated signals with shaping functions of duration $T$. It can be seen that $B_{99}T_b = 1.17$ for binary SSB-ASK, quaternary QASK, and OQASK with HS shaping function and binary MSK with NRZ shaping function. The number is very close to the optimal value for the ASK, which is 1.117. It can be seen from this table that the bandwidth of baseband with NRZ shaping function is 9.65, of LSK is 19.3, and for FSK (with $h = 0.5$) only 1.17. This contradicts our conceptions from analog communication, where the bandwidth of the

**Table 3.6 $f_0T$ for Butterworth and Chebyshev filters for a channel bandwidth of 30 MHz in the 6-GHz band**

| $B_cT$ | NRZ | | | | | | | HS | | | | | | | SFSK | | | | | | |
|---|---|---|---|---|---|---|---|---|---|---|---|---|---|---|---|---|---|---|---|---|---|
| | BUTTERWORTH FILTER | | | CHEBYSHEV FILTER | | | | BUTTERWORTH FILTER | | | CHEBYSHEV FILTER | | | | BUTTERWORTH FILTER | | | CHEBYSHEV FILTER | | | |
| | | | | $r$ = .1 dB | | $r$ = .5 dB | | | | | $r$ = .1 dB | | $r$ = .5 dB | | | | | $r$ = .1 dB | | $r$ = .5 dB | |
| | $n=4$ | $n=6$ | $n=8$ | $n=4$ | $n=6$ | $n=4$ | $n=6$ | $n=4$ | $n=6$ | $n=8$ | $n=4$ | $n=6$ | $n=4$ | $n=6$ | $n=4$ | $n=6$ | $n=8$ | $n=4$ | $n=6$ | $n=4$ | $n=6$ |
| .8 | .26 | .33 | .35 | .27 | .34 | .31 | .36 | .23 | .33 | .34 | .24 | .33 | .29 | .36 | .28 | .38 | .40 | .29 | .38 | .35 | .40 |
| .9 | .32 | .38 | .40 | .31 | .38 | .36 | .41 | .27 | .37 | .39 | .37 | .36 | .34 | .40 | .34 | .43 | .46 | .34 | .43 | .40 | .46 |
| 1.0 | .39 | .43 | .44 | .35 | .43 | .40 | .45 | .31 | .41 | .43 | .32 | .42 | .39 | .45 | .41 | .47 | .49 | .39 | .45 | .45 | .47 |
| 1.1 | .44 | .48 | .50 | .40 | .47 | .45 | .50 | .36 | .46 | .48 | .37 | .46 | .43 | .49 | .45 | .51 | .52 | .42 | .49 | .48 | .51 |
| 1.2 | .50 | .53 | .55 | .44 | .52 | .50 | .55 | .41 | .50 | .53 | .42 | .51 | .48 | .54 | .50 | .55 | .56 | .46 | .53 | .52 | .58 |
| 1.3 | .55 | .59 | .61 | .49 | .57 | .55 | .60 | .48 | .55 | .58 | .46 | .55 | .52 | .59 | .57 | .61 | .62 | .50 | .58 | .56 | .61 |
| 1.4 | .54 | .66 | .67 | .55 | .63 | .61 | .66 | .55 | .60 | .63 | .50 | .60 | .57 | .64 | .65 | .68 | .68 | .56 | .63 | .62 | .66 |
| 1.5 | .56 | .74 | .75 | .57 | .68 | .68 | .72 | .60 | .65 | .68 | .54 | .64 | .62 | .69 | .73 | .78 | .77 | .64 | .70 | .70 | .73 |
| 1.6 | .58 | .78 | .86 | .59 | .76 | .70 | .78 | .66 | .71 | .73 | .59 | .69 | .67 | .74 | .81 | .87 | .89 | .72 | .82 | .81 | .87 |
| 1.7 | .62 | .83 | .96 | .62 | .95 | .75 | 1.03 | .72 | .76 | .79 | .63 | .74 | .72 | .79 | .90 | .93 | .95 | .77 | .87 | .86 | .91 |
| 1.8 | .67 | .89 | 1.01 | .67 | .99 | .80 | 1.06 | .78 | .82 | .84 | .68 | .79 | .77 | .84 | 1.00 | 1.01 | 1.01 | .83 | .91 | .91 | .94 |
| 1.9 | .72 | .95 | 1.05 | .72 | 1.02 | .86 | 1.08 | .86 | .89 | .91 | .74 | .85 | .83 | .89 | 1.11 | 1.12 | 1.13 | .92 | .98 | .97 | 1.00 |
| 2.0 | .80 | 1.00 | 1.09 | .79 | 1.05 | .93 | 1.11 | .95 | .97 | .97 | .80 | .90 | .89 | .95 | 1.16 | 1.33 | 1.43 | 1.00 | 1.20 | 1.08 | 1.07 |

modulated signal cannot be less than the bandwidth of the baseband signal and the bandwidth of a frequency modulated signal is not smaller than the bandwidth of an amplitude modulated signal.

**Table 3.7 Normalised 99% bandwidth ($B_{99} T_b \log_2 M$) of various signals**

| MODULATION TYPE \ SIGNAL SHAPING | | RECTANGLE R | HALF SINE HS | RAISED COSINE RC | TRIANGLE TR |
|---|---|---|---|---|---|
| Baseband and ASK-SSB all $M$ | | 9.65 | 1.17 | 1.43 | 1.33 |
| ASK-DSB all $M$ | | 19.30 | 2.34 | 2.86 | 2.66 |
| QASK, OQASK all | $M \geqq 4$ | 19.30 | 2.34 | 2.86 | 2.66 |
| PSK and DPSK | $M = 2$ | 19.30 | 3.74 | 2.96 | 3.28 |
| PSK and DPSK | $M = 4$ | 19.30 | 3.84 | 4.00 | 3.65 |
| MSK | $M = 2$ | 1.17 | 1.50 | 2.20 | 1.92 |
| MSK | $M = 4$ | 2.52 | – | – | – |

## 3.13 PROBLEMS

3.2

a. Show that if $s(t)$ is a real, wide-sense stationary random process then the autocorrelation is a real and even function of $\tau$, i.e.

$$R_s(\tau) = R_s^*(\tau) = R_s(-\tau)$$

b. Show that if $R_s(\tau)$ is real and even then the PSD, $S_s(f)$ is a real and even function of $f$.

3.3.1 Show that

$$\sum_i \delta(f - k/R) = T \sum_i \exp(-j\, 2\, \pi f i T)$$

where $R = 1/T$.

3.3.2

a. Show that if the symbols are equiprobable

$$\overline{|B(f, a_0)|^2} - |\overline{B(f, a_0)}|^2 = \sum_{i=1}^{M} \sum_{k=1}^{M} \{B(f, a(i)) - B(f, a(k))\}/M^2$$

for $a_0 \in \{a(1), a(2), \ldots, a(M)\}$.

b. Compute the value of part (a) for $M = 2$.

3.3.3 Let

$$S_g(f) = \int_0^T \int_0^T R_g(t, t') \exp(-j\, 2\, \pi f(t - t')\, dt\, dt'$$

a. Show that changing variables $x = t'$, $z = t - t'$ the area of integration has changed from $(0 \leqq t \leqq T, 0 \leqq t' \leqq T)$ to $(-x \leqq z \leqq T - x, 0 \leqq x \leqq T)$ and

$$S_g(f) = \int_0^T \left\{ \int_{-x}^{T-x} R_g(z + x, x) \exp(-2\, \pi f z)\, dz \right.$$

b. Show that by changing the order of integration

$$S_g(f) = \int_0^T \left\{ \int_0^{T-z} R_g(x + z, x)\, dx \right\} \exp(-j\, 2\, \pi f z)\, fz$$

$$+ \int_{-T}^{0} \left\{ \int_{-z}^{T} R_g(z + x, x)\, dx \right\} \exp(-j\, 2\, \pi f z)\, dz$$

c. Change, in the second term of (b), variables $z' = -z$ and then $x' = x - z'$ and obtain

$$\int_0^T \left\{ \int_0^{T-z'} R_g(x', x', + z')\, dx' \right\} \exp(j\, 2\, \pi f z')\, dz'$$

d. Show that if $R_g(x, y) = R_g^*(y, x)$, then

$$S_g(f) = 2 \int_0^T \text{Re} \left\{ \int_0^{T-z} R_g(z + x, x)\, dx \right\} \exp(-j\, 2\, \pi f z)\, dz$$

e. Show that if in addition to (d) $R_g(x, y)$ is real, then

$$S_g(f) = 2 \int_0^T \left\{ \int_0^{T-z} R_g(z + x, x)\, dx \right\} \cos(2\, \pi f z)\, dz$$

3.4.1 Assume independent, equiprobable symbols from the set $\mathring{A}_{\pm} = \{\pm 1, \pm 3, \ldots \pm (M - 1)\}$.

a. Compute the PSD of a baseband signal with NRZ, RZ, HS, RC, and TR shaping functions.

b. Compute the out-of-band power $P_{OB}(B)$, $0 \leqq B \leqq 5\,R$.

3.4.2 Compute the PSD of a baseband signal with common NRZ shaping function and correlated binary symbols with correlation

$$\overline{a_i a_0} = \rho^{|i|}$$

3.4.3 Compute the PSD of a baseband signal with common NRZ shaping function and ternary symbols $a_i = \{0, \pm 1\}$. The ternary symbols are produced from equiprobable binary symbols $b_i = \{\pm 1\}$ by the following rule

$$\text{If } b_i = -1, \text{ then } a_i = 0$$

$$\text{If } b_i = +1, \text{ then } a_i = \pm 1 \text{ alternatively, so that } \sum_{-\infty}^{K} a_i = 0, \pm 1$$

3.4.4 Compute the PSD of a baseband signal with shaping functions

$$h(t, a(i)) = h_1(t - iT/M) \qquad i = 0, 1, \ldots, M - 1$$

$$h_1(t) = \sin(M\pi t/T)u_{T/M}(t)$$

and independent, equiprobable symbols.

3.5.1

a. Show that a 2-RC shaping function is obtained by processing a 1-NRZ shaping function by a linear filter with a 1-HS impulse response.

b. Compute the PSD of OQASK and QASK with 2-RC shaping function and independent, equiprobable symbols from the set $\mathring{A}_{\pm}$.

3.5.2 Let $h(t)$ be the common shaping function of duration $T$, and let $S_h(f)$ be the PSD of an LSK signal with this shaping function and independent, equiprobable symbols from the set $\mathring{A}_{\pm}$. Let

$$g(t) = h(t/K)$$

and let $S_g(f)$ be the PSD assuming this shaping function.

a. Show that $g(t)$ has duration $KT$.

b. Find $S_g(f)$ in terms of $S_h(f)$.

c. Let $B_{h,x}$ and $B_{g,x}$ be the $x$% bandwidth of the signals with shaping functions $h(t)$ and $g(t)$, respectively. Show that $B_{g,x} = B_{h,x}/K$.

d. Comment on the meaning and implications of (c).

3.6 Show that if $h(t)$ of duration $T$ has $N$ continuous derivatives, i.e., $dh^i(t)/dt^i$ is continuous in $0 \leq t \leq T$ for $i = 0, 1, \ldots, N$, then for large frequencies the asymptotic behavior of $H(f)$ is as in eq. (3.6.6).

3.7.1 Show that if

$$b(t) = \exp(ja_0 f(t))$$

and $a_0$ is an equiprobable random symbol from the set $\mathring{A}_{\pm}$, then the average is given by

$$m_b(t) = \sum_{n=0}^{M-1} \exp\{j(2n + 1 - M)f(t)\}/M = \frac{\sin(Mf(t))}{M \sin(f(t))}$$

3.7.2 Compute the PSD of quaternary PSK with HS shaping function of duration $T$.

3.7.3 Compute the PSD of quaternary PSK with RC shaping function of duration $2T$.

3.7.4 Compute the PSD of binary PSK with modified duobinary shaping function.

3.8.1 Compute the PSD of quaternary FSK with HS shaping function. Assume (a) $\beta(T) = 0.5\pi$, (b) $\beta(T) = \pi$.

3.8.2 Compute the PSD of binary FSK with duobinary and 2-RC shaping functions. Assume (a) $\beta(2T) = 0.5\pi$, (b) $\beta(2T) = \pi$.

3.8.3 We are given a summation over two indices

$$y = \sum_{n=0}^{N} \sum_{k=0}^{K} f_k(a_{n-k})$$

so that $0 \leq n \leq N$, $0 \leq k \leq K$.

a. Assume that $N < K$. Change indices $z = n - k$, $k = k$. Show that the summation is over the three domains

| (1) | (2) | (3) |
|---|---|---|
| $-K \leq z \leq N - K$ | $N - K + 1 \leq z \leq 0$ | $1 \leq z \leq N$ |
| $-z \leq k \leq K$ | $-z \leq k \leq N - z$ | $0 \leq k \leq N - z$ |

Sketch these domains.

b. Assume that $N \geqq K$. Change indices as in (a). Show that the three domains now are

| (1) | (2) | (3) |
|---|---|---|
| $-K \leqq z \leqq 0$ | $1 \leqq z \leqq N - K$ | $N - K + 1 \leqq z \leqq N$ |
| $-z \leqq k \leqq K$ | $0 \leqq k \leqq K$ | $0 \leqq k \leqq N - z$ |

Sketch these domains.

3.9.1

a. Show that MSK with shaping functions $h(t, a_0)$, $a_0 \in A_{\pm}$ has an OQASK representation with shaping function as in eq. (3.9.9).

b. Show that the PSD of general MSK has the form of (3.9.7).

c. Show that if (3.9.10) is satisfied, then the PSD has the form of (3.9.11).

3.9.2 Compute the PSD of quaternary MSK with shaping functions as in (3.9.14).

3.9.3 Compute the PSD of quaternary MSK with shaping function as in (3.9.15).

3.10.1

a. Sketch the input-output characteristics for the following nonlinear devices

$$z = \begin{cases} \text{sign } x & \text{Hard limiter} \\ \left.\begin{cases} x & |x| \leqq c \\ c \text{ sign } x & |x| \geqq c \end{cases}\right\} & \text{Clipper} \\ C\{1 - 2\,Q(|x|)\} \text{ sign } x & \text{Soft limiter} \end{cases}$$

and

$$Q(x) = (2\,\pi)^{-1/2} \int_x^\infty \exp\,(-t^2/2)\,dt$$

b. Assume $x = A \cos \theta$. Compute ths AM-AM conversion factor $g(A)$ for these nonlinear devices.

3.10.2 Compute the PSD of QASK with HS shaping function of duration 2 $T$ and hard limiter.

3.10.3 Draw real-time models of the bandpass nonlinearities whose complex models are given in Fig. 3.30.

3.11 Compute the 3-dB bandwidth of a fourth-order Butterworth filter that is required for shaping an LSK signal with NRZ shaping function in order to fit the 30-MHz mask in the 6-GHz band. Assume $B_c T = 1$.

## 3.14 REFERENCES


3.1 V. K. Prabhu, "Spectral Occupancy of Digital Angle Modulation Signals," *BSTJ*, Vol. 59, April 1976, pp. 429–453.

3.2 D. Slepian and H. O. Pollak, "Prolate Spheroidal Wave Functions, Fourier Analysis and Uncertainty, Part 1," *BSTJ*, Vol. 40, Jan. 1961, pp. 43–63.

3.3 H. J. Landau and H. O. Pollak, "Prolate Spheroidal Wave Functions, Fourier Analysis and Uncertaintity, Part 2," *BSTJ*, Vol. 40, Jan 1961, pp. 65–84.

3.4 W. R. Bennett, *Introduction to Signal Transmission*, McGraw-Hill Book Company, New York, 1970, p. 17.

3.5 D. H. Nuttal and F. Amoroso, "Minimum Gabor Bandwidth of M-Orthogonal Signals," *IEEE Tr. Inf. Theory*, Vol. IT-11, July 1965, pp. 440–444.

3.6 V. K. Prabhu and H. E. Rowe, "Spectra of Digital Phase Modulation by Matrix Methods," *BSTJ*, Vol. 53, May–June 1974, pp. 899–935.

3.7 L. J. Greenstein, "Spectra of PSK with Overlapping Baseband Pulses," *IEEE Tr. Comm.*, Vol. COM-25, May 1977, pp. 523–530.

3.8 R. R. Anderson and J. Salz, "Spectra of Digital FM," *BSTJ*, Vol. 44, Jul.–Aug. 1965, pp. 1165–1189.

3.9 T. Tjhung, "Band Occupancy of Digital FM Signals," *IEEE Tr. Comm. Techn.*, Vol. COM-12, Dec. 1964, pp. 211–216.

3.10 H. E. Rowe and V. K. Prabhu, "Power Spectrum of a Digital Frequency Modulation Signal," *BSTJ*, Vol. 54, July–Aug. 1975, pp. 1095–1125.

3.11 F. Amoroso, "The Use of Bandlimited Pulses in MSK Transmission," *IEEE Tr. Comm.*, Vol. COM-27, Oct. 1979, pp. 1616–1623.

3.12 M. C. Austin and M. V. Chang, "Quadrature Overlapped Raised Cosine Modulation," *IEEE Tr. Comm.*, Vol. COM-29, Mar. 1981, pp. 237–249.

3.13 C. Y. Garrison, "A Power Spectral Density Analysis for Digital FM," *IEEE Tr. Comm.*, Vol. COM-23, Nov. 1975, pp. 1228–1243.

3.14 T. Tjeng and T. Tjhung, "Power Spectra and Power Distribution of Random Binary FM Signals with Premodulation Shaping," *Electronic Letters*, Vol. 1, Aug. 1965, pp. 176–178.

3.15 H. J. Von Bayer and T. Tjhung, "Effect of Pulse Shaping on Digital FM Spectra," *Proc. NEC.*, 1965, pp. 363–368.

3.16 M. K. Simon, "A Generalisation of Minimum Shift Keying (MSK)–Type Signalling Based upon Input Data Symbol Pulse Shaping," *IEEE Tr. Comm.*, Vol. COM-24, Aug. 1976, pp. 845–856.

3.17 I. Korn, "Generalised Minimum Shift Keying," *IEEE Tr. Inf. Theory*, Vol, IT-26, Mar. 1980, pp. 234–238.

3.18 D. Muilwijk, "Correlative Phase Shift Keying—A Class of Constant Envelope Modulation Techniques," *IEEE Tr. Comm.*, Vol. COM-29, Mar. 1981, pp. 226–236.

3.19 S. G. Wilson and R. C. Gauss, "Power Spectra of Multi-*h* Phase Codes," *IEEE Tr. Comm.*, Vol. COM-29, March 1981, pp. 250–256.

3.20 T. Aulin, N. Rydbeck, and C. E. W. Sundberg, "Continuous Phase Modulation—Part 2: Partial Response Signalling," *IEEE Tr. Comm.*, Vol. COM-29, Mar. 1981, pp. 210–225.

3.21 A. A. M. Saleh, "Frequency Independent and Frequency Dependent Nonlinear Models of TWT Amplifiers," *IEEE Tr. Comm.*, Vol. COM-29, Nov. 1981, pp. 1715–1720.

3.22 D. Divsalar and M. K. Simon, "The Power Spectral Density of Digital Modulation

Transmitted over Nonlinear Channels," *IEEE Tr. Comm.*, Vol. COM-30, Jan. 1982, pp. 142–151.
3.23 FCC Docket 19311, FCC 74–985, adopted Sept. 19, 1974, released Sept. 27, 1974, revised Jan. 75.
3.24 L. J. Greenstein and D. Vitello, "Required Transmit Filter Bandwidths in Digital Radio Systems," *IEEE Tr. Comm.*, Vol. COM-29, Sept. 1981, pp. 1405–1408.
3.25 I. Korn, "Error Probability and Bandwidth of Digital Modulation," *IEEE Tr. Comm.*, Vol. COM-28, Feb, 1980, pp. 287–290.
3.26 G. L. Pierobon, S. G. Pupolin, G. P. Tronca, "Power spectrum of angle modulated correlated digital signals", *IEEE Tr. Comm.*, Vol. COM-30, Feb 82, pp. 389–396.
3.27 T. Aulin, C. E. Sundberg, "Calculating digital FM spectra by means of autocorrelation", *IEEE Tr. Comm.*, Vol. COM-30, May 82, pp. 1199–1280.
3.28 T. Aulin, C. E. Sundberg, "Exact asymptotic behaviour of digital FM spectra", *IEEE Tr. Comm.*, Vol. COM-30, Nov. 82, pp. 2438–2449.
3.29 T. Aulin, C. E. Sundberg, "An easy way to calculate power spectra for digital FM", *IEE Proc.* part F, Vol. 130, Oct. 83, pp. 519–527.

# 4 ASK BASEBAND SYSTEM

## 4.1 Introduction

A model of an ASK baseband system is presented in Fig. 4.1a and a simplified model in Fig. 4.1b. In this figure $\{a_i\}$ is a sequence of independent $M$-ary symbols from the set $\mathring{A} = \{\pm 1, \pm 3, \ldots \pm (M - 1)\} = \{2m - M - 1, m = 1, \ldots M\}$, generated by a symbol source at the rate of $R = 1/T$ symbols per second (bauds). Thus at time $iT$ the symbol $a_i$ is transmitted in the form of a shaping function $h_S(t - iT)$. $h_S(t)$, $h_T(t)$, $h_C(t)$, $h_R(t)$, and $h_D(t)$ are, respectively, the impulse responses of the shaping filter, transmitter filter, channel filter, receiver filter, and detector filter. The detector filter may represent here an equalizing filter. We assume that all these filters are baseband filters with Fourier transforms (FT), $H_S(f)$, $H_T(f)$, $H_C(f)$, $H_R(f)$, and $H_D(f)$, respectively. To simplify notation, we denote

$$g_C(t) = h_S(t) * h_T(t) * h_C(t) \tag{4.1.1}$$

$$h_{RD}(t) = h_R(t) * h_D(t) \tag{4.1.2}$$

$$g(t) = g_C(t) * h_{RD}(t) \tag{4.1.3}$$

where * denotes convolution, $g_C(t)$ represents all filters in the transmitter and channel, and $h_{RD}(t)$ represents all filters in the receiver. $n_C(t)$ is zero-mean,

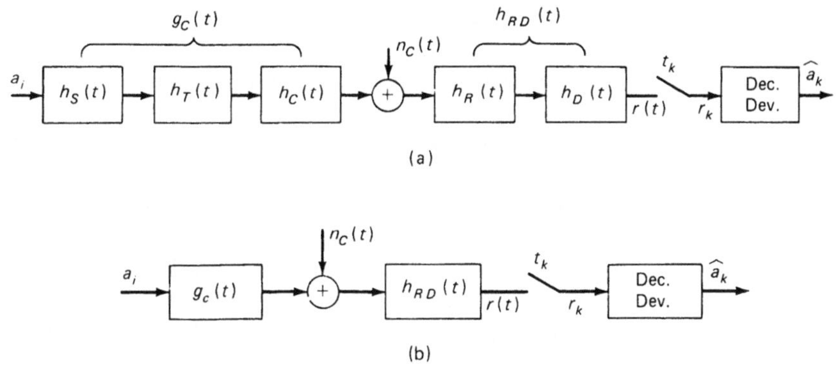


Fig. 4.1. (a) Model of baseband ASK system. (b) Simplified model.

Gaussian, white noise with power spectral density (PSD) $(1/2)N_0$. The output of the detector filter is

$$r(t) = \sum_i a_i g(t - iT) + n(t) \tag{4.1.4}$$

where $n(t)$ is zero mean, Gaussian noise with PSD

$$S_n(f) = 0.5\, N_0 |H_{RD}(f)|^2 \tag{4.1.5}$$

and variance

$$\sigma_n^2 = \int_{-\infty}^{\infty} S_n(f)\, df = 0.5\, N_0 \int_{-\infty}^{\infty} |H_{RD}(f)|^2\, df \tag{4.1.6}$$

and $H_{RD}(f)$ is the FT of $h_{RD}(t)$. Samples are taken at times

$$t_k = t_0 + kT \tag{4.1.7}$$

Thus the input to the decision device is

$$r_k = \sum_i a_i g_{k-i} + n_k \tag{4.1.8}$$

where

$$r_k = r(t_k), \qquad g_k = g(t_k), \qquad n_k = n(t_k) \tag{4.1.9}$$

In a symbol-by-symbol detection method, the decision device produces an estimated value of the symbol $a_k$, denoted by $\hat{a}_k$ from the sample $r_k$, i.e.

$$\hat{a}_k = d(r_k) \tag{4.1.10}$$

which may or not be the same as $a_k$. The probability of symbol error is

$$P(e) = P(\hat{a}_k \neq a_k) \tag{4.1.11}$$

Because an LSK bandpass system can be represented by an equivalent baseband system, many results of the analysis of the ASK baseband system will also be relevant to a bandpass system. In particular, it will be shown that a QASK (and OQASK) system is equivalent to two parallel baseband ASK systems, and most of the analysis will apply to QASK even without modifications. The understanding and analysis of many topics, such as intersymbol interference, equalization, matched filters, and optimal decision regions, are simplified if taken in the context of an ASK baseband system.

This chapter has the following outline. In Section 4.2 we obtain the optimal maximal likelihood decision rule, decision regions, and an expression for error probability. We discuss matched filters and signal-to-noise ratios. In Section 4.3 we present Nyquist conditions of no intersymbol interference and particularly discuss the raised cosine family with excess bandwidth, β, and the spectral efficiency of these signals. Section 4.4 is dedicated to presentation of bounds to error probability in the presence of ISI. In Section 4.5 we compute the error probability of systems with NRZ, HS, and SP shaping functions, Butterworth filters in transmitter and receiver, and various detector filters. In a short section, 4.6, we refer to approximation of raised cosine functions by functions with a finite number of poles, and finally in Section 4.7 we present a brief summary, followed by problems and a list of references.

## 4.2 OPTIMAL DECISION REGION AND ERROR PROBABILITY

### 4.2.1 Maximum likelihood decision rule

We obtain from (4.1.8)

$$r_k = a_k g_0 + \sum_{i \neq k} a_i g_{k-i} + n_K \tag{4.2.1}$$

Only the first term in (4.2.1) carries information about the symbol $a_k$. The second term

$$I = \sum_{i \neq k} a_i g_{k-i} = \sum_i{}' a_{k-i} g_i \tag{4.2.2}$$

is intersymbol interference (ISI), i.e., interference from symbols $\{a_i\}$ $i \neq k$ on $a_k$. In (4.2.2) $\sum'$ denotes a summation with the term $i = 0$ missing. The last term is zero-mean, Gaussian noise with variance, as given in (4.1.6). There is no ISI if

$$g_n = 0 \qquad n \neq 0 \tag{4.2.3}$$

and in this case (4.2.1) is simplified to

$$r_k = a_k g_0 + n_k \tag{4.2.4}$$

We shall derive the decision function $d(r_k)$ for the case of no ISI, but the same rule is used even when ISI is present. We shall use here a maximum likelihood (ML) rule, which does not depend on the symbol probabilities and which minimizes the error probability. This rule is

$$\hat{a}_k = a(m) \text{ if } p(r_k|a_k = a(m)) = \max\{p(r_k|a_k = a(i))\} \qquad i = 1, \ldots, M \tag{4.2.5}$$

and if for a certain value of $r_k$ the maximum is achieved by several $a(i)$ we can arbitrarily select only one of them, say with the lowest value of $i$. For Gaussian, zero-mean noise we obtain from (4.2.4)

$$\begin{aligned} p(r_k|a_k = a(i)) &= p_n(r_k - a(i)g_0) \\ &= (2\pi\sigma_n^2)^{-1/2} \exp\left\{-\frac{1}{2}\frac{(r_k - a(i)g_0)^2}{\sigma_n^2}\right\} \end{aligned} \tag{4.2.6}$$

Hence (4.2.5) implies

$$\hat{a}_k = a(m) \text{ if } \{r_k - a(m)g_0\}^2 = \min\{r_k - a(i)g_0\}^2 \qquad i = 1, \ldots, M \tag{4.2.7}$$

Let us define the decision region

$$DR_m = \{r_k: |r_k - a(m)g_0| = \min\{|r_k - a(i)g_0|\} \qquad i = 1, \ldots, M \tag{4.2.8}$$

i.e., $r_k$ belongs to $DR_M$ if the Euclidian distance between $r_k$ and $a(m)g_0$ is shorter than between $r_k$ and all other points. Thus (4.2.7) implies

$$\hat{a}_k = a(m) \ldots \text{ if } r_k \in DR_m \tag{4.2.9}$$

If a point $r_k$ belongs, according to (4.2.8), simultaneously to two or more sets, we can arbitrarily modify the rule so that it belongs to one set only (say the one with the lowest subscript); however, this is not consequential because the probability that this happens is zero. Thus the real line $DR = \{r_k: -\infty < r_k < \infty\}$ is subdivided into nonoverlapping decision regions such that

$$DR = \bigcup_{m=1}^{M} DR_m \tag{4.2.10}$$

Assuming that

$$-\infty = a(0) < a(1) < a(2) < \ldots < a(M) < a(M+1) = \infty \tag{4.2.11}$$

and there is no loss in generality in this assumption, we obtain from (4.2.8)

$$DR_m = \{d_{m-1} < r_k < d_m\} \tag{4.2.12}$$

where

$$d_m = 0.5\{a(m) + a(m+1)\}g_0 \tag{4.2.13}$$

This is illustrated in Fig. 4.2. The decision function is thus

$$\hat{a}_k = d(r_k) = \begin{cases} a(1) & \text{if } r_k \leqq d_1 \\ a(m) & \text{if } d_{m-1} < r_k \leqq d_m,\ m = 2, \ldots, M-1 \\ a(M) & d_{M-1} < r_k \end{cases} \tag{4.2.14}$$

which is illustrated in Fig. 4.3 for $M = 6$. If the symbol set is such that

$$a(i) - a(i-1) = 2\,d \tag{4.2.15}$$

then we obtain from (4.2.12) and (4.2.13)

$$DR_m = \begin{cases} \{r_k - a(1)g_0 < dg_0\} & m = 1 \\ \{|r_k - a(m)g_0| < dg_0\} & m = 2, \ldots, M-1 \\ \{r_k - a(M)g_0 > -dg_0\} & m = M \end{cases} \tag{4.2.16}$$

The set $\mathring{A}_{\pm}$ satisfies condition (4.2.15) with $a(1) = 1 - M$ and $d = 1$. The decision region for this set and $M = 6$ are shown in Fig. 4.4. The set $\mathring{A}_0 = \{0, 1, \ldots, M-1\}$ also satisfies condition (4.2.15) with $a(1) = 0$, $d = 0.5$. The symbol error probability is given by

$$P(e) = \sum_{m=1}^{M} P(e|m)\,P_m \tag{4.2.17}$$

where the conditional error probability is

$$P(e|m) = P(\hat{a}_k \neq a(m)|a_k = a(m)) \tag{4.2.18}$$

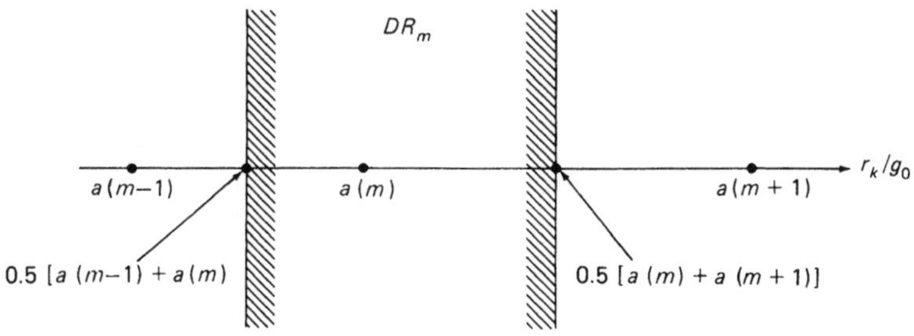


Fig. 4.2. Decision regions for ML decision rule.

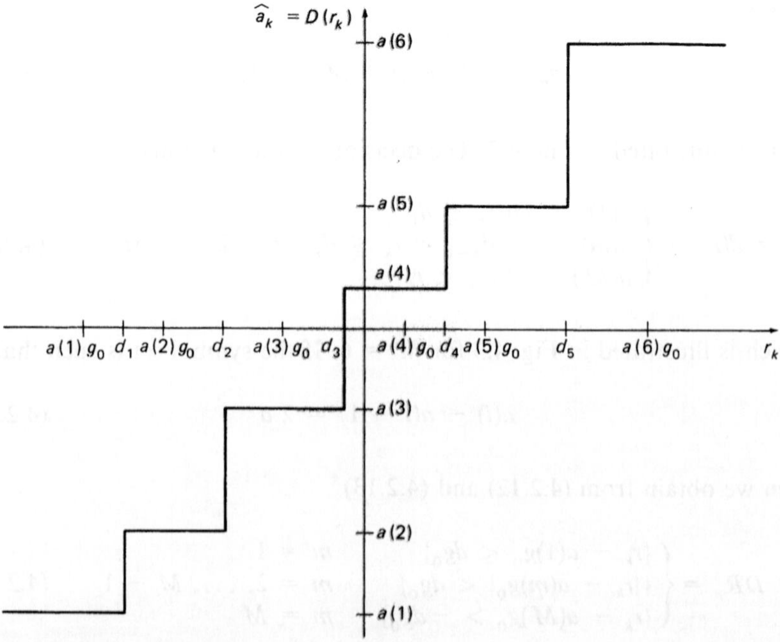


Fig. 4.3. Decision function for ML decision rule.

and we shall assume that

$$P_m = 1/M \tag{4.2.19}$$

An error occurs when $a_k = a(m)$ only if $r_k \notin DR_m$, i.e.

$$P(e|m) = P(r_k \notin DR_m | a_k = a(m)) \tag{4.2.20}$$

and using (4.2.16) we have

$$P(e|m) = \begin{cases} P(r_k - a(1)g_0 > dg_0 | a_k = a(1)) & m = 1 \\ P(|r_k - a(m)g_0| > dg_0 | a_k = a(m)) & m = 2, \ldots, M-1 \\ P(r_k - a(M)g_0 < -dg_0 | a_k = a(M)) & m = M \end{cases} \tag{4.2.21}$$

Using (4.2.4) in (4.2.21) and remembering that the noise is independent of the symbols

$$P(e|m) = \begin{cases} P(n_k \geqq dg_0) & m = 1 \\ P(|n_k| \geqq dg_0) & m = 2, \ldots, M-1 \\ P(n_k \leqq -dg_0) & m = M \end{cases} \tag{4.2.22}$$

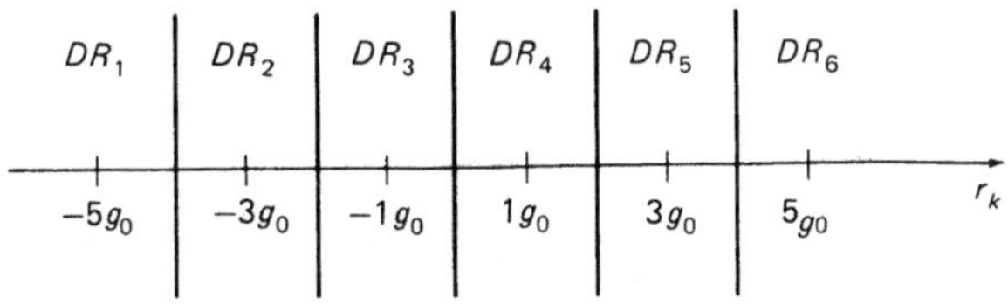


Fig.4.4 Decision regions for symbols from set $\mathring{A}_{\pm}$.

In fact eq. (4.2.22) can be obtained directly by the following simple reasoning. The only reason $r_k$ does not belong to the correct region is due to excessive noise, i.e., the noise $n_k$ drives $r_k$ beyond the decision boundaries. This happens when $|n_k| > dg_0$ for symbols $m = 2, \ldots, M - 1$, $n_k > dg_0$ for $m = 1$ and $n_k < -dg_0$ for $m = M$.

In the binary case, (4.2.16) is simplified to

$$DR_m = \begin{cases} \{r_k - a(1)g_0 < dg_0\} & m = 1 \\ \{r_k - (a(1) + 2\, d_0)g_0 > -dg_0\} & m = 2 \end{cases} \tag{4.2.23}$$

which is the same as

$$DR_m = \begin{cases} \{r_k < dg_0 + a(1)g_0\} & m = 1 \\ \{r_k > dg_0 + a(1)g_0\} & m = 2 \end{cases} \tag{4.2.24}$$

Hence

$$\hat{a}_k = d(r_k) = \begin{cases} a(1) \text{ if } r_k < dg_0 + a(1)g_0 \\ a(2) \text{ if } r_k > dg_0 + a(1)g_0 \end{cases} \tag{4.2.25}$$

If the symbols are $\pm 1$ (i.e., $d = 1$, $a(1) = -1$)

$$\hat{a}_k = \operatorname{sign} r_k \tag{4.2.26}$$

In the binary case, (4.2.22) is also simplified to

$$P(e|m) = \begin{cases} P(n_k \geqq dg_0) & m = 1 \\ P(n_k \leqq -dg_0) & m = 2 \end{cases} \tag{4.2.27}$$

$n_k$, being zero-mean and Gaussian is an even (symmetric) random variable, i.e., for any $C$

$$P(n_k > C) = P(n_k < -C) \tag{4.2.28}$$

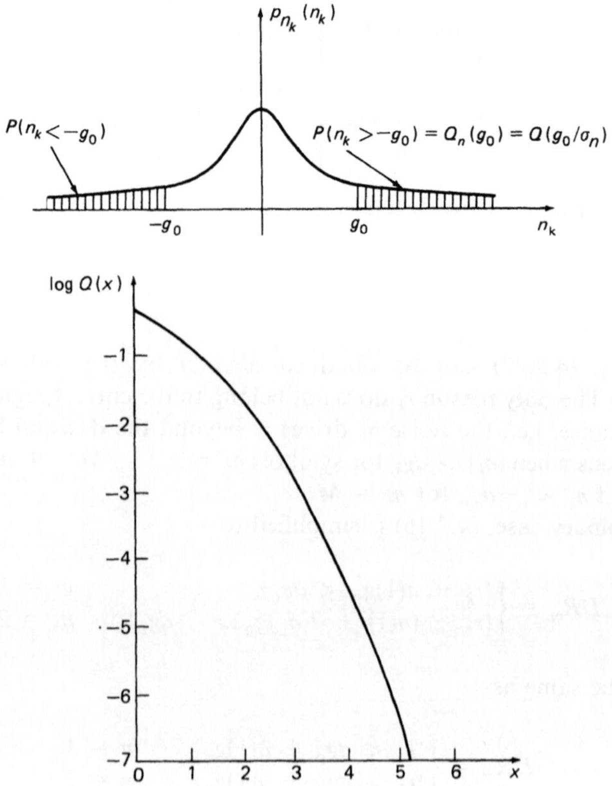


Fig. 4.5. Gaussian probability density and $Q(x)$ function.

Thus we obtain

$$P(n_k < -g_0) = P(n_k > g_0) \tag{4.2.29}$$

$$P(|n_k| > g_0) = 2\,P(n_k > g_0) \tag{4.2.30}$$

where

$$P(n_k > g_0) = \int_{g_0}^{\infty} (2\,\pi\sigma_n^2)^{-1/2} \exp\left(-(1/2)n^2/\sigma_n^{\,2}\right) dn = Q(g_0/\sigma_n) \tag{4.2.31}$$

and $Q(x)$ is the area of the tail of the normal probability density

$$Q(x) = (2\,\pi)^{-1/2} \int_{x}^{\infty} \exp\left(-(1/2)n^2\right) dn \tag{4.2.32}$$

When we substitute (4.2.29)–(4.2.32) into (4.2.17), we obtain

$$P(e) = 2\,(1 - M^{-1})Q(g_0/\sigma_n) \tag{4.2.33}$$

If the noise is not Gaussian, but is a symmetric rv, (4.2.33) is also valid provided we replace $Q(g_0/\sigma_n)$ by

$$Q_n(g_0) = P(n_k > g_0) \tag{4.2.34}$$

In Fig. 4.5 we illustrate the evenness of the Gaussian random variable and the meaning of the $Q(x)$ function. The $Q(x)$ function is related to the $erf(x)$ and $erfc(x)$ functions often mentioned in the literature by

$$erf(x) = 2\,\pi^{-1/2}\int_0^x \exp\,(-n^2)\,dn \tag{4.2.35}$$

$$erfc(x) = 1 - erf(x) \tag{4.2.36}$$

$$Q(x) = \tfrac{1}{2}\,erfc\,(\sqrt{1/2}\,x) \tag{4.2.37}$$

The $Q(x)$ function is presented in Table 4.1. Excellent approximations to $Q(x)$ by simpler functions can be found in Ref. 4.1. The $Q(x)$ function has the following properties, which can be observed from eq. (4.2.32) or Fig. 4.5

1. $Q(-\infty) = 1$, $Q(0) = 0.5$, $Q(\infty) = 0$.
2. $Q(x)$ is a continuous, decreasing function of $x$. It follows from the second property that the error probability in (4.2.33) is minimized if we maximize the ratio $g_0/\sigma_n$. Using the inverse FT we obtain from (4.1.3)

$$\begin{aligned} g_0 &= \int_{-\infty}^{\infty} G(f)\exp\,(j\,2\,\pi f t_0)\,df \\ &= \int_{-\infty}^{\infty} G_C(f)H_{RD}(f)\exp\,(j\,2\,\pi f t_0)\,df \end{aligned} \tag{4.2.38}$$

and using (4.1.6) we obtain

$$g_0/\sigma_n = (\eta\,2\,E_C/N_0)^{0.5} \tag{4.2.39}$$

where $E_C$ is the energy in the function $g_C(t)$, i.e.

$$E_C = \int_{-\infty}^{\infty} |G_C(f)|^2\,df = \int_{-\infty}^{\infty} g_C^2(t)\,dt \tag{4.2.40}$$

and

$$\eta = \left\{ \int_{-\infty}^{\infty} G_C(f) H_{RD}(f) \exp(j\, 2\, \pi f t_0)\, df \right\}^2 \Big/ (E_C E_{RD}) \qquad (4.2.41)$$

where $E_{RD}$ is defined as in (4.2.40) with $G_C(f)$ replaced by $H_{RD}(f)$.

**Table 4.1 The $Q(x)$ function**

| $x = \sqrt{\gamma_b}$ | $E_b/N_o$ (dB) | $\gamma_b = 2\, E_b/N_o$ (dB) | log $Q(x)$ |
|---|---|---|---|
| 1.0000 | −3.0103 | .0000 | −.7995 |
| 1.1000 | −2.1824 | .8279 | −.8675 |
| 1.2000 | −1.4267 | 1.5836 | −.9390 |
| 1.3000 | −.7314 | 2.2789 | −1.0141 |
| 1.4000 | −.0877 | 2.9226 | −1.0928 |
| 1.5000 | .5115 | 3.5218 | −1.1752 |
| 1.6000 | 1.0721 | 4.0824 | −1.2612 |
| 1.7000 | 1.5987 | 4.6090 | −1.3510 |
| 1.8000 | 2.0952 | 5.1055 | −1.4445 |
| 1.9000 | 2.5648 | 5.5751 | −1.5419 |
| 2.0000 | 3.0103 | 6.0206 | −1.6430 |
| 2.1000 | 3.4341 | 6.4444 | −1.7480 |
| 2.2000 | 3.8382 | 6.8485 | −1.8569 |
| 2.3000 | 4.2243 | 7.2346 | −1.9696 |
| 2.4000 | 4.5939 | 7.6042 | −2.0863 |
| 2.5000 | 4.9485 | 7.9588 | −2.2069 |
| 2.6000 | 5.2892 | 8.2995 | −2.3315 |
| 2.7000 | 5.6170 | 8.6273 | −2.4600 |
| 2.8000 | 5.9329 | 8.9432 | −2.5926 |
| 2.9000 | 6.2377 | 9.2480 | −2.7291 |
| 3.0000 | 6.5321 | 9.5424 | −2.8697 |
| 3.1000 | 6.8169 | 9.8272 | −3.0143 |
| 3.2000 | 7.0927 | 10.1030 | −3.1630 |
| 3.3000 | 7.3600 | 10.3703 | −3.3157 |
| 3.4000 | 7.6193 | 10.6296 | −3.4725 |
| 3.5000 | 7.8711 | 10.8814 | −3.6333 |
| 3.6000 | 8.1158 | 11.1261 | −3.7983 |
| 3.7000 | 8.3537 | 11.3640 | −3.9674 |
| 3.8000 | 8.5854 | 11.5957 | −4.1406 |
| 3.9000 | 8.8110 | 11.8213 | −4.3179 |
| 4.0000 | 9.0309 | 12.0412 | −4.4993 |
| 4.1000 | 9.2454 | 12.2557 | −4.6849 |
| 4.2000 | 9.4547 | 12.4650 | −4.8747 |
| 4.3000 | 9.6591 | 12.6694 | −5.0685 |
| 4.4000 | 9.8588 | 12.8691 | −5.2666 |
| 4.5000 | 10.0540 | 13.0643 | −5.4688 |
| 4.6000 | 10.2449 | 13.2552 | −5.6752 |
| 4.7000 | 10.4317 | 13.4420 | −5.8858 |
| 4.8000 | 10.6145 | 13.6248 | −6.1005 |

| | | | |
|---|---|---|---|
| 4.9000 | 10.7936 | 13.8039 | −6.3195 |
| 5.0000 | 10.9691 | 13.9794 | −6.5426 |
| 5.1000 | 11.1411 | 14.1514 | −6.7700 |
| 5.2000 | 11.3098 | 14.3201 | −7.0015 |
| 5.3000 | 11.4752 | 14.4855 | −7.2373 |
| 5.4000 | 11.6376 | 14.6479 | −7.4773 |
| 5.5000 | 11.7970 | 14.8073 | −7.7215 |
| 5.6000 | 11.9535 | 14.9638 | −7.9699 |
| 5.7000 | 12.1072 | 15.1175 | −8.2225 |
| 5.8000 | 12.2583 | 15.2686 | −8.4794 |
| 5.9000 | 12.4067 | 15.4170 | −8.7405 |
| 6.0000 | 12.5527 | 15.5630 | −9.0059 |
| 6.1000 | 12.6963 | 15.7066 | −9.2754 |
| 6.2000 | 12.8375 | 15.8478 | −9.5493 |
| 6.3000 | 12.9765 | 15.9868 | −9.8273 |
| 6.4000 | 13.1133 | 16.1236 | −10.1096 |
| 6.5000 | 13.2480 | 16.2583 | −10.3962 |
| 6.6000 | 13.3806 | 16.3909 | −10.6870 |
| 6.7000 | 13.5112 | 16.5215 | −10.9820 |
| 6.8000 | 13.6399 | 16.6502 | −11.2812 |
| 6.9000 | 13.7667 | 16.7770 | −11.5849 |
| 7.0000 | 13.8917 | 16.9020 | −11.8919 |
| 7.1000 | 14.0149 | 17.0252 | −12.2039 |
| 7.2000 | 14.1363 | 17.1466 | −12.5200 |
| 7.3000 | 14.2562 | 17.2665 | −12.8367 |

### 4.2.2 Matched filters

We obtain from (4.2.39) and (4.2.33)

$$P(e) = 2(1 - 1/M)Q(\sqrt{\eta\, 2\, E_C/N_0}) \tag{4.2.42}$$

To minimize the error probability, we have to maximize $\eta$. From Schwartz's inequality

$$\eta \leq \int_{-\infty}^{\infty} |G_C(f)^2|\, df \int_{-\infty}^{\infty} |H_{RD}(f) \exp(j\, 2\, \pi f t_0)|^2\, df/(E_C E_{RD}) = 1 \tag{4.2.43}$$

with equality if and only if

$$H_{RD}(f) \exp(j\, 2\, \pi f t_0) = K G_C^*(f) \tag{4.2.44}$$

i.e.

$$H_{RD}(f) = K G_C^*(f) \exp(-j\, 2\, \pi f t_0) \tag{4.2.45}$$

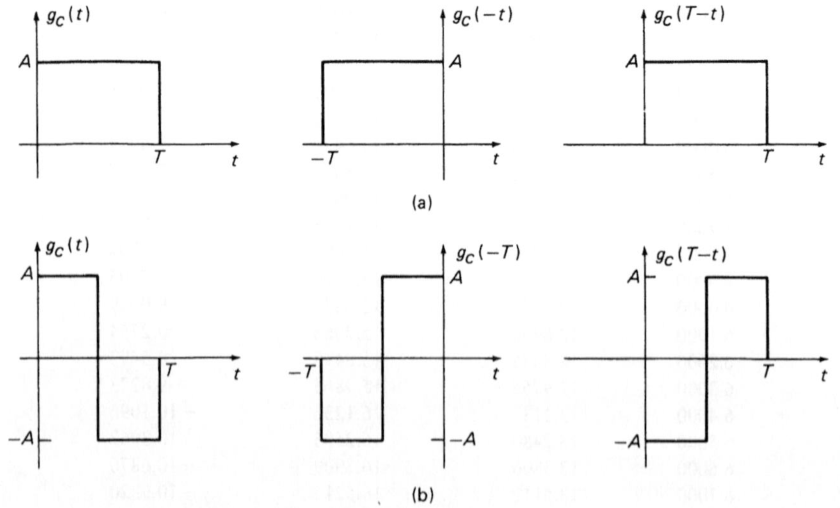


Fig. 4.6. Example of matched filters: (a) NRZ, (b) SP.

or in the time domain

$$h_{RD}(t) = Kg_C(t_0 - t) \tag{4.2.46}$$

where $K$ is an arbitrary constant, which we assume for convenience to be equal to 1.

The receiver filter described by (4.2.45) or (4.2.46) is called a *matched filter* to the signal $g_C(t)$. With a matched filter the symbol error probability is

$$P(e) = 2(1 - 1/M)Q(\sqrt{2\, E_C/N_0}) \tag{4.2.47}$$

With any other filter, the probability of error is larger, and we have to use eq. (4.2.42) with $0 \leq \eta \leq 1$. In order to obtain the matched filter we first take $g_C(t)$ in reversed time, i.e. $g_C(-t)$, and shift the function to the right by $t_0$, i.e., obtain $g_C(-(t - t_0)) = g(t_0 - t)$. This is illustrated for the NRZ and SP functions in Fig. 4.6, where we also assumed that $t_0 = T$. Note that from (4.2.46) we obtain the following properties of matched filters:

a. If $g_C(t)$ has duration $KT$, $h_{RD}(t)$ also has duration $KT$, and $g(t)$ in (4.1.3), being a convolution, has duration 2 $KT$.

b. Assuming $K = 1$ in (a) we obtain explicitly

$$g(t) = \int_{-\infty}^{\infty} h_{RD}(t - \tau)g_C(\tau)\, d\tau = \int_{-\infty}^{\infty} g_C(t_0 - t + \tau)g_C(\tau)\, d\tau \tag{4.2.48}$$

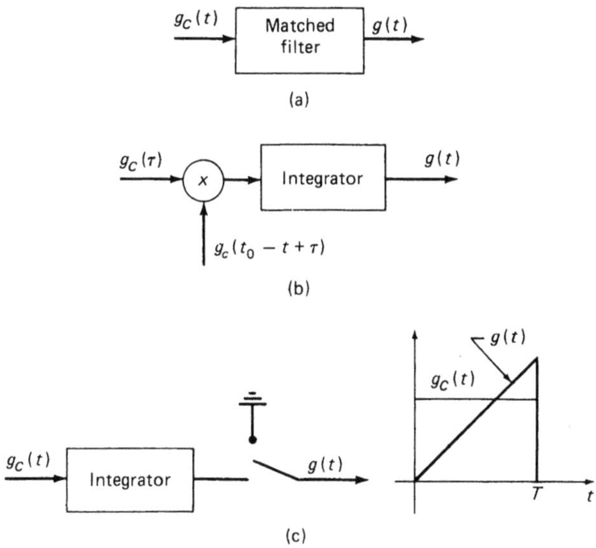


Fig. 4.7. Realization of matched filters: (a) filter, (b) correlator, (c) integrate and dump circuit for NRZ.

The maximal value is obtained at time $t = t_0$ with

$$g(t_0) = g_0 = E_C \tag{4.2.49}$$

and $g(t)$ is zero when $|t_0 - t| > T$. When $g_C(t)$ does not contain impulses, which is normally the case, $g(t)$ is zero for $|t - t_0| \geqq T$; thus $g_i = g(t_0 + iT) = 0$ for all $i \neq 0$, and there is no ISI. The function $g_C(t)$ has duration $T$, if the shaping function has duration $T$, and both $h_T(t)$ and $h_C(t)$ are impulses, i.e., do not distort the shaping function. In other words $H_T(f)$ and $H_C(f)$ must be constant over the range of frequencies for which $H_S(f)$ is not zero.

c. If $t_0 = 0$ and $g_C(t)$ is an even function of time, then

$$h_{RD}(t) = g_C(t) \tag{4.2.50}$$

Equation (4.2.50) is also true for a function $g_C(t)$, which is symmetric around $t_0/2$. The NRZ function in Fig. 4.6 has this property for $t_0 = T$.

d. If $g_C(t)$ is a causal function (i.e., $g_C(t) = 0$ for $t < 0$) and finite duration $KT$, then $H_{RD}(t)$ is causal if $t_0 \geqq KT$.

e. It follows from (4.2.48) that the matched filter can be implemented by a correlator, as shown in Fig. 4.7b. Because, in digital modulation, only the value $g(t_0)$ is of interest, the integrator output can be dumped (i.e., reduced to 0) immediately after $t_0$. Particularly, if $g_C(t)$ is the NRZ function (which is a constant), there is no need for the multiplier, and the integrate and dump circuit for this case is shown in Fig. 4.7c. We also show there the output, which is a ramp function of duration $T$. Without dumping the output, $g(t)$, is a triangle of duration 2 $T$, which coincides with the ramp for $0 \leq t \leq T$.

### 4.2.3 Signal-to-noise ratio

Equations (4.2.42) and (4.2.47) are not yet in their final form. We would like to relate the error probability to the average signal energy at the receiver input. We have shown in Chapter 3 that the average power in the signal

$$s(t) = \sum_i a_i g_C(t - iT) \tag{4.2.51}$$

is

$$P = \overline{a_i^2} E_C / T \tag{4.2.52}$$

and the average energy per symbol in this signal is

$$E_s = PT = \overline{a_i^2} E_C \tag{4.2.53}$$

For the set $\mathring{A}_\pm$ we obtain

$$\overline{a_i^2} = (M^2 - 1)/3 \tag{4.2.54}$$

Hence if the symbols belong to this set the error probability is

$$P(e) = 2(1 - 1/M) Q(\sqrt{\eta (2\, E_s/N_0) 3/(M^2 - 1)}) \tag{4.2.55}$$

For other symbol sets, replace $(M^2 - 1)/3$ by $\overline{a_i^2}$. The rest of this chapter deals mainly with the set $\mathring{A}_\pm$. In Section 4.8 several problems are devoted to other symbol sets.

The term $E_s/N_0$ is the ratio of average symbol energy and noise, or in short the signal-to-noise ratio, which will be denoted by

$$\gamma = 2\, E_s/N_0 \tag{4.2.56}$$

which is usually expressed in decibels (dB), i.e.

$$(\gamma)_{dB} = 10 \log (2\, E_s/N_0) \tag{4.2.57}$$

Because

$$2\, E_s/N_0 = \frac{PT}{N_0/2} = \frac{P}{N} \tag{4.2.58}$$

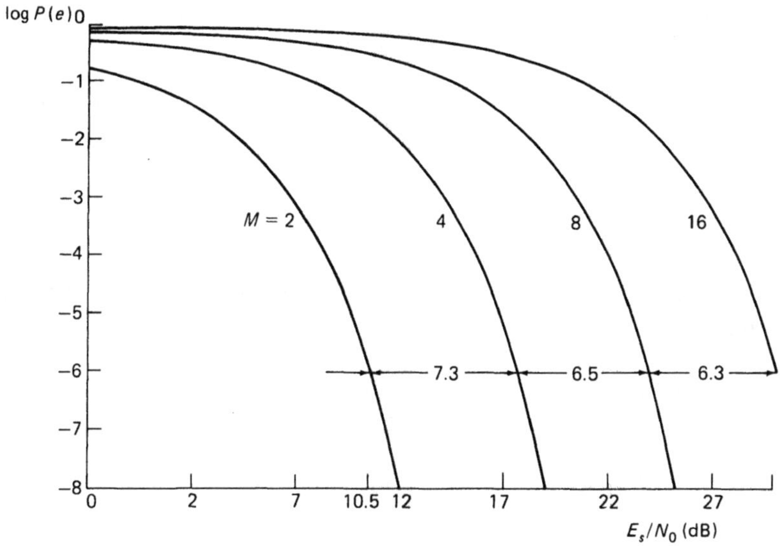


Fig. 4.9. Bit error probability of $M$-ary ASK as a function of signal-to-noise ratio.

where $N$ is the noise power at the output of an ideal filter with bandwidth $1/(2\ T)$ when the input is white noise with PSD $N_0/2$, this term is also the ratio of average signal power to noise power. For the binary case eq. (4.2.55) is simplified to

$$P_b(e) = Q(\sqrt{\eta(2\ E_b/N_0)}) \tag{4.2.59}$$

where the subscript $b$ indicates the binary case, i.e., $P_b(e)$ is the bit error probability or bit error rate (BER), and $E_b$ is the average energy per bit. Equations (4.2.55) and (4.2.59) are shown in Fig. 4.8 for $M = 2, 4, 8$, and 16. Because an $M$-ary symbol represents $\log_2 M$ bits, the average energy per bit is related to the average symbol energy by

$$E_b = E_s/\log_2 M \tag{4.2.60}$$

If we encode sequences of $\log_2 M$, into an $M$-ary symbol using a *Gray code*, symbols $a(m)$ and $a(m + 1)$ differ in one bit only. Gray codes for $M = 4, 8$, and 16 are shown in Table 4.2. Thus if $a(m)$ is in error received as $a(m + 1)$ or $a(m - 1)$, only one out of the $\log_2 M$ bits is in error; hence in this case the bit error probability is

$$P_b(e) = P(e)/\log_2 M \tag{4.2.61}$$

For not too small values of $\gamma$, only such errors will usually occur; hence

(4.2.61) is an excellent approximation to the bit error probability. Combining (4.2.55), (4.2.60), and (4.2.61), we obtain

$$P_b(e) = \{2(1 - 1/M)/\log_2 M)Q(\sqrt{\eta\gamma_b \, 3 \log_2 M/(M^2 - 1)}) \quad (4.2.62)$$

where

$$\gamma_b = 2\, E_b/N_0 \quad (4.2.63)$$

For binary symbols, eq. (4.2.62) is reduced to (4.2.59). Equation (4.2.62) is presented in Fig. 4.9 for $M = 2, 4, 8, 16$, and $\eta = 1$.

**Table 4.2 Gray codes for $M$ = 4, 8, and 16**

| $M$-ARY SYMBOL $a(i)$ | BINARY SEQUENCE | | |
|---|---|---|---|
| $i$ | $M = 4$ | $M = 8$ | $M = 16$ |
| 1 | 00 | 000 | 0000 |
| 2 | 01 | 001 | 0001 |
| 3 | 11 | 011 | 0011 |
| 4 | 10 | 010 | 0010 |
| 5 | | 110 | 0110 |
| 6 | | 111 | 0111 |
| 7 | | 101 | 0101 |
| 8 | | 100 | 0100 |
| 9 | | | 1100 |
| 10 | | | 1101 |
| 11 | | | 1111 |
| 12 | | | 1110 |
| 13 | | | 1010 |
| 14 | | | 1011 |
| 15 | | | 1001 |
| 16 | | | 1000 |

*Example* 4.3.1 Bit rate and signal-to-noise ratio
Compute the signal-to-noise ratio required to achieve a bit error probability of $10^{-6}$ in an $M$-ary ASK system with matched filter and $M = 2, 4, 8$, and 16.

*Solution* From Fig. 4.9 we find $\gamma_b$ = 13.5 dB for $M = 2$, 17.4 dB for $M = 4$, 21.5 dB for $M = 8$, and 26 dB for $M = 16$. As the bit rate in this system is

$$R_b = R \log_2 M$$

the higher bit rate is obtained with a penalty in the required signal-to-noise ratio.

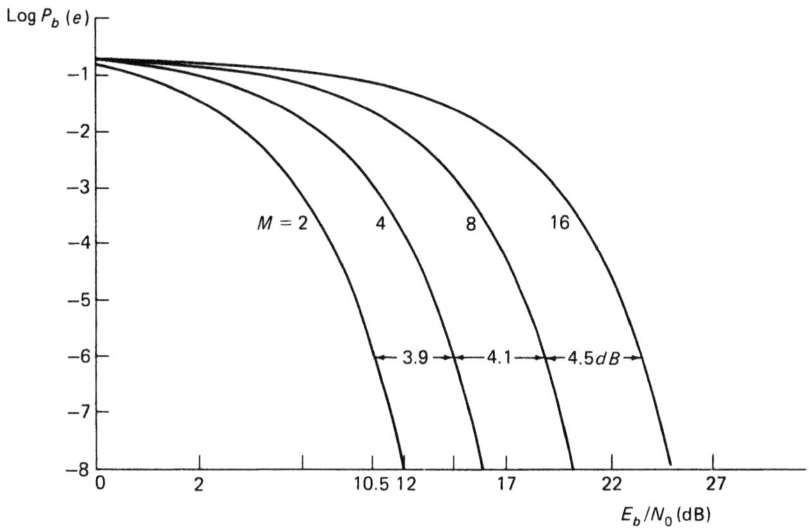


Fig. 4.9. Bit error probability of $M$-ary ASK as a function of signal-to-noise ratio.

## 4.3 NYQUIST CONDITION FOR NO ISI

We have already shown in Section 4.2 that if $g_C(t)$ has duration $T$ and a matched filter is used, then $g(t)$ satisfies eq. (4.2.3) and there is no ISI. However, the PSD of the signal $s(t)$ in (4.2.51) is $a_i^2|G_C(f)|^2/T$, and the bandwidth depends on the form of $G_C(f)$ as explained in Chapter 3. Our aim in this section is to find a function that satisfies eq. (4.2.3) and has the minimum possible bandwidth or is very close to the minimum bandwidth. We also have to establish the value of the minimum bandwidth.

### 4.3.1 Intuitive approach

Intuitively, since we are looking for a function that has a value of 0 at points $iT$, $i \neq 0$, we can start with a sinusoid

$$g(t) = \sin(\pi t/T) \tag{4.3.1}$$

which satisfies eq. (4.2.3); unfortunately, however, $g(0)$ is also 0. We can modify slightly (4.3.1) to obtain

$$g_N(t) = g_0 \sin(\pi t/T)/(\pi t/T) = g_0 \operatorname{sinc}(t/T) \tag{4.3.2}$$

which also satisfies (4.2.3) and $g_N(0) = g_0 \neq 0$. The FT of (4.3.2) is

$$G_N(f) = g_0 T u_R(f + f_N) \tag{4.3.3}$$

where

$$f_N = 1/(2\,T) = R/2 \tag{4.3.4}$$

is called the *Nyquist frequency*, and $u_R(f)$ is a unit value rectangular pulse

$$u_R(f) = \begin{cases} 1 & 0 \leqq f \leqq R \\ 0 & \text{otherwise} \end{cases} \tag{4.3.5}$$

Thus the bandwidth of $g_N(t)$ and therefore also the bandwidth of the signal

$$s(t) = \sum_i a_i g_N(t - iT) \tag{4.3.6}$$

is $f_N$, i.e., half the symbol rate. This bandwidth is related to the bit rate by

$$f_N = R/2 = R_b/\{2 \log_2 M\} \tag{4.3.7}$$

The sinc function is not the only one that satisfies (4.2.3). In fact any function of the form

$$g_N(t) = g_0\, h(t) \operatorname{sinc}(t/T),\ h(0) \neq 0 \tag{4.3.8}$$

also satisfies (4.2.3); however since

$$G_N(f) = H(f) * g_0 T u_R(f + f_N) \tag{4.3.9}$$

the bandwidth of the signal in (4.3.8) will exceed $f_N$. Any function that satisfies eq. (4.2.3) is called here a Nyquist function. We have already specified a whole family of such functions (eq. (4.3.8)), but we have not shown yet that $f_N$ is indeed the minimum possible bandwidth and that (4.3.2) is the only such function with the minimum bandwidth. To do exactly that we need a more rigorous, analytic approach.

### 4.3.2 Analytic approach

The sampled value is given by

$$g_n = \int_{-\infty}^{\infty} G(f) \exp(j\,2\,\pi f n T)\, df \tag{4.3.10}$$

which can also be written as

$$g_n = \sum_{k=-\infty}^{\infty} \int_{-f_N+kR}^{f_N+kR} G(f) \exp(j\,2\,\pi f n T)\, df \tag{4.3.10a}$$

We change variables

$$f' = f - kR$$

so that

$$g_n = \sum_k \int_{-f_N}^{f_N} G(f' + kR) \exp \{j\, 2\, \pi(f' + kR)nT\}\, df' \qquad (4.3.11)$$

Since both $k$ and $n$ are integers

$$\exp (j\, 2\, \pi knRT) = \exp (j\, 2\, \pi kn) = 1 \qquad (4.3.12)$$

Replacing $f'$ by $f$ and changing the order of summation and integration, we obtain from (4.3.11) and (4.3.12)

$$g_n = \int_{-f_N}^{f_N} G_\Sigma(f) \exp (j\, 2\, \pi fnT)\, df \qquad (4.3.13)$$

where

$$G_\Sigma(f) = \sum_k G(f + kR) \qquad (4.3.14)$$

Note that $G_\Sigma(f)$ is a periodic function with period $R$. Note also that $g_n$ is uniquely determined by $G_\Sigma(f)$ in the first period only ($|f| \leqq f_N$) and not by $G(f)$ directly. Many functions $G(f)$ lead to the same $G_\Sigma(f)$, hence the same set $\{g_n\}$. Several such functions, which have a triangular $G_\Sigma(f)$ are shown in Fig. 4.10. From $\{g_n\}$ we can determine $G_\Sigma(f)$, but not $G(f)$. $\{g_n\}$ and $G_\Sigma(f)$ form a Fourier series pair with

$$G_\Sigma(f) = T \sum_i g_n \exp (-j\, 2\, \pi nf/R) \qquad (4.3.15)$$

When $g_n = 0$, $n \neq 0$, we obtain

$$G_\Sigma(f) = g_0 T \qquad (4.3.16)$$

which is the same as (4.3.3) when confined to $|f| \leqq f_N$.

Thus any function $G(f)$ that generates a periodic function $G_\Sigma(f)$ that is a constant $g_0 T$ is a Nyquist function $G_N(f)$. Its main property is

$$G_{N\Sigma}(f) = \sum_k G_N(f + kR) = g_0 T \qquad (4.3.17)$$

We shall consider several Nyquist functions.

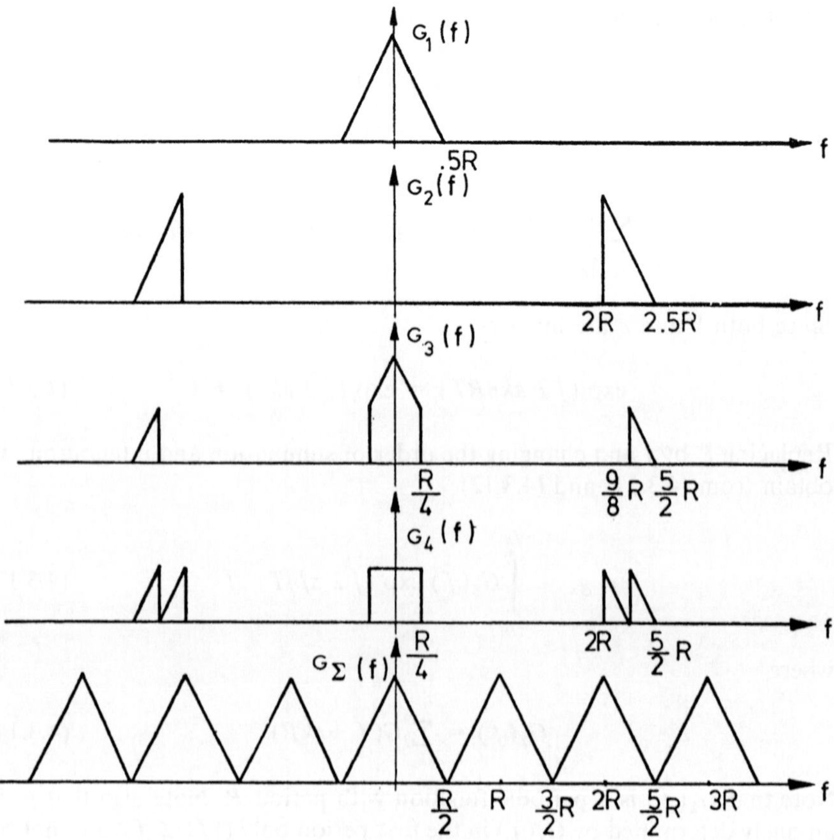


Fig. 4.10. Several functions $G_i(f)$, $i$ = 1, 2, 3, 4, with identical samples $\{g_n\}$.

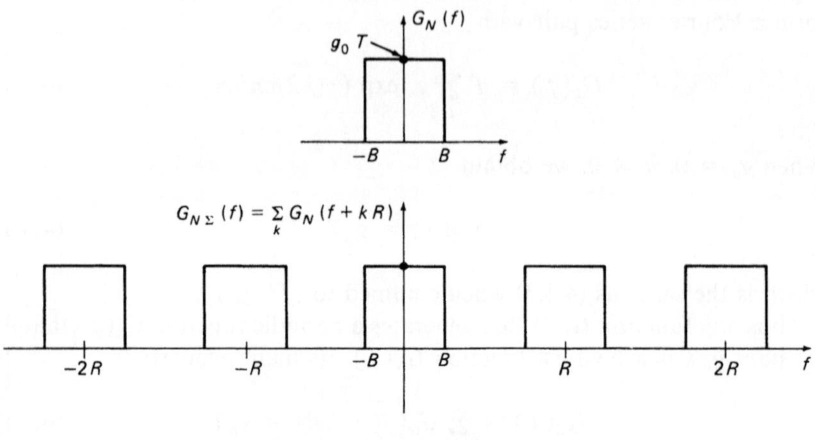


Fig. 4.11. Function with one-half the Nyquist bandwidth.

### 4.3.3 Minimum bandwidth

Let $G_N(f)$ be as in (4.3.3). The terms $\{G_N(f + kR)\}$ do not overlap, and (4.3.17) is satisfied. The bandwidth of this is $f_N$. The bandwidth cannot be less than $f_N$, because if

$$G_N(f) = g_0 T u_{2B}(f + B), \qquad B < f_N \tag{4.3.18}$$

eq. (4.3.17) is not satisfied. This is demonstrated in Fig. 4.11 for $B = f_N/2$. We thus conclude that the minimum bandwidth of signal with no ISI is $f_N$, the Nyquist bandwidth. The function (4.3.1) is the only function that satisfies (4.2.3) and (4.3.17) and has bandwidth $f_N$.

### 4.3.4 Bandwidth not exceeding *R*

Assume that $G_N(f) = 0$ for $|f| \geqq R = 2f_N$. It follows from (4.3.17) that in the first period

$$G_{N\Sigma}(f) = G_N(f + R) + G_N(f) + G_N(f - R) = g_0 T \tag{4.3.19}$$

Because $G_{N\Sigma}(f)$ in (4.3.19) is an even function, it is sufficient to specify its values for $0 \leqq f \leqq f_N$. For such $f$, $G_N(f + R) = 0$; hence

$$G_N(f) + G_N(f - R) = g_0 T \tag{4.3.20}$$

We change variables

$$f = f_N - f' \tag{4.3.21}$$

and write

$$G_N(f) = G_{\text{od}}(f) + 0.5\, g_0 T \tag{4.3.22}$$

so that (4.3.20) is simplified to

$$G_{\text{od}}(f_N - f') + G_{\text{od}}(-f_N - f') = 0 \qquad 0 \leqq f' \leqq f_N \tag{4.3.23}$$

Since $g_N(t)$ is a real function

$$G_{\text{od}}(-f) = G^*_{\text{od}}(f) \tag{4.3.24}$$

and (4.3.23) can be written as

$$G_{\text{od}}(f_N - f') = -G^*_{\text{od}}(f_N + f') \qquad 0 \leqq f' \leqq f_N \tag{4.3.25}$$

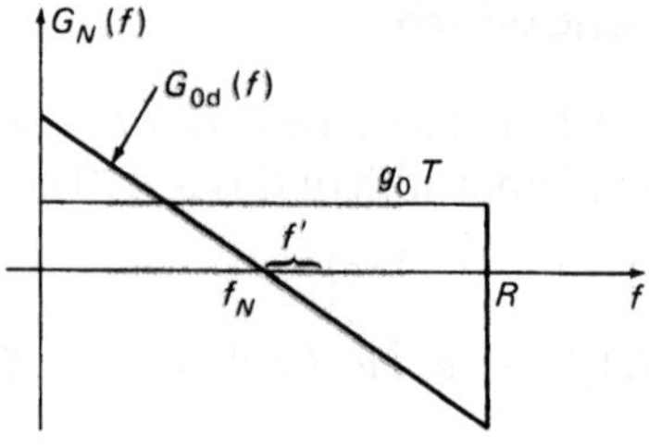


Fig. 4.12. Example of Nyquist function.

with

$$\mathrm{Re}\,\{G_{od}(f_N)\} = 0 \qquad (4.3.26)$$

which means that $G_N(f)$ is composed of a constant ($0.5\,g_0T$) and an odd function around $f_N$. This is illustrated in Fig. 4.12, assuming that $G_{od}(f)$ is real.

### 4.3.5 Raised cosine family

A special but most practical function that satisfies (4.3.19) is the raised cosine family in the frequency domain with parameter β defined by

$$G_N(f) = \begin{cases} g_0T & 0 \leqq |f/f_N| \leqq 1 - \beta \\ g_0T\cos^2\{0.25\,\pi(|f/f_N| - 1 + \beta)/\beta\} & 1 - \beta \leqq |f/f_N| \leqq 1 + \beta \\ 0 & 1 + \beta \leqq |f/f_N| \end{cases} \qquad (4.3.27)$$

The bandwidth of this function is

$$B = f_N(1 + \beta) \qquad (4.3.28)$$

Hence the parameter β is the excess bandwidth beyond the minimal, Nyquist bandwidth and $0 \leqq \beta \leqq 1$. In the time domain

$$g_N(t) = g_0\,\mathrm{sinc}\,(t/T)\cos(\beta\pi t/T)/\{1 - (2\,\beta t/T)^2\} \qquad (4.3.29)$$

$G_N(f)$ and $g_N(t)$ are presented for several values of β in Fig. 4.13. The name *raised cosine* stems from the fact that for $\beta = 1$ (i.e., 100% excess bandwidth)

$$G_N(f) = 0.5\,g_0T\{1 + \cos(\pi|f|/R)\}u_{2R}(f + R) \qquad (4.3.30)$$

which is a raised cosine.

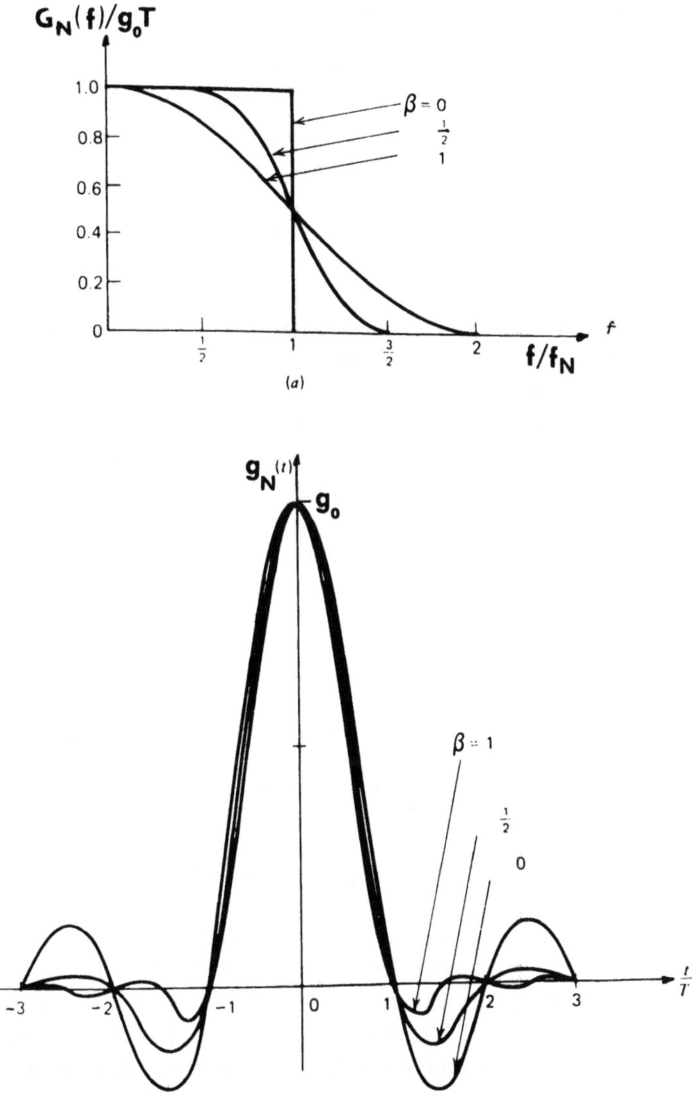


Fig. 4.13. The raised cosine family: (a) in the frequency domain, (b) in the time domain.

## 4.3.6 Spectral efficiency

The bandwidth is related to the bit rate from (4.3.28) and (4.3.7) by

$$B = R_b(1 + \beta)/\{2 \log_2 M\} \tag{4.3.31}$$

Thus, given a certain bandwidth, the possible bit rate, without ISI is given by

$$R_b = 2\ B\ log_2\ M/(1 + \beta) \tag{4.3.32}$$

The spectral efficiency is defined as the number of bits per second (bps) per hertz (Hz), i.e.

$$\eta_B = R_b/B = 2 \log_2 M/(1 + \beta) \text{ bps/Hz} \tag{4.3.33}$$

which is shown in Fig. 4.14.

In practice the value of $\beta$ is limited to $0.25 \leqq \beta \leqq 0.5$. A larger value of $\beta$ is inefficient in the utilization of the available bandwidth, while a smaller value of $\beta$ leads to difficulties in filter realization and to a smaller tolerance to sampling time jitter. The latter statement needs some clarification. The sampling times $\{t_i\}$ are determined by a nonlinear timing synchronization circuit in the receiver. Ideally, $t_i = iT$ for the Nyquist function; however, in practice $t_i = t_0 + iT$ where $t_0$ is an offset or jitter. If we compute now the values of $g_N(t_i)$ from (4.3.29), we obtain

$$g_N(t_i) = g_0 \sin(\pi t_i/T) \frac{\cos(\beta\pi t_i/T)}{(\pi t_i/T)\{1 - (2\ \beta t_i/T)^2\}} \tag{4.3.34}$$

with a maximal value of ISI given by

$$I_{\max} = (M - 1) \sum_i{}' |g_N(t_i)| \tag{4.3.35}$$

which will increase with decreasing values of $\beta$. In fact when $\beta = 0$, $I_{\max} = \infty$.

The system performance is adversely affected by ISI, i.e., the error probability is increased when ISI is increased. We have not yet proved this statement. It will be proved in the next section where the effect of ISI is analyzed and computed. Therefore, we can only state in anticipation of the next section that the quality of the system is inversely related to the value of $I_{\max}$.

*Example* 4.3.2 Bandwidth and bit rate

In a digital communications system the available bandwidth is 40 $M$ Hz. Assume that $0.25 \leqq \beta$ and the required bit rate is 140 $M$ bps. Compute the minimal value of $M$.

*Solution* The spectral efficiency is here

$$\eta_B = 140/40 = 3.5 \text{ bps/Hz}$$

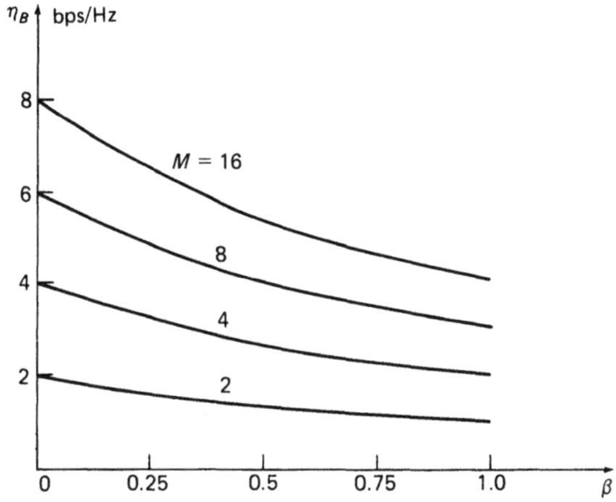


Fig. 4.14. Bandwidth efficiency of $M$-ary ASK system with Nyquist function and excess bandwidth $\beta$.

Using either (4.3.33) or Fig. 4.14, we come to the conclusion that $M = 4$ is not sufficient, but $M = 8$ is sufficient with $0.25 \leqq \beta \leqq 0.7$. In this case, the value $\beta = 0.7$ would have been selected.

All results for the matched filter case of Section 4.2 (i.e., $\eta = 1$) are valid for the system with the Nyquist function (4.3.27), provided $G_C(f)$ and $H_{RD}(f)$ are matched.

Let

$$H_N(f) = \sqrt{G_N(f)} = \begin{cases} \sqrt{g_0 T} & 0 \leqq |f/f_N| \leqq 1 - \beta \\ \sqrt{g_0 T} \cos\{0.25\,\pi(|f/f_N| - 1 + \beta)/\beta\} & 1 - \beta \leqq |f/f_N| \leqq 1 + \beta \\ 0 & 1 + \beta \leqq |f/f_N| \end{cases} \tag{4.3.36}$$

with IFT

$$h_N(t) = 4\,\beta \frac{\cos\{(1 + \beta)\pi t/T\} + \sin\{(1 - \beta)\pi t/T\}(4\,\beta t/T)^{-1}}{(\pi T^{1/2})\{(4\,\beta t/T)^2 - 1\}} \tag{4.3.37}$$

If we let

$$G_C(f) = H_N(f) \tag{4.3.38}$$

and

$$H_{RD}(f) = H_N(f) \exp(-j\,2\,\pi f t_0) \tag{4.3.39}$$

we obtain the matched filter pair as required.

In some papers other filter pairs have been considered, namely

a.
$$G_C(f) = G_N(f) \qquad (4.3.40a)$$

$$H_{RD}(f) = u_{R(1+\beta)}\{f + f_N(1 + \beta)\} \qquad (4.3.40b)$$

b.
$$G_C(f) = u_{R(1+\beta)}\{f + f_N(1 + \beta)\} \qquad (4.3.41a)$$

$$H_{RD}(f) = G_N(f) \exp(-j\,2\,\pi f t_0) \qquad (4.3.41b)$$

In these two cases one of the filters is an ideal lowpass filter with bandwidth $f_N(1 + \beta)$, and the other filter is the Nyquist filter. In both cases we obtain from (4.2.41)

$$\eta = 1/(1 + \beta) \qquad (4.3.42)$$

which is less than 1 for $0 < \beta \leqq 1$.

### 4.3.7 Equalization

In order to obtain (4.3.38), we have, according to (4.1.1)

$$H_S(f)H_T(f)H_C(f) = H_N(f) \qquad (4.3.43)$$

If the channel and shaping functions are given, we design the transmitter filter so that

$$H_T(f) = H_N(f)/\{H_C(f)H_S(f)\} \qquad (4.3.44)$$

In many cases we may assume that the channel does not introduce any distortion, i.e., $H_C(f) = 1$ in the frequency band $|f| \leqq f_N(1 + \beta)$. In many other cases, however, $H_C(f)$ is not known exactly, is varying with time, and also may contain random parameters. For example the telephone channel has this property. Any time a connection between two subscribers is made, a different route in the telephone network is selected with different channel transfer function $H_C(f)$. In these cases we have to abandon condition (4.3.43) and to be satisfied with the overall condition

$$H_{RD}(f) = G_N(f) \exp(-j\,2\,\pi f t_0)/\{H_S(f)H_T(f)H_C(f)\} \qquad (4.3.45)$$

The receiver filter may be composed of a fixed filter and a variable filter, called an *equalizer*, and denoted by $H_E(f)$, i.e.

$$H_{RD}(f) = H_R(f)H_E(f) \tag{4.3.46}$$

(here $H_R(f)$ is in fact $H_R(f)H_D(f)$, i.e., represents all fixed filtering in the receiver) with

$$H_R(f) = G_N(f) \exp(-j\,2\,\pi f t_0)/\{H_S(f)H_T(f)\} \tag{4.3.47}$$

and

$$H_E(f) = 1/H_C(f) \tag{4.3.48}$$

We have dedicated a special chapter in this book to equalization; therefore at this point we state only that the equalizer is automatic and adaptive and is realized by a tapped delay line with variable tap gains.

## 4.4 EFFECT OF ISI

When the interference term in (4.2.2) is nonzero, we have to modify in Section 4.2 the noise term to include $I$, i.e., replace $n_k$ by $n_k + I$. If the symbols belong to a symmetric set (for example, $\mathring{A}_{\pm}$) and the symbols are equiprobable, then $I$ is a symmetric random variable. These conditions are only sufficient conditions for symmetry of $I$; the necessary conditions are weaker. Because $n_k$ is also a symmetric random variable, the sum $n_k + I$ is also such. Assuming that the decision rule remains unchanged when ISI is present, eq. (4.2.33) remains valid, provided we replace $Q(g_0/\sigma_n)$, which is defined in (4.2.31) by $P(n_k + I > g_0)$. Using the properties of conditional random variables, the fact that the noise $n_k$ and the interference $I$ are independent, and the definition of statistical average, we obtain

$$\begin{aligned} P(n_k + I > g_0) &= \int_{-\infty}^{\infty} P(n_k + I > g_0 | I = y)p_I(y)\,dy \\ &= \int_{-\infty}^{\infty} P(n_k > g_0 - y)p_I(y)\,dy = \int_{-\infty}^{\infty} Q\{(g_0 - y)/\sigma_n\}p_I(y)dy \\ &= \overline{Q\{(g_0 - I)/\sigma_n\}} \end{aligned} \tag{4.4.1}$$

where $p_I(y)$ is the probability density of $I$ (which may contain impulses), and the bar denotes the statistical average over $I$. Since $I$ is symmetric we may replace in (4.4.1) $-I$ by $I$. We can also normalize $I$ by $g_0$ and obtain

$$I' = I/g_0 = \sum_i{}' a_{k-i}g_i' \tag{4.4.2}$$

where

$$g_i' = g_i/g_0 \tag{4.4.3}$$

Thus the error probability in the presence of ISI is, from (4.4.1) and (4.2.33)

$$P(e) = 2(1 - 1/M)\overline{Q\{(g_0/\sigma_n)(1 + I')\}} \tag{4.4.4}$$

This equation remains valid for non-Gaussian symmetric noise if we replace the $Q(x)$ function by $Q_n(x)$ as defined in (4.2.34), and the average is over $I'$. Similarly, eqs. (4.2.55) and (4.2.62) are replaced by

$$P(e) = 2(1 - 1/M)\overline{Q\{\sqrt{\eta(2\,E_S/N_0)3/(M^2 - 1)}\,(1 + I')\}} \tag{4.4.5}$$

and

$$P_b(e) = \{2(1 - 1/M)/\log_2 M\}\overline{Q\{\sqrt{\eta\gamma_b 3 \log_2 M/(M^2 - 1)}\,(1 + I')\}} \tag{4.4.6}$$

Before we actually compute the error probabilities we shall state some properties of the interference term $I'$ (or $I$) and obtain some intuitive familiarity.

### 4.4.1 Properties of interference

a. $I$ is a finite or infinite sum of independent random variables if $\{a_i\}$ are independent.

b. We can replace $g_i(g_i')$ by $|g_i|(|g_i'|)$ without affecting the probability distribution of $I(I')$.

c. We can reorder the terms in (4.4.2) without affecting the probability distribution of $I(I')$.

d. Applying (b) and (c) to (4.4.2), we can write

$$I = \sum_{k=1}^{\infty} a_k' h_k,\; I' = \sum_{k=1}^{\infty} a_k' h_k/g_0 \tag{4.4.7}$$

where $\{h_k\}$ is an ordered, according to the rank, nonincreasing sequence (i.e., $h_k \geqq h_{k+1}$) from the set $\{|g_i|, i \neq 0\}$, and $a_k'$ is the corresponding $a_i$.

e. If $\{a_i\}$ are independent, we can set in (4.4.7) $a_k' = a_i$ because the probability distribution is not affected by changing the name of the random variable $a_k'$. If $M = 2^\mu$ and $a_k$ are independent and equiprobable from the set $\mathring{A}_\pm$, we can write

$$a_k = \sum_{j=1}^{\mu} a_{kj} 2^j \tag{4.4.8}$$

where $a_{kj}$ are independent, equiprobable binary ($\pm 1$) random variables. Thus we can rewrite

$$I = \sum_i{}' a_{k-i}g_i = \sum_i{}' \sum_{j=1}^{\mu} a_{kj}(2^j g_i) \qquad (4.4.9)$$

and reorder $I$ so that

$$I = \sum_{k=1}^{\infty} a_k h_k \qquad (4.4.10)$$

with $h_k \geqq h_{k+1}$ from the set $\{|2^j g_i|,\ i \neq 0,\ j = 1, \ldots, m\}$ and $a_k$ are independent binary random variables. It follows that we have to find means to compute the error probability for the binary case only, if $\{a_k\}$ are independent, equiprobable, and from the set $\mathring{A}_{\pm}$. These statements are best clarified by a specific example.

*Example* 4.4.1 Ranking of ISI terms
Let $\{a_i\}$ be independent, and let the values of $\{g_i\}$ be as follows:

$$g_0 = 1,\ g_1 = 0.2,\ g_2 = 0.3,\ g_3 = -0.15,\ g_{-1} = -0.4,\ g_{-2} = 0.1$$

and other values are zero. Taking the absolute value and ranking, we obtain

$$I' = I = \sum_{k=1}^{5} a'_k h_k = \sum_{k=1}^{5} a_k h_k$$

with

$$h_1 = |g'_{-1}| = 0.4,\ h_2 = |g'_2| = 0.3,\ h_3 = |g'_1| = 0.2,$$
$$h_4 = |g'_3| = 0.15,\ h_5 = |g'_{-2}| = 0.1$$

$$a'_1 = a_{k+1},\ a'_2 = a_{-2+k},\ a'_3 = a_{-1+k},\ a'_4 = a_{-3+k},\ a'_5 = a_{2+k}$$

In Fig. 4.15 we show a function $g(t)$ from which these samples $\{g_i\}$ may have been taken.

The interference term (4.4.2) shows the effect of both past symbols $\{a_i,\ i < k\}$ and also future symbols $\{a_i,\ i > k\}$ on the present symbol $a_k$. The fact that past symbols affect the decision about the present symbol is not a great surprise if the system response $g(t)$ has a memory with nonzero values at the sampling times. The fact that future symbols can affect the decision about the present symbol needs an explanation and sounds initially strange. The

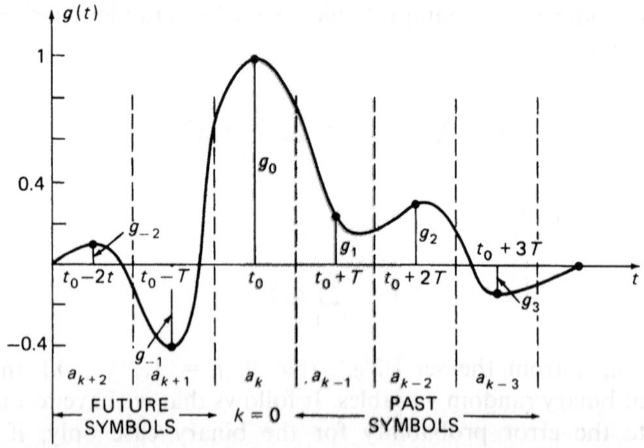


Fig. 4.15. A signal with ISI.

explanation is quite simple. Assume that $g(t)$ is a causal function and the sampling time $t_0$ is $KT < t_0 \leqq (K + 1)T$. That means that when we decide about $a_k$ the symbols $a_{k+1}, \ldots, a_{k+K}$ have already been transmitted and since they are in the system we may expect that they affect the performance. In Fig. 4.15, $2\,T < t_0 < 3\,T$. Hence two future symbols $a_{k+1}$ and $a_{k+2}$ affect the performance through the nonzero values $g_{-1}$ and $g_{-2}$, respectively. If $0 \leqq t_0 \leqq T$, future symbols have no effect on $a_k$, because future symbols have not yet been transmitted. In eq. (4.4.2) the number of past symbols may be infinite, but the number of future symbols is not greater than $K$ if $KT < t_0 \leqq (K + 1)T$ and $g(t)$ is causal.

### 4.4.2 Eye diagram

In practice ISI can be observed on an oscilloscope. If we trigger the oscilloscope at the rate of $R = 1/T$ in synchronization with the symbol and signal rate, the signal

$$s(t) = \sum_i a_i g(t - iT) \tag{4.4.11}$$

will persist on the screen and will collapse into a window of duration $T$, called the eye diagram. This is shown in Fig. 4.16 for a binary signal with no ISI. The eye diagram is completely open, and the signal transition timing is sharp. In Fig. 4.17 the binary signal contains ISI, and the eye diagram is partially closed. The transition region is blurred. The sampling time is selected in the middle of the eye diagram where the margin to noise (which may reduce the eye opening) is largest. The margin to noise is reduced if jitter in the timing circuit will move the sampling time from the middle position. The amplitude

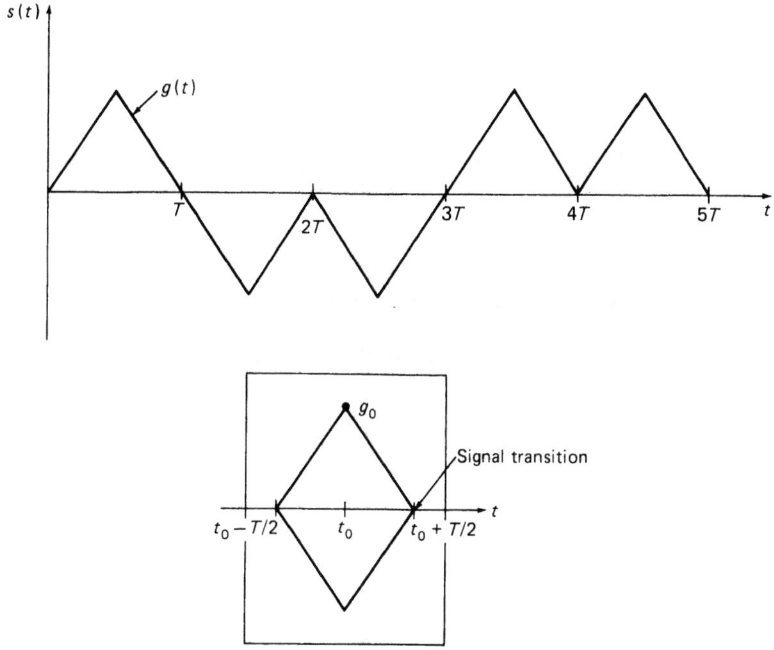


Fig. 4.16. Signal with no ISI and eye diagram.

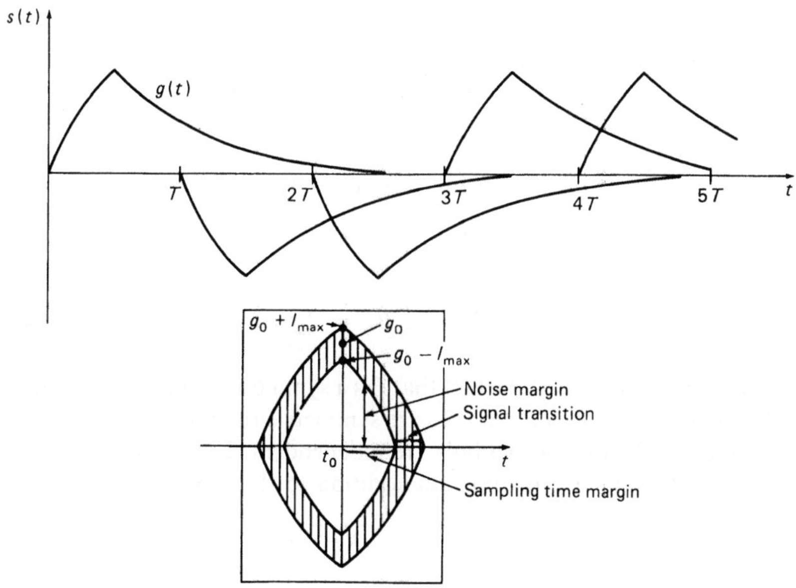


Fig. 4.17. Signal with ISI and eye diagram.

of permissable jitter is also reduced because of the increased signal transition region. Note that when

$$I_{\max} = (M - 1)\sum{}' |g_i| > g_0 \tag{4.4.12}$$

the eye is closed even without noise. In this case errors occur even in the absence of noise. More information about eye diagrams can be found in Ref. 4.2.

### 4.4.3 Computation of error probability

In order to compute the error probability it is essential to compute the value of

$$P = \overline{Q_n(g_0 + I)} = \overline{P(n > g_0 + I)} \tag{4.4.13}$$

which for Gaussian noise is

$$P = \overline{Q\{(g_0 + I)/\sigma_n\}} \tag{4.4.14}$$

Here we wrote $n = n_k$ to simplify the notation. We assume that $I$ has already been reordered according to rank, i.e.

$$I = \sum_{i=1}^{\infty} a_i h_i,\ h_i \geq h_{i+1} \geq 0 \tag{4.4.15}$$

and the symbols are independent and equiprobable from the set $\mathring{A}_{\pm}$. In fact the results are valid for any symmetric set, and the required modification for nonsymmetric sets and not equiprobable symbols, being simple, will not be discussed further.

Let us decompose $I$ into a significant and remainder part

$$I = I_N + R_N \tag{4.4.16}$$

$$I_N = \sum_{1}^{N} a_i h_i,\ R_N = \sum_{N+1}^{\infty} a_i h_i \tag{4.4.17}$$

We have already discussed the fact that $I$ is a symmetric random variable and for the same reason both $I_N$ and $R_N$ are symmetric random variables. $I_N$ and $R_N$ are independent if the symbols are independent. From these statements we have the following properties, in addition to those mentioned before

a. $$\overline{I^{2k+1}} = \overline{I_N^{2k+1}} = \overline{R_N^{2k+1}} = 0 \tag{4.4.18}$$

b. $$\overline{I_N^{2k}} = \overline{(I_{N-1} + a_N h_N)^{2k}} = \sum_{i=0}^{k} \binom{2k}{2i} \overline{I_{N-1}^{2i}}\ \overline{a_N^{2(k-i)}} h_N^{2(k-i)} \tag{4.4.19}$$

where

$$\binom{k}{i} = \frac{k!}{i!(k-i)!} \tag{4.4.20}$$

c. $$\overline{Q_n(g_0 + I)} = \overline{Q_n(g_0 - I)} = 0.5\,\overline{\{Q_n(g_0 + I) + Q_n(g_0 - I)\}} \tag{4.4.21}$$

d. $$-\rho_N \leqq R_N \leqq \rho_N = (M-1)\sum_{N+1}^{\infty} h_i \tag{4.4.22}$$

Equation (4.4.18) states that all odd moments are zero. Equation (4.4.19) shows how to obtain the moments in an iterative way. Equation (4.4.22) states that $R_N$ can be upper bounded by $\rho_N$ and lower bounded by $-\rho_N$ and

$$\lim_{N\to\infty} \rho_N = 0 \tag{4.4.23}$$

for all function $g(t)$ which decay sufficiently with time. In order to compute (4.4.13) we need the probability density of $I$. When the number of interfering terms is infinite, this probability density can be computed in very few cases,[4.3] and even these cases are impractical. For example, if we assume that

$$h_i = h^i,\ h = 2^{-K} \tag{4.4.24}$$

and $K$ is an integer, the probability density can be found. When $h = 1/2$, $I$ is uniformly distributed in $-1$——$1$. When the number of interfering terms is finite, we can compute (4.4.13) exactly, at least in principle, although the computation time may be prohibitive: thus assume that

$$I = I_N,\ R_N = 0 \tag{4.4.25}$$

then

$$P = \overline{Q_n(g_0 + I_N)} = \sum_{j=1}^{L} Q_n(g_0 + I_N|\mathbf{a}_N = \mathbf{a}(j))P(\mathbf{a} = \mathbf{a}(j))$$

$$= \sum_{j=1}^{L} Q_n(g_0 + I_N(j))/L \tag{4.4.26}$$

where

$$\mathbf{a} = \{a_1, a_2, \ldots, a_N\} \tag{4.4.27}$$

$$\mathbf{a}(j) = \{a_1(j), \ldots, a_N(j)\} \tag{4.4.28}$$

$$I_N(j) = \sum_{i=1}^{N} a_i(j)h_i \tag{4.4.29}$$

and

$$L = M^N \tag{4.4.30}$$

$\mathbf{a}(j)$ is the $j$th realization of the sequence $\mathbf{a}$. There are $L$ such sequences, all of which are equiprobable, with probability $1/L$. The meaning of (4.4.29) is best shown by an example.

*Example* 4.4.2 Values of ISI
Find the values of $I_N(j)$ assuming binary symbols ($M = 2$) and three interfering terms $N = 3$.

*Solution* In this case $a_i = \pm 1$ and $L = 8$. The various $I_3(j), j = 1, \ldots, 8$ terms are

$$\begin{aligned}
I_3(1) &= -h_1 - h_2 - h_3 \\
I_3(2) &= -h_1 - h_2 + h_3 \\
I_3(3) &= -h_1 + h_2 - h_3 \\
I_3(4) &= -h_1 + h_2 + h_3 \\
I_3(5) &= \phantom{-}h_1 - h_2 - h_3 \\
I_3(6) &= \phantom{-}h_1 - h_2 + h_3 \\
I_3(7) &= \phantom{-}h_1 + h_2 - h_3 \\
I_3(8) &= \phantom{-}h_1 + h_2 + h_3
\end{aligned}$$

It may happen that two (or more) terms $I_N(j)$ are equal, but this does not affect (4.4.26). So long as $L$ is a manageable integer, say about a million, (4.4.26) can be programmed on a computer, and results may be obtained in a reasonable time. For example, for binary symbols this limits $N$ to 20, for quaternary symbols $N$ is limited to 10, for $M = 8$ $N \leqq 7$, and for $M = 16$ $N \leqq 5$. In most cases the number of significant interfering terms is less than 20, and hence eq. (4.4.27) is very useful in practice at least in the binary case.

If $N$ is too large we have to resort to bounds or approximations to $P$. Many such bounds are available, and we shall state and derive briefly some of them.

**4.4.3.1 Worst-case bound** Because

$$-\rho_0 \leqq I \leqq \rho_0 \tag{4.4.31}$$

and $Q_n(x)$ is a decreasing function of $x$ (this is obvious when the noise is Gaussian, for non-Gaussian noise we assume in addition to symmetry that $p_n(x)$ is a nonincreasing function of $x$ for $x \geqq 0$), we obtain

$$Q_n(g_0 + \rho_0) \leqq Q_n(g_0 + I) \leqq Q_n(g_0 - \rho_0) \tag{4.4.32}$$

Hence from (4.4.13)

$$Q_n(g_0 + \rho_0) \leqq P \leqq Q_n(g_0 - \rho_0) \tag{4.4.33}$$

This case is called the *worst-case bound,* because equality in (4.4.31) happens only if all symbols are either $M - 1$ (upper bound) or $1 - M$ (lower bound), which has a very low probability. In fact in the eye diagram, $I_{\max} = \rho_0$, and this seems to be the only case when this bound is used in practice. Because of the rarity of the event $I = \rho_0$, the eye diagram, although a handy tool in estimating the distortion in the system, is not reliable in the determination of the error probability.

**4.4.3.2 Bounds by finite number of terms**[4.12] Combining (4.4.13), (4.4.17), and (4.4.26), we obtain

$$P = \sum_{j=1}^{L} \overline{Q_n(g_0 + I_N + R_N | \mathbf{a} = \mathbf{a}(j))}/L = \sum_{j=1}^{L} \overline{Q_n(g_0 + I_N(j) + R_N)}/L \tag{4.4.34}$$

and the average is now only over $R_N$. Apply now (4.4.21) with $g_0$ replaced by $g_0 + I_N(j)$ and $I$ replaced by $R_N$ to each term in (4.4.34). Since $Q_n(x)$ is decreasing with $x$ and $R_N$ is bounded by $\rho_N$, we obtain

$$Q_n(g_0 + I_N(j) + \rho_N) \leqq \overline{Q_n(g_0 + I_N(j) + R_N)} \leqq Q_n(g_0 + I_N(j)) \tag{4.4.35}$$

$$Q_n(g_0 + I_N(j)) \leqq \overline{Q_N(g_0 + I_N(j) - R_N)} \leqq Q_n(g_0 + I_N(j) - \rho_N) \tag{4.4.36}$$

This is illustrated in Fig. 4.18. Thus

$$\begin{aligned} P_L &= 0.5\,\{\overline{Q_n(g_0 + I_N)} + \overline{Q_n(g_0 + I_N + \rho_N)}\} \\ &\leqq P \leqq 0.5\,\{\overline{Q_n(g_0 + I_N)} + \overline{Q_n(g_0 + I_N - \rho_N)}\} = P_U \end{aligned} \tag{4.4.37}$$

where the average is now over $I_N$ only and is given in (4.4.26). The difference between the upper and lower bounds

$$\Delta P = P_U - P_L = 0.5\,\{\overline{Q_n(g_0 + I_N - \rho_N)} - \overline{Q_n(g_0 + I_N + \rho_N)}\} \tag{4.4.38}$$

goes to zero because $Q_n(x)$ is a continuous function of $x$ and (4.4.23)

We can slightly improve the lower bound. $Q_n(x)$ is a concave function (i.e., $Q_n(x + a) + Q_n(x - a) \geqq 2\,Q_n(x)$), for all $x > 0$; thus eq. (4.4.21) is bounded below by $Q_n(g_0)$. Hence

$$P_L = \overline{Q_N(g_0 + I_N)} \tag{4.4.39}$$

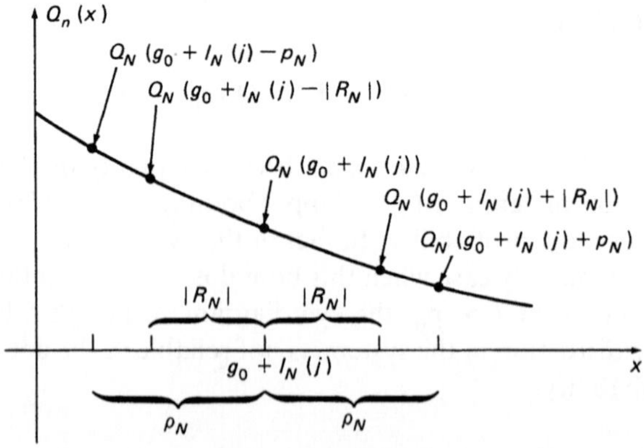


Fig. 4.18. Illustration of bounds (eqs. (4.4.35), (4.4.36)).

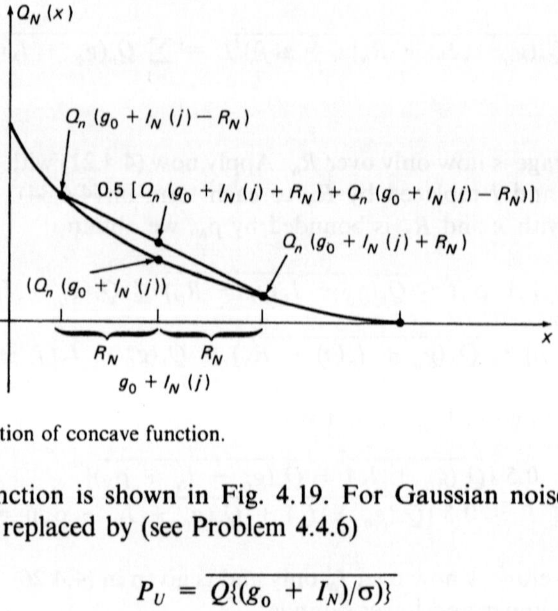


Fig. 4.19. Illustration of concave function.

A concave function is shown in Fig. 4.19. For Gaussian noise the upper bound can be replaced by (see Problem 4.4.6)

$$P_U = \overline{Q\{(g_o + I_N)/\sigma)\}} \tag{4.4.40}$$

where

$$\sigma^2 = \sigma_n^2/\{1 - (\sigma_{RN}/\sigma_n)^2\} \tag{4.4.41}$$

and

$$\sigma_{RN}^2 = \overline{R_N^2} = \overline{a_i^2} \sum_{N+1}^{\infty} h_i^2 < \sigma_n^2 \tag{4.4.42}$$

Equation (4.4.41) can always be satisfied by a proper selection of $N$. Thus for Gaussian noise

$$\overline{Q\{(g_0 + I_N/\sigma_n\}} \leqq P \leqq \overline{Q\{(g_0 + I_N/\sigma\}} \qquad (4.4.37a)$$

**4.4.3.3 Taylor series expansion**[4.5, 4.7–4.10] If the number of terms $L = M^N$ is too large to compute (4.4.26), we expand the function into a Taylor series. In the Gaussian case

$$P = \overline{Q\{(g_0 + I_N)/\sigma_n\}} = Q(g_0/\sigma_n) + \sum_{k=1}^{\infty} P_{2k} \qquad (4.4.43)$$

where

$$P_k = \frac{\overline{I_N^k}}{\sigma_n^k k!} \frac{d^k Q(x)}{dx^k}\bigg|_{x=g_0/\sigma_n} = \frac{\overline{I_N^k} G_a(g_0) H_{k-1}(0.5^{1/2} g_0/\sigma_n)}{k!(2^{1/2}\sigma)^{k-1}} \qquad (4.4.44)$$

$G_a(x)$ is the Gaussian function

$$G_a(x) = (2\,\pi\sigma_n)^{-1/2} \exp\{-(1/2)x^2/\sigma_n^2\} \qquad (4.4.45)$$

and $H_k(x)$ is a Hermite polynomial of order $k$ that satisfy the recursive equation

$$H_{k+1}(x) = -\frac{dH_k(x)}{dx} + 2xH_k(x) \qquad (4.4.46)$$

$$\frac{dH_k(x)}{dx} = 2\,kH_{k-1}(x),\; H_0(x) = 1,\; H_1(x) = 2\,x \qquad (4.4.47)$$

There are no odd terms in (4.4.43) because of (4.4.18). Since[4.4]

$$|H_k(x)| < 2^{k/2+1}(k!)^{1/2} \exp(x^2/2) \qquad (4.4.48)$$

and

$$\overline{I_N^{2k+h}} = \overline{I_N^{2k} I_N^h} \leqq \overline{I_N^{2k}} \rho_{1N}^h \qquad (4.4.49)$$

where

$$\rho_{1N} = (M - 1) \sum_{1}^{N} h_i \qquad (4.4.50)$$

the remainder of the series in (4.4.43) is bounded by[4.10]

$$|T_{2K}| = \left| \sum_{k=K}^{\infty} P_{2k} \right| < G_a(1/2\ g_0)\rho_1^2 \overline{I_N^{2K}}/(A_K B_K) \tag{4.4.51}$$

$$A_K = \sigma_n^{2K+1}(K+1)\sqrt{(2\ K+1)!} \tag{4.4.52}$$

$$B_K = 1 - (\rho_1/\sigma)^2\sqrt{2\ (K+1)(K+3)} > 0 \tag{4.4.53}$$

If we use the bound[4.4]

$$|H_{2k+1}(x)| \leqq |x| \exp\,(x^2/2)(2\ k+2)!/(k+1)! \tag{4.4.54}$$

then

$$|T_{2K}| \leqq g_0 G_a(1/2\ g_0)(\rho_1/\sigma_n)^2 \overline{I_N^{2K}}/(C_K D_K) \tag{4.4.55}$$

where

$$C_K = \sigma_n^{2K}(K+1)! \tag{4.4.56}$$

$$D_K = 1 - (\rho_1/\sigma_n)^2/(K+2) > 0 \tag{4.4.57}$$

Thus we can always find a $K$ such that $|T_{2K}| < \varepsilon$ for any arbitrary $\varepsilon$, and thus (4.4.43) is approximated up to $\varepsilon$ by a final sum

$$P = Q(g_0/\sigma_n) + \sum_{k=1}^{K-1} P_{2K} \tag{4.4.58}$$

with $P_k$ given in (4.4.44). The moments $\overline{I_N^{2k}}$ can be obtained by the method of (4.4.19).

**4.4.3.4 Legendre series expansion[4.12]** The starting point is again (4.4.13) in the form

$$P = (1/2)\{\overline{Q_n(g_0 + I_N)} + \overline{Q_N(g_0 - I_N)}\} = \overline{P(I_N)} \tag{4.4.59}$$

It will be more convenient to normalize the random variable, so that its range lies within $|x| \leqq 1$. To that end we write

$$\begin{aligned} g_0 \pm I_N &= g_0\{1 \pm \sum_{i=1}^{N} a_i h_i/g_0\} \\ &= g_0\{1 \pm (\rho_{1N}/g_0) \sum_{i=1}^{N} a_i h_i/\rho_{1N}\} \end{aligned} \tag{4.4.60}$$

Denote

$$x = \sum_{i=1}^{N} a_i h_i / \rho_{1N} \tag{4.4.61}$$

$$\lambda = \rho_{1N} / g_0 \tag{4.4.62}$$

Thus defining

$$f(x) = 0.5 \{Q_n\{g_0(1 + \lambda x)\} + Q_n\{g_0(1 - \lambda x)\}\} \tag{4.4.63}$$

we have

$$P = \overline{f(x)} = \int_{-1}^{1} f(a) p_x(a)\, da \tag{4.4.64}$$

where $p_x(a)$ is the probability density of the random variable $x$. We note that $f(x)$ is an even function, and hence all odd moments of both $f(x)$ and $x$ are zero.

The Legendre polynomials

$$L_n(x) = (2^n n!)^{-1} \frac{d^n(x^2 - 1)^n}{dx^n}$$

$$= \sum_{k=0}^{n} \iota_k x^k, \quad L_0(x) = 1 \tag{4.4.65}$$

are orthogonal functions, i.e.

$$\int_{-1}^{1} L_n(x) L_m(x)\, dx = \begin{cases} (n + 0.5)^{-1} & m = n \\ 0 & m \neq n \end{cases} \tag{4.4.66}$$

and $\{\iota_k\}$ are its coefficients.

We expand $f(x)$ into a Legendre series (this is the same as a Fourier series, but instead of cosines, sines, or exponentials, we use the Legendre polynomials)

$$f(x) = \sum_{n=0}^{\infty} f_{2n} L_{2n}(x) \tag{4.4.67}$$

with the (Legendre) coefficients obtained from

$$f_{2n} = (2\,n + 0.5) \int_{-1}^{1} L_{2n}(x) f(x)\, dx \tag{4.4.68}$$

we truncate (4.4.67) to $K$ terms, and the remainder is

$$T_K(x) = \sum_{K+1}^{\infty} f_{2n} L_{2n}(x) \tag{4.4.69}$$

Thus

$$P = \sum_{n=0}^{K} f_{2n} \overline{L_{2n}(x)} + \overline{T_K(x)}$$

$$= \sum_{n=0}^{K} f_{2n} \sum_{k=0}^{n} \iota_{2k} \overline{x^{2k}} + \overline{T_K(x)} \tag{4.4.70}$$

We have already dropped here the odd indexed terms in anticipation of $\overline{x^i} = 0$ for $i$ odd. The coefficients $\{\iota_k\}$ are available from (4.4.65). $\overline{x^{2k}}$ can be obtained using the method of (4.4.19). The coefficients $\{f_n\}$ are found from (4.4.68). It can be shown that $T_K(x)$ is bounded by

$$\bar{T}_K(x) < 2 \max_{|x| \leq 1} \left| \frac{d^{K+2} f(x)}{dx^{K+2}} \right| \Big/ (K+2)! \tag{4.4.71}$$

The Legendre series expansions leads to a better approximation of $P$ for the same number of terms $K$ than the Taylor series expansions.

**4.4.3.5 Quadrature formulas**[4.13–4.15, 4.23] We approximate (4.4.63) by a linear combination of values of the function $f(x)$

$$P = \sum_{i=1}^{K} w_i f(x_i) + T_K(x) \tag{4.4.72}$$

The abscissas $\{x_i\}$ and weights $\{w_i\}$ can be obtained from polynomials $\{f_n(x)\}$, which are orthonormal with respect to the probability density $p_x(x)$, i.e.

$$\int_{-1}^{1} f_n(x) f_m(x) p_x(x)\, dx = \begin{cases} 1 & m = n \\ 0 & m \neq 0 \end{cases} \tag{4.4.73}$$

The method is as follows:

1. $\{x_i\}$ are the roots of $f_K(x)$.
2.

$$w_i = -C_{K+1} \left[ C_K f_{K+1}(x_i) \frac{df_K(x_i)}{dx} \right]^{-1} \tag{4.4.74}$$

where $C_K$ is the highest coefficient of polynomial $f_K(x)$, i.e.

$$f_K(x) = C_K x^K + \ldots \tag{4.4.75}$$

With this relation the remainder is

$$T_K(x) = \left[C_K^2(2\,K)!\right]^{-1} \frac{d^{2K}f(x)}{dx^{2K}} \tag{4.4.76}$$

Note that the remainder is zero if $f(x)$ is a polynomial of degree less then 2 $K$. Thus the main problem is to find the polynomial, especially since $p_x(x)$ is not known. It is known, however that the polynomials satisfy the recursive equation

$$xf_{n-1}(x) = \beta_{n-1}f_{n-2}(x) + \alpha_n f_{n-1}(x) + \beta_n f_n(x) \tag{4.4.77}$$

with

$$f_{-1}(x) = 0, \qquad f_0(x) = 1$$

Thus the problem is to find the coefficients $\{\alpha_n, \beta_n\}$. These are found from the moments of

$$\overline{x^k} = \overline{I_N^k}/\rho_{1N}^k \tag{4.4.78}$$

as follows:

3. Compute

$$\left.\begin{aligned} r_{i,i} &= \left(x^{2(i-1)} - \sum_{k=1}^{i-1} r_{k,i}\right)^{1/2} \\ r_{i,j} &= \left(x^{i+j-2} - \sum_{k=1}^{i-1} r_{k,i}r_{k,j}\right) \Big/ r_{i,i} \end{aligned}\right. \qquad 1 \leqq i \leqq j \leqq K+1 \tag{4.4.79}$$

4. Compute

$$\begin{cases} \alpha_j = r_{j,j+1}/r_{j,j} - r_{j-1,j}/r_{j-1,j-1} & j = 1, 2, \ldots, K \\ \beta_j = r_{j+1,j+1}/r_{j,j},\ r_{0,0} = 1,\ r_{0,1} = 0 & j = 1, 2, \ldots, K-1 \end{cases} \tag{4.4.80}$$

Now we can apply steps (1) and (2) to find $\{x_i\}$ and $\{w_i\}$. Alternatively, we can write the Jacobian matrix

$$J = \begin{pmatrix} \alpha_1 & \beta_1 & 0 & \cdots & 0 & 0 \\ \beta_1 & \alpha_2 & \ddots & & & \\ 0 & \ddots & \ddots & \ddots & & 0 \\ & & & & & \\ 0 & & & & \alpha_{K-1} & \beta_{K-1} \\ 0 & \cdots & & 0 & \alpha_{K-1} & \alpha_K \end{pmatrix} \tag{4.4.81}$$

The eigenvalues of $J$ are the abscissas $\{x_i\}$, and the squares of the first component of the eigenvectors are the weights $\{w_i\}$. For those who do not remember the meaning of these terms the following is sufficient.

A vector $\mathbf{v} = (v_1, v_2, \ldots, v_k)^T$ is an eigenvector of the matrix $J$, and $\lambda$ is an eigenvalue of the eigenvector if

$$J\mathbf{v} = \lambda\mathbf{v} \tag{4.4.82}$$

For a Gaussian noise the error term can be bounded by

$$|T_K(x)| \leq \begin{cases} E_K \exp\{-0.25\,(g_0/\rho_{IN} - 1)^2/\sigma_n^2\} & g_0 > \rho_{IN} \\ E_K & g_0 < \rho_{IN} \end{cases} \tag{4.4.83}$$

where

$$E_K = \{\sqrt{\pi K}(2\,K)!\; C_K^2 \sigma^{2K}\}^{-1} \tag{4.4.84}$$

**4.4.3.6 Bounds to probability densities**[4.20–4.23] Let $p_L(x)$ and $p_U(x)$ be probability densities such that

$$P_L = \int_{-\rho}^{\rho} P(I) p_L(I)\, dI \leq P \leq \int_{-\rho}^{\rho} P(I) p_U(I)\, dI = P_U \tag{4.4.85}$$

and the second moment is preserved, i.e.

$$\int_{-\rho}^{\rho} I^2 p_L(I)\, dI = \int_{-\rho}^{\rho} I^2 p_U(I)\, dI = \overline{I^2} = \sigma_I^2 \tag{4.4.86}$$

Indeed such probability densities can be found, and they depend on the relation between $\sigma_n$, $g_0$, $\rho_1$, and $\sigma_I$. For a certain set of these values,[4.2.1] the result is

$$P(\sigma_I) \leq P \leq \{1 - (\sigma_I/\rho_1)^2\} P(0) + (\sigma_I/\rho_1)^2 P(\rho_1) \tag{4.4.87}$$

Further improvements to these bounds can be found in Ref. 4.22.

**4.4.3.7 Chernoff bound**[4.16] According to (4.4.13) and (4.4.21), we have to compute

$$P = P(I + n > g_0) \tag{4.4.88}$$

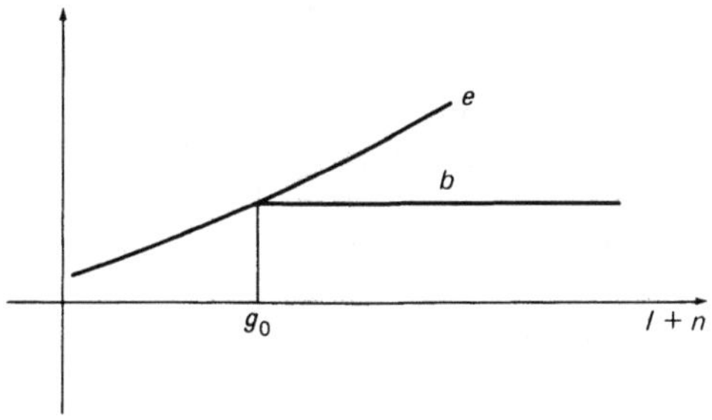


Fig. 4.20. Illustration of Chernoff bound.

Let us define two random variables, a binary random variable, $b$

$$b = u(I + n - g_0) = \begin{cases} 1 & I + n \geqq g_0 \\ 0 & I + n < g_0 \end{cases} \quad (4.4.89)$$

and an exponential random variable, $e$

$$e = \exp\{\lambda(I + n - g_0)\}, \qquad \lambda \geqq 0 \quad (4.4.90)$$

These random variables are illustrated in Fig. 4.20. Note that, because $b \leqq e$, we also have

$$\overline{b} < \overline{e} \quad (4.4.91)$$

In addition note that the average of $b$ is

$$\overline{b} = 1\, P(b = 1) + 0\, P(b = 0) = P(b = 1) = P(I + n \geqq g_0) = P \quad (4.4.92)$$

Thus combining (4.4.90) and (4.4.91)

$$P \leqq \overline{\exp\{\lambda(I + n - g_0)\}} = \exp(-\lambda g_0)\, \overline{\exp(\lambda n)}\, \overline{\exp(\lambda I)} \quad (4.4.93)$$

For Gaussian noise, $n$

$$\overline{\exp(\lambda n)} = \exp(0.5\, \lambda^2 \sigma_n^2) \quad (4.4.94)$$

and for the interference

$$\overline{\exp(\lambda I)} = \prod_{i=1}^{\infty} \overline{\exp(\lambda a_i h_i)} \quad (4.4.95)$$

Each term in (4.4.95) can be bounded by

$$\overline{\exp(\lambda a_i h_i)} = \frac{\sinh(\lambda h_i M)}{M \sinh(\lambda h_i)} \leqq \exp\{\lambda h_i(M - 1)\} \tag{4.4.96}$$

Another bound is (see Problem 4.4.6)

$$\overline{\exp(\lambda a_i h_i)} \leqq \exp\{\lambda^2 h_i^2(M^2 - 1)/6\} \tag{4.4.97}$$

The first bound is tighter so long as

$$h_i \geqq 6/\{\lambda(M + 1)\} \tag{4.4.98}$$

Let $i = K$ be the largest index for which this is true. Thus for $i > K$, we shall use (4.4.97). Combining (4.4.93) through (4.4.98), we obtain

$$P \leqq \exp\{\lambda(-g_0 + 0.5\,\lambda\sigma_n^2 + \rho_{IK} + 0.5\,\lambda\sigma_{IK}^2)\} \tag{4.4.99}$$

where

$$\sigma_{IK}^2 = (M^2 - 1)\sum_{K+1}^{\infty} h_i^2/3 \tag{4.4.100}$$

Since $\lambda \geqq 0$ is arbitrary, we shall find the optimal $\lambda$ that tightens the bound in (4.4.99). Taking the derivative with respect to $\lambda$, we obtain

$$\lambda_{0p} = (g_0 - \rho_{IK})/(\sigma_n^2 + \sigma_{IK}^2) \tag{4.4.101}$$

and the tighter bound is

$$P \leqq \exp\{-0.5\,(g_0 - \rho_{IK})^2/(\sigma_n^2 + \sigma_{IK}^2)\} \tag{4.4.102}$$

Other bounds can be found in Refs. 4.9, 4.18–4.20, and 4.24.

**4.4.3.8 Bounds and approximation of Jenq et al.**[4.25,4.26] The error probability is from (4.4.1) or (4.4.13)

$$P = \int_{-\infty}^{\infty} Q_n(g_0 - y)p_I(y)\,dy \tag{4.4.103}$$

where $p_I(y)$ is the probability density of the interference. We divide the range of $y$ into intervals $\{y_k, y_{k+1}\}$ such that

$$y_k = \sum_{i=1}^{k} h_i, \; y_0 = 0, \; y_{-1} = -\infty \tag{4.4.104}$$

We assume that the symbols are equiprobable and binary ($\pm 1$), but, as explained in Section 4.4.1, this is not a restriction on the application of the results so long as the symbols are from the set $\mathring{A}_{\pm}$ and $M$ is a power of 2. Thus

$$P = \sum_{k=0}^{\infty} \int_{y_{k-1}}^{y_k} Q_n(g_0 - y) p_I(y)\, dy \tag{4.4.105}$$

Since $Q_n(x)$ is a decreasing function of $x$, we have for $y_{k-1} \leqq y \leqq y_k$

$$Q_n(g_0 - y_{k-1}) \leqq Q_n(g_0 - y) \leqq Q_n(g_0 - y_k) \tag{4.4.106}$$

Denoting

$$q_k = \int_{y_{k-1}}^{y_k} p_I(y)\, dy \tag{4.4.107}$$

$$Q_n(g_0 - y_k) = S_k \tag{4.4.108}$$

we obtain

$$P_L = \sum_{k=0}^{\infty} S_{k-1} q_k \leqq P \leqq \sum_{k=0}^{\infty} S_k q_k = P_U \tag{4.4.109}$$

Because

$$S_{-1} = P(n > g_0 - y_{-1}) = P(n > \infty) = 0 \tag{4.4.110}$$

the lower bound in (4.4.109) is in fact

$$P_L = \sum_{k=0}^{\infty} S_k q_{k+1} \tag{4.4.111}$$

Denoting

$$Q_I(x) = P(I \geqq x) \tag{4.4.112}$$

we have from (4.4.107)

$$q_k = Q_I(y_{k-1}) - Q_I(y_k) \tag{4.4.113}$$

and

$$Q_l(y_k) = L^{-1} \sum_{j=1}^{L} P(I_k(j) + R_k \geqq y_k)$$

$$= L^{-1} \sum_{j=1}^{L} P\left(\sum_{i=1}^{k} a_i(j)h_i + R_k \geqq y_k\right) \qquad (4.4.114)$$

where

$$L = 2^k \qquad (4.4.115)$$

is the number of sequences $\mathbf{a}(j) = \{a_1(j), \ldots, a_k(j)\}$.

There is one sequence for which all symbols are $a_i = 1$. For this sequence.

$$P(I_k(j) + R_k \geqq y_k) = P(y_k + R_k \geqq y_k) = P(R_k \geqq 0) = 0.5 \qquad (4.4.116)$$

where the last equality follows from the symmetry of $R_k$. There are $\binom{k}{1} = k$ sequences, such that all symbols are $a_i = 1$, except, say, symbol $a_j$, which is $-1$. For these sequences

$$P(I_k(j) + R_k \geqq y_k) = P(R_k \geqq 2\, h_i), \qquad i = 1, \ldots, k \qquad (4.4.117)$$

There are $\binom{k}{2} = (k - 1)k/2$ sequences, such that all except two symbols are 1; thus for them

$$P(I_k(j) + R_k \geqq y_k) = P(R_k \geqq 2\, h_i + 2\, h_m),\ i, m = 1, \ldots, k \qquad (4.4.118)$$

Generally we have $\binom{k}{r}$ sequences with $r$ 1 s and $(k - r)$ $-1$ s. Finally we have one sequence for which all symbols are $-1$, and for for this sequence

$$P(I_k(j) + R_k \geqq y_k) = P(R_k \geqq 2\, y_k) \qquad (4.4.119)$$

Let

$$e_k = \sum_{i=1}^{k} P(R_k \geqq 2\, h_i) + \sum_{i=1}^{k} \sum_{\substack{m=1 \\ m \neq 1}}^{k} P(R_k \geqq 2\, h_i + 2\, h_m)$$

$$+ \ldots + P(R_k \geqq 2\, y_k) \qquad (4.4.120)$$

and $e_k = 0$ for $k \leqq 0$. When we substitute (4.4.120) and (4.4.116) into (4.4.114) and (4.4.113), we obtain

$$Q_I(k_k) = 2^{-(k+1)} + 2^{-k} e_k \tag{4.4.121}$$

$$q_k = 2^{-(k+1)} + 2^{-k}(2\, e_{k-1} - e_k) \tag{4.4.122}$$

Applying (4.4.122) to eqs. (4.4.109) and (4.4.111), we obtain

$$P_L = \sum_{k=0}^{\infty} S_k\{2^{-(k+2)} + 2^{-(k+1)}(2\, e_k - e_{k+1})\} \tag{4.4.123}$$

$$P_U = \sum_{k=0}^{\infty} S_k\{2^{-(k+1)} + 2^{-k}(2\, e_{k-1} - e_k)\} \tag{4.4.124}$$

Denote

$$P_a = \sum_{k=0}^{\infty} S_k 2^{-(k+1)} \tag{4.4.125}$$

$$\Delta_L = \sum_{k=0}^{\infty} 2^{-k}(2\, e_k - e_{k+1}) S_k \tag{4.4.126}$$

$$\Delta_U = \sum_{k=0}^{\infty} 2^{-k}(2\, e_{k-1} - e_k) S_k = \sum_{k=1}^{\infty} 2^{-k}(2\, e_{k-1} - e_k) S_k$$

$$= \sum_{k=0}^{\infty} 2^{-(k+1)}(2\, e_k - e_{k+1})) S_{k+1} \tag{4.4.127}$$

Thus

$$0.5\,(P_a + \Delta_L) \leqq P \leqq P_a + \Delta_U \tag{4.4.128}$$

Because

$$\Delta_L = \sum_{k=0}^{\infty} 2^{-(k-1)} S_k e_k - \sum_{k=0}^{\infty} 2^{-k} S_k e_{k+1}$$

$$= \sum_{k=0}^{\infty} 2^{-k} S_{k+1} e_{k+1} - \sum_{k=0}^{\infty} 2^{-k} S_k e_{k+1} = \sum_{k=0}^{\infty} 2^{-k} e_{k+1}(S_{k+1} - S_k) \tag{4.4.129}$$

and both $e_{k+1} \geqq 0$ and $S_{k+1} - S_k \geqq 0$ also $\Delta_L \geqq 0$. Therefore

$$0.5\, P_a \leqq P \leqq P_a + \Delta_U \tag{4.4.130}$$

In many cases $\Delta_U \to 0$; hence

$$0.5\, P_a \leqq P \leqq P_a \tag{4.4.131}$$

$P_a$ can be approximated in Practice by a finite number of terms in (4.4.125), say $K = 20$; hence up to a ratio of 2

$$P = \sum_{k=0}^{K} S_k 2^{-(k+1)} = \sum_{k=0}^{K} Q_n\left(g_0 - \sum_{i=1}^{k} h_i\right) 2^{-(k+1)} \tag{4.4.132}$$

and we have the convention that $\sum_{i=1}^{0} = 0$.

### 4.4.4 Bounds in systems with dependent symbols

When the symbols are dependent we cannot use property (e) of Section 4.4.1 or the bounds presented before that rely on the independence of the symbols. The readers interested in this topic are referred to Refs. 4.11, 4.20, 4.27, and 4.28.

### 4.4.5 Applications of bounds to systems with Nyquist function response

I have found that the most convenient bound are those in Sections 4.4.3.2 and 4.4.3.8. The quadrature rule bounds suffer from numerical instability. Both the Taylor and Legendre series expansions also have numerical difficulties that may lead in some cases to divergence of the series and even to negative values for the error probability.

In Section 4.3.6 we promised to find the effect of jitter on error probability. Thus we apply the bounds of Sections 4.4.3.2 and 4.4.3.8 to an $M$-ary ASK digital communication system with a matched filter and overall Nyquist system response with excess bandwidth $\beta$ for which $g(t) = g_N(t)$ and $g_N(t)$ is given in (4.3.29). The samples are taken at times $t_i = t_0 + iT$, with offset $t_0 \neq 0$. Since

$$g(t_0) = g_N(t_0)$$

when we use (4.4.6), we have to substitute

$$\sqrt{\eta} = g_N(t_0)/g_0$$

and when we compute I we reorder according to rank the set $\{g_i' = |g_N(t_i)/g(t_0)|, i \neq 0\}$ for $M = 2$, the set $\{g_i', 2\, g_i'\}$ for $M = 4$, and the set $\{g_i', 2$

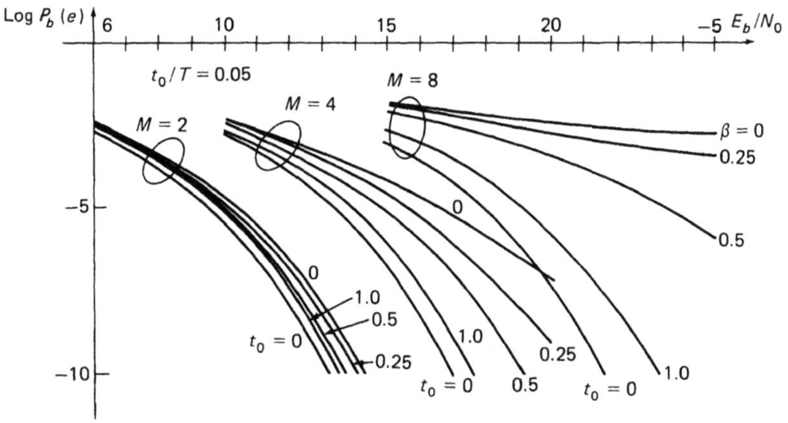


Fig. 4.21. Bit error probability as a function of signal-to-noise ratio per bit for an $M$-ary ASK system with raised cosine response and excess bandwidth β in the presence of sampling time offset.

$g_i', 4g_i'\}$ for $M = 8$. In fact it was sufficient to do the reordering for only $N = 8$ terms in the binary case, i.e., $I_N$ had only eight terms. We also tried $N = 12$ terms, but this has no effect on the error probability. Thus only eight ISI terms are here significant. In approximating $P_a$ it was sufficient to use $K = 15$ terms only. We also tried $K = 20$, but this again has no effect on the error probability. The results are shown in Figs. 4.21, 4.22, and 4.23. In Fig. 4.21 we show the error probability as a function of signal-to-noise ratio with β as a parameter and $t_0/T$ either 0 or 0.05. In Fig. 4.22 we show the bit error probability as a function of sampling time offset with β as a parameter and fixed signal-to-noise ratio. In Fig. 4.23 we show the bit error probability as a function of excess bandwidth and fixed signal-to-noise ratio and $t_0/T = 0.05$. It is clear from these figures that the effect of sampling time offset (which causes the ISI here) on the error probability is as follows:

a. $P_b(e)$ is an increasing function of sampling time offset.
b. For a given sampling time offset the bit error probability is a decreasing function of β.
c. For a given sampling time offset, bit error probability, and excess bandwidth, the bit error probability is more affected for multilevel symbols than for binary symbols. Thus when designing a quaternary ASK system (which is equivalent to a 16-ary QASK or OQASK, as explained in the section on these systems) either the offset must be reduced or the excess bandwidth must be increased. This is even more pronounced if we intend to design an octal ASK system (equivalent to 64-ary QASK or OQASK systems). Because the rationale for multilevel system is an improvement in spectral efficiency, increasing β is partially self-defeating.

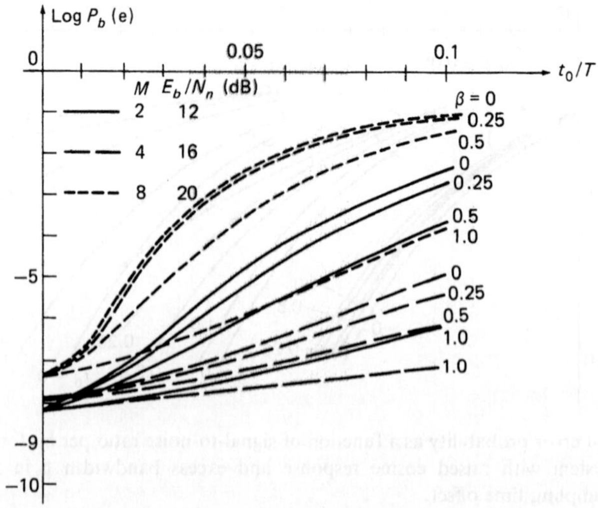


Fig. 4.22. Bit error probability as a function of sampling time for an $M$-ary ASK system with raised cosine response and excess bandwidth β.

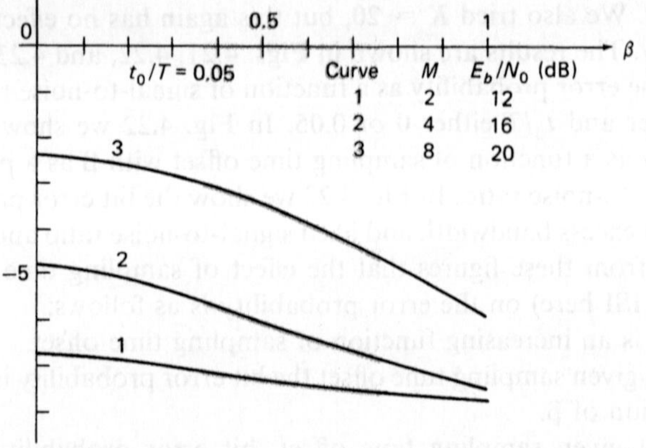


Fig. 4.23. Bit error probability as a function of excess bandwidth for an $M$-ary ASK system with raised cosine response.

Note also from these figures, that even when $\beta = 0$, so that $I_{\max} = \rho_1 = \infty$ (i.e., the eye diagram is closed) the error probability is not 0.5 as may have been expected only from the eye diagram. Thus, as already stated, the eye diagram does not supply quantitative information on the error probability.

## 4.5 SYSTEM WITH NRZ, HS, AND SP SHAPING FUNCTIONS[4.29–4.35]

The model of the system is the same as in Fig. 4.1; for convenience, however, and the necessity of additional notation, it is presented again in Fig. 4.24. In this section, the shaping functions are NRZ, HS, or SP, i.e.

$$h_S(t) = \begin{cases} h_N(t) = u_T(t) & \text{NRZ} \\ h_H(t) = \sin(\pi t/T)u_T(t) & \text{HS} \\ h_{SP}(t) = u_{0.5T}(t) - u_{0.5T}(t - T) & \text{SP} \end{cases} \quad (4.5.1)$$

where

$$u_T(t) = u(t) - u(t - T) \quad (4.5.2)$$

and $u(t)$ is the unit step function

$$u(t) = \begin{cases} 1 & t \geqq 0 \\ 0 & t < 0 \end{cases} \quad (4.5.3)$$

All these functions have already been defined in Chapter 2, but are presented here again for convenience.

We shall assume, without loss in generality that filters $H_T(f)$ and $H_C(f)$ are lumped together to form the filter $H_{TC}(f)$. We shall also assume that the detector filter is either matched to the shaping function or variously mismatched. We already know that if $H_{TC}(f) = H_R(f) = 1$, the matched filter is the optimal filter. However, when $H_{TC}(f)$ and (or) $H_R(f)$ are not ideal, the matched filter is not matched any more to the incoming signal, and hence we can expect that it will not be any more optimal. In fact, it will be shown that a very simple detector, namely a sample detector, in which the detector filter is eliminated and the decisions are made directly on the samples at the receiver filter output outperforms (i.e., leads to a smaller error probability) in some cases the matched filter. Which filter is better depends on the amount of distortion introduced by the transmitter filter, channels, and receiver filters. The amount of distortion depends on the bandwidth of

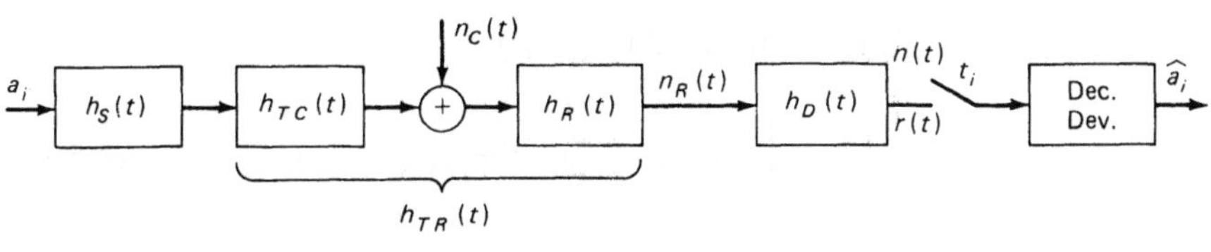


Fig. 4.24. Model of ASK baseband system.

the filters. We shall indeed show that when the bandwidth is large the matched filter is better, and when the bandwidth is small, and this is the more practical case, the sample detector is better.

We assume that $H_{TC}(f)$ and $H_R(f)$ are causal filters with a finite number of distinct poles. The method presented here can be extended and was in fact extended to filters with multiple poles.[4.29, 4.30, 4.34] However, this only complicates the formulas without contributing to a deeper insight into the problem. In fact, in practice, the poles are never identical, due to component tolerances. If in theory, say $p_1$ and $p_2$ are identical poles, we can replace $p_2$ by $p_1 + \varepsilon$ with $|\varepsilon| \ll |p_1|$, and the problem is reduced to the case of simple poles. Thus there is no significant restriction in the assumption of simple poles only.

We have to compute

$$g(t) = h_S(t) * h_{TC}(t) * h_R(t) * h_D(t) \tag{4.5.4}$$

and

$$\sigma_n^2 = \overline{n^2(t)} = 0.5\, N_0 \int_{-\infty}^{\infty} |H_R(f)H_D(f)|^2\, df \tag{4.5.5}$$

for the eight systems, which differ in the shaping function and detector filter, as defined in Table 4.3. Systems NN, HH, and SPSP have matched filters. The systems in which $h_D(t) = \delta(t)$ have a sample detector. We shall use the following notation

$$h_{TR}(t) = h_{TC}(t) * h_R(t) = h_T(t) * h_C(t) * h_R(t) \tag{4.5.6}$$

$$g_R(t) = h_S(t) * h_{TR}(t) \tag{4.5.7}$$

$$n_R(t) = n_C(t) * h_R(t) \tag{4.5.8}$$

$$g_N(t) = u(t) * h_{TR}(t) = \int_0^t h_{TR}(\tau)\, d\tau u(t) \tag{4.5.9}$$

$$\begin{aligned} g_H(t) &= \sin(\pi t/T) * h_{TR}(t) \\ &= \int_0^t \sin(\pi(t-\tau)/T) h_{TR}(\tau)\, d\tau u(t) \end{aligned} \tag{4.5.10}$$

$$n(t) = n_R(t) * h_D(t) = \int_0^{\infty} n_R(t-\tau) h_D(\tau)\, d\tau \tag{4.5.11}$$

**Table 4.3 Systems with various shaping functions and detector filters**

| SYSTEM | $h_S(t)$ | $h_D(t)$ | TYPE OF DETECTOR |
|---|---|---|---|
| NN | $h_N(t)$ | $h_N(t)$ | Matched filter |
| NS | $h_N(t)$ | $\delta(t)$ | Sample detector |
| HH | $h_H(t)$ | $h_H(t)$ | Matched filter |
| HS | $h_H(t)$ | $\delta(t)$ | Sample detector |
| HN | $h_H(t)$ | $h_N(t)$ | Integrate and dump (ID) |
| HR | $h_H(t)$ | $u_{0.5T}(t)$ | ID with half integration time |
| SPSP | $h_{SP}(t)$ | $h_{SP}(t)$ | Matched filter |
| SPS | $h_{SP}(t)$ | $\delta(t)$ | Sample detector |

These functions have the following physical meaning; $h_{TR}(t)$ is the impulse response of transmitter, channel, and receiver filter when lumped into a single filter, $g_R(t)$ is the impulse response of the system up to detector filter, $n_R(t)$ is the noise at the receiver filter output, $g_N(t)$ is the response of $h_{TR}(t)$ to a unit step function, $g_H(t)$ is the reponse of $h_{TR}(t)$ to a sinusoid with frequency $f = R/2$, which is applied at time $t = 0$, and finally, $n(t)$ is the noise at detector filter output. We shall derive separately $g(t)$ and the noise variance $\sigma_n^2$.

### 4.5.1 Derivation of system reponse $g(t)$

#### 4.5.1.1 Causal filters

Because (see Fig. 4.25)

$$h_N(t) = u(t) - u(t - T) \tag{4.5.12}$$

$$h_H(t) = \sin(\pi t/T)u(t) + \sin\{\pi(t - T)/T\}u(t - T) \tag{4.5.13}$$

$$h_{SP}(t) = u(t) - 2\,u(t - 0.5\,T) + u(t + T) \tag{4.5.14}$$

we obtain

$$g_R(t) = \begin{cases} g_N(t) - g_N(t - T) & \text{NN, NS} \\ g_H(t) + g_H(t - T) & \text{HH, HS, HN, HR} \\ g_N(t) - 2\,g_N(t - 0.5\,T) + g_N(t - T) & \text{SPSP, SPS} \end{cases} \tag{4.5.15}$$

Since from (4.5.4), (4.5.6), and (4.5.7)

$$g(t) = g_R(t) * h_D(t) \tag{4.5.16}$$

when we use $g_R(t)$ from (4.5.15) and $h_D(t)$ from Table 4.3, we obtain for the eight systems in the table

$$g(t) = \begin{cases} g_{NN}(t) - 2\,g_{NN}(t-T) + g_{NN}(t-2\,T) \\ g_N(t) - g_N(t-T) \\ g_{HH}(t) + 2\,g_{HH}(t-T) + g_{HH}(t-2\,T) \\ g_H(t) + g_H(t-T) \\ g_{HN}(t) - g_{HN}(t-2\,T) \\ g_{HN}(t) + g_{HN}(t-T) - g_{HN}(t-0.5\,T) - g_{HN}(t-1.5\,T) \\ g_{NN}(t) - 4\,g_{NN}(t-0.5\,T) + 6\,g_{NN}(t-T) \\ \qquad - 4\,g_{NN}(t-1.5\,T) + g_{NN}(t-2\,T) \\ g_N(t) - 2\,g_N(t-0.5\,T) + g_N(t-T) \end{cases} \tag{4.5.17}$$

where

$$g_{NN}(t) = \int_0^t g_N(y)\,dyu(t) \tag{4.5.18}$$

$$g_{HH}(t) = \int_0^t \sin\{\pi(t-y)/T\}g_H(y)\,dyu(t) \tag{4.5.19}$$

$$g_{HN}(t) = \int_0^t g_H(y)\,dyu(t) \tag{4.5.20}$$

**4.5.1.2 Filters with a finite number of distinct poles** Let $H'_{TC}(s)$ and $H_R'(s)$ be the Laplace transform (LT) of $h_{TC}(t)$ and $h_R(t)$, respectively. The LT and Fourier transform (FT) are related by

$$H_R(f) = H'_R(s = j\,2\,\pi f) \tag{4.5.21}$$

From now on we shall drop the subscript $C$ in $h_{TC}(t)$ and $H'_{TC}(s)$. Let $N_T$ and $N_R$ be the number of poles in transmitter (including channel) and receiver filters, respectively. Each filter can be described by

$$H'_x(s) = T_x(s)\Big/\prod_1^{N_x}(s + p_{x,i}) = \sum_1^{N_x} \rho_{x,i}/(s + p_{x,i}), \qquad x = T, R \tag{4.5.22}$$

where $T_x(s)$ is a polynomial of degree less than $N_x$, $\{-p_{x,i}\}$ are the poles, and $\{\rho_{x,i}\}$ are the residues at the poles, i.e.

$$\rho_{x,i} = \lim_{s\to -p_{x,i}} H'_x(s)(s + p_{x,i}) \tag{4.5.23}$$

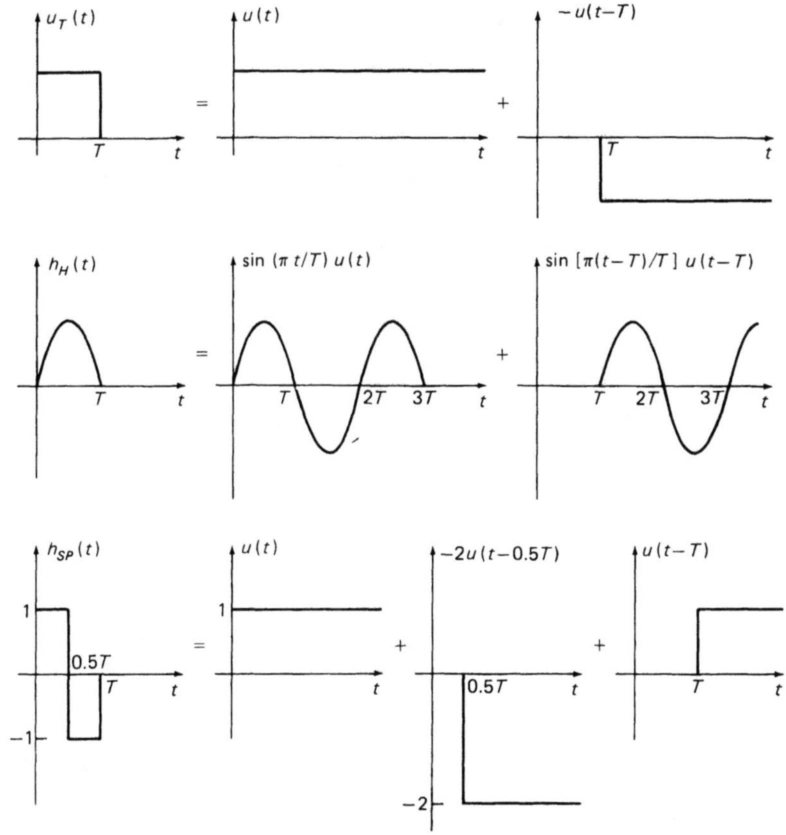


Fig. 4.25. NRZ, HS, and SP shaping fuctions as sums of other elementary functions.

We shall find the poles and residues of the lumped filter

$$\begin{aligned} H'_{TR}(s) &= H_T'(s)H_R'(s) = T_T(s)T_R(s) \Big/ \prod_1^{N_T} (s + p_{T,i}) \prod_1^{N_R} (s + p_{R,i}) \\ &= T_T(s)T_R(s) \prod_{i=1}^{N_{TR}} (s + p_{TR,i})^{-1} = \sum_1^{N_{TR}} \rho_{TR,i}/(s + p_{TR,i}) \end{aligned} \tag{4.5.24}$$

where

$$N_{TR} = N_T + N_R \tag{4.5.25}$$

$$p_{TR,i} = \begin{cases} p_{R,i} & i = 1, \ldots, N_R \\ p_{T,i-N_R} & i = N_R + 1, \ldots, N_{TR} \end{cases} \tag{4.5.26}$$

and

$$\begin{aligned}\rho_{TR,i} &= \lim_{s \to -p_{TR,i}} H'_{TR}(s)(s + p_{TR,i}) \\ &= \begin{cases} \rho_{R,i} H'_T(-p_{R,i}) & i = 1, \ldots, N_R \\ \rho_{T,i-N} H'_R(-p_{T,i-N_R}) & i = N_R + 1 \ldots, N_{TR} \end{cases}\end{aligned} \tag{4.5.27}$$

Taking the inverse LT of (4.5.24), we obtain

$$h_{TR}(t) = \sum_{i=1}^{N_{TR}} \rho_{TR,i} \exp(-p_{TR,i} t) u(t) \tag{4.5.28}$$

When we substitute (4.5.28) into (4.5.9) and (4.5.10), we obtain

$$g_N(t) = \sum_{i=1}^{N_{TR}} \rho_{TR,i} T\{1 - \exp(-p_{TR,i} t)\} u(t)/(p_{TR,i} T) \tag{4.5.29}$$

and

$$g_H(t) = \sum_{i=1}^{N_{TR}} \rho_{TR,i} T \frac{p_{TR,i} T \sin(\pi t/T) - \pi \cos(\pi t/T) + \pi \exp(-p_{TR,i} t)}{(p_{TR,i} T)^2 + \pi^2} u(t) \tag{4.5.30}$$

Now, we substitute (4.5.29) and (4.5.30) into (4.5.18)–(4.5.20) and obtain

$$g_{NN}(t) = T \sum_{i=1}^{N_{TR}} \rho_{TR,i} T\{p_{TR,i} t + \exp(-p_{TR,i} t) - 1\} u(t)/(p_{TR,i} T)^2 \tag{4.5.31}$$

$$g_{HN}(t) = T \sum_{i=1}^{N_{TR}} \rho_{TR,i} T \frac{\{1 - \cos(\pi t/T)\} p_{TR,i} T/\pi - \sin(\pi t/T) + \{1 - \exp(-p_{TR,i} t)\}(p_{TR,i} T/\pi)^{-1}}{(p_{TR,i} T)^2 + \pi^2} u(t) \tag{4.5.32}$$

$$g_{HH}(t) = T \sum_{i=1}^{N_{TR}} \rho_{TR,i} T f_i(t) u(t)/\{(p_{TR,i} T)^2 + \pi^2\} \tag{4.5.33}$$

where

$$\begin{aligned} f_i(t) &= (0.5\, \pi t/T)\{(\mathrm{sinc}\,(t/T) - \cos(\pi t/T)) p_{TR,i} T/\pi - \sin(\pi t/T)\} \\ &\quad + \frac{\exp(-p_{TR,i} t) - \cos(\pi t/T) + (p_{TR,i} T/\pi) \sin(\pi t/T)}{(p_{TR,i} T/\pi)^2 + 1} \end{aligned} \tag{4.5.34}$$

**4.5.1.3 Butterworth filters**[4.36] A Butterworth filter of order $N_B$ has a transfer function

$$|H_B(f)|^2 = \{1 + (f/f_{B0})^{2N_B}\}^{-1}, \; B = T, R \tag{4.5.35}$$

where $f_{B0}$ is the 3-dB bandwidth of the filters, i.e.

$$10 \log \{|H_B(f_{B0})|^2/|H_B(0)|^2\} = 10 \log (1/2) = -3 \text{ dB} \tag{4.5.36}$$

The impulse response and the LT of this filter are

$$h_B(t) = \sum_{i=1}^{N_B} \rho_{B,i} \exp(-p_{B,i}t) \tag{4.5.37}$$

$$H'_B(s) = \sum_{i=1}^{N_B} \rho_{B,i}/(s + p_{B,i}) = \omega_{B0}^{N_B} \Big/ \prod_{i}^{N_B} (s + p_{B,i}) \tag{4.5.38}$$

with

$$p_{B,i} = \omega_{B0} \exp(j\psi_{B,i}) \tag{4.5.39}$$

$$\psi_{B,i} = 0.5\,\pi(2\,i - 1)/N_B - \pi/2 \tag{4.5.40}$$

$$\omega_{B0} = 2\,\pi f_{B0} \tag{4.5.41}$$

$$\rho_{B,i} = \omega_{B0} \left| \prod_{\substack{j=1 \\ j\neq 1}}^{N_B} 2 \sin\{(0.5(\psi_{B,i} - \psi_{B,j})\} \right|^{-1} \exp\{j(1 + N_B/2)\psi_{B,i}\} \tag{4.5.42}$$

Note that

$$\psi_{B,i} = -\psi_{B,N-i}$$

hence

$$p_{B,i} = p^*_{B,N-i}, \; \rho_{B,i} = \rho^*_{B,N-i} \tag{4.5.43}$$

and it is thus sufficient to know these values for $i = 1, 2, \ldots, N_B/2$ ($N_B$ even) and $i = 1, \ldots, (N_B + 1)/2$ ($N_B$ odd). In Table 4.4 we present the values of $|\rho_{B,i}/\omega_{B0}|$ for Butterworth filters of order up to 10. The phase of the residua can be easily computed from (4.5.40).

In Fig. 4.26 we show the response $g(t)$ (in fact $g(t)$ may be normalized by a constant, $\sigma_n$, which we compute in the next subsection) of some of the systems defined in Table 4.3 and with Butterworth filters in transmitter and receiver. The 3-dB bandwidth $f_{B0}$ is either the same for both filters or the transmitter filter is wideband and the receiver filter has 3-dB bandwidth $f_{R0}$.

**Table 4.4 Values of residue for Butterworth filters**

| $N_B/i$ | 1 | 2 | 3 | 4 | 5 |
|---|---|---|---|---|---|
| 1 | 1.000000 | | | | |
| 2 | 0.707107 | | | | |
| 3 | 1.000000 | 0.577350 | | | |
| 4 | 1.207107 | 0.500000 | | | |
| 5 | 1.894427 | 1.376382 | 0.447214 | | |
| 6 | 2.638959 | 1.523603 | 0.408248 | | |
| 7 | 4.311941 | 3.438658 | 1.655971 | 0.377964 | |
| 8 | 6.422089 | 4.291103 | 1.777433 | 0.353553 | |
| 9 | 10.721146 | 8.996110 | 5.193907 | 1.890427 | 0.333333 |
| 10 | 16.599100 | 12.059952 | 6.144852 | 1.996584 | 0.316228 |

Note that the response decreases rapidly with time, due to the exponential decay; hence in the sequel not more than eight interfering terms must be taken into account when the error probability is computed. Note that when the detector is a matched filter (see Fig. 4.26 for system HH) the response improves with bandwidth, and in the system with the sampling detector (see Fig. 4.26 for system HS) the best response is for a 3-dB bandwidth of about $R$. From these figures we can intuitively determine the optimal sampling time, $t_0$, in each case. The optimal sampling time is by definition the sampling time that gives the least error probability. This sampling time is close to the position of the peak value of $g(t)$, but it is not identical with that position because of the effect of ISI. We elaborate on this statement. Without ISI the best sampling time is without question the position of the peak. In the presence of ISI, the ISI terms may also have large values at times $t_0 + iT$ when $t_0 = t_{peak}$, while if $t_0 = t_{peak} + \varepsilon$ the ISI terms may have reduced values. For that reason the optimal sampling time is found by varying $\varepsilon$.

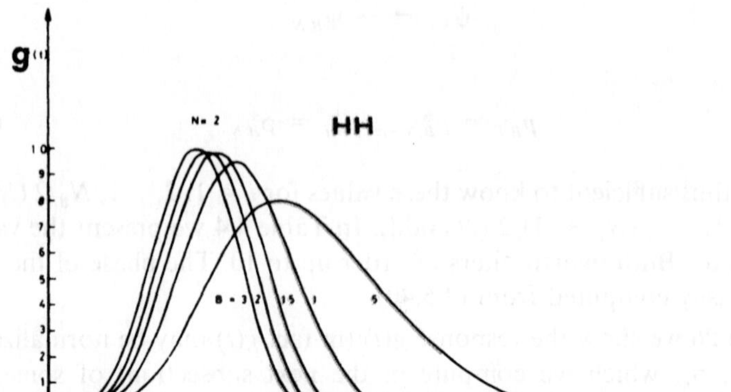


Fig. 4.26. Response of systems defined in Table 4.3. The transmitter and receive filters are identical Butterworth filters of order $N$. The bandwidth is either the same or the transmitter filter is wideband. I. Korn, "Probability of Error in Binary Communication Systems with Causal Bandlimiting Filters," *IEEE Tr. Comm.*, Vol. COM-21, August 1973, pp. 878–898. Copyright © 1973 IEEE).

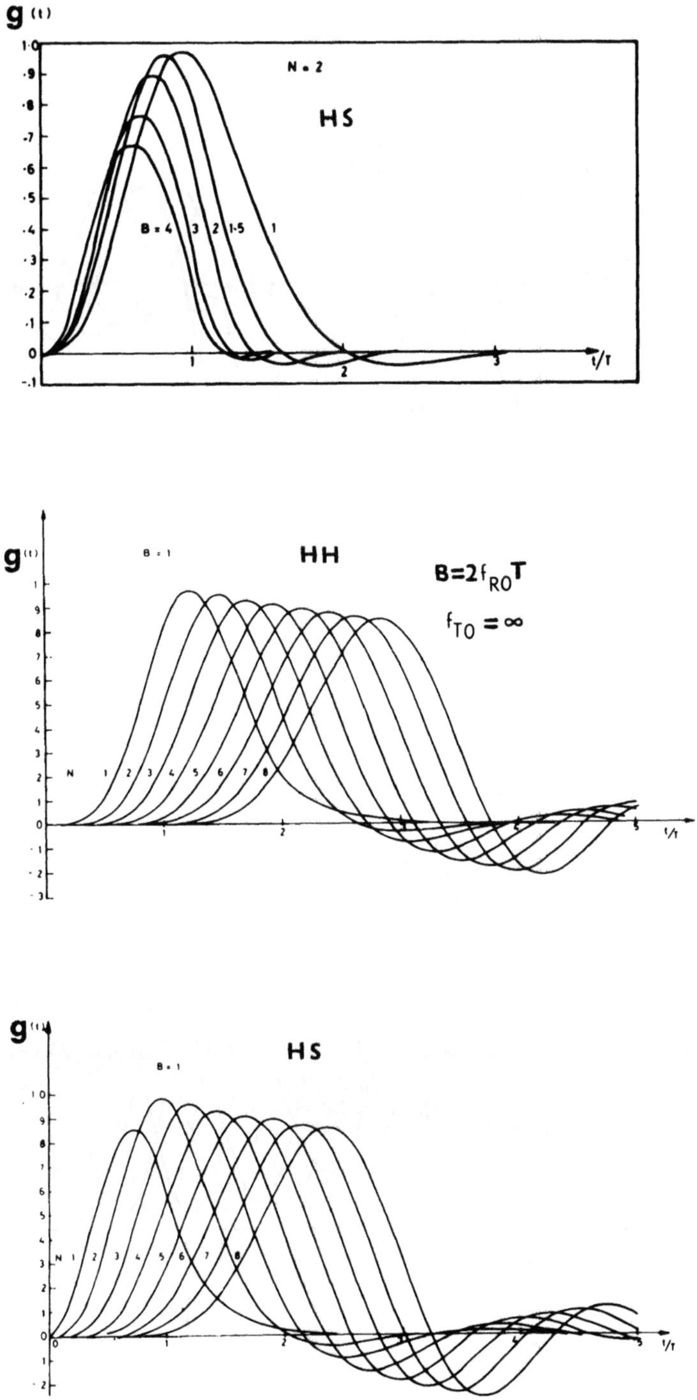
g (t)
N = 2
HS
B = 4 3 2 1·5 1
t/T
g (t)
B = 1
HH
B=2f_RO T
f_TO = ∞
N 1 2 3 4 5 6 7 8
t/T
g (t)
HS
B = 1
N 1 2 3 4 5 6 7 8
t/T

Fig. 4.26. (*con't.*)

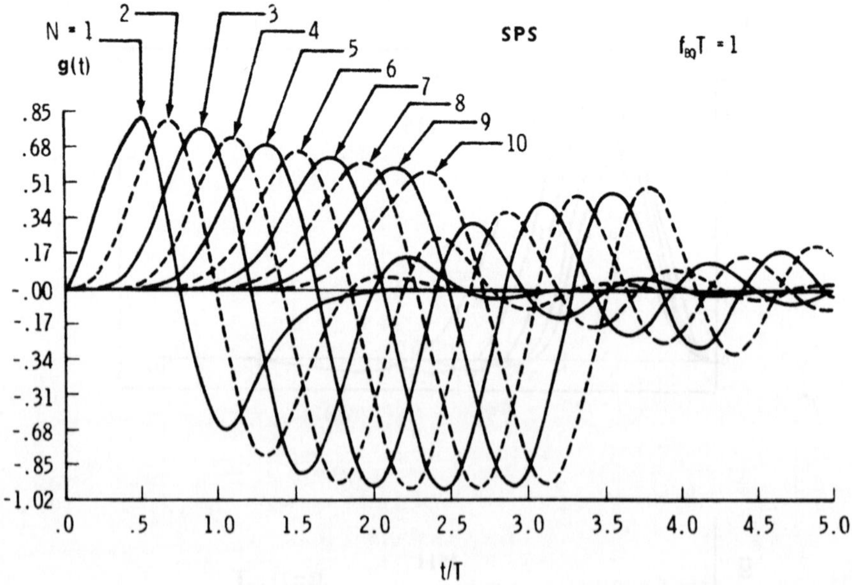
N = 1
2
3
4
5
6
7
8
9
10
g(t)
SPS
$f_{B0}T = 1$
.85
.68
.51
.34
.17
-.00
-.17
-.34
-.31
-.68
-.85
-1.02
.0
.5
1.0
1.5
2.0
2.5
3.0
3.5
4.0
4.5
5.0
t/T

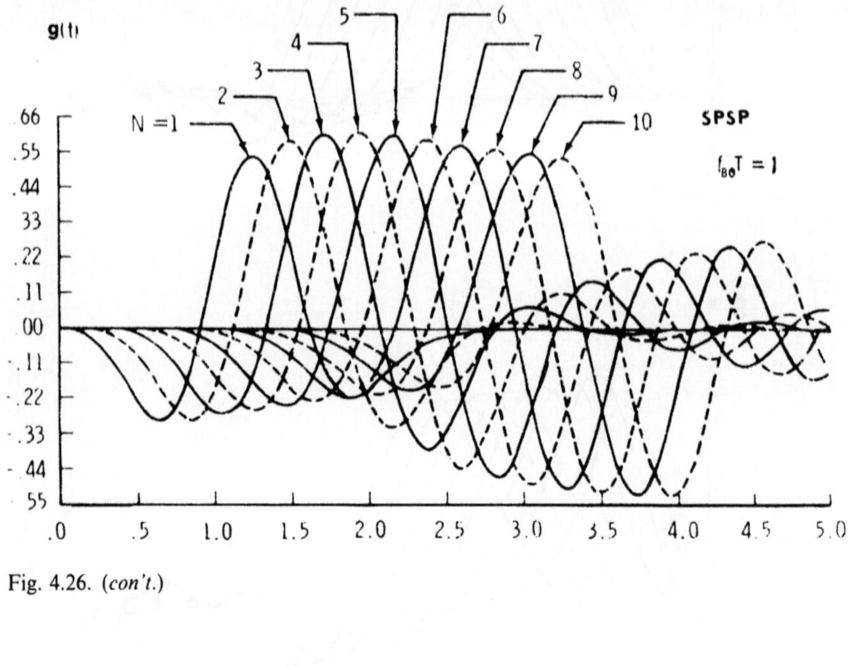
g(t)
N = 1
2
3
4
5
6
7
8
9
10
SPSP
$f_{B0}T = 1$
.66
.55
.44
.33
.22
.11
.00
-.11
-.22
-.33
-.44
-.55
.0
.5
1.0
1.5
2.0
2.5
3.0
3.5
4.0
4.5
5.0

Fig. 4.26. (*con't.*)

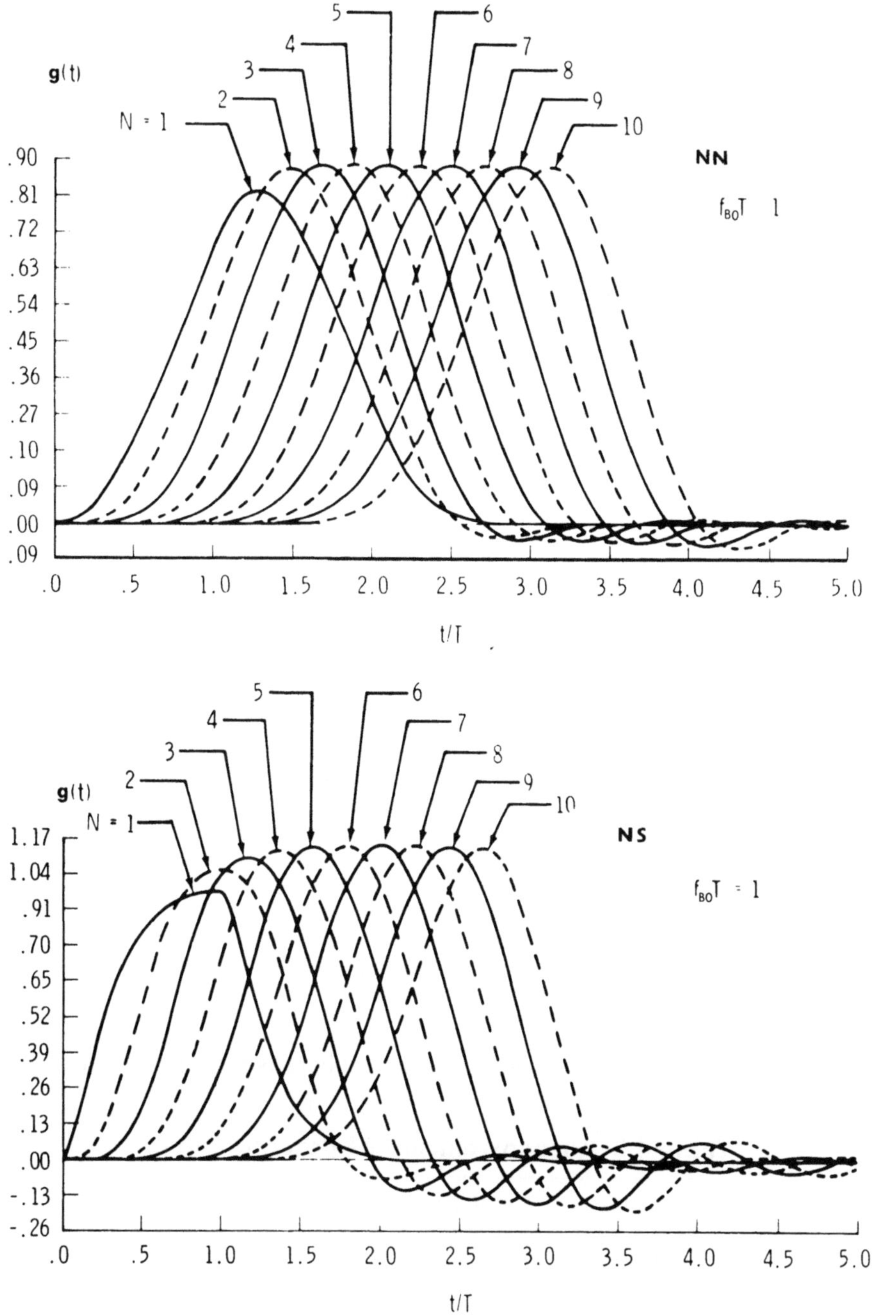
g(t)
N = 1
2
3
4
5
6
7
8
9
10
NN
f_BO T 1
.90
.81
.72
.63
.54
.45
.36
.27
.10
.09
.00
.09
.0 .5 1.0 1.5 2.0 2.5 3.0 3.5 4.0 4.5 5.0
t/T
g(t)
N = 1
2
3
4
5
6
7
8
9
10
NS
f_BO T = 1
1.17
1.04
.91
.70
.65
.52
.39
.26
.13
.00
-.13
-.26
.0 .5 1.0 1.5 2.0 2.5 3.0 3.5 4.0 4.5 5.0
t/T

Fig. 4.26. (*con't.*)

### 4.5.2 Derivation of noise variance

For the sampling detector, the noise variance is

$$\sigma_n^2 = \overline{n^2(t)} = \overline{n_R^2(t)} = R_{nR}(0) \tag{4.5.44}$$

while for other detectors we compute from (4.5.11)

$$\sigma_n^2 = \overline{n^2(t)} = \int_0^T\int_0^T \overline{n_R(t-\tau_1)n_R(t-\tau_2)h_D(\tau_1)h_D(\tau_2)}\, d\tau_1\, d\tau_2$$

$$= \int_0^T\int_0^T R_{nR}(\tau_2-\tau_1)h_D(\tau_1)h_D(\tau_2)\, d\tau_1\, d\tau_2 \tag{4.5.45}$$

where $R_{nR}(\tau)$ is the autocorrelation of the noise $n_R(t)$. Changing variables

$$\tau = \tau_2 - \tau_1 \tag{4.5.46}$$

and the order of intergration, it is shown in the problem section (see Problem 4.5.3) that

$$\sigma_n^2 = \int_0^T R_{nR}(\tau)R_D(\tau)\, d\tau \tag{4.5.47}$$

where $R_D(\tau)$, the autocorrelation of the detector filter, is

$$R_D(\tau) = 2\int_0^{T-\tau} h_D(t-\tau)h_D(t)\, dt \tag{4.5.48}$$

The autocorrelation depends on the detector filter, as shown in Table 4.5

**Table 4.5 Autocorrelation of detector filter**

| DETECTOR | $h_D(t)$ | $R_D(\tau)$ $\quad 0 \leqq \tau \leqq T$ |
|---|---|---|
| 1 | $h_N(t)$ | $2(T-\tau)$ |
| 2 | $u_{0.5T}(t)$ | $(T-2\tau)u_{0.5T}(t)$ |
| 3 | $h_{SP}(t)$ | $2(T-3\tau)u_{0.5T}(\tau) - 2(T-\tau)u_{0.5T}(\tau-0.5T)$ |
| 4 | $h_H(t)$ | $(T-\tau)\cos(\pi\tau/T) + (T/\pi)\sin(\pi\tau/T)$ |

Thus, to derive the variance, we need only $R_{nR}(\tau)$ for $\tau \geqq 0$ only. Because the autocorrelation is an even function, we know that $R_{nR}(-\tau) = R_{nR}(\tau)$.

**4.5.2.1 Causal filter** We obtain from (4.5.8) the PSD (power spectral density) of receiver filter output, assuming that the channel noise is white with PSD 0.5 $N_0$

$$S_{nR}(f) = (1/2)N_0|H_R(f)|^2 \qquad (4.5.49)$$

The autocorrelation is therefore

$$R_{nR}(\tau) = (1/2)N_0 \int_{-\infty}^{\infty} |H_R(f)|^2 \exp(j\,2\,\pi f\tau)\, df \qquad (4.5.50)$$

Changing variables

$$s = j\,2\,\pi f \qquad (4.5.51)$$

we obtain

$$R_{nR}(\tau) = (1/2)N_0(j\,2\,\pi)^{-1} \int_{-\infty}^{\infty} H'_R(s)H'_R(-s) \exp(s\tau)\, ds \qquad (4.5.52)$$

**4.5.2.2 Filters with a finite number of distinct poles** Applying Cauchy's residue theorem,[4.36] we obtain from (4.5.52)

$$R_{nR}(\tau) = (1/2)N_0 \sum_{i=1}^{N_R} \rho_{R,i}H'_R(p_{R,i}) \exp(-p_{R,i}\tau) \qquad (4.5.53)$$

For a sampling detector we obtain from (4.5.44) and (4.5.50)

$$\sigma_n^2 = (1/2)N_0 \int_{-\infty}^{\infty} |H_R(f)|^2\, df \qquad (4.5.54)$$

For the other detectors, we substitute eq. (4.5.53) and the entries of Table 4.5 into eq. (4.5.47), and the results are, after straightforward but sometimes tedious manipulations

$$\sigma_n^2 = N_0T^2 \sum_{i=1}^{N_R} \rho_{R,i}H'_R(p_{R,i})V_i \qquad (4.5.55)$$

$V_i =$

$\{p_{R,i}T + \exp(-p_{R,i}T) - 1\}(p_{R,i}T)^{-2}$ 1

$\{0.5\, p_{R,i}T + \exp(-p_{R,i}T) - 1\}(p_{R,i}T)^{-2}$ 2

$\{p_{R,i}T - 3 + 4\exp(-0.5\, p_{R,i}T) - \exp(-p_{R,i}T)\}(p_{R,i}T)^{-2}$ 3

$\{1 + \exp(-p_{R,i}T) + 0.5\, p_{R,i}T(1 + (p_{R,i}T/\pi)^2)\}(1 + (p_{R,i}T/\pi)^2)^{-2}\pi^{-2}$ 4

(4.5.56)

**4.5.2.3 Butterworth filters** For a sampling detector we obtain from (4.5.54) and (4.5.35) with $B = R$

$$\sigma_n^2 = 0.5\, N_0 \int_{-\infty}^{\infty} \{1 + (f/f_{R0})^{2N_R}\}^{-1}\, df = N_0\omega_{R0}\{4\, N_R \sin(0.5\,\pi/N_R)\}^{-1} \tag{4.5.57}$$

The autocorrelation can be obtained from the general formula (4.5.53) and substitution of the values in Section 4.5.1.3 or directly

$$R_{nR}(\tau)$$

$$= (0.5)N_0 \int_{-\infty}^{\infty} \{1 + (f/f_{R0})^{2N_R}\}^{-1} \exp(j\,2\,\pi f\tau)\, df$$

$$= 0.25\,(N_0\omega_0/N_R) \sum_{i=1}^{N_R} \cos(\omega_{R0}\tau \sin\psi_{R,i} - \psi_{R,i}) \exp(-\omega_{R0}\tau\cos\psi_{R,i})u(\tau)$$

$$= 0.25\,(N_0/N_R) \sum_{i=1}^{N_R} p_{R,i} \exp(-p_{R,i}\tau)u(\tau) \tag{4.5.58}$$

with the $\{p_{R,i}\}$ as given in (4.5.39). Note that, although in (4.5.58) and (4.5.55), the terms are complex, the final result is real, because the term with index $i$ is the complex conjugate of the term with index $N_R - i$. In fact, if we want, we can precede the summations in these two equations by the operation Re { }.

When we substitute (4.5.58) and the entries of Table 4.5, we obtain

$$\sigma_n^2 = (1/2)N_0T \sum_{i=1}^{N_R} p_{R,i}TV_i/N_R \tag{4.5.59}$$

With $V_i$ as in (4.5.56). When we substitute the pole values

$$p_{R,i} = \omega_{R0} \exp(j\psi_{R,i}) \tag{4.5.60}$$

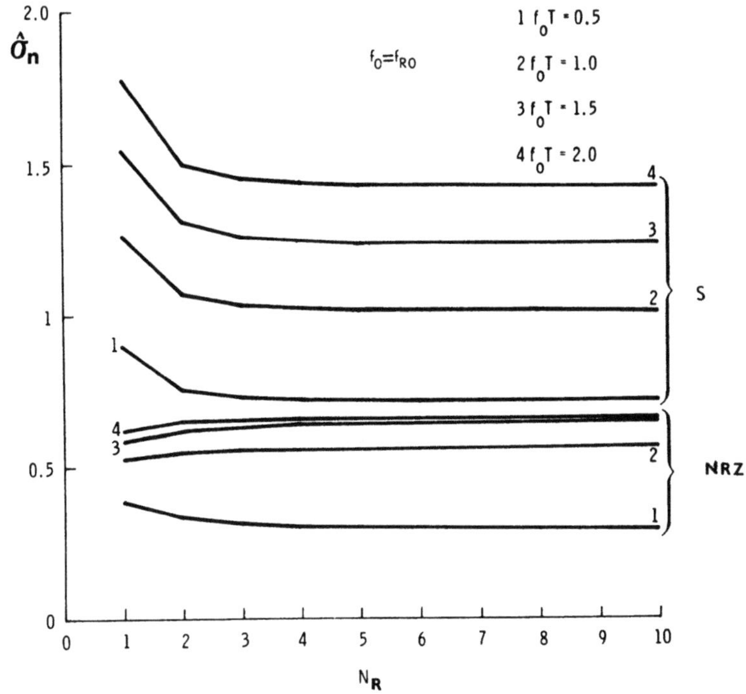


Fig. 4.27. The variance of noise for systems with Butterworth receiver filter of order $N$ and 3-dB bandwidth $f_{R0}$ and NRZ or sample detector filters. I. Korn, "Probability of Error in Binary Communication System with Causal Bandlimiting Filters. Part I: Nonreturn to Zero Signals," *IEEE Tr. Comm.*, Vol. COM-21, August 1973, pp. 878–890. Copyright © 1973 IEEE).

we can obtain the explicit final form for the noise variance. Thus for example if $h_D(t) = h_N(t)$, we obtain

$$\sigma_n^2 = (1/2)(N_0/\omega_{R0})\{\omega_{R0}T - (\sin(0.5\,\pi/N_R))^{-1} - \sum_{i=1}^{N_R} \cos(\omega_{R0}T \sin\psi_{R,i} + \psi_{R,i}) \exp(-\omega_{R0}T\cos\psi_{R,i})\} \qquad (4.5.61)$$

In Fig. 4.27 we show the normalized variance, $\hat{\sigma}_n$

$$\hat{\sigma}_n = \begin{cases} \sigma_n(T/N_0)^{1/2} & \text{Sample} \\ \sigma_n(N_0T)^{-1/2} & \text{NRZ} \end{cases}$$

for systems with sample and NRZ detectors as a function of number of poles in the Butterworth filter and with $f_{R0}/R$ as a parameter. Note that the variance does not change much for $N \geqq 3$.

### 4.5.3 Error probability

After we have computed $g(t)$ and $\sigma_n$, we can also compute their ratio $g(t)/\sigma_n$, which we can call the *normalized system response* to the shaping function. In fact for some systems in Fig. 4.26 we have indeed sketched the normalized system response. The normalized system response is proportional in all cases to $(T/N_0)^{1/2}$, which is proportional to the signal-to-noise ratio. This is explained in the next few lines.

The energy in the shaping function is

$$E = \int_0^T h_S^2(t)\, dt = \delta T \tag{4.5.62}$$

with $\delta = 1$ for NRZ and SP and $\delta = 0.5$ for HS. The average energy per bit is

$$E_b = (M^2 - 1)\delta T/(3 \log_2 M) \tag{4.5.63}$$

thus

$$T/N_0 = \frac{3 \log_2 M}{\delta(M^2 - 1)} E_b/N_0 \tag{4.5.64}$$

Note that the energy per bit, $E_b$, here is defined at the transmitter filter input, not at the receiver filter input as was done in section 4.2. They are related by

$$E = E_C \int_{-\infty}^{\infty} |H_S(f)|^2\, df \Big/ \int_{-\infty}^{\infty} |H_S(f)H_{TC}(f)|^2\, df \tag{4.5.65}$$

Thus when the bandwidth of the transmitter-channel filter is not too narrow, most of the shaping function energy passes this filter. Hence $E$ is very close to $E_C$, and the difference between the two definitions is not significant.

We applied the bounds of 4.4.3.2 and 4.4.3.8 and obtained the bit error probability as a function of signal-to-noise ratio per bit, filter bandwidth, and other parameters. In Fig. 4.28 we show the bit error probability for six of the systems in Table 4.3 with binary symbols as a function of 3-dB bandwidth. In this figure it was assumed that the filters in receiver and transmitter are identical Butterworth filters of order $N_B = 2, 3, 4$, and the signal-to-noise ratio was fixed to 10 dB. Note that the systems in which the detector filter is matched to the shaping function (systems NN and HH) improve with bandwidth, though other systems, particularly the systems with a sample detector (NS and HS), have an optimal bandwidth. Note also that when the bandwidth is narrow (about $f_{B0} \leq 0.65\, R$) the systems with the sample

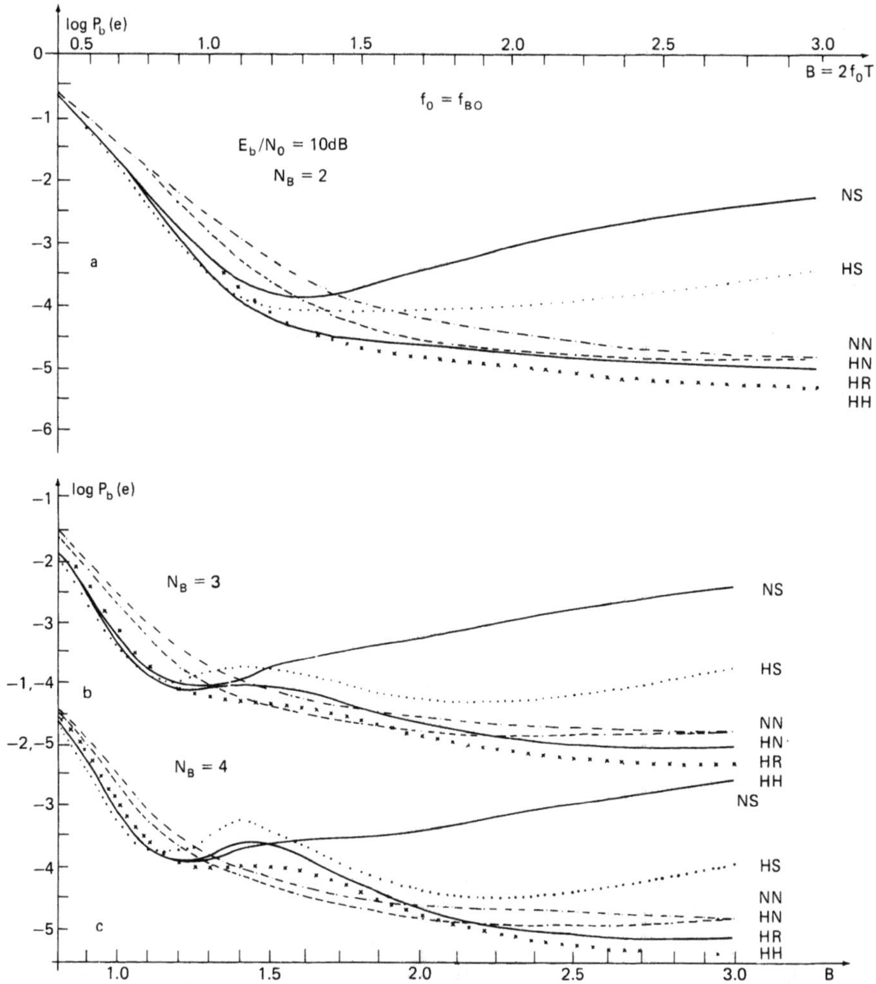


Fig. 4.28. Bit error probability of binary ASK for systems NN, NS, HH, HS, HR, and HN as a function of normalised 3-dB bandwidth (I. Korn, "OQASK and MSK Systems with Bandlimiting Filters in Transmitter and Receiver and Various Detector Filters," *IEE Proc.*, Vol. 127, Pt. F, December 1980, pp. 439–447).

detector are not worse than the systems with matched filters or other detectors. In addition, in this range of bandwidth, systems NS and HS have an almost identical error probability. This has a simple intuitive explanation. When the filters are narrowband, it does not matter what the shaping function is; the output is determined by the filters only. Figure 4.29 is similar to Fig. 4.28 with two differences: the symbols are quaternary, and the systems are NS and HS.

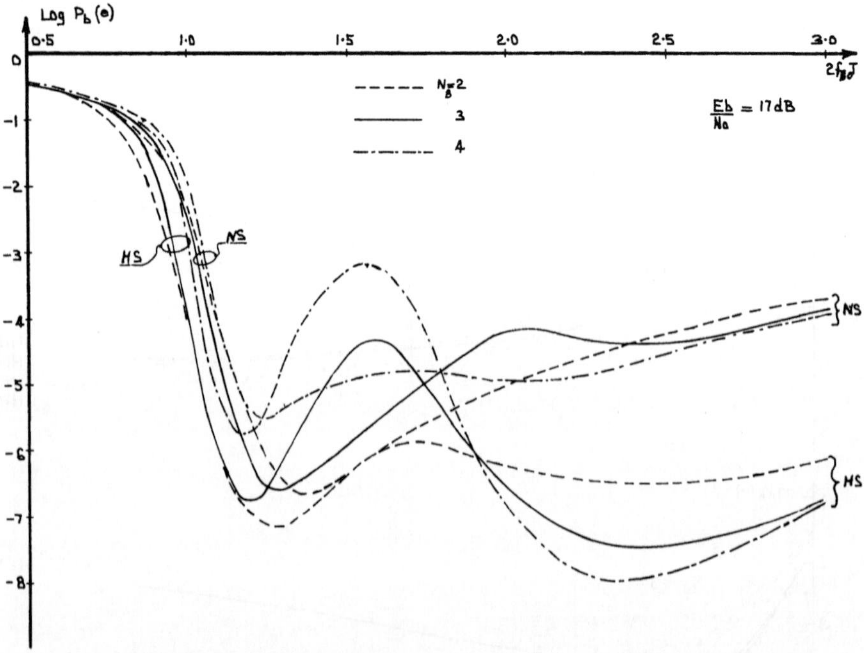


Fig. 4.29. Bit error probability of quaternary ASK for systems NS and HS as a function of normalized bandwidth (I. Korn, Y. Tsang, "Effect of Intersymbol and Quadrature Channel Interference on Error Probability of 16-ary Offset Quadrature Amplitude Modulation with Sinusoidal and Rectangular Shaping," IEEE *Tr. Comm.*, Vol. COM-31, February 1983, pp. 264–269. Copyright © 1983 IEEE).

In Figs. 4.30 and 4.31 we present the bit error probability of binary systems as a function of signal-to-noise ratio. The parameters are the filter bandwidth and filter order. The curve optimal corresponds to the matched filter case and wideband transmitter-channel-receiver filters. The horizontal difference between the curve marked optimal and any other curve is the additional energy in dB required in the nonoptimal systems to achieve the same error probability as in the optimal system.

*Example* 4.5.1 Error probability in a system with Butterworth filters
Find the signal-to-noise ratio required to achieve a bit error probability of $10^{-7}$ in the NN system with identical Butterworth filters in transmitter and receiver of order 4 and bandwidth $f_{B0} = R$.

*Solution* From Fig. 4.31 we obtain that the signal-to-noise ratio is about 12.4 dB. In the optimal case the required signal-to-noise ratio is 11.3 dB. Therefore the system with the Butterworth filters requires 1.1 dB more energy than the optimal system.

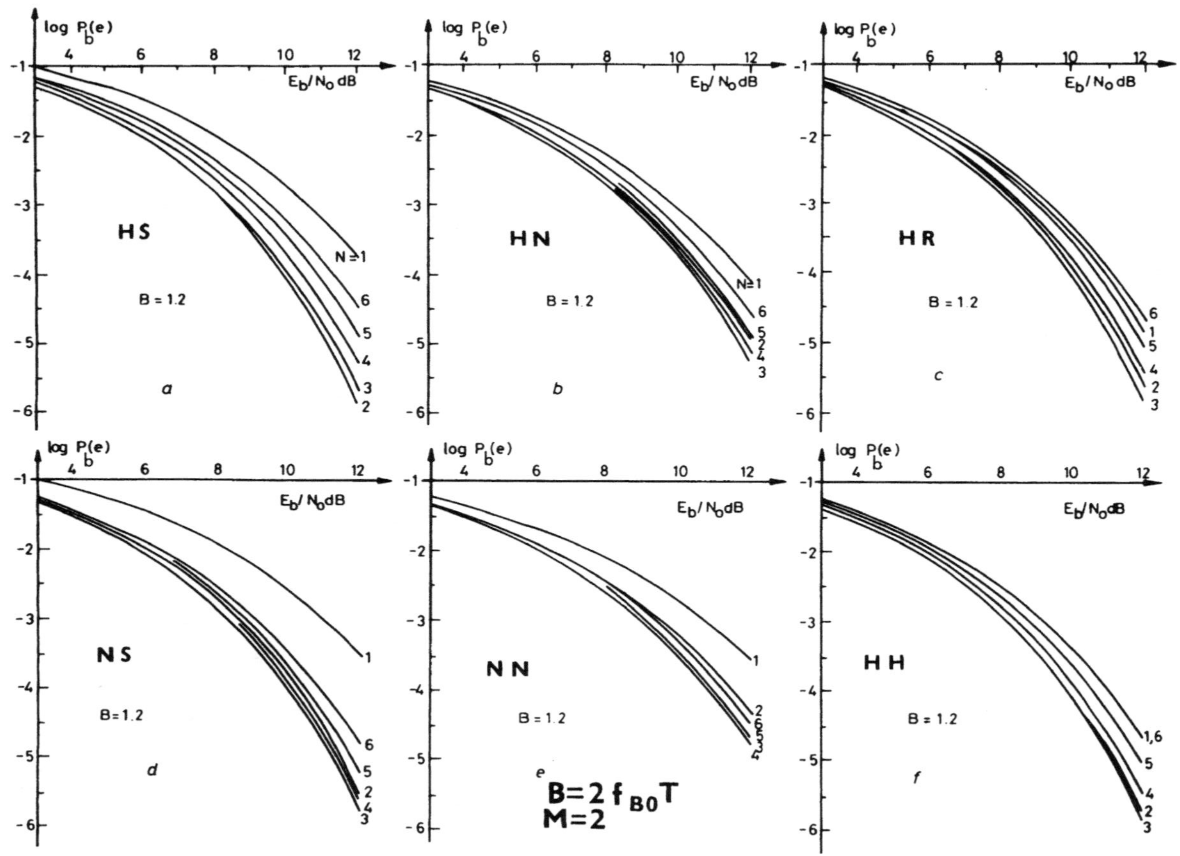


Fig. 4.30. Bit error probability of binary ASK for systems NN, NS, HH, HS, HR and HN as a function of signal-to-noise ratio per bit (I. Korn, "OQASK and MSK systems with Bandlimiting Filters in Transmitter and Receiver and Various Detector Filters," *IEE Proc.*, Vol. 127, Pt. F, December 1980, pp. 439–447).

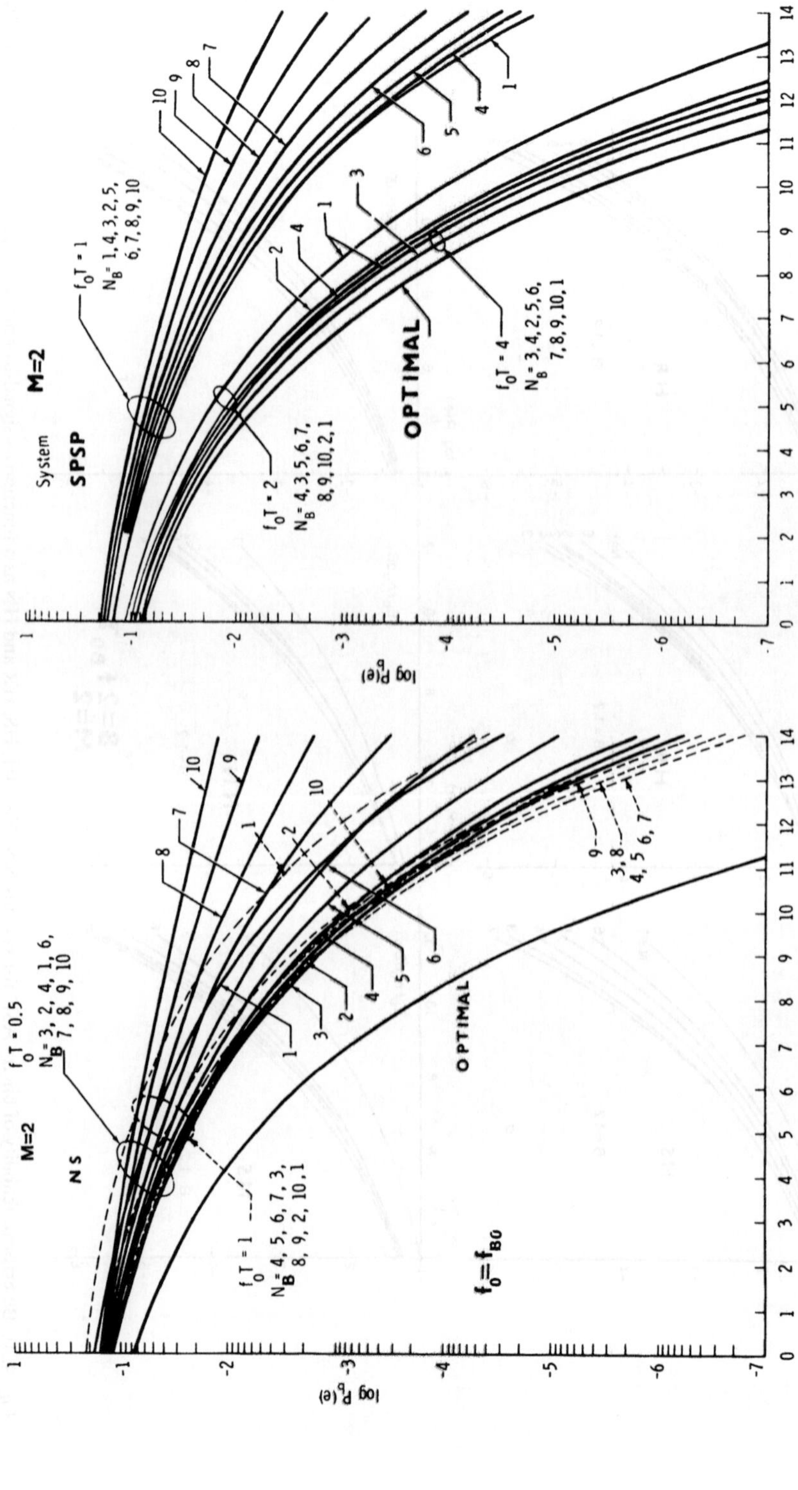
System
SPSP
M=2
$f_0T = 1$
$N_B = 1, 4, 3, 2, 5, 6, 7, 8, 9, 10$
$f_0T = 2$
$N_B = 4, 3, 5, 6, 7, 8, 9, 10, 2, 1$
$f_0T = 4$
$N_B = 3, 4, 2, 5, 6, 7, 8, 9, 10, 1$
OPTIMAL
log $P_b(e)$
$E_b/No$ (dB)
M=2
N S
$f_0 = f_{BO}$
$f_0T = 0.5$
$N_B = 3, 2, 4, 1, 6, 7, 8, 9, 10$
$f_0T = 1$
$N_B = 4, 5, 6, 7, 3, 8, 9, 2, 10, 1$
OPTIMAL
log $P_b(e)$
$E_b/No$ (dB)

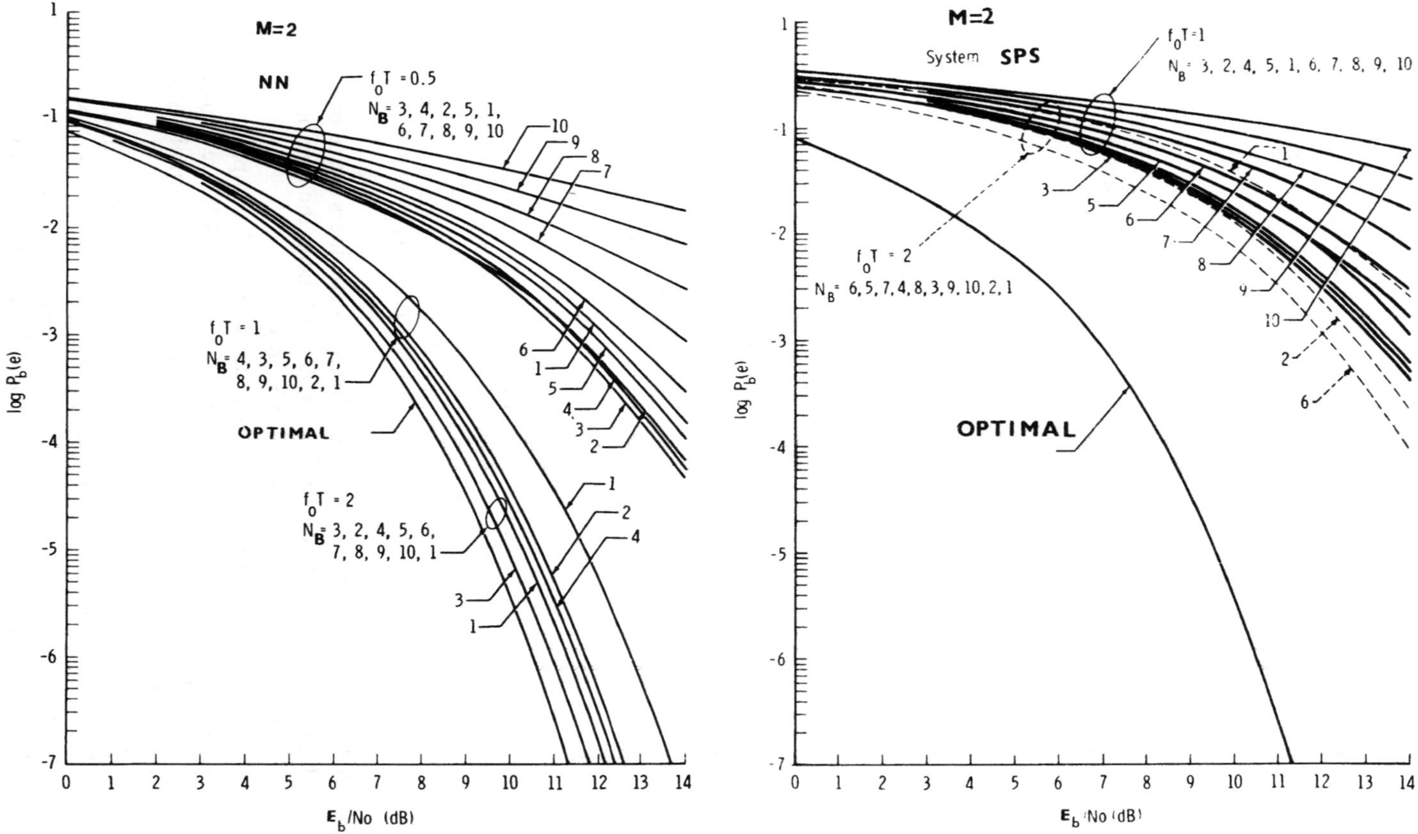


Fig. 4.31. Bit error probability of binary ASK for systems SPS, SPSP, NS, and NN as function of signal-to-noise ratio per bit (I. Korn, "Probability of Error in Binary Communication Systems with Causal Bandlimiting Filters," *IEEE Tr. Comm.*, Vol. COM-21, August 1973, pp. 878–898. Copyright © 1973 IEEE).

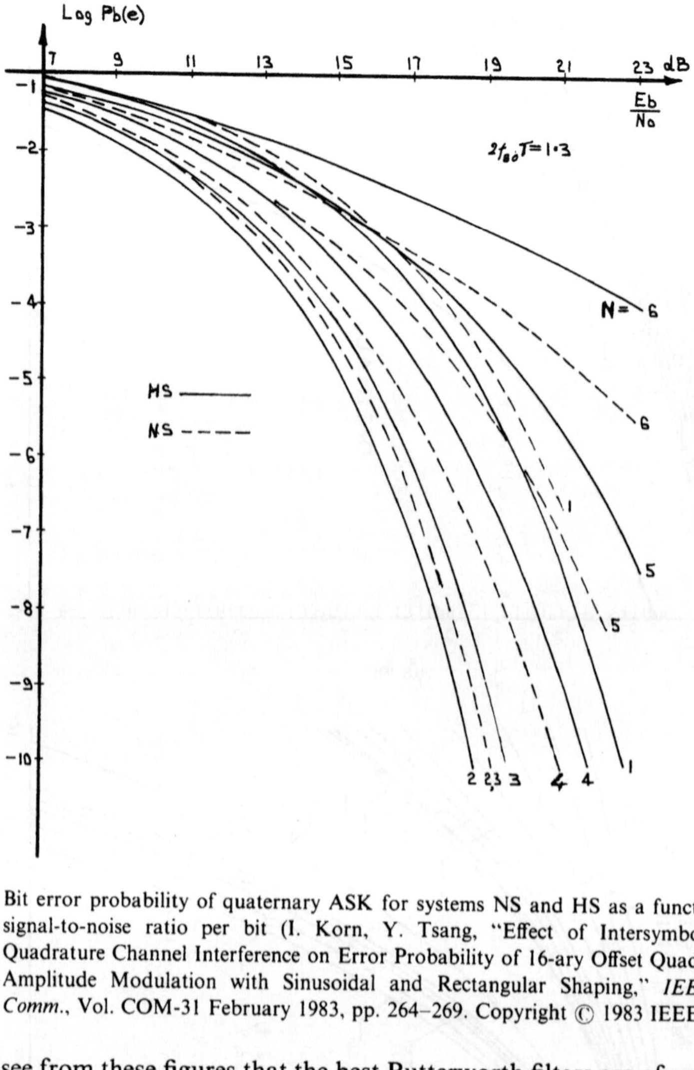


Fig. 4.32. Bit error probability of quaternary ASK for systems NS and HS as a function of signal-to-noise ratio per bit (I. Korn, Y. Tsang, "Effect of Intersymbol and Quadrature Channel Interference on Error Probability of 16-ary Offset Quadrature Amplitude Modulation with Sinusoidal and Rectangular Shaping," *IEEE Tr. Comm.*, Vol. COM-31 February 1983, pp. 264–269. Copyright © 1983 IEEE).

We can see from these figures that the best Butterworth filters are of order 2, 3, or 4. Figure 4.32 is similar to Fig. 4.30, but here the symbols are quaternary, and the systems are HS and NS only.

In computing the error probability, we used optimal sampling times. Optimal sampling times for systems HS, NN, SPSP, and SPS are shown in Table 4.6. The effect of offset in sampling time from its optimal value is demonstrated in Fig. 4.33.

In Table 4.7 we show the actual values of the upper and lower bounds from eqs. (4.4.37) and (4.4.39) for the following case: the system is NN, the transmitter and receiver filters are identical Butterworth filters of order $N_B = 5$ and bandwidth $f_{B0}T = 1$, or the bandwith of transmitter filter is $\infty$,

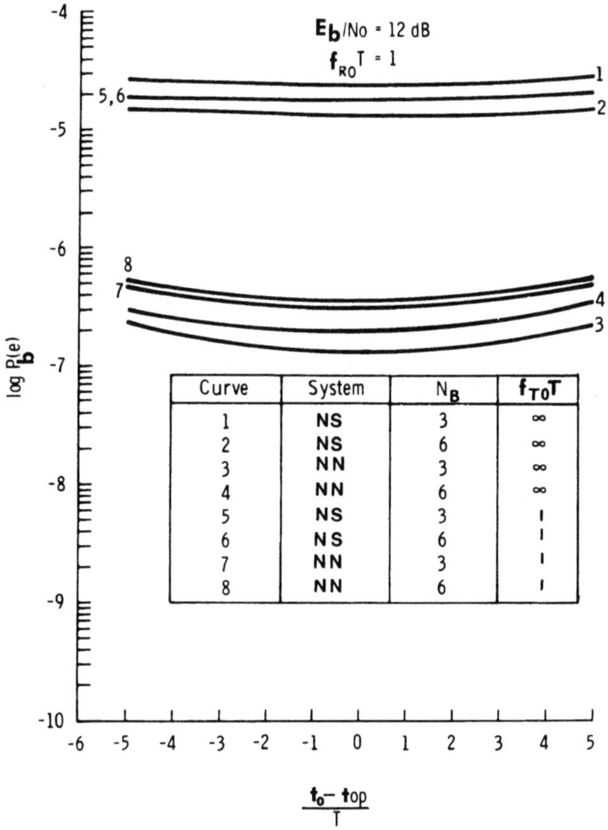


| Curve | System | $N_B$ | $f_{TO}T$ |
|---|---|---|---|
| 1 | NS | 3 | ∞ |
| 2 | NS | 6 | ∞ |
| 3 | NN | 3 | ∞ |
| 4 | NN | 6 | ∞ |
| 5 | NS | 3 | 1 |
| 6 | NS | 6 | 1 |
| 7 | NN | 3 | 1 |
| 8 | NN | 6 | 1 |

Fig. 4.33. Effect of offset in sampling time on bit error probability of systems NS and NN (I. Korn, "Probability of Error in Binary Communication system with Causal Bandlimiting Filters. Part I: Nonreturn to Zero Signals," *IEEE Tr. Comm.*, Vol. COM-21, August 1973, pp. 878–890. Copyright © 1973 IEEE).

the optimal sampling times are $t_0 = 2.053$ and 1.532, the number of significant interfering terms is $N = 4$ (three from the past and one from the future), and the number of terms in the remainder $R_N$ was selected so that additional terms have not changed the fourth significant figure in $P_U(e)$. As can be seen the bounds practically coincide; hence either the lower or upper bound can be used as the true value.

Similar, practically coinciding bounds have been obtained in all other cases, but the number of required significant interfering terms increased with increasing filter order, $N_B$, and decreasing bandwidth, $f_{BO}T$, but in no case that we considered has the number exceeded 8.

In applying the approximation of Section 4.4.3.8 we used $N \leqq 8$ and $K = 15$. We tried larger numbers, but this has not changed the error probability.

## Table 4.6 Optimal sampling time $t_{op}/T$

| $f_{T0}T$ | $f_{R0}T$ | SYSTEM | $N_B$ 1 | 2 | 3 | 4 | 5 | 6 | 7 | 8 | 9 | 10 |
|---|---|---|---|---|---|---|---|---|---|---|---|---|
| ∞ | 0.5 | NS | 1.000 | 1.045 | 1.204 | 1.402 | 1.615 | 1.834 | 2.057 | 2.281 | 2.507 | 2.734 |
| ∞ | 0.5 | NN | 1.215 | 1.483 | 1.731 | 1.959 | 2.178 | 2.396 | 2.616 | 2.836 | 3.057 | 3.280 |
| 0.5 | 0.5 | NS | 1.069 | 1.489 | 1.933 | 2.359 | 2.793 | 3.233 | 3.675 | 4.120 | 4.565 | 5.002 |
| 0.5 | 0.5 | NN | 1.501 | 1.999 | 2.466 | 2.903 | 3.334 | 3.767 | 4.202 | 4.637 | 5.071 | 5.503 |
| ∞ | 1.0 | NS | 1.000 | 0.710 | 0.810 | 0.920 | 1.040 | 1.140 | 1.240 | 1.340 | 1.440 | 1.551 |
| ∞ | 1.0 | NN | 1.118 | 1.228 | 1.328 | 1.431 | 1.532 | 1.634 | 1.735 | 1.836 | 1.937 | 2.038 |
| 1.0 | 1.0 | NS | 1.002 | 1.020 | 1.184 | 1.366 | 1.569 | 1.780 | 1.989 | 2.202 | 2.414 | 2.626 |
| 1.0 | 1.0 | NN | 1.270 | 1.469 | 1.659 | 1.855 | 2.053 | 2.253 | 2.453 | 2.655 | 2.857 | 3.061 |
| ∞ | 2.0 | NS | 1.062 | 1.114 | 1.166 | 1.218 | 1.269 | 1.321 | 1.372 | 1.423 | 1.474 | 1.525 |
| 2.0 | 2.0 | NN | 1.140 | 1.233 | 1.332 | 1.432 | 1.533 | 1.634 | 1.735 | 1.837 | 1.940 | 2.042 |

## Table 4.7 Upper and lower bounds to probability of error system NN $f_{R0}T = 1$

| $E_b/N_0$ (dB) | $f_{T0}T = \infty$ | | $f_{T0}T = 1$ | |
|---|---|---|---|---|
| | $P_L(e)$ | $P_U(e)$ | $P_L(e)$ | $P_U(e)$ |
| 0 | $8.935 \cdot 10^{-2}$ | $8.936 \cdot 10^{-2}$ | $9.233 \cdot 10^{-2}$ | $9.238 \cdot 10^{-2}$ |
| 1 | $6.590 \cdot 10^{-2}$ | $6.592 \cdot 10^{-2}$ | $6.863 \cdot 10^{-2}$ | $6.867 \cdot 10^{-2}$ |
| 2 | $4.567 \cdot 10^{-2}$ | $4.568 \cdot 10^{-2}$ | $4.804 \cdot 10^{-2}$ | $4.808 \cdot 10^{-2}$ |
| 3 | $2.933 \cdot 10^{-2}$ | $2.934 \cdot 10^{-2}$ | $3.125 \cdot 10^{-2}$ | $3.128 \cdot 10^{-2}$ |
| 4 | $1.716 \cdot 10^{-2}$ | $1.717 \cdot 10^{-2}$ | $1.859 \cdot 10^{-2}$ | $1.861 \cdot 10^{-2}$ |
| 5 | $8.950 \cdot 10^{-3}$ | $8.953 \cdot 10^{-3}$ | $9.920 \cdot 10^{-3}$ | $9.934 \cdot 10^{-3}$ |
| 6 | $4.060 \cdot 10^{-3}$ | $4.062 \cdot 10^{-3}$ | $4.635 \cdot 10^{-3}$ | $4.643 \cdot 10^{-3}$ |
| 7 | $1.553 \cdot 10^{-3}$ | $1.554 \cdot 10^{-3}$ | $1.842 \cdot 10^{-3}$ | $1.846 \cdot 10^{-3}$ |
| 8 | $4.821 \cdot 10^{-4}$ | $4.825 \cdot 10^{-4}$ | $6.012 \cdot 10^{-4}$ | $6.028 \cdot 10^{-4}$ |
| 9 | $1.160 \cdot 10^{-4}$ | $1.161 \cdot 10^{-4}$ | $1.540 \cdot 10^{-4}$ | $1.545 \cdot 10^{-4}$ |
| 10 | $2.043 \cdot 10^{-5}$ | $2.045 \cdot 10^{-5}$ | $2.924 \cdot 10^{-5}$ | $2.936 \cdot 10^{-5}$ |
| 11 | $2.442 \cdot 10^{-6}$ | $2.446 \cdot 10^{-6}$ | $3.821 \cdot 10^{-6}$ | $3.840 \cdot 10^{-6}$ |
| 12 | $1.802 \cdot 10^{-7}$ | $1.805 \cdot 10^{-7}$ | $3.125 \cdot 10^{-7}$ | $3.144 \cdot 10^{-7}$ |
| 13 | $7.243 \cdot 10^{-9}$ | $7.260 \cdot 10^{-9}$ | $1.416 \cdot 10^{-8}$ | $1.427 \cdot 10^{-8}$ |
| 14 | $1.350 \cdot 10^{-10}$ | $1.354 \cdot 10^{-10}$ | $3.058 \cdot 10^{-10}$ | $3.088 \cdot 10^{-10}$ |

## 4.6 APPROXIMATION OF NYQUIST FUNCTION[4.37–4.38]

In Section 4.3 we showed that Nyquist functions of the raised cosine family with excess bandwidth $0 \leq \beta \leq 1$ cause no ISI, and with a matched filter in transmitter and receiver we obtain the least error probability. Expressions

(4.3.27) and (4.3.36) are not in the form of filters with a finite number of poles. Hence a problem arises in approximating these formulas by filters with a finite number of poles. This problem is treated in depth in Refs. 4.37 and 4.38.

## 4.7 SUMMARY

We have derived an expression of the error probability for an ASK system with and without ISI. We have found the condition of no ISI and treated in some detail the raised cosine family with excess bandwidth $\beta$, beyond the minimum Nyquist bandwidth. We have presented various bounds and an approximation to the error probability in the presence of no ISI. We have applied two of these bounds to a system with a Nyquist function, but with offset in sampling time, and to systems with NRZ, HS, and SP shaping functions, various detector filters, and Butterworth filters in receiver and transmitter. We have shown that for narrow filter bandwidth (and this is the most practical case) the simplest system, i.e., a system with a sample detector, is the best system, and it does not matter whether the shaping function is HS or NRZ. Because systems with NRZ and HS shaping function represent what is known as QPSK (or OQASK) and MSK systems (the ASK system is one of two identical branches of these system), all results of this section are valid for these systems also.

## 4.8 PROBLEMS

4.2.1 A maximum a posteriori (MAP) decision rule is

$$\hat{a}_k = a(m) \text{ if } P(a_k = a(m)|r_k) = \max_{i=1,\ldots M} P(a_k = a(i)|r_k)$$

Show that if the symbols are equiprobable, the MAP rule is the same as the maximum likelihood rule.

4.2.2 Derive the ML rule assuming that the noise has a double exponential probability density

$$p_n(x) = 0.5\,\lambda \exp(-\lambda|x|)$$

4.2.3 Compute the bit error probability in an $M$-ary ASK system with matched filter as a function of signal-to-noise ratio per bit if the symbols are from the set $\mathring{A}_0 = \{0, 1, \ldots, M-1\}$. If $M = 2$, this system is called *on-off-keying* (OOK). Compare the energy required to achieve an error probability of $10^{-6}$ in OOK and in binary system with symbols $\pm 1$.

4.2.4 Show that if we double the number of symbols in an $M$-ary ASK system with matched filters and $M$ is large, we need 6 dB more energy per symbol to achieve the same symbol error probability.

4.2.5

a. Derive and sketch the matched filters for NRZ, RZ, and HS shaping functions ($t_0 = T$).

b. Compute the output of these filters when the input is the NRZ pulse.

c. Compute the values of $\eta$ if the input is the NRZ pulse. (Assume $h_T(t) = h_C(t) = h_R(t) = \delta(t)$).

4.2.6 Compute the signal-to-noise ratio per bit, $\gamma_b$, to achieve a bit error probability of $10^{-4}$ in an $M$-ary ASK system with matched filter and $M = 2$ $k$, $k = 1, 2, \ldots, 8$.

4.3.1 A function $G(f)$ has the form

$$G(f) = (0.5\,A/R)(2\,R - |f|) \qquad |f| \leqq 2\,R$$

Compute and sketch $G_\Sigma(f)$.

4.3.2 The complex function

$$G(f) = G_I(f) + jG_Q(f)$$

is 0 for $|f| \geqq R$. Show that this function has no ISI if $G_I(f)$ is an even function and $G_Q(f)$ is an odd function around $f = R/2$ for $f \geqq 0$.

4.3.3 Let

$$H(f) = (2\,A/R)(R/2 - f)u_{0.5R}(f)$$

Let $G_1(f)$ and $G_2(f)$ be even functions of $f$, such that for $f \geqq 0$

$$G_1(f) = H(f) + H(f - 2\,R)$$

$$G_2(f) = H(f) + H(-f + 2.5\,R)$$

a. Sketch $H(f)$, $G_1(f)$, and $G_2(f)$.

b. Will $g_1(t)$ and $g_2(t)$ cause ISI?

4.3.4 In an ASK system, the samples of the system response are

$$g_0 = 2,\ g_1 = g_{-1} = -1,\ g_i = 0\ |i| > 1$$

Find the function $G(f)$ with minimum bandwidth.

4.3.5 Let $g(t)$ be the system response of an ASK system. Let $h(t)$ be the derivative of $g(t)$. Let $g_k$ and $h_k$ be the samples of $g(t)$ and $h(t)$, respectively, at times $t_k = kT$. Note that $h_k = 0$ for all $k$ means that a small amount of offset or jitter in the sampling times does not affect the value of $g_k$.

a. Show that

$$g_k = \int_{-f_N}^{f_N} G_\Sigma(f) \exp(j\, 2\, \pi f k T)\, df$$

b. Show that

$$G_\Sigma(f) = T \sum_k g_k \exp(-j\, 2\, \pi f k T)$$

c. Show that

$$h_k = \int_{-f_N}^{f_N} H_\Sigma(f) \exp(j\, 2\, \pi k T)\, df$$

where

$$H_\Sigma(f) = \sum_k j\, 2\, \pi(f - kR) G(f - kR)$$

d. Show that $h_k = 0$ all $k$ is equivalent to

$$\sum_k kG(f - kR) = f T^2 \sum_k g_k \exp(-j\, 2\, \pi f k T)$$

e. Show that (d) cannot be achieved by a function $G(f)$ with bandwidth less than $R$.

f. Show that the function

$$G(f) = T(1 - |f|T) \sum_k g_k \exp(-j\, 2\, \pi f k T) U_{2R}(f + R)$$

satisfies both (b) and (d).

g. Find a function $G(f)$ for which $h_k = 0$ all $k$ and $g_k = 0$, $k \neq 0$. This function has no ISI and is tolerant to sampling time jitter.

4.4.1 $g(t)$ is obtained from the response of a first-order Butterworth filter to an NRZ shaping function. Assume $\omega_{B0} T = 4$.

a. Compute and sketch $g(t)$.
b. Assuming that $t_0 = T$, compute the values of $g_i$ for $-5 \leq i \leq 5$.
c. Repeat (b) if $t_0 = 2.5\,T$.
d. Which of the samples in (c) are associated with past symbols and which with future symbols? How many past and future symbols affect the performance?
e. Reorder the samples in (c) according to nonincreasing value.
f. Reorder the samples in (c) to obtain

$$I = \sum_{1}^{10} a_i h_i \qquad \text{with } a_i = \pm 1$$

if the system has quaternary symbols ($\pm 1, \pm 3$).

4.4.2 In three ASK systems the noise variance is the same, but the samples of the system response are

| SYSTEM | $g_0$ | $g_{-1}$ | $g_{-2}$ | $g_1$ | $g_2$ | $g_3$ |
|---|---|---|---|---|---|---|
| 1 | 10 | 2 | −1 | 0.5 | 0.25 | 1 |
| 2 | 10 | −2 | −0.25 | −0.5 | −1 | 1 |
| 3 | 5 | 2 | −1 | 0.5 | 0.25 | 1 |

Rank the three systems according to error probability.

4.4.3
a. Compute the probability density of

$$I = \sum_{i=1}^{\infty} a_i h^i, \; a_i = \pm 1$$

if $h = 1/2$ and $h = 1/4$.
b. Assume you have the probability density of $I$ when $h = A$. Compute the probability density when $h = A^2$, $h = A^{1/2}$, and $h = A^{1/3}$.

4.4.4 Compute the values of $I_N(j)$ if only $h_1$ and $h_2$ are nonzero and the symbols are quaternary ($-1, \pm 3$).

4.4.5 Write a computer program for the computation of the bounds in (4.4.37). Assume that the total number of samples is $K$ and the number of terms in $I_N$ is $N < K$.

4.4.6

a. Show that

$$P(n \geqq g_0 + I_N(j) + R_n) = \int_0^\infty (2\pi\sigma_n^2)^{-1/2}$$

$$\exp\{-0.5(n - g_0 - I_N(j) - R_N)/\sigma_n^2\}\, dn$$

b. Show that if $a \in \mathring{A}_\pm$

$$\exp(\lambda a_i h_i) \leqq \exp\{\lambda^2 \sigma_a^2 h^2{}_i/2\}$$

(Hint: expand both sides into Taylor series, and show that each term of the series on the left-hand side is not greater than the corresponding term on the right-hand side.)

c. Using (b) show that

$$\exp(-\lambda R_N) \leqq \exp(\lambda^2 \sigma_{RN}^2/2)$$

$$\sigma_{RN}^2 = \sigma_a^2 \sum_{N+1}^{\infty} h_i^2,\ \sigma_a^2 = (M^2 - 1)/3$$

d. Using (c) with $\lambda = n - g_0 - I_N(j)$, show that

$$\overline{P(n \geqq g_0 + I_N(j) + R_N)} \leqq \{1 - (\sigma_{RN}/\sigma_n)^2\}^{-1/2} Q\{(g_0 + I_N(j))/\sigma\}$$

where $\sigma$ is given in eq. (4.4.41).

e. Show that

$$P(I + n > g_0) \leqq Q\{(g_0 + I_N)/\sigma\}$$

4.4.7

a. Using Schwartz's inequality for real functions

$$\left\{\int_{-\infty}^{\infty} f(x)g(x)\, dx\right\}^2 \leqq \int_{-\infty}^{\infty} f^2(x)\, dx \int_{-\infty}^{\infty} g^2(x)\, dx$$

show that if $x$ is a zero-mean random variable, then

$$\overline{(|x|^n)^2} \leqq \overline{|x|^{n+k}}\ \overline{|x|^{n-k}},\ n \geqq k \geqq 0$$

b. Show that

$$(\overline{|x|})^2 \leqq \overline{x^2} = \sigma_x^2$$

$$\overline{|x|} \geqq \sigma_x^4/\overline{|x|^3}$$

$$\overline{|x|} \geqq \sigma_x^3/\overline{x^4}$$

c. Using Jensen's inequality for concave functions

$$\overline{f(x)} \geqq f(\overline{x})$$

show that if $g_0 \geqq \rho_0$ and $Q_n(x)$ is concave for $x \geqq 0$, $P$ is bounded by

$$P \leqq Q_n(g_0 + \sigma_I) + Q_n(g_0 - \sigma_I^3/(\overline{I^4})^{1/2}$$

d. Show that if $g_0 \geqq 3\,\sigma_n$, $\rho_0 < \sigma_n/2$, then

$$P_L \leqq P \leqq cP_L$$

where

$$P_L = Q_n(g_0) + (1/2)\rho_0^2 Q_n''(g_0)$$

$$c = (1/2)\{Q_n(g_0 - \rho_0) + Q_n(g_0 + \rho_0)\}/\{Q_n(g_0) + (1/2)\rho_0^2 Q_n''(g_0)\}$$

and $Q_n''(g_0)$ is the second derivative of $Q_n(x)$ at $x = g_0$.

4.4.8 Write a computer program for the computation of $P_a$ (eq. (4.4.125) or (4.4.132)) assuming the number of interfering terms is $N$ and $K < N$.

4.5.1 Derive eq. (4.5.24).

4.5.2 Derive eqs. (4.5.29)–(4.5.34).

4.5.3 Derive eqs. (4.5.47) and (4.5.48) and the entries in Table 4.5.

4.5.4 Derive eq. (4.5.56).

4.5.5 Derive eq. (4.5.58).

4.5.6

a. Compute the variance $\sigma_n^2$ of eq. (4.5.59), assuming a Butterworth filter of order $N$.

b. Sketch $\sigma_n^2$ as a function of $N$ for $N = 1, 2, \ldots, 10$ and $f_0 T = 0.5, 1.0$.

4.5.7 The noise bandwidth of a filter is

$$B_n = \int_0^\infty |H(f)|^2 \, df$$

Compute the relation between noise bandwidth and 3-dB bandwidth of a Butterworth filter.

4.5.8 Use your computer program in Problem (4.4.5) to compute the error probability of system NS with second-order Butterworth filters in receiver and transmitter.

4.5.9 Use your computer program in Problem 4.4.8 to compute the error probability of system NS with second-order Butterworth filters in receiver and transmitter.

## 4.9 REFERENCES

4.1 P. O. Borjesson and C. E. W. Sundberg, "Simple Approximations of the Error Function $Q(x)$ for Communications Applications," *IEEE Tr. Comm.*, Vol. COM-27, March 1979, pp. 639–642.

4.2 E. A. Newcombe and S. Pasupathy, "Error Rate Monitoring for Digital Communications," *Proc. IEEE*, Vol. 70. August 1982, pp. 805–828.

4.3 F. S. Hill and M. A. Blanco, "Random Geometric Series and Intersymbol Interference," *IEEE Tr. Inf. Theory*, Vol. IT-19, May 1973, pp. 326–335.

4.4 M. Abramowitz and I. A. Stegun, *Handbook of Mathematical Functions*, National Bureau of Standards, Washington D.C., 1967, p. 287.

4.5 Y. W. Yeh and E. Y. Ho, "Improved Interference Error Bounds in Digital Systems," *BSTJ*, Vol. 50, Oct. 1971, p. 2585–2598.

4.6 M. R. Aaron and D. W. Tufts, "Intersymbol Interference and Error Probability," *IEEE Tr. Inf. Theory*, Vol. II-12, Jan. 1966, pp. 26–34.

4.7 E. Y. Ho and Y. S. Yeh, "A New Approach for Evaluating the Error Probability in the Presence of Intersymbol Interference and Additive Gaussian Noise," *BSTJ*, Vol. 49, Nov. 1970, pp. 2249–2266.

4.8 E. Y. Ho and Y. S. Yeh, "Error probability of Multilevel Digital System and Intersymbol Interference and Gaussian Noise," *BSTJ*, Vol. 50, March 1971, pp. 1017–1023.

4.9 O. Shimbo and M. I. Celebiler, "The Probability of Error due to Intersymbol Interference and Gaussian Noise in Digital Communication Systems," *IEEE Tr. Comm. Tech.*, Vol. COM-19, April 1971, pp. 113–119.

4.10 V. K. Prabhu, "Some Considerations of Error Bounds in Digital Systems," *BSTJ*, Vol. 50, Dec. 1971, pp. 3127–3151.

4.11 I. Korn, "Bounds to Probability of Error in Binary Communication Systems with Intersymbol Interference with Dependent or Independent Symbols," *IEEE Tr. Comm.*, Vol. COM-22, Feb. 1974, pp. 251–254.

4.12 J. V. Murphy, "Binary Error Rate Caused by Intersymbol Interference and Gaussian Noise," *IEEE Tr. Comm.*, Vol. COM-21, Sept. 1973, pp. 1039–1046.
4.13 G. H. Golub and J. H. Welsh, "Calculation of Gauss Quadrature Rules," *Math Comput.*, Vol. 23, April 1969, pp. 221–230.
4.14 S. Benedetto, G. De Vincentis, and A. Luvison, "Error Probability in the Presence of Intersymbol Interference and additive Noise for Multilevel Digital Signals," *IEEE Tr. Comm. Tech.*, Vol. COM-21, March 1973, pp. 181–190.
4.15 S. Benedetto, G. De Vincentis, and A. Luvison, "Application of Gaussian Quadrature Rules to Digital Communication Problems," *IEEE Tr. Comm.*, Vol. COM-21, Oct. 1973, pp. 1159–165.
4.16 B. S. Saltzberg, "Intersymbol Interference Error Bounds with Application to Ideal Bandlimited Signals," *IEEE Tr. Inf. Theory*, Vol. IT-14, July 1968, pp. 563–568.
4.17 J. W. Smith, "A Simple Approximation of Data System Error Rate," *IEEE Tr. Comm. Tech.*, Vol. COM-17, June 1969, pp. 415–417.
4.18 R. Lugannani, "Intersymbol Interference and Probability of Error in Digital Systems," *IEEE Tr. Inf. Theory*, Vol. IT-15, Nov. 1970, pp. 686–688.
4.19 P. J. Mclane, "Lower Bounds for Finite Intersymbol Interference Error Rates," *IEEE Tr. Comm.*, Vol. COM-22, June 1974, pp. 853–857.
4.20 F. E. Glave, "An Upper Bound to the Probability of Error due to Intersymbol Interference for Uncorrelated Digital Signals," *IEEE Tr. Inf. Theory*, Vol. IT-18, May 1972, pp. 356–363.
4.21 J. W. Matthews, "Sharp Error Bounds for Intersymbol Interference," *IEEE Tr. Inf. Theory*, Vol. IT-19, July 1973, pp. 440–447.
4.22 I. Korn, "Improvement to Sharp Error Bounds for Intersymbol Interference," *Proc. IEE*, Vol. 122, March 1975, pp. 265–267.
4.23 K. Yao and E. M. Biglieri, "Multidimensional Moment Error Bounds for Digital Communication Systems," *IEEE Tr. Inf. Theory*, Vol. IT-26, July 1980, pp. 454–464.
4.24 K. Yao and R. M. Tobin, "Moment Space Upper and Lower Error Bounds for Digital Systems with Intersymbol Interference," *IEEE Tr. Inf. Theory*, Vol. IT-22, Jan. 1976, pp. 65–74.
4.25 Y. C. Jenq, B. Liu, and J. B. Thomas, "Probability of Error in PAM Systems with Intersymbol Interference and Additive Noise," *IEEE Tr. Inf. Theory*, Vol. IT-23, Sept. 1977, pp. 575–582.
4.26 Y. C. Jenq, B. Liu, and J. B. Thomas, "Threshold Effect on Error Probability in QAM Systems," *IEEE Tr. Comm.*, Vol. COM-28, July 1980, pp. 1047–1051.
4.27 V. K. Prabhu, "Intersymbol Interference Performance of Systems with Correlated Digital Signals," *IEEE Tr. Comm.*, Vol. COM-21, Oct. 1973., pp. 1147–1152.
4.28 I. Korn, "Probability of Error in Digital Communication Systems with Intersymbol Interference and Dependent Symbols," *IEEE Tr. Inf. Theory*, Vol. IT-20, Sept. 1972, pp. 663–668.
4.29 I. Korn, "Intersymbol Interference in Binary Communication System with Single Pole Bandlimiting Filters," *IEEE Tr. Comm.*, Vol. COM-21, March 1973, pp. 238–243.
4.30 I. Korn, "Probability of Error in Binary Communication System with Causal Bandlimiting Filters. Part 1: Nonreturn to Zero Signals," *IEEE Tr. Comm.*, Vol. COM-21, August 1973, pp. 878–890.
4.31 I. Korn, "Probability of Error in Binary Communication Systems with Causal Bandlimiting Filters. Part 2: Split Phase Signals," *IEEE Tr. Comm.*, Vol. COM-21, August 1973, pp. 891–898.
4.32 I. Korn, "Performance of Several Digital Communication Systems," *Proc. IEE*, Vol. 126, August 1979, pp. 724–728.
4.33 I. Korn, "The Effect of Bandlimiting Filters on Probability of Error of MSK," *IEEE Tr. Comm.*, Vol. COM-27, Sept. 1979, pp. 1348–1353.

4.34 I. Korn, "OQASK and MSK Systems with Bandlimiting Filters in Transmitter and Receiver and Various Detector Filters," *IEE Proc.*, Vol. 127, Pt. F, Dec. 1980, pp. 439–447.

4.35 I. Korn and Y. Tsang, "Effect of Intersymbol and Quadrature Channel Interference on Error Probability of 16-ary Offset Quadrature Amplitude Modulation with Sinusoidal and Rectangular Shaping," *IEEE Tr. Comm.*, Vol. COM-31, Feb. 1983, pp. 264–269.

4.36 F. K. Kuo, *Network Analysis and Synthesis*, John Wiley & Sons, New York, 1962.

4.37 S. E. Nader and L. F. Lind, "Optimal Data Transmission Filters," *IEEE Tr. Circ. Syst.*, Vol. CAS-26, Jan. 1979, pp. 36–45.

4.38 J. W. Bayless, A. A. Collins, and R. D. Pederson, "The Specification and Design of Bandlimited Digital Radio Systems," *IEEE Tr. Comm.*, Vol. COM-27, Dec. 1979, pp. 1763–1770.

# 5 ASK BANDPASS SYSTEM

## 5.1 INTRODUCTION

In this chapter we are concerned with ASK-DSB, ASK-SSB, and ASK-VSB, which were defined in Chapter 2 and are depicted Fig. 5.1. This is a short chapter, because, after showing that the model of Fig. 5.1 is reduced to the baseband model of Fig. 5.2, we can use all the results from Chapter 4.

The chapter has the following outline. In Section 5.2 we show the equivalence of the bandpass and baseband model. In Section 5.3 we compute the error probability for the baseband model, assuming the filters are symmetric. In Section 5.4 we consider a bandpass system with a nonsymmetric filter in the receiver. In Section 5.5 we have the summary and conclusions.

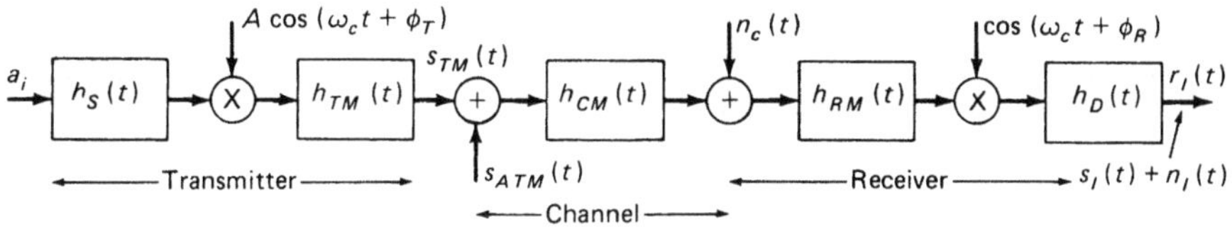


Fig. 5.1. Model of bandpass ASK system.

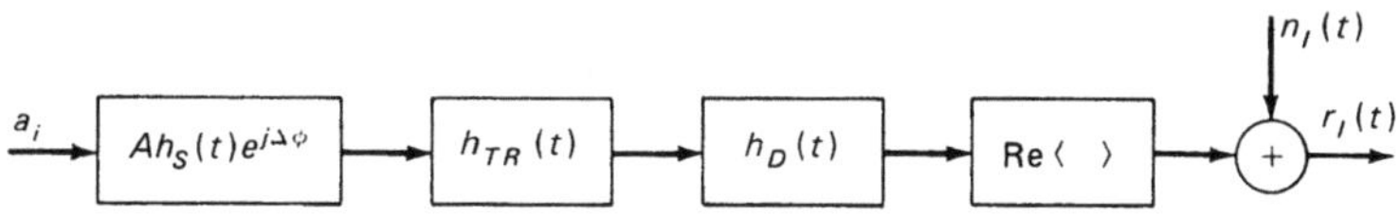


Fig. 5.2. Equivalent baseband model of bandpass ASK system.

## 5.2 BANDPASS AND BASEBAND ASK

The modulated signal in ASK is

$$s_M(t) = \mathrm{Re}\,\{s(t)\exp(j(\omega_C t + \phi_T))\} \tag{5.2.1}$$

where $f_C = \omega_C/(2\pi)$ is the carrier frequency, $\phi_T$ is the transmitter phase, and

$$s(t) = A\sum_i a_i h_S(t - iT) * h_B(t) \tag{5.2.2}$$

Here $A$ is the amplitude, which is related to the average signal energy as shown later; $h_S(t)$ is the common shaping function (the case of noncommon shaping function $h_S(t, a_i)$ is a trivial extention); $a_i$ is a symbol from the set $\mathring{A}_{\pm}$ (in the binary case, $a_i$ may be from the set {0, 1}; and $h_B(t)$ is a band shaping filter

$$h_B(t) = \begin{cases} \delta(t) & \text{DSB} \\ h_{\text{SSB}}(t) & \text{SSB} \\ h_{\text{VSB}} & \text{VSB} \end{cases} \tag{5.2.3}$$

and $h_{\text{SSB}}(t)$, $h_{\text{VSB}}(t)$ are defined in Chapter 2, Section 2. The main property of this filter is

$$H_B(f) + H_B^*(-f) = 2 \tag{5.2.4}$$

where both here and later a capital letter denotes the Fourier transform (FT) of the corresponding lower-case time function. This filter may be realized in baseband with quadrature modulators or as a bandpass filter that is a part of the transmitter filter. The latter was indeed assumed in the model of Fig. 5.1. The modulated signal is distorted and shaped by the bandpass filters in transmitter, channel, and receiver, the center frequency of which is $f_C$ and whose transfer functions are $H_{TM}(f)$, $H_{CM}(f)$, and $H_{RM}(f)$, respectively. The signal is coherently demodulated, using the locally produced carrier $\cos(\omega_C t + \phi_R)$, the phase of which $\phi_R$ may not be identical with the transmitter phase, $\phi_T$, because of imperfections in the carrier tracking circuits that are not shown in Fig. 5.1. The reader is referred to Refs. 5.1 and 5.2 for treatment of carrier and phase synchronization circuits. The difference between the phases

$$\Delta\phi = \phi_T - \phi_R \tag{5.2.5}$$

has a probability density function (pdf)[5.1]

$$p_{\Delta\phi}(x) = (2\pi I_0(\gamma_p))^{-1} \exp(\gamma_p \cos x) \tag{5.2.6}$$

where

$$I_0(\gamma_p) = (2\pi)^{-1} \int_{-\pi}^{\pi} \exp(\gamma_p \cos x)\, dx \tag{5.2.7}$$

is the zero-order Bessel function, and $\gamma_p$ is the signal-to-noise ratio at the phase-locked loop (PLL) synchronization circuit. For large values of $\gamma_p$

$$I_0(\gamma_p) = \exp(\gamma_p)(2\pi\gamma_p)^{-1/2} \tag{5.2.8}$$

Hence $p_{\Delta\phi}(x)$ is approximately Gaussian

$$p_{\Delta\phi}(x) = (2\pi/\gamma_p)^{-1/2} \exp(-\gamma_p x^2/2) \tag{5.2.9}$$

with variance

$$(\Delta\phi)^2 = \gamma_p^{-1} \tag{5.2.10}$$

In addition to the main signal, an interfering signal $s_{AM}(t)$, which is similar to the main signal except for the carrier frequency, which is $f_C + f_A$, is affecting the performance of the system if $f_C + f_A$ is within the bandwidth of the receiver filter. The matter of adjacent channel interference will be dealt with in Chapter 6; hence this will not be considered any more here.

The demodulated signal is low pass-filtered by the detector filter, $h_D(t)$, whose main task is to eliminate double carrier frequency terms, but can also be used for signal shaping. The noise, $n_C(t)$, is zero mean, Gaussian, white with power spectral density (PSD), $N_0/2$.

The output of the detector filter is

$$r_l(t) = A \sum_i a_i g_l(t - iT) + n_l(t) \tag{5.2.11}$$

where

$$g_l(t) = \text{Re}\{g(t)\} \tag{5.2.12}$$

$$g(t) = h_S(t) * h_B(t) * h_T(t) * h_C(t) * h_R(t) * h_D(t) \exp(j\Delta\phi) \tag{5.2.13}$$

$$H_L(f) = H_{LM}(f + f_C)u(f + f_C),\ L = T, C, R \tag{5.2.14}$$

is the baseband equivalent filter of the corresponding bandpass filter, and $n_l(t)$ is zero mean, Gaussian noise with variance

$$\sigma_n^2 = N_0 \int_{-\infty}^{\infty} |H_{RD}(f)|^2\, df \tag{5.2.15}$$

$$H_{RD}(f) = H_R(f)H_D(f) \tag{5.2.16}$$

Thus we derive the baseband model of the system, which is shown in Fig. 5.2.

## 5.3 ERROR PROBABILITY

To make a decision about symbol $a_k$, a sample is taken at time $t_k = t_0 + kT$, and the result is from (5.2.11)

$$r_{I,k} = a_k A g_{I,0} + A \sum_i{}' a_i g_{I,k-i} + n_{I,k} \tag{5.3.1}$$

where, as in Chapter 4

$$z_k = z(t_k),\ z = r_I,\ g_I,\ n_I \tag{5.3.2}$$

and $\sum'$ means the summation without the $k$th term. The only difference between (5.3.1) and (4.2.1) is the notation. Therefore all results of Chapter 4 are valid here, particularly eq. (4.4.4) with $g_0/\sigma_n$ replaced by $Ag_{I,0}/\sigma_n$ and

$$I' = \sum_i a_i g_{I,k-i}/g_{I,0} \tag{5.3.3}$$

Now, because

$$g_I(t) = (1/2)\{g(t) + g^*(t)\} \tag{5.3.4}$$

we obtain

$$g_{I,0} = \frac{1}{2}\int_{-\infty}^{\infty} \{G(f) + G^*(-f)\} \exp(j\, 2\, \pi f t_0)\, df \tag{5.3.5}$$

where, from (5.2.13)

$$G(f) = H_S(f)H_B(f)H_T(f)H_C(f)H_R(f)H_D(f) \exp(j\Delta\phi) \tag{5.3.6}$$

Denoting

$$G_C(f) = H_S(f)H_B(f)H_T(f)H_C(f) \tag{5.3.7}$$

and using (5.2.16), we obtain

$$g_{I,0} = \frac{1}{2}\int_{-\infty}^{\infty} \{G_C(f)H_{RD}(f) \exp(j\Delta\phi) + G_C^*(-f)H_{RD}^*(-f) \exp(-j\Delta\phi)\} \exp(j\, 2\, \pi f t_0)\, df \tag{5.3.8}$$

we define

$$\eta = \frac{g_{I,0}^2}{E_C E_{RD}} \tag{5.3.9}$$

where

$$E_C = \int_{-\infty}^{\infty} |G_C(f)|^2 \, df \tag{5.3.10}$$

$$E_{RD} = \int_{-\infty}^{\infty} |H_{RD}(f)|^2 \, df \tag{5.3.11}$$

Thus from (5.3.9) and (5.2.15) we obtain the ratio

$$Ag_{I,0}/\sigma_n = \left(\frac{A^2 E_C E_{RD} \eta}{N_0 E_{RD}}\right)^{1/2} = (A^2 E_C \eta / N_0)^{1/2} \tag{5.3.12}$$

The bandpass signal at the receiver input is

$$s_{RM}(t) = \text{Re}\,\{A \sum_i a_i g_C(t - iT) \exp\,(j(\omega_C t + \phi_T))\} \tag{5.3.13}$$

It was shown in Chapter 3 that if the symbols are independent the average power of this signal is

$$P = 0.5\, A^2 E_C \overline{a_i^2}/T \tag{5.3.14}$$

Hence the average energy per symbol is

$$E_S = PT = A^2 E_C \overline{a_i^2}/2 \tag{5.3.15}$$

When we substitute (5.3.15) into (5.3.12), we obtain

$$Ag_{I,0}/\sigma_n = \left(\frac{\eta\, 2\, E_S}{N_0 \overline{a_i^2}}\right)^{1/2} \tag{5.3.16}$$

which is the same as for baseband, although the power in (5.3.14) contains a factor of 1/2, and the variance of noise in (5.2.13) is lacking this factor. In baseband it is other way round, but the ratio (5.3.16) is the same. If we have a matched filter situation

$$H_{RD}(f) = G_C^*(f) \exp(-j\, 2\, \pi f t_0) \tag{5.3.17}$$

then

$$E_{RD} = E_C \tag{5.3.18}$$

and (5.3.9) is

$$\eta = \cos^2 \Delta\phi \tag{5.3.19}$$

If the symbols belong to the set $\mathring{A}_{\pm}$ and they are equiprobable, we can use eq. (4.2.62) with $\eta$ as in (5.3.19) to compute the bit error probability. The results for Nyquist filters are valid here, provided

$$G_C(f) = H_{RD}(f) = H_N(f) \tag{5.3.20}$$

where $H_N(f)$ is given in (4.3.36). The results in Chapter 4 for the systems defined in Table 4.3 are also valid here provided

$$h_{TC}(t) = h_B(t) * h_T(t) * h_C(t) \tag{5.3.21}$$

and $h_R(t)$ are real functions. This will certainly be true for ASK-DSB where $H_B(f) = 1$ if $H_{TM}(f)$, $H_{CM}(f)$, and $H_{RM}(f)$ are symmetric around $f_C$ for $f \pm f_C \geqq 0$. The model for such a system is shown in Fig. 5.3, where

$$h_{TR}(t) = h_T(t) * h_C(t) * h_R(t) \tag{5.3.22}$$

and we assumed that $\Delta\phi = 0$. To use the graphs in Chapter 4 when $\Delta\phi \neq 0$, we have to modify the signal-to-noise ratio $E_b/N_0$ by 20 log cos $\Delta\phi$. A more detailed discussion of the effect of phase offset is presented in Chapter 6.

*Example* 5.3.1
Compute the required signal-to-noise ratio $E_b/N_0$ in order to achieve a bit error probability of $10^{-4}$ for system NS in Table 4.3, assuming identical third-order Butterworth filters in transmitter and receiver with 3-dB

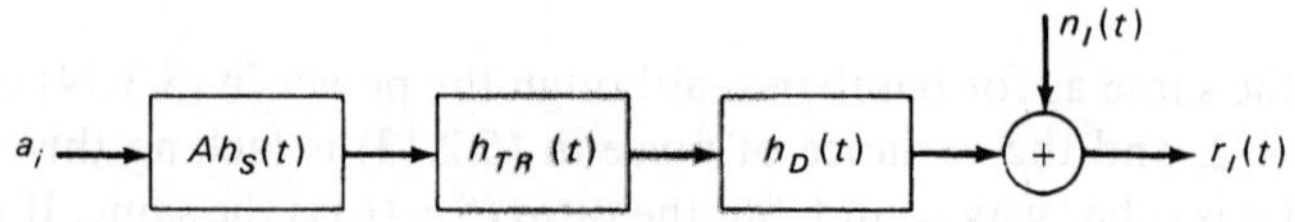


Fig. 5.3. Baseband model of ASK-DSB system.

bandwidth $f_0 = 0.65\,R$ and quaternary symbols. The phase offset is $\Delta\phi = 5°$.

The solution is found in Fig. 4.32, where we find that if $\Delta\phi = 0$, $E_b/N_0 = 15$ dB. Because

$$20 \log \cos 5° = -0.03$$

the required signal-to-noise ratio is increased by 0.03, which is just negligible.

## 5.4 ERROR PROBABILITY FOR ASK-DSB WITH NONSYMMETRIC BANDPASS FILTER[5.4–5.6]

Let $2f_0$ be the 3-dB bandwidth of a bandpass filter, and let $f_C$ be the center frequency. The bandpass filter is obtained from a low pass filter by the transformation[5.3]

$$s \rightarrow \tfrac{1}{2}\,\omega_C(s/\omega_C + \omega_C/s) \tag{5.4.1}$$

Thus a lowpass filter with 3-dB bandwidth $f_0$

$$H'_R(s) = \sum_{i=1}^{N} \rho_i/(s/\omega_0 + p_i) \tag{5.4.2}$$

where $\{p_i\}$ are the poles and $\{\rho_i\}$ are the residua, is transformed into

$$H'_{RM}(s) = 2\,k_f \sum_{i=1}^{N} \rho_i \frac{s/\omega_C}{(s/\omega_C)^2 + 2\,k_f p_i(s/\omega_C) + 1} \tag{5.4.3}$$

where

$$k_f = f_0/f_C \tag{5.4.4}$$

is the ratio of bandwidth to center frequency. The bandpass filter passes frequencies between $f_L$ and $f_H$ where

$$f_L f_H = f_0^2 \qquad f_H - f_L = 2\,f_0 \tag{5.4.5}$$

and the filter is not symmetric around $f_C$, unless $k_f \rightarrow 0$. In many practical systems, $k_f$ may be close to 1; therefore it is worthwhile to investigate the effect of $k_f$ on the system performance. For example, in one of the Intelsat modems the bandwidth is about 30 MHz, and the intermediate frequency, which corresponds here to $f_C$, is only 70 MHz.

Instead of reducing the bandpass system to an equivalent baseband system here, we shall analyze the bandpass system directly, since for $k_f \leqq 1$, the system is in fact a baseband system. We shall follow here Ref. 5.4 and make the following assumptions.

a. The system is NN of Table 4.3, i.e., the shaping filter is NRZ, and the detector filter is matched to this pulse, which means that it is an ideal integrator for a period $T$.

b. The carrier frequency is such that $f_C T$ is an integer.

c. The symbols are binary, $\pm 1$ and equiprobable.

d. The channel and transmitter filters are wideband.

e. $0 < k_f < 1$.

The system is shown in Fig. 5.4. The input to the receiver filter is

$$A \sum_i a_i f(t - iT) + n_C(t) \tag{5.4.6}$$

where

$$f(t) = u_T(t) \cos \omega_C t = \cos \omega_C t u(t) - \cos (\omega_C(t - T))u(t - T) \tag{5.4.7}$$

The output of the receiver filter is

$$A \sum_i a_i g_R(t - iT) + n_R(t) \tag{5.4.8}$$

where

$$g_R(t) = G_R(t) - G_R(t - T) \tag{5.4.9}$$

$$G_R(t) = \int_0^t h_{RM}(t - y) \cos (\omega_C y) \, dy u(t) \tag{5.4.10}$$

and

$$n_R(t) = \int_{-\infty}^t h_{RM}(t - y) n_C(y) \, dy \tag{5.4.11}$$

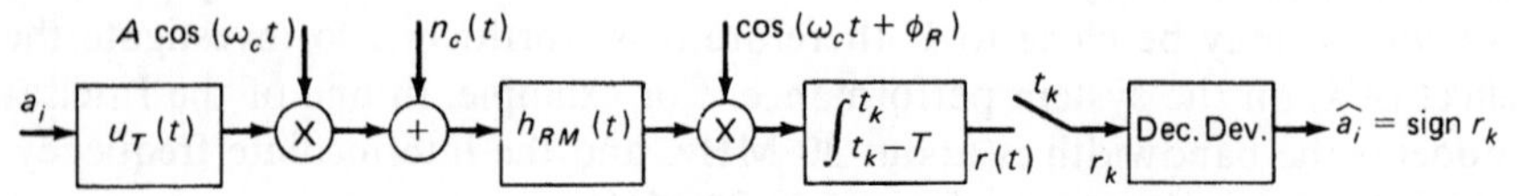


Fig. 5.4. Baseband ASK-DSB system with NRZ shaping function and matched filter.

The output of the integrator at time $t_k$ is

$$r_k = Aa_k g_0 + A \sum_i{}' a_i g_{k-i} + n_k \tag{5.4.12}$$

where

$$z_k = z(t_k),\ z = r, g, n \tag{5.4.13}$$

$$g(x) = G(x) - 2\,G(x - T) + G(x - 2\,T) \tag{5.4.14}$$

$$G(x) = \int_0^x G_R(t) \cos(\omega_C t + \phi_R)\, dt \tag{5.4.15}$$

$$n(x) = \int_{x-T}^x n_R(t) \cos(\omega_C t + \phi_R)\, dt \tag{5.4.16}$$

The error probability is

$$\begin{aligned} P_b(e) &= \underline{P(r_k > 0 | a_k = -1) = P(n_k > Ag_0(1 - I'))} \\ &= \overline{Q(\eta(2\,E_b/N_0)^{1/2})(1 + I'))} \end{aligned} \tag{5.4.17}$$

where

$$I' = \sum_i{}' a_i g_{k-i}/g_0 \tag{5.4.18}$$

$$\eta = (Ag_0/\sigma_n)(2\,E_b/N_0)^{-1/2} \tag{5.4.19}$$

and $\sigma_n$ is the variance of $n(x)$, which can be computed from (5.4.16)

$$\sigma_n^2 = \int_0^T R_{nR}(\tau)\{(T - \tau) \cos(\omega_C \tau) - \sin(\omega_C \tau) \cos(2\,\omega_C \tau + 2\,\phi_R)/\omega_C\}\, d\tau \tag{5.4.20}$$

and

$$R_{nR}(\tau) = \frac{1}{2} N_0 \int_{-\infty}^{\infty} h_{RM}(y + \tau) h_{RM}(y)\, dy \tag{5.4.21}$$

From (5.4.6) and (5.4.7), the average energy per bit is

$$E_b = A^2 T/2 \tag{5.4.22}$$

Hence (5.4.19) is simplified to

$$\eta = g_0(\sigma_n^2 T/N_0)^{-1/2} \tag{5.4.23}$$

The details of the derivation of $g(x)$ and $\sigma_n^2$ are given in Ref. 5.4 for the transfer function of (5.4.3). The results for a Butterworth filter of order 5 are

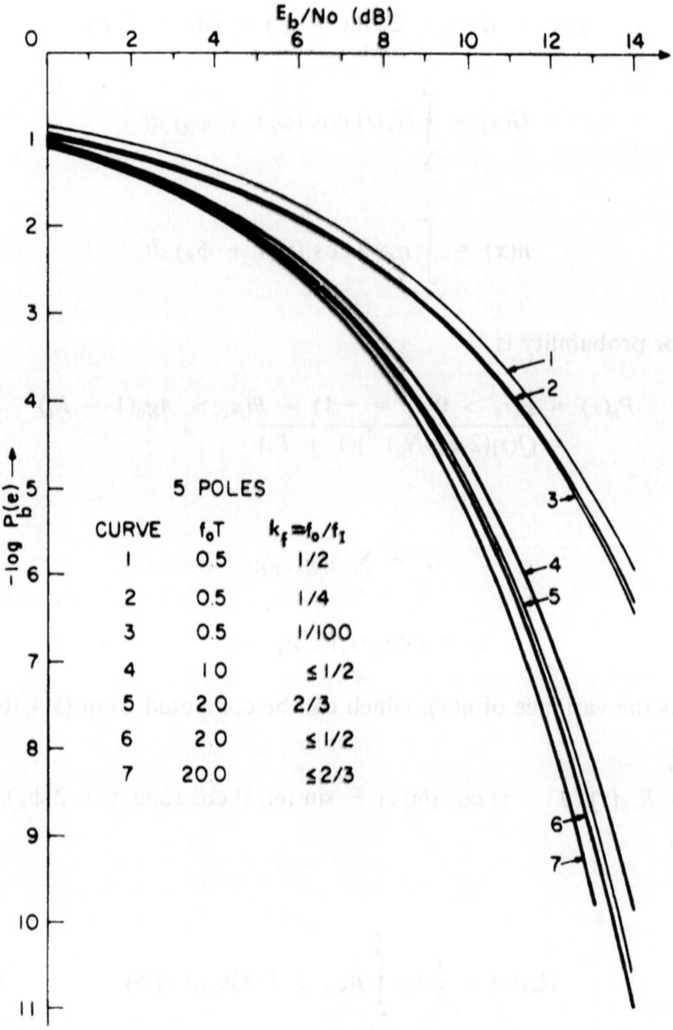


Fig. 5.5. Bit error probability as a function of signal-to-noise ration with 3-dB bandwidth $f_0T$ and bandwidth-to-carrier frequency ratio $k_f$ as a parameter (I. Korn, M. Namet, "Performance of Biphase Bandpass Communication System," *IEEE Tr. Comm.*, Vol. COM-23, July 1975, pp. 757–761. Copyright © 1975 IEEE).

shown in Fig. 5.5 for various values of 3-dB bandwidth $f_0T = f_0/R_b$ and $k_f$ (for optimal $t_0$ and $\phi_R$). The typical form of $P_b(e)$ as a function of $k_f$ is shown in Fig. 5.6. The curve is flatter for increasing values of $f_0T$. For example if $f_0T \geqq 1$, $k_f$ does not affect $P_b(e)$ for $k_f \leqq 1/2$.

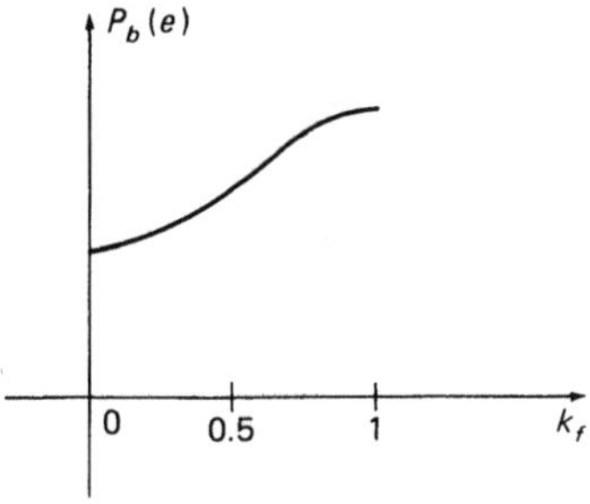


Fig. 5.6. Bit error probability as a function of bandwidth-to-carrier frequency ratio.

## 5.5 SUMMARY AND CONCLUSIONS

We have shown that ASK-DSB, SSB, and VSB bandpass systems can be represented by equivalent baseband systems. We have also shown that if the resulting baseband equivalent filters are symmetric (the impulse response is real), then we can use the results of Chapter 4. A bandpass system introduces a new factor, namely, a phase offset that increases the error probability. We have also considered a binary ASK-DSB system in which the bandpass receiver filter is not symmetric and for which the ratio of carrier frequency to bandwidth is not large. We have shown that this ratio affects badly the error probability, particularly for small bandwidth.

Although this chapter is concerned with ASK, the results apply equally well to binary PSK with NRZ shaping function, because in this case it is identical to binary ASK-DSB. The results, however, do not apply to DPSK.

## 5.6 PROBLEMS

5.2.1 Derive eq. (5.2.9).

5.3.1 Show that if $H_T(f)$, $H_C(f)$, $H_R(f)$ are symmetric filters, then $G(f)$ in (5.3.6) is also a symmetric filter.

5.3.2 Derive eq. (5.3.19).

5.3.3 Compute the average error probability of binary ASK-DSB with Nyquist overall transfer function and receiver matched to transmitter, assuming that $\Delta\phi$ is a random variable with pdf as in (5.2.6) with $\gamma_p = 20$ dB.

5.4.1 Compute the impulse response $h_{RM}(t)$ from eq. (5.4.3).

5.4.2 Prove eq. (5.4.20).

5.4.3 Compute the effect of $k_f$, relaxing some or all of the assumptions (a), (b), (c), (d), and (e) in Section 5.4.

5.4.4 Compute the effect of $k_f$ if the nonsymmetric filter is in transmitter instead of receiver.

## 5.7 REFERENCES


5.1 J. J. Spilker, *Digital Communications by Satellite*, Prentice-Hall, Inc., Englewood Cliffs, N.J., 1977.

5.2 W. C. Lindsey and M. K. Simon, *Telecommunication Systems Engineering*, Prentice-Hall, Inc., Englewood Cliffs, N.J., 1973.

5.3 F. K. Kuo, *Network Analysis and Synthesis*, John Wiley & Sons, Inc., New York, 1962, chapter 12.

5.4 I. Korn and M. Namet, 'Performance of Biphase Bandpass Communication System," *IEEE Tr. Comm.*, Vol. COM-23, July 1975, pp. 757–761.

5.5 I. Korn, "Degradation of Probability of Error due to IF Filtering," *IEEE Tr. AES*, Vol. AES-9, July 1973, pp. 544–547.

5.6 I. Korn and M. Namet, "Binary Communication with Large Bandwidth to IF Frequency Ratios," *IEEE Tr. AES*, Vol. AES-11, March 1975, pp. 162–168.

# 6 QASK AND OQASK

## 6.1 INTRODUCTION

In the previous chapter we dealt with ASK-DSB, SSB, VSB, which is one family within linear shift keying (LSK). In this chapter we analyze QASK and OQASK, which also are part of LSK. A model of QASK and OQASK is shown in Fig. 6.1. The modulated signal in the main channel is

$$s_M(t) = \text{Re}\,\{s(t) \exp\,(j(\omega_C t + \phi_T))\} \tag{6.1.1}$$

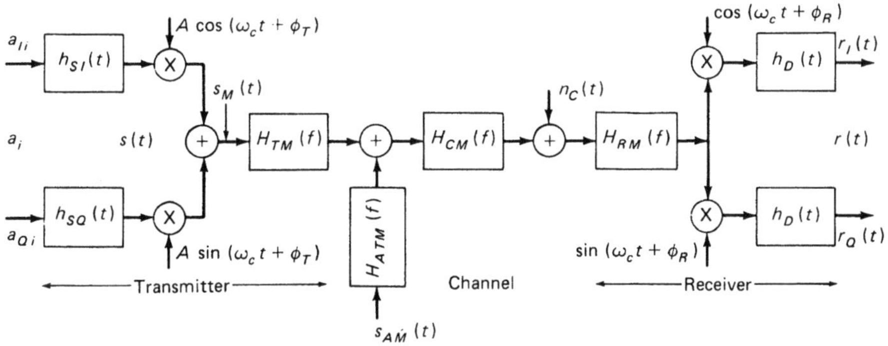


Fig. 6.1. Model of bandpass QASK and OQASK digital communication systems.

where

$$f_C = \omega_C/(2\,\pi) \tag{6.1.2}$$

is the carrier frequency, $\phi_T$ is the transmitter phase, and

$$s(t) = A\left(\sum_i a_{Ii} h_{SI}(t - iT) + j \sum_i a_{Qi} h_{SQ}(t - iT)\right) \tag{6.1.3}$$

is the complex envelope. Here $A$ is the amplitude, which is related to the average symbol energy; $h_{SI}(t)$ and $h_{SQ}(t)$ are shaping functions (these functions may not be common, but rather symbol-dependent, but we shall not discuss this matter here), and

$$a_i = a_{Ii} + ja_{Qi} \tag{6.1.4}$$

is a complex or two-dimensional symbol, the set of which forms a symbol constellation, as shown in Fig. 6.2. In all practical QASK systems

$$h_{SI}(t) = h_{SQ}(t) = h_S(t) \tag{6.1.5}$$

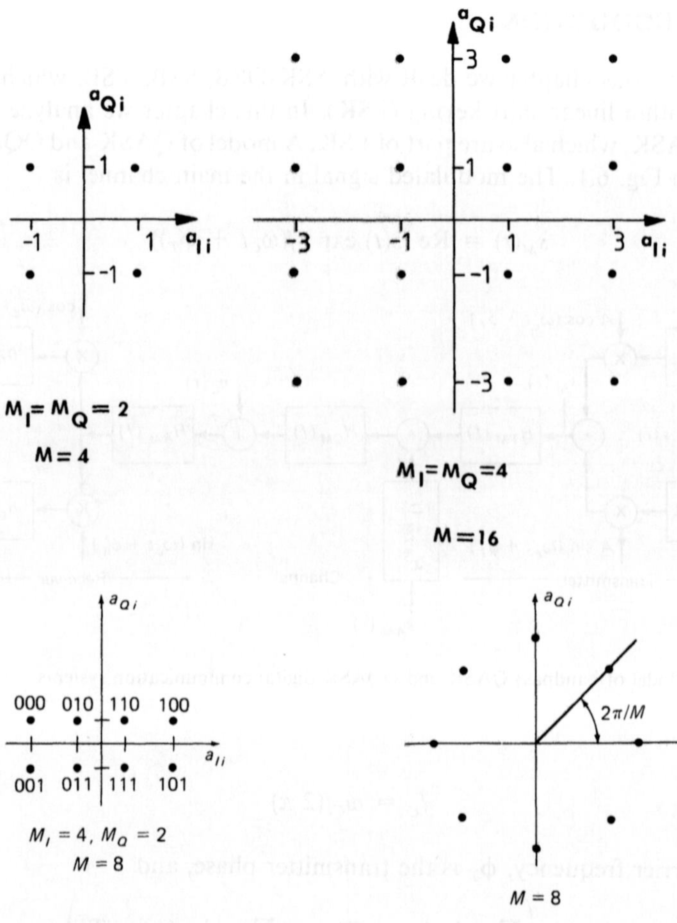


Fig. 6.2. Symbol constellations.

while in OQASK

$$h_{SI}(t) = h_S(t), \qquad h_{SQ}(t) = h_S(t - 0.5\,T) \tag{6.1.6}$$

i.e., the quadrature shaping function is delayed by half the symbol duration. Therefore, from now on, (6.1.3) is replaced by

$$s(t) = A\left(\sum_i a_{Ii}h_S(t - iT) + j\sum_i a_{Qi}h_S(t - iT - \varepsilon T)\right) \qquad (6.1.7)$$

where $\varepsilon = 0$ for QASK and $\varepsilon = 1/2$ for OQASK. In QASK and OQASK with a rectangular constellation, the symbols $\{a_{Ii}\}$ and $\{a_{Qi}\}$ are taken from the same set $\mathring{A}_{\pm}$ or from two sets $\mathring{A}_{\pm}$, one with $M_I$ symbols and the other with $M_Q$ symbols to form a set with

$$M = M_I M_Q \qquad (6.1.8)$$

symbols. For example in Fig. 6.2 there is a constellation with $M_I = 4$ and $M_Q = 2$. The symbols $\{a_{Ii}\}$ and $\{a_{Qi}\}$ are independent for these constellations. In a circular constellation

$$a_i = \exp\,(j\pi a_i'/M) \qquad (6.1.9)$$

where $a_i' \in \{0, 2, \ldots, 2\,M - 2\}$ or $a_i' \in \{\pm 1, \pm 3, \ldots, \pm\,(M - 1)\}$.

QASK with a circular constellation and NRZ shaping function is identical to PSK with the NRZ shaping function, which is the universally used shaping function for PSK.

The signal is distorted and shaped by the transmitter, channel, and receiver bandpass filters with center frequency $f_C$ and whose transfer functions are $H_{TM}(f)$, $H_{CM}(f)$, and $H_{RM}(f)$, respectively (the impulse responses are $h_{TM}(t)$, $h_{CM}(t)$, $h_{RM}(t)$). The signal is demodulated by a coherent detector with locally generated carriers $\cos\,(\omega_C t + \phi_R)$, $\sin\,(\omega_C t + \phi_R)$, the phase of which, $\phi_R$, drifts around $\phi_T$ causing a random phase error

$$\Delta\phi = \phi_T - \phi_R \qquad (6.1.10)$$

the probability density function (pdf) of which may be as in eq. (5.2.6). The demodulated signal is lowpass-filtered by the detector filter with transfer function $H_D(f)$ (impulse response $h_D(t)$) whose main task is to eliminate double carrier frequency terms, but is also used to provide a final shaping of the resulting baseband signal. The transmitter filter is used to contain the signal within a certain bandwidth, while the receiver filter eliminates noise and interfering signals that fall outside the signal bandwidth.

In addition to the desired signal, the channel carries other signals that may affect the performance of the system if their bandwidth overlaps the bandwidth of the receiver filter. Such signals cause *adjacent channel interference* (ACI). One such typical signal is shown in Fig. 6.1. This signal has the same form as the main signal with the following differences:

a. The carrier frequency is $f_C + f_A$, and the phase is $\phi_{TA}$.

b. The amplitude is $A_A$.

c. The symbols are $b_i = b_{Ii} + jb_{Qi}$ and, although they are from the same set as the symbols $a_i$, $\{b_i\}$, are independent of $\{a_i\}$.

d. There is a delay, $\tau$, in the generation of $\{b_i\}$ relative to $\{a_i\}$. Thus

$$s_{AM}(t) = \text{Re}\,\{s_A(t) \exp\,(j(\omega_C + \omega_A)t + \phi_{AT}))\qquad (6.1.11)$$

with

$$s_A(t) = A_A\left(\sum_i b_{Ii}h_S(t - iT - \tau) + j\sum_i b_{Qi}h_S(t - iT - \varepsilon T - \tau)\right)\qquad (6.1.12)$$

In fact we may assume that the shaping functions in the adjacent channel differ from the shaping function in the main channel or that, at least, the symbol duration $T$ is different, but these are simple generalizations that will not be considered here. The power spectral density (PSD) of two typical adjacent signals is shown in Fig. 6.3. The signal $s_{AM}(t)$ is shaped by the transmitter filter in adjacent channel $H_{ATM}(f)$, which we assume to be identical to $H_{TM}(f)$ except for the center frequency, which is $f_C + f_A$.

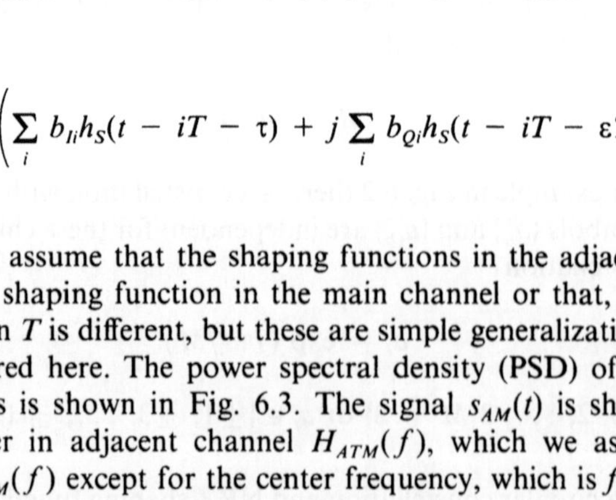


Fig. 6.3. Power spectral density of main and interfering signal.

The noise in the system is assumed to be zero mean, Gaussian, and white with PSD, $N_0/2$. It is represented by a single term, $n_C(t)$, at the receiver filter input.

Figure 6.4 shows the baseband equivalent system, derived from the bandpass system in Fig. 6.1. The validity of this equivalence was established in Chapter 1, Section 4 (for the signal) and Section 8 (for the noise). In the baseband model the signals are replaced by their complex envelopes and the filters by their baseband equivalent filters, all referred to the receiver center frequency, $f_C$. The transfer functions of the baseband equivalent filters are

$$H_L(f) = H_{LM}(f + f_C)u(f + f_C),\ L = T, C, R\qquad (6.1.13)$$

$$H_{AT}(f) = H_T(f - f_A)\qquad (6.1.14)$$

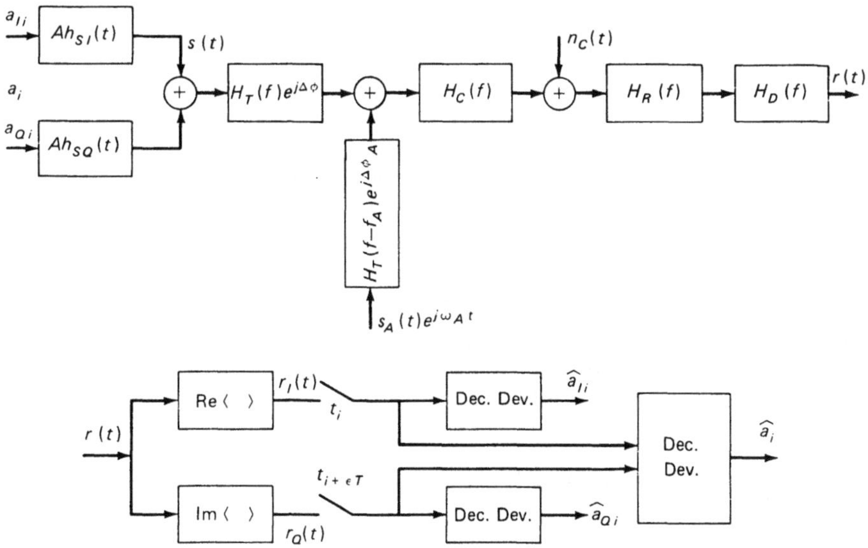


Fig. 6.4. Baseband equivalent model of QASK and OQASK systems.

with impulse response $h_L(t)$ and

$$h_{AT}(t) = h_T(t) \exp(j\omega_A t) \tag{6.1.15}$$

the detector filter output is given thus by

$$\begin{aligned} r(t) = {} & s(t) * h_T(t) * h_C(t) * h_R(t) * h_D(t) \exp(j\Delta\phi) + n_C(t) * h_R(t) * h_D(t) \\ & + s_A(t) \exp(j\omega_A t) * h_T(t) \exp(j\omega_A t) * h_C(t) * h_R(t) * h_D(t) \\ & \exp(j\Delta\phi_A) \end{aligned} \tag{6.1.16}$$

where

$$\Delta\phi_A = \phi_{AT} - \phi_R \tag{6.1.17}$$

has a uniform psd in $-\pi$—$\pi$, and

$$\omega_A = 2\pi f_A t \tag{6.1.18}$$

From $r(t)$ the detector decides about the values of $\{a_i\}$. The rest of this chapter is dedicated to the analysis of various systems described by eq. (6.1.16).

In Section 6.2 we derive the conditions on the filters of the system for the presence and absence of ACI, quadrature channel interference (QCI), and intersymbol interference (ISI). In Section 6.3 we assume that there is no interference, and we compute the error probability for systems with rectangular, circular, and general constellations. We conclude there that rectangular and circular signal constellations are either optimal or close to optimal; hence the effect of interference is computed only for systems with these constellations. In Section 6.4 we compute the error probability in the presence of interference with rectangular constellations. The systems have either a Nyquist function response or have Butterworth or Gaussian filters in their receiver and transmitter. In Section 6.5 we compute the error probability in the presence of interference for systems with circular constellations. The systems have a Nyquist function response or have Butterworth filters. In Section 6.6 we assume that the channel has frequency selective fading, and we present formulas for the computation of the error probability. Section 6.7 is a summary followed by problems and a list of references.

## 6.2 CONDITIONS OF NO INTERFERENCE

Let

$$g(t, f_A) = h_S(t) \exp(j\omega_A t) * h_T(t) \exp(j\omega_A t) * h_C(t) * h_R(t) * h_D(t) \quad (6.2.1)$$

Thus

$$g(t) = g(t, 0) \quad (6.2.2)$$

Hence it is sufficient to compute $g(t, f_A)$ only. When we substitute (6.1.7), (6.1.12), (6.2.1), and (6.2.2) into (6.1.16), we obtain

$$\begin{aligned} r(t) = {} & \sum_i a_{Ii} y(t - iT) + j \sum_i a_{Qi} y(t - iT - \varepsilon T) \\ & + \sum_i b_{Ii} y(t - iT - \tau, f_A) + j \sum_i b_{Qi} y(t - iT - \varepsilon T - \tau, f_A) \\ & + n_I(t) + j n_Q(t) \end{aligned} \quad (6.2.3)$$

where

$$y(t) = A g(t) \exp(j\Delta\phi) \quad (6.2.4)$$

$$y(t, f_A) = A_A g(t, f_A) \exp(j\Delta\phi_A) \quad (6.2.5)$$

and $n_I(t)$, $n_Q(t)$ are zero mean, independent Gaussian random processes with the same PSD

$$S_{nI}(f) = S_{nQ}(f) = N_0 |H_{RD}(f)|^2 \quad (6.2.6)$$

where

$$H_{RD}(f) = H_R(f)H_D(f) \tag{6.2.7}$$

Because $h_S(t)$ and $h_D(t)$ are real functions, $y(t)$ will be real only if

$$h_T(t) * h_C(t) * h_R(t) \exp(j\Delta\phi) \tag{6.2.8}$$

is real. This will indeed happen if

$$H_{TR}(f) = H_T(f)H_C(f)H_R(f) \tag{6.2.9}$$

is a symmetric function, i.e.

$$H_{TR}(f) = H^*_{TR}(-f) \tag{6.2.10}$$

(i.e., the bandpass filters are symmetric around $f_C$) and $\Delta\phi = 0$.

Let $r_I(t)$ ($y_I(t)$, $y_I(t, f_A)$) be the real part and $r_Q(t)$($y_Q(t)$, $y_Q(t, f_A)$) be the imaginary part of $r(t)$ ($y(t)$, $y(t, f_A)$). Thus

$$\begin{aligned} r_I(t) = {} & \sum_i a_{Ii} y_I(t - iT) - \sum_i a_{Qi} y_Q(t - iT - \varepsilon T) \\ & + \sum_i b_{Ii} y_I(t - iT - \tau, f_A) - \sum_i b_{Qi} y_Q(t - iT - \varepsilon T - \tau, f_A) + n_I(t) \end{aligned} \tag{6.2.11}$$

$$\begin{aligned} r_Q(t) = {} & \sum_i a_{Qi} y_I(t - iT - \varepsilon T) + \sum_i a_{Ii} y_Q(t - iT) \\ & + \sum_i b_{Qi} y_I(t - iT - \varepsilon T - \tau, f_A) + \sum_i b_{Ii} y_Q(t - iT - \tau, f_A) + n_Q(t) \end{aligned} \tag{6.2.12}$$

The inphase signal is sampled at times $t_k = t_0 + kT$, and the quadrature signal at times $t_k + \varepsilon T$. The sampled values are

$$\begin{aligned} r_{I,k} = {} & a_{Ik} y_{I,0} + \sum_i{}' a_{Ii} y_{I,k-i} - \sum_i a_{Qi} y_{Q,k-i}(\varepsilon) \\ & + \sum_i b_{Ii} y_{I,k-i}(\tau, f_A) - \sum_i b_{Qi} y_{Q,k-i}(\varepsilon, \tau, f_A) + n_{I,k} \end{aligned} \tag{6.2.13}$$

$$\begin{aligned} r_{Q,k} = {} & a_{Qk} y_{I,0} + \sum_i{}' a_{Qi} y_{I,k-i} + \sum_i a_{Ii} y_{Q,k-i}(-\varepsilon) \\ & + \sum_i b_{Qi} y_{I,k-i}(\tau, f_A) + \sum_i b_{Ii} y_{Q,k-i}(-\varepsilon, \tau, f_A) + n_{Q,k}(-\varepsilon) \end{aligned} \tag{6.2.14}$$

where $\sum'$ denotes the summation with the term $i = k$ missing

$$y_{I,k} = y_I(t_k), \qquad y_{Q,k}(\pm\varepsilon) = y_Q(t_k \mp \varepsilon T) \tag{6.2.15}$$

$$n_{I,k} = n_I(t_k), \qquad n_{Q,k}(-\varepsilon) = n_Q(t_k + \varepsilon T) \tag{6.2.16}$$

$$y_{I,k-i}(\tau, f_A) = y_I(t_{k-i} - \tau, f_A) = \mathrm{Re}\,\{y(t_0 + (k-i)T - \tau)\} \tag{6.2.17}$$

$$\begin{aligned} y_{Q,k-i}(\pm\varepsilon, \tau, f_A) &= y_Q(t_{k-i} \mp \varepsilon T - \tau, f_A) \\ &= \mathrm{Im}\,\{y(t_0 + (k-i)T \mp \varepsilon T - \tau)\} \end{aligned} \tag{6.2.18}$$

A model that implements these equations is shown in Fig. 6.5. From $r_{I,k}$ we make decisions about the value of $a_{I,k}$, from $r_{Q,k}$ we make decisions about the value of $a_{Q,k}$; or from

$$r_k = r_{I,k} + jr_{Q,k} \tag{6.2.19}$$

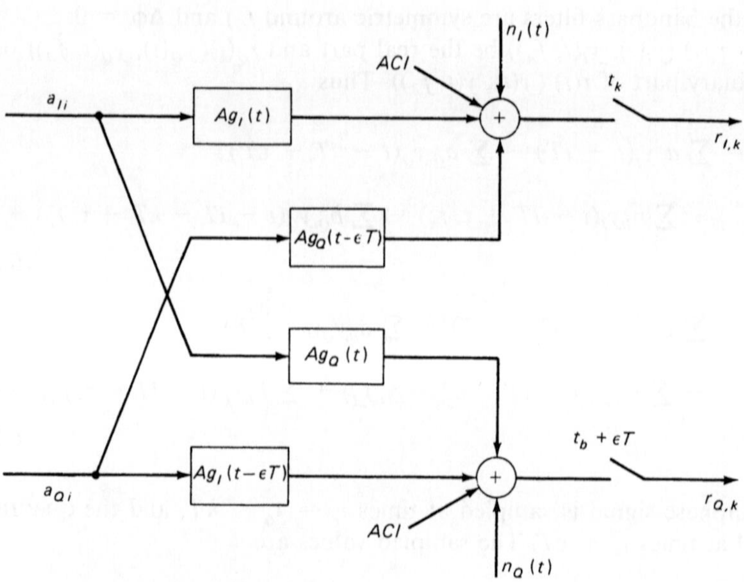


Fig. 6.5. Simplified model of Fig. 6.4.

we can decide about the value of $a_k$.

We can see from (6.2.13) and (6.2.14) that only the first term depends on the symbol of interest. The second term is ISI, which was already discussed in Chapter 4. There is no ISI if

$$y_{I,k} = 0 \tag{6.2.20}$$

for all $k \neq 0$. The third term is QCI, because the symbols in the quadrature channel (quadrature carrier) affect the decisions about the symbols in the inphase channel and vice versa. This term is zero only if

$$y_{Q,k}(\varepsilon) = 0 \tag{6.2.21}$$

for all $k$. This will be satisfied if

$$y_Q(t) = 0 \tag{6.2.22}$$

The fourth and fifth terms form ACI, because here the symbols in the adjacent channel (in the signal of adjacent channel) affect the decisions about the symbols in the main signal. These terms are 0 if either $A_A = 0$ or $f_A$ is such that

$$g(t, f_A) = 0 \tag{6.2.23}$$

The last terms are zero mean, Gaussian random variables with the same variance

$$\sigma_n^2 = N_0 \int_{-\infty}^{\infty} |H_{RD}(f)|^2 \, df \tag{6.2.24}$$

$n_{I,k}$ and $n_{Q,k}(-\varepsilon)$ are independent if $\varepsilon = 0$. If $H_{RD}(f)$ is a symmetric function, $\{n_{I,k}\}$ and $\{n_{Q,k}(-\varepsilon)\}$ are independent for any $\varepsilon$. We thus can see from Fig. 6.5 that when $h_Q(t) = 0$, the system is reduced to two parallel ASK systems, as shown in Fig. 6.6, that are independent unless the symbols $a_{Ii}$ and $a_{Qi}$ are dependent.

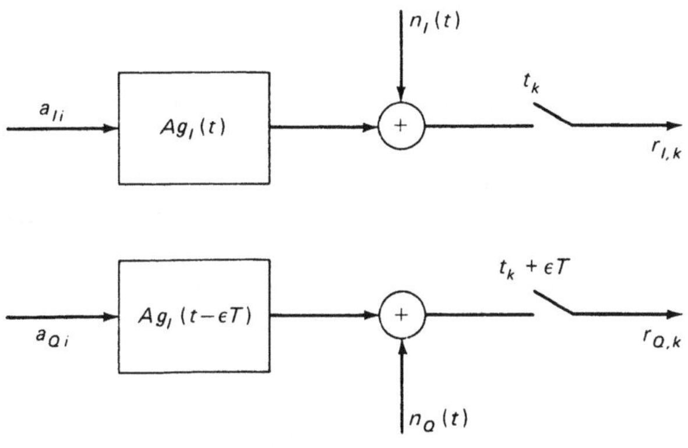


Fig. 6.6. The equivalence of QASK and OQASK to two parallel ASK systems.

## 6.3 SYSTEMS WITH NO INTERFERENCE

In this section we assume that there is no ISI, QCI, and ACI; hence (6.2.13) and (6.2.14) are simplified to

$$r_{I,k} = a_{Ik} y_0 + n_{I,k} \tag{6.3.1}$$

$$r_{Q,k} = a_{Qk} y_0 + n_{Q,k} \tag{6.3.2}$$

where here, because $\Delta\phi = 0 = g_Q(t)$

$$y_0 = A g_{I,0} = A g_0 \tag{6.3.3}$$

We can combine (6.3.1) and (6.3.2) into a single equation

$$r_k = a_k y_0 + n_k \tag{6.3.4}$$

where $a_k$ belongs to a complex set of $M$ symbols $\mathring{A} = \{a(1), a(2), \ldots, a(M)\}$, where

$$a(i) = a_I(i) + j a_Q(i), \qquad i = 1, 2, \ldots, M \tag{6.3.5}$$

Let $DR_i$, $i = 1, \ldots, M$ be a partition of the two-dimensional (or complex) plane into decision regions, so that if $r_k \in DR_m$, the decision is that $a_k = a(m)$. The partition is determined by the maximum likelihood rule, which we have already applied in Chapter 4 to a one-dimensional problem. This rule states here that $r_k \in DR_m$ if

$$p_{r_k|a_k}(r|a(m)) = \max_{i=1,\ldots,M} p_{r_k|a_k}(r|a(i)) \tag{6.3.6}$$

where $p_{r_k|a_k}(\cdot|\cdot)$ is the conditional pdf of $r_k$, given $a_k$.

It follows from (6.3.4) and the independence of the noise and the symbols that

$$p_{r_k|a_k}(r|a(i)) = p_{n_k}(r - a(i)y_0) = p_{n_{I,k}, n_{Q,k}}(r_I - a_I(i), r_Q - a_Q(i)) \tag{6.3.7}$$

If the noises are independent, (6.3.7) is simplified to

$$\begin{aligned} p_{r_k|a_k}(r|a(i)) &= p_{n_{I,k}}(r_I - a_I(i)y_0) p_{n_{Q,k}}(r_Q - a_Q(i)y_0) \\ &= (2\pi\sigma_n^2)^{-1} \exp\{-\tfrac{1}{2}\{(r_I - a_I(i)y_0)^2 + (r_Q - a_Q(i)y_0)^2\}/\sigma_n^2\} \\ &= (2\pi\sigma_n^2)^{-1} \exp\{-\tfrac{1}{2}|r - a(i)y_0|^2/\sigma_n^2\} \end{aligned} \tag{6.3.8}$$

and the maximal value is achieved when $|r - a(i)y_0|$ is minimum. Thus the ML decision region is in this instance

$$DR_m = \{r_k: |r_k - a(m)y_0| \leqq |r_k - a(i)y_0|, \qquad i = 1, \ldots, M\} \quad (6.3.9)$$

If there is equality for two or more symbols, we can assign $r_k$ arbitrarily to the symbol with the lowest index, but this is not of any importance because the probability of this event is zero. Equation (6.3.9) has the following physical meaning: all points $r_k$ which are closer in the conventional Euclidian sense to the point $a(m)y_0$ than to any other point, belong to the region $DR_m$, where the decision is $a_k = a(m)$. For the rectangular and circular symbol constellations the decision regions are rectangles and sections of a circle, respectively, as illustrated in Figs. 6.7 and 6.8. When symbol $a_k = a(i)$ is transmitted, $r_k$ may or may not belong to $DR_i$, depending on where the tip of the noise vector lies, as shown in the figure. An error occurs if the noise vector causes $r_k$ to lie outside the boundary of region $DR_i$. Alternatively, a correct decision is taken if the noise is such that $r_k$ falls within $DR_i$. Let the conditional probability of a correct decision, given that the transmitted symbol is $a(i)$, be

$$\begin{aligned} P(c|i) &= P(r_k \in DR_i|a_k = a(i)) \\ &= P(a(i)y_0 + n_k \in DR_i) = P(n_k \in R_i) \end{aligned} \qquad (6.3.10)$$

where $R_i$ is the set $\{DR_i - a(i)y_0\}$, i.e.

$$R_i = \{n_k: n_k + a(i)y_0 \in DR_i\} \qquad (6.3.11)$$

which is the set $DR_i$ shifted to the origin so that $a(i)y_0$ is pivoted on the origin. This is illustrated in Fig. 6.7 for three regions. The average probability of a correct decision is thus

$$P(c) = \sum_{i=1}^{M} P(c|i)P_i = \sum_{i=1}^{M} P(n_k \in R_i)P_i \qquad (6.3.12)$$

The error probability is computed from (6.3.12) simply by

$$P(e) = 1 - P(c) \qquad (6.3.13)$$

*Example* 6.3.1 Quaternary symbols
Assume that $M = 4$ and the symbols are $a(1) = 1 + j$, $a(2) = -1 + j$, $a(3) = -1 - j$, $a(4) = 1 - j$, as in Fig. 6.2. Because here $r_k = (\pm 1 \pm j)y_0 + n_k$. The decision regions are here

$$
\begin{aligned}
DR_1 &= \{r_k: r_{I,k} \geqq 0, \quad r_{Q,k} \geqq 0\} \\
DR_2 &= \{r_k: r_{I,k} \leqq 0, \quad r_{Q,k} \geqq 0\} \\
DR_3 &= \{r_k: r_{I,k} \leqq 0, \quad r_{Q,k} \leqq 0\} \\
DR_4 &= \{r_k: r_{I,k} \geqq 0, \quad r_{Q,k} \leqq 0\}
\end{aligned}
$$

i.e., the four quarters of the plane.

### 6.3.1 Rectangular constellation

In a rectangular constellation we may assume, without any loss in generality, that

$$a_{Ii} \in \{\pm 1, \pm 3, \ldots \pm (M_I - 1)\} \text{ and } a_{Qi} \in \{\pm 1, \pm 3, \ldots, \pm (M_Q - 1)\}$$

The symbols are independent, and we can view the system as two ASK systems with $M_I$ and $M_Q$ symbols, respectively. We showed in Chapters 4 and 5 that the bit error probability is related to the signal-to-noise ratio per bit by

$$P_b(e) = \frac{2\,(1 - M_L^{-1})}{\log_2 M_L} Q\left(\eta \frac{2\,E_S}{N_0 a_i^2}\right) = \frac{2\,(1 - M_L^{-1})}{\log_2 M_L} Q\left(\eta \frac{3 \log_2 M_L}{M_L^2 - 1} \frac{2\,E_b}{N_0}\right) \tag{6.3.14}$$

where $M_L$ here is $M_I$ or $M_Q$, $a_i$ is $a_{Ii}$ or $a_{Qi}$, and $E_S$ is the average energy per symbol. Alternatively, we can view the system as having two-dimensional symbols. The three regions $R_1$, $R_2$, $R_3$ are typical for this constellation. For example, in quaternary system with symbols $\pm 1 \pm j$ all regions are similar to $R_1$, except for a rotation. This rotation has no effect on the computation of error probability, because, as was shown in Chapter 1, Gaussian noise is immune to rotation, i.e., $n$ and $n \exp(j\alpha)$ have the same pdf. Similarly, the case $M = 8$ in which $a_{Ii} = \pm 1, \pm 3$ and $a_{Qi} = \pm 1$ leads to four regions of type $R_1$ and four regions of type $R_2$. The case $M = 16$, where $a_{Ii}, a_{Qi} = \pm 1, \pm 3$ has four regions of type $R_1$, four regions of type $R_3$, and eight of type $R_2$. Finally, the case $M = 64$, where $a_{Ii}, a_{Qi} = \pm 1, \pm 3, \pm 5, \pm 7$ has four regions of type $R_1$, 24 regions of type $R_2$, and 36 regions of type $R_3$. It thus follows from (6.3.12) that, assuming equiprobable symbols

$$P(c) = \begin{cases} P(1) & M = 4 \\ \frac{1}{2}\,(P(1) + P(2)) & M = 8 \\ \frac{1}{4}\,(P(1) + P(3) + 2\,P(2)) & M = 16 \\ \frac{1}{16}\,(P(1) + 6\,P(2) + 9\,P(3)) & M = 64 \end{cases} \tag{6.3.15}$$

where

$$P(i) = P(n \in R_i), \qquad i = 1, 2, 3 \tag{6.3.16}$$

We can see from Fig. 6.7 that

$$P(1) = P(n_{I,k} > -y_0)P(n_{Q,k} > -y_0) = \{1 - Q(y_0/\sigma_n)\}^2 \quad (6.3.17)$$

$$P(2) = P(|n_{I,k}| < y_0)P(n_{Q,k} > -y_0) = (1 - 2\,Q(y_0/\sigma_n)(1 - Q(y_0/\sigma_n)) \quad (6.3.18)$$

$$P(3) = P(|n_{I,k}| < y_0)P(|n_{Q,k}| < y_0) = \{1 - 2\,Q(y_0/\sigma_n)\}^2 \quad (6.3.19)$$

When we substitute (6.3.19) and (6.3.15) into (6.3.13), we obtain

$$P(e) = \begin{cases} 2\,Q(y_0/\sigma_n)\{1 - 0.5\,Q(y_0/\sigma_n)\} & M = 4 \\ 2.5\,Q(y_0/\sigma_n)\{1 - 0.6\,Q(y_0/\sigma_n)\} & M = 8 \\ 3\,Q(y_0/\sigma_n)\{1 - 0.75\,Q(y_0/\sigma_n)\} & M = 16 \\ 3.5\,Q(y_0/\sigma_n)\{1 - \frac{49}{56}\,Q(y_0/\sigma_n)\} & M = 64 \end{cases} \quad (6.3.20)$$

We shall relate now the ratio $y_0/\sigma_n$ to the signal-to-noise ratio. We have already defined, in Section 4, the filter efficiency factor

$$\eta = \frac{g^2(t_0)}{E_C E_{RD}} = \frac{\left(\int_{-\infty}^{\infty} G_C(f)H_{RD}(f)\exp(j\,2\,\pi f t_0)\,df\right)^2}{E_C E_{RD}}$$

where $E_C$ is the energy in $G_C(f)$, and $E_{RD}$ is the energy in $H_{RD}(f)$. When $H_{RD}(f)$ is matched to $G_C(f)$, $\eta = 1$; otherwise $0 \leqq \eta < 1$. Thus

$$y_0 = Ag_0 = A(\eta E_C E_{RD})^{1/2} \quad (6.3.21)$$

and since

$$\sigma_n^2 = N_0 E_{RD} \quad (6.2.22)$$

the ratio is

$$y_0/\sigma_n = (\eta A^2 E_C/N_0)^{1/2} \quad (6.3.23)$$

It was shown in Chapter 3 that the average energy per symbol (the average power multiplied by the symbol duration, $T$) at the receiver input (the signal is the same as in (6.1.1) and (6.1.7) with $h_S(t)$ replaced by $g_C(t)$) is

$$E_S = A^2\sigma_a^2 E_C/2 \quad (6.3.24)$$

where

$$\sigma_a^2 = \overline{|a_i|^2} \tag{6.3.25}$$

Thus

$$y_0/\sigma_n = \left(\eta \frac{2\,E_S}{N_0\sigma_a^2}\right)^{1/2} \tag{6.3.26}$$

For rectangular constellations in Fig. 5.2, we obtain

$$\sigma_a^2 = \begin{cases} 2 & M = 4 \\ 5.5 & M = 8 \\ 9.75 & M = 16 \\ 41.93 & M = 64 \end{cases} \tag{6.3.27}$$

The two-dimensional symbols can be generated from sequences of

$$\mu = \log_2 M \tag{6.3.28}$$

binary symbols. If the mapping is a two-dimensional Gray code, as shown, for example, in Fig. 6.2 for $M = 8$, an error in a symbol will cause only one bit error out of the $\mu$ bits. Therefore the bit error probability is

$$P_b(e) = P(e)/\log_2 M \tag{6.3.29}$$

The symbol energy is related similarly to the energy per bit

$$E_b = E_S/\mu \tag{6.3.30}$$

If the error probability is not too high (less than $10^{-2}$), we can ignore in (6.3.20) the terms in the bracket, and combining (6.3.20) and (6.3.26) through (6.3.30), we obtain

$$P_b(e) = k_1 Q(\eta k_2\, 2\, E_b/N_0)^{1/2} \tag{6.3.31}$$

where

$$k_1 = k/\mu \tag{6.3.32}$$

$$k_2 = \mu/\sigma_a^2 \tag{6.3.33}$$

and $k$ is 2 for $M = 4$, 2.5 for $M = 8$, 3 for $M = 16$, and 3.5 for $M = 64$. The values of $k_1$ and $k_2$ are given in Table 6.1

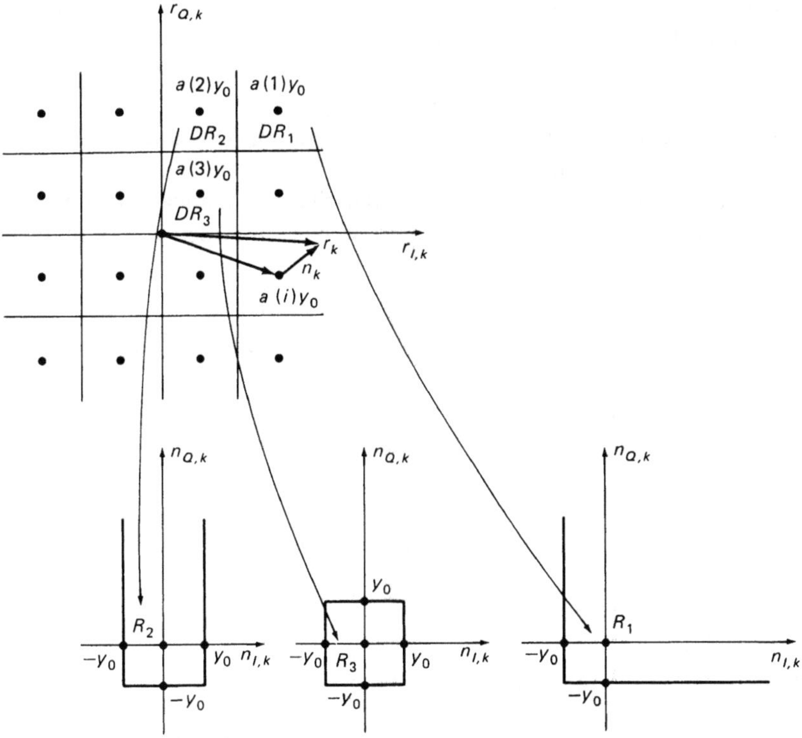


Fig. 6.7. Decision regions for a rectangular constellation.

**Table 6.1 Values of $k_1$ and $k_2$**

| $M$ | $k_1$ | $k_2$ |
|---|---|---|
| 4 | 1.0 | 1.0 |
| 8 | 0.833 | 0.545 |
| 16 | 0.75 | 0.41 |
| 64 | 0.5833 | 0.143 |

When we compare $k_1$ and $k_2$ with the coefficients

$$\frac{2\,(1 - M_L^{-1})}{\log_2 M_L} \text{ and } \frac{3\log_2 M_L}{M_L^2 - 1}$$

of eq. (6.3.14), taking $M_L = M^{1/2}$, the results are almost identical, the small discrepancies being caused by ignoring the terms in the brackets in (6.3.20). This enforces our previous statement that QASK and OQASK with a rectangular constellation can be treated as two ASK systems. Thus all results that have been obtained in Chapter 4 for ASK with a matched filter are valid here also if $M$ is replaced by $M_L = M^{1/2}$.

*Example* 6.3.2 Quaternary QASK and OQASK
Compute the bit error probability of quaternary QASK and OQASK with matched filter detector if $E_S/N_0 = 13.5$ dB.

Because quaternary QASK (and OQASK) is identical to two binary ASK systems, we can use Fig. 4.9 with $M = 2$, provided we compute first the signal-to-noise ratio per bit, which is

$$\frac{E_b}{N_0} = \frac{E_S}{N_0\mu} = \frac{1}{2}\frac{E_S}{N_0} = (13.5 - 3)\text{ dB} = 10.5\text{ dB}$$

Thus from Fig. 4.9

$$P_b(e) = 10^{-6}$$

The symbol error probability is from (6.3.29)

$$P(e) = 2 \times 10^{-6}$$

### 6.3.2 Circular constellation

When the symbols $a_i$ are located uniformly on a circle, all regions $DR_i$ are identical except for a rotation; hence the error probability is the same for all symbols and

$$P(e) = P(e|a_k = a(1) = 0) \tag{6.3.34}$$

This is illustrated, assuming that $a_i \in \{0, 2, \ldots, 2M - 2\}$, in Fig. 6.8. The case $M = 2$ is the same as binary ASK, and the case $M = 4$ is the same as the rectangular constellation with the same number of symbols. Thus in this section we have to compute the error probability only for $M > 4$ and $M = 3$. We shall present two methods: one is an exact method, but very difficult to generalize to include interference; the second method is an approximation that is excellent for reasonably high signal-to-noise ratios.

*Exact method* Because

$$r_k = y_0 + n_{I,k} + jn_{Q,k} = A_r \exp(j\phi_r) \tag{6.3.35}$$

$$n_{Q,k} = A_r \sin\phi_r \tag{6.3.36}$$

$$n_{I,k} = A_r \cos\phi_r - y_0 \tag{6.3.37}$$

there is an error, independent of the value of $A_r$, provide $\pi \geqq |\phi_r| > \pi/M$. Since

$$\tan \phi_r = \frac{n_{Q,k}}{y_0 + n_{I,k}} \tag{6.3.38}$$

$\phi_r$ is a symmetric *rv*, and thus

$$P(e) = 2 \int_{\pi/M}^{\pi} p_{\phi r}(\phi)\, d\phi \tag{6.3.39}$$

First we find the joint pdf, using the method of Chapter 1, Section 6.

$$\begin{aligned} p_{A_r,\phi_r}(A_r, \phi_r) &= p_{n_{I,k},n_{Q,k}}(A_r \sin \phi_r, A_r \cos \phi_r - y_0)A_r \\ &= (2\,\pi\sigma_n^2)^{-1} A_r \exp\left(-\frac{1}{2}\left(\frac{A_r \sin \phi_r}{\sigma_n}\right)^2\right) \\ &\quad \exp\left(-\frac{1}{2}\left(\frac{y_0 - A_r \cos \phi_r}{\sigma_n}\right)^2\right) \end{aligned} \tag{6.3.40}$$

After integration with respect to $A_r$, we obtain

$$\begin{aligned} p_{\phi r}(\phi_r) &= \int_0^{\infty} p_{A_r,\phi_r}(A_r, \phi_r)\, dA_r = (2\,\pi)^{-1} \exp\left(-0.5\,(y_0/\sigma_n)^2\right) \\ &\quad + (2\,\pi)^{-1/2}(y_0 \cos \phi_r/\sigma_n) \exp\left(-\frac{1}{2}\left(\frac{y_0 \sin \phi_r}{\sigma_n}\right)^2\right) \\ &\quad (1 - Q(y_0 \cos \phi_r/\sigma_n)) \end{aligned} \tag{6.3.41}$$

which, for reasonable value of $y_0/\sigma_n$, is simplified to

$$p_{\phi r}(\phi_r) \geqq (2\,\pi)^{-1/2}(y_0 \cos \phi_r/\sigma_n) \exp\left(-0.5\,(y_0 \sin \phi_r/\sigma_n)^2\right) \tag{6.3.42}$$

which leads to a closed form result after substitution into (6.3.39). This was first derived in Ref. 6.1. The relation (6.3.26) is valid here also, but in this constellation

$$\sigma_a^2 = 1 \tag{6.3.43}$$

Hence

$$y_0/\sigma_n = (\eta\, 2\, E_S/N_0)^{1/2} = (\eta\mu\, 2\, E_b/N_0)^{1/2} \tag{6.3.44}$$

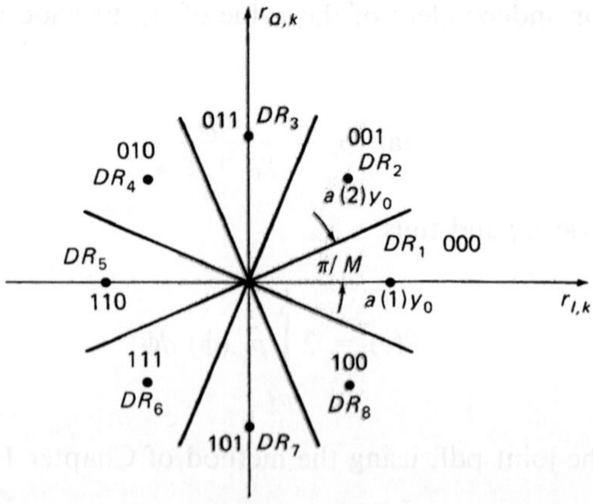


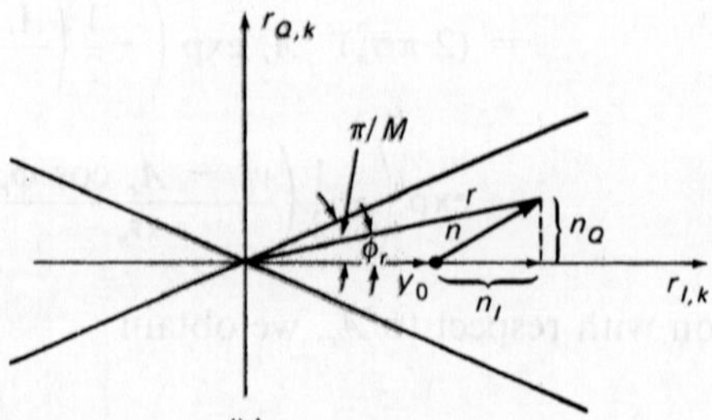


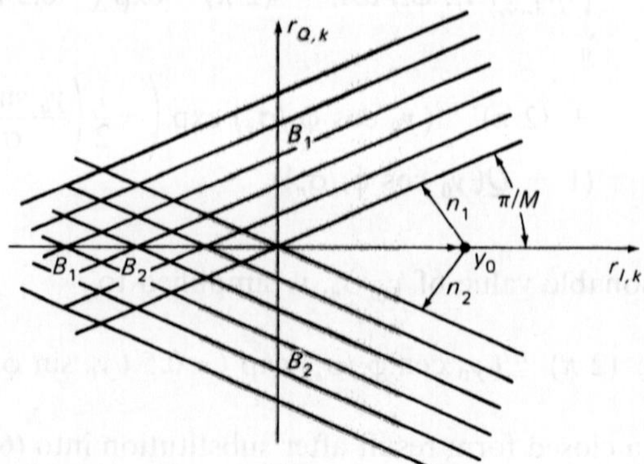


Fig. 6.8. Decision regions for a circular constellation.

Finally, if we encode $\mu$ binary symbols into the $M$-ary symbol, using a Gray code as shown in Fig. 6.8, we obtain the bit error probability

$$P_b(e) = P(e)/\mu \tag{6.3.45}$$

*Approximation* We can see from Fig. 6.8(c) that

$$P(e) = P(r_k \in B_1 \cup B_2) \tag{6.3.46}$$

Thus

$$\text{Max}\,\{P(r_k \in B_1), P(r_k \in B_2)\} \leqq P(r_k \in B_1 \cup B_2) \leqq P(r_k \in B_1) + P(r_k \in B_2)$$

and

$$\begin{aligned} P(r_k \in B_i) &= P(n_i > y_0 \sin(\pi/M)) \\ &= Q\left(\frac{y_0 \sin(\pi/M)}{\sigma_n}\right), \qquad i = 1, 2 \end{aligned} \tag{6.3.47}$$

$n_1$ and $n_2$ are shown in Fig. 6.8c and, because of rotational invariance, they have the same pdf as $n_I$ and $n_Q$. It thus follows from (6.3.45) and (6.3.46)

$$P_L(e) \leqq P(e) \leqq 2\, P_L(e) \tag{6.3.48}$$

$$P_L(e) = Q(y_0 \sin(\pi/M)/\sigma_n) \tag{6.3.49}$$

Using expression (6.3.45) and a Gray code, the bit error probability is bounded as in (6.3.48), with

$$P_L(e) = Q((\eta\mu\, 2\, E_b/N_0)^{1/2} \sin(\pi/M))/\mu \tag{6.3.50}$$

For $M \geqq 4$ and not too low signal-to-noise ratio, the upper bound is very close to the true value.

*Example* 6.3.3
Compute the error probability of $M$-ary PSK as a function of signal-to-noise ratio per bit, assuming a matched filter in the receiver.

For $M = 2$ we can use the result for binary ASK

$$P(e) = Q((2\, E_b/N_0)^{1/2})$$

which is also the lower bound in (6.3.49).

For $M = 4$ the result is the same as for quaternary QASK, which is

$$P(e) = 2\,Q((2\,E_b/N_0)^{1/2})$$

which is the same as the upper bound in (6.3.48).

For $M = 2^\mu$, $\mu > 2$, we use the upper bound in (6.3.48)

$$P(e) = 2\,Q((\mu\,2\,E_b\,\sin^2(\pi/M)/N_0)^{1/2})$$

The results are presented in Figs. 6.9 and 6.10.

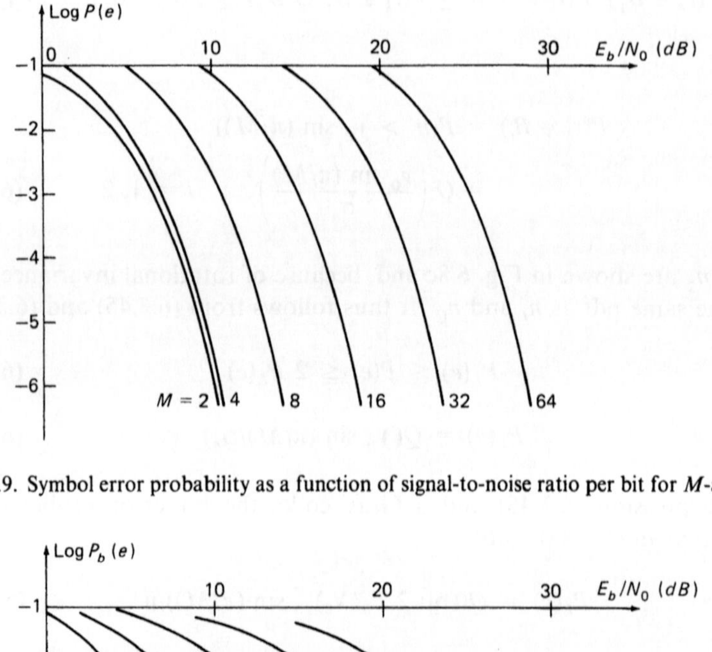


Fig. 6.9. Symbol error probability as a function of signal-to-noise ratio per bit for $M$-ary PSK.

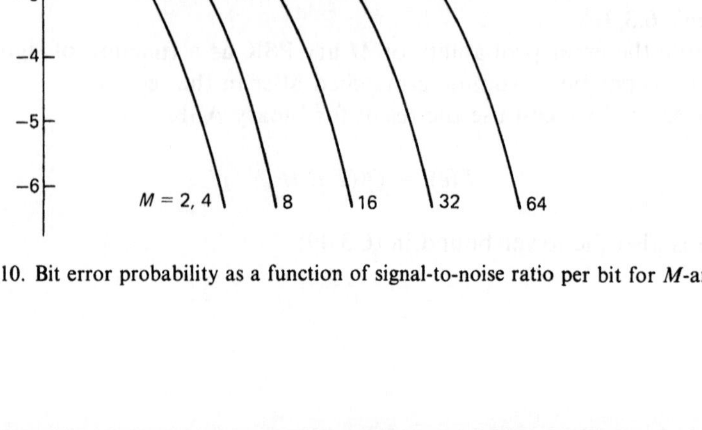


Fig. 6.10. Bit error probability as a function of signal-to-noise ratio per bit for $M$-ary PSK.

### 6.3.3 General constellation

In a general constellation the conditional error probability when symbol $a_k = a(i)$ is transmitted is

$$P(e|a_k = a(i)) = \sum_{m \neq i} P(r_k \in DR_m | a_k = a(i)) \tag{6.3.51}$$

Let $DR_{m,i}$ be the set of points in the plane that are closer to $a(m)y_0$ than $a(i)y_0$

$$DR_{m,i} = \{r_k: |r_k - a(m)y_0| \leqq |r_k - a(i)y_0|\} \tag{6.3.52}$$

Since

$$DR_m \subset DR_{m,i} \tag{6.3.53}$$

we obtain

$$\begin{aligned} P(e|a_k = a(i)) &\leqq \sum_{m \neq i} P(r_k \in DR_{m,i}|a_k = a(i)) \\ &= \sum_{m \neq i} P(n_k \in R_{m,i}) \end{aligned} \tag{6.3.54}$$

where

$$R_{m,i} = \{n_k: n_k + a(i)y_0 \in DR_{m,i}\} \tag{6.3.55}$$

i.e., the set $DR_{m,i}$ shifted to the origin. This is illustrated in Fig. 6.11. The noise, $n_k$, will belong to $R_{m,i}$ if its projection on the line connecting the points $a(i)y_0$ and $a(m)y_0$, denoted in Fig. 6.10 by $n_1$, exceeds half the distance between these points, which is $d_{i,m}y_0$, where

$$d_{i,m} = \tfrac{1}{2} |a(m) - a(i)| \tag{6.3.56}$$

Since the noise is invariant to a rotation, $n_1$ is also zero mean, Gaussian with variance $\sigma^2{}_n$; thus

$$P(n_k \in R_{m,i}) = P(n_1 > d_{i,m}y_0) = Q(d_{i,m}y_0/\sigma_n) \tag{6.3.57}$$

Thus

$$P(e|a_k = a(i)) \leqq \sum_{m \neq i} Q(d_{i,m}y_0/\sigma_n) \tag{6.3.58}$$

and assuming equiprobable symbols

$$P(e) \leqq M^{-1} \sum_i \sum_{m \neq i} Q(d_{i,m}y_0/\sigma_n) \tag{6.3.59}$$

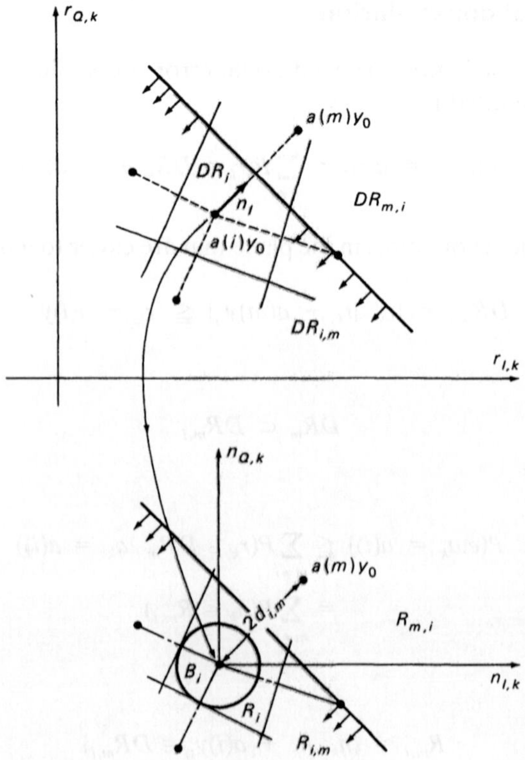


Fig. 6.11. Decision regions for general constellation.

$y_0/\sigma_n$ is related to the average energy per symbol as in (6.3.26); hence

$$P(e) \leqq M^{-1} \sum_{i} \sum_{m \neq i} Q((\eta \; 2 \; E_S/N_0)^{1/2} \; d_{i,m}/\sigma_a) \tag{6.3.60}$$

The last equation leads to an optimization problem: find the set of points on the plane $\{a(i), i = 1, \ldots, M\}$ so that $\{d_{i,m}/\sigma_a\}$ is maximized. Because, for not too low signal-to-noise ratios, the dominant term in (6.3.58) is the term with the smallest value of $d_{i,m}$, the optimization problem is equivalent to maximizing the minimal value of $d_{i,m}/\sigma_a$. Such an optimization was performed in Ref. 6.2. It was shown there that the optimal constellation consists of points that form almost equilateral triangles as shown in Fig. 6.12.

Although (6.3.61) is a useful expression, we can find for high signal-to-noise ratios (used in practice) a simpler bound. Let

$$B_i = \{n_k \colon |n_k| \leqq y_0 d_i\} \tag{6.3.61}$$

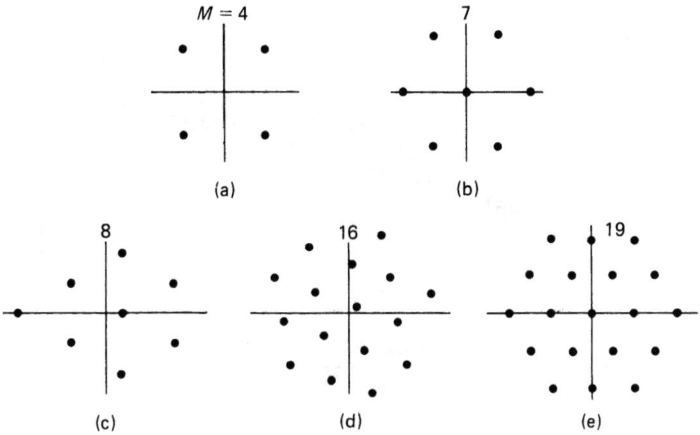


Fig. 6.12. Optimal constellations.

where $d_i$ is the minimal distance to the boundary of $R_i$, i.e.

$$d_i = \min_{m=1,\ldots,M} d_{i,m} \tag{6.3.62}$$

Because

$$B_i \subset R_i \tag{6.3.63}$$

$$P(e|a_k = a(\mathrm{i})) = P(n_k \notin R_i) \leqq P(n_k \notin B_i) = P(|n_k| > d_i y_0) \tag{6.3.64}$$

It was shown in Chapter 1 (Example 1.6.4) that the pdf of $|n_k|$ is

$$p_{|nk|}(n) = (n/\sigma_n^2) \exp(-0.5\, n^2/\sigma_n^2) u(n) \tag{6.3.65}$$

Therefore

$$P(e) \leqq M^{-1} \sum_{i=1}^{M} \exp(-d_i^2 y_0^2/\sigma^2{}_n) \leqq \exp(-d^2 y_0^2/\sigma^2{}_n) \tag{6.3.66}$$

where

$$d = \min_i d_i \tag{6.3.67}$$

After substitution of (6.3.26), we obtain

$$P(e) \leqq \exp\left(-d^2 \eta \frac{2\, E_S}{N_0 \sigma_a^2}\right) \tag{6.3.68}$$

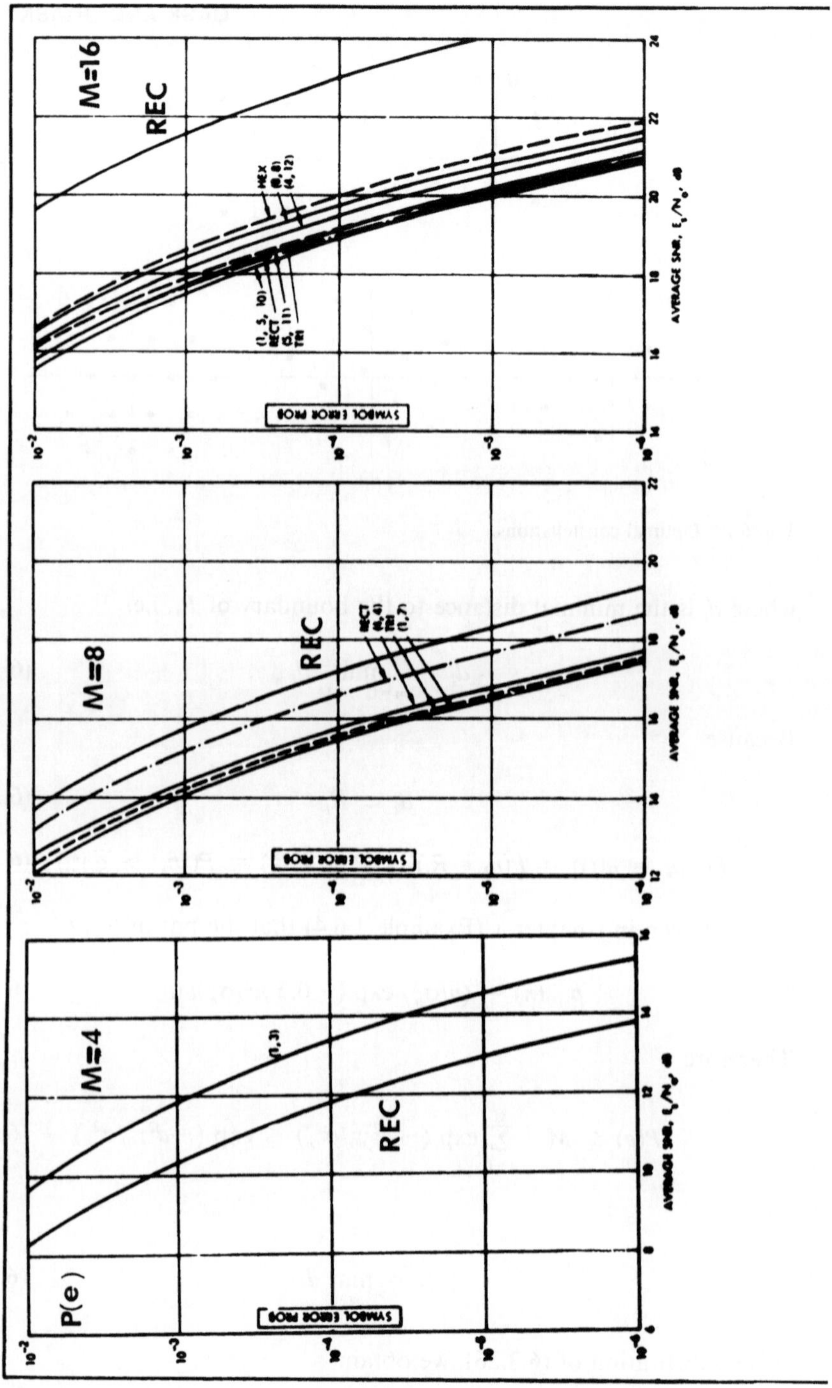
M=16
REC
HEX
(8, 8)
(4, 12)
(1, 5, 10)
RECT
(5, 11)
TRI
SYMBOL ERROR PROB
AVERAGE SNR, E_s/N_0, dB
M=8
REC
RECT
TRI
(1, 7)
SYMBOL ERROR PROB
AVERAGE SNR, E_s/N_0, dB
M=4
(1, 3)
REC
P(e)
SYMBOL ERROR PROB
AVERAGE SNR, E_s/N_0, dB

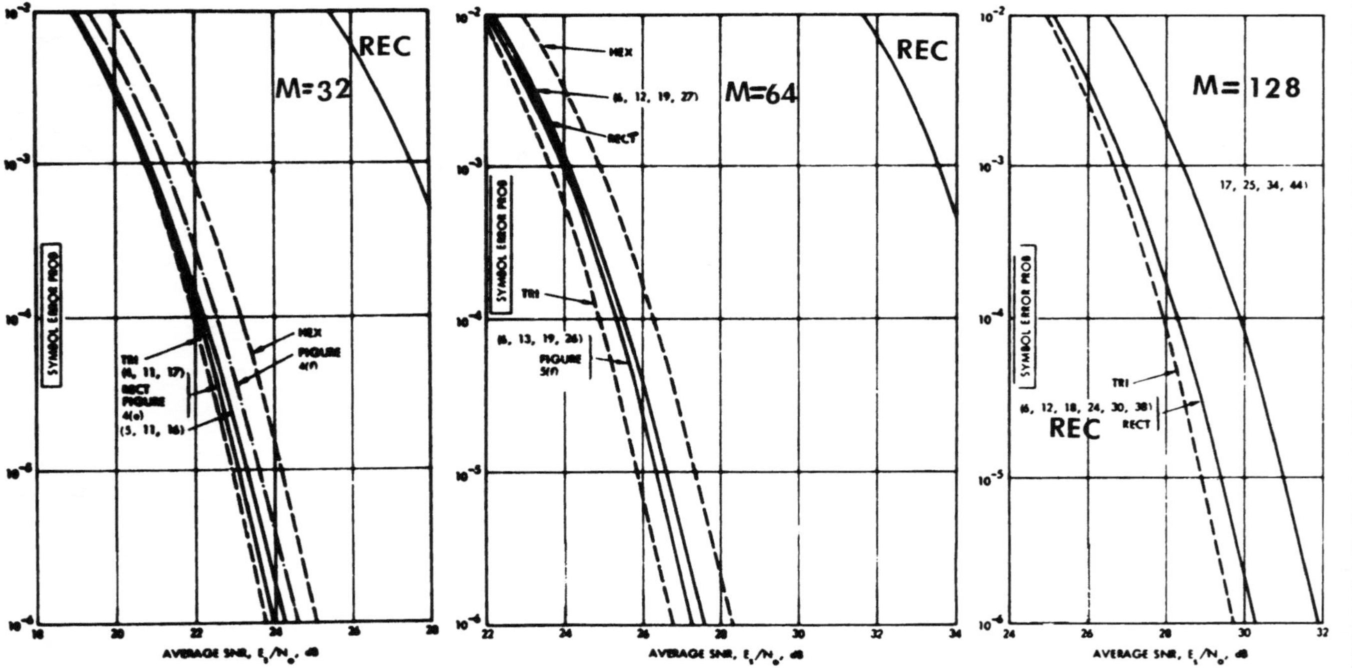


Fig. 6.13. Symbol error probability as a function of signal-to-noise for symbol for various symbol constellations (C. M. Thomas, M. Y. Weidner, S. H. Durani, "Digital Amplitude-Phase Keying with *M*-ary Alphabets," *IEEE Tr. Comm.*, Vol. COM-22, February 1974, pp. 28–38. Copyright © 1974 IEEE).

In Fig. 6.13 is shown the symbol error probability as a function of $E_S/N_0$ for various symbol constellations, which are defined in Fig. 6.14. We can see from Fig. 6.13 that the rectangular constellation is either the best or not far away from the best. Let $(E_S/N_0)_{min}$ be the minimum signal-to-noise ratio to achieve a certain error probability with the best constellation, and let

$$E_S/N_0 = (E_S/N_0)_{min} + \Delta E_S/N_0 \tag{6.3.69}$$

be the signal-to-noise ratio for the rectangular constellation. Table 6.2 shows $\Delta E_S/N_0$ for various $M$ and $P(e) = 10^{-5}$.

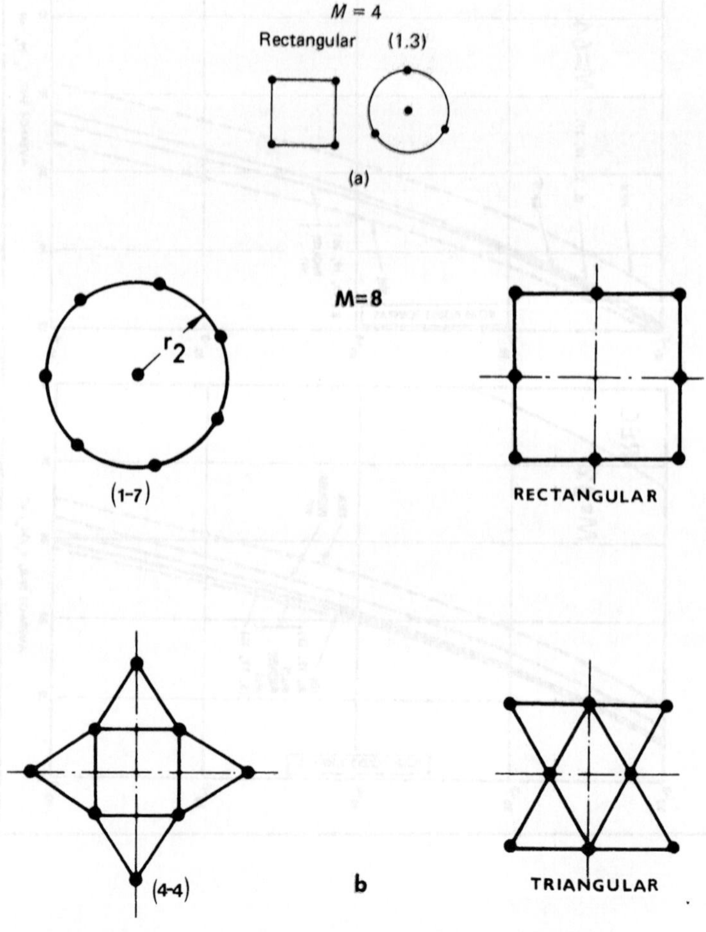


Fig. 6.14. Symbol constellations for $M = 4$, 8, 16, 32, and 64 symbols (C. M. Thomas, M. Y. Weidner, S. H. Durani, "Digital amplitude-Phase Keying with $M$-ary Alphabets," *IEEE Tr. Comm.*, Vol. COM-22, February 1974, pp. 28–38. Copyright © 1974 IEEE).

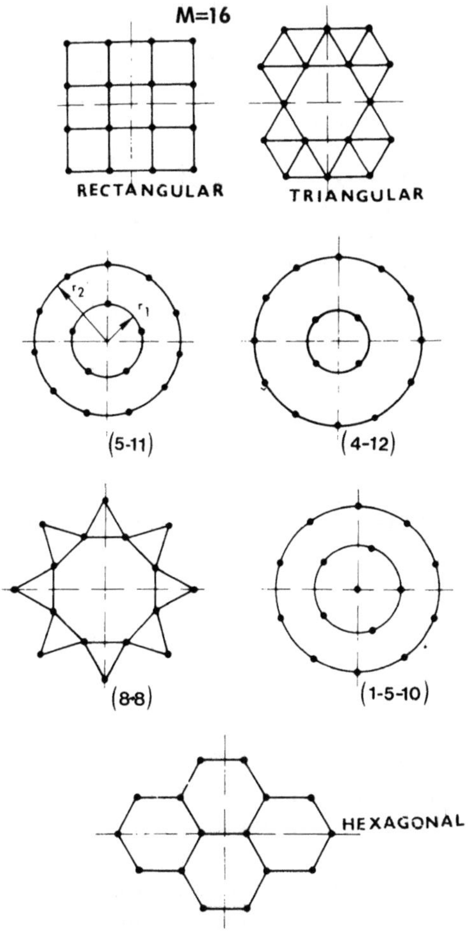


c

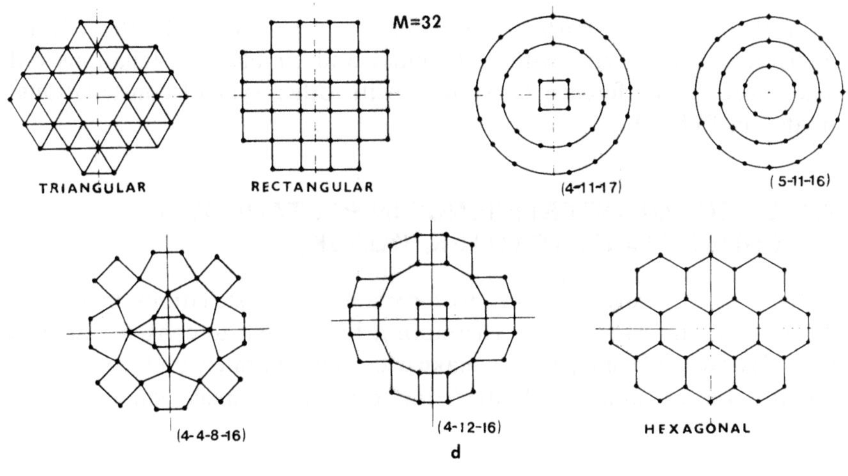


d

Fig. 6.14. (*con't.*)

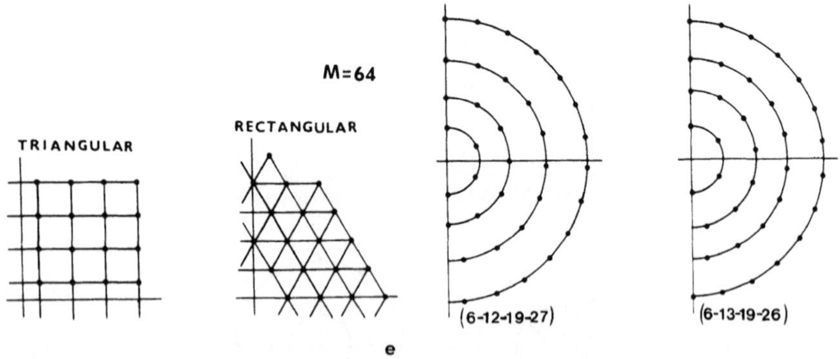


Fig. 6.14. (*con't.*)

**Table 6.2 Best and rectangular constellation**

| $M$ | 4 | 8 | 16 | 32 | 64 | 128 |
|---|---|---|---|---|---|---|
| $\Delta E_S/N_0$ (dB) | 0 | 1.2 | 0.1 | 0.2 | 0.4 | 0.5 |

We thus conclude that the penalty in signal-to-noise ratio of using a rectangular constellation instead of the best constellation is rather small, while the simplicity of implementation of the rectangular constellation is rather outstanding.

In many application, in which the system contains a nonlinear amplifier (for example a traveling wave tube (TWT)) signals with constant envelopes are preferred. In this case we would use a circular constellation denoted by PSK in Fig. 6.13.

In the remaining parts of this chapter we shall study the effect of interference on systems with rectangular and circular constellations only. The effect of interference on systems with other symbol constellations is treated in Ref. 6.17.

## 6.4 EFFECT OF INTERFERENCE IN RECTANGULAR CONSTELLATIONS (QASK, OQASK)

In this section we are concerned with rectangular constellations, mainly with $M = 4$, 16 and 64 symbols. Therefore it is sufficient to consider either eq. (6.2.13) or (6.2.14) only, and we make decisions separately on the value of $a_{Ik}$ and $a_{Qk}$. Let us combine all interfering terms into a single equation

$$I = \sum_i{}' a_{Ii} y_{I,k-i} - \sum_i a_{Qi} y_{Q,k-i}(\varepsilon) + \sum_i b_{Ii} y_{I,k-i}(\tau, f_A) - \sum_i b_{Qi} y_{Q,k-i}(\varepsilon, \tau, f_A) \tag{6.4.1}$$

Thus

$$r_{I,k} = a_{Ik} y_{I,0} + I + n_{I,k} \tag{6.4.2}$$

The interference term can be reordered according to rank, as explained in Section 4.4.1, to obtain

$$I = \sum_{i=1}^{\infty} a_i h_i, \qquad h_i \geqq h_{i+1} \tag{6.4.3}$$

where $\{a_i = \pm 1\}$ are binary, independent, equiprobable symbols, and $h_i$ is a member from the set

$$\{2^{m_I} |y_{Ii}| \; i \neq 0, \; 2^{m_Q} |y_{Q,i}(\varepsilon)|, \; 2^{m_I} |y_{I,i}(\tau, f_A)|, \; 2^{m_Q} |y_{Q,i}(\varepsilon, \tau, f_A)|\} \tag{6.4.4}$$

where

$$m_I = 0, 1, 2, \ldots, \log_2 M_I - 1, \; m_Q = 0, 1, 2, \ldots, \log_2 M_Q - 1 \tag{6.4.5}$$

*Example* 6.4.1

Assume a system with only one ISI and one ACI nonzero terms

$$|y_{I,1}| = x_1 \qquad |y_{Q,0}| = x_2 > 2\, x_1$$

Assume that the symbols are $a_{Ii} \in \{\pm 1, \pm 3\}$ and $a_{Qi} \in \{\pm 1, \pm 3, \pm 5, \pm 7\}$; thus $M_I = 4$, and $M_Q = 8$. In this case $h_i$ will take its values from

$$\{x_1, 2\, x_1, x_2, 2\, x_2, 4\, x_2\}$$

$$\text{and } h_1 = 4\, x_2, \; h_2 = 2\, x_2, \; h_3 = x_2, \; h_4 = 2\, x_1, \; h_5 = x_1$$

Equation (6.4.2) is identical to (4.2.1); hence we may be tempted to use uncritically the expressions for symbol and error probabilities derived in Chapter 4 (for example, eqs. (4.4.4) through (4.4.6)). However, this will be correct only if the symbol-dependent term in (6.4.2)

$$y_{I,0} = A \operatorname{Re} \{g_0 \exp(j\Delta\phi)\} \tag{6.4.6}$$

is identical to the same term in the absence of any interference in eq. (6.3.1)

$$y_0 = A g_{I,0} \tag{6.4.7}$$

because the decision rule has been made under this assumption, and all formulas in Chapter 4 have been derived under this assumption. Let

$$\delta = \text{Re}\,\{g_0 \exp(j\Delta\phi)\}/g_{I,0} \tag{6.4.8}$$

Thus

$$y_{I,0} = \delta y_0 \tag{6.4.9}$$

If $\delta = 1$, we can use the formulas of Chapter 4 with $M$ replaced by $M_I$ and $g_0/\sigma_n$ replaced by $y_{I,0}/\sigma_n$. This implies that if $M_I = M_Q = (M)^{1/2}$, the bit error probability of QASK and OQASK with $M = 4, 16, 64$ is identical to the bit error probability of ASK with $M = 2, 4, 8$, respectively, if the interference term $I$ is the same.

If $\delta \neq 1$, and this will happen mainly because of phase offset, which causes QCI, we shall need new formulas, which will be derived in subsection 6.4.1.

### 6.4.1 Effect of QCI and ISI[6.4–6.8]

In this section we shall assume that there is no ACI; hence the last two sums in (6.4.1) are missing. This assumption is not required for the derivation of the formulas; we use it only in the numerical examples, because we have not yet derived expressions for $g(t, f_A)$. It will be also convenient if we normalize the interference term; thus

$$I' = I/y_{I,0} \tag{6.4.10}$$

and

$$r_{I,k} = (a_{I,k} + I')\delta y_0 + n_{I,k} \tag{6.4.11}$$

Because the symbols belong to the set $\mathring{A}_{\pm} = \{\pm 1, \pm 3, \ldots, \pm(M_I - 1)\}$, the decision rule is as in (4.2.14), with

$$d_m = (-M_I + 2\,m)y_0 \tag{6.4.12}$$

Thus

$$\hat{a}_{ik} = \begin{cases} 1 - M_I & \text{if } -\infty < r_k \leqq (2 - M_I)y_0 \\ i & (i - 1)y_0 \leqq r_k \leqq (i + 1)y_0 \\ M_I - 1 & \text{if } (M_I - 2)y_0 \leqq r_k < \infty \end{cases} \tag{6.4.13}$$

and $i = \pm 1, \pm 3, \ldots, \pm(M_I - 3)$.

The conditional error probabilities are thus

$$\begin{aligned} P(e|a_{Ik} = 1 - M_I, I') &= P(r_{Ik} > (2 - M_I)y_0|a_{Ik} = 1 - M_I, I') \\ &= P((1 - M_I + I')\delta y_0 + n_{I,k} \geqq -(M_I - 2)y_0) \\ &= P(n_{I,k} \geqq ((M_I - I' - 1)\delta - M_I + 2)y_0)) \\ &= Q\{((M_I - I' - 1)\delta - M_I + 2)y_0/\sigma_n\} \end{aligned} \tag{6.4.14}$$

$$\begin{aligned} P(e|a_{Ik} = M_I - 1, I') &= P((M_I - 1 + I')\delta y_0 + n_{I,k} \leqq (M_I - 2)y_0) \\ &= Q\{((M_I - 1 + I')\delta - M_I + 2)y_0/\sigma_n)\} \end{aligned} \tag{6.4.15}$$

and for $i \neq \pm(M_I - 1)$

$$\begin{aligned} P(e|a_{Ik} = i, I') &= P((i + I')\delta y_0 + n_{I,k} < (i - 1)y_0) \\ &\quad + P((i + I')\delta y_0 + n_{I,k} > (i + 1)y_0) \\ &= Q\{((i + I')\delta - i + 1))y_0/\sigma_n\} \\ &\quad + Q\{(i + 1 - (i + I')\delta)y_0/\sigma_n\} \end{aligned} \tag{6.4.16}$$

The average error probability, assuming equiprobable symbols, is

$$\begin{aligned} P(e) = M_I^{-1}\Bigg\{&\overline{Q\{((M_I - 1 + I')\delta - M_I + 2)y_0/\sigma_n\}} \\ &+ \overline{Q\{((M_I - 1 - I')\delta - M_I + 2)y_0/\sigma_n\}} \\ &+ \sum_{i \neq \pm(M_I - 1)} \overline{Q\{((i + I')\delta - i + 1)y_0/\sigma_n\}} \\ &+ \overline{Q\{(i + 1 - (i + I')\delta)y_0/\sigma_n\}}\Bigg\} \end{aligned} \tag{6.4.17}$$

where the bar denotes the average over $I'$. Since $I'$ is a symmetric rv, we can replace in (6.4.17) $I'$ by $-I'$ whenever this is required. Note also that the two parts of the summation are equal; therefore

$$\begin{aligned} P(e) = (2/M_I)\Bigg\{&\overline{Q\{((M_I - 1 + I')\delta - M_I + 2)y_0/\sigma_n\}} \\ &+ \sum_{i \neq \pm(M_I - 1)} \overline{Q\{((i + I')\delta - i + 1)y_0/\sigma_n\}}\Bigg\} \end{aligned} \tag{6.4.18}$$

When $\delta = 1$, eq. (6.4.18) is simplified to

$$P(e) = 2(1 - M_I^{-1})\overline{Q\{(1 + I')y_0/\sigma_n\}} \tag{6.4.19}$$

which is the same as (4.4.4) with the notation $M \to M_I$, $g_0 \to y_0$.

*Example* 6.4.2
Specify the formula for the error probability for $M_I = 2, 4, 6, 8$. Using

(6.4.16), we obtain

$\underline{M_I = 2}$

$$P_2(e) = \overline{Q\{(1 + I')\delta y_0/\sigma_n\}} \tag{6.4.20}$$

$\underline{M_I = 4}$

$$P_4(e) = \tfrac{1}{2}\,\{\overline{Q\{((3 + I')\delta - 2)y_0/\sigma_n\}} + P_2(e) + \overline{Q\{((I' - 1)\delta + 2)y_0/\sigma_n\}}\} \tag{6.4.21}$$

$\underline{M_I = 6}$

$$P_6(e) = \tfrac{1}{3}\{\overline{Q\{((5 + I')\delta - 4)y_0/\sigma_n\}} + 2\,P_4(e) + \overline{Q\{((I' - 3)\delta + 4)y_0/\sigma_n\}}\} \tag{6.4.22}$$

$\underline{M_I = 8}$

$$P_8(e) = \tfrac{1}{4}\{\overline{Q\{((7 + I')\delta - 6)y_0/\sigma_n\}} + 3\,P_6(e) + \overline{Q\{((I' - 5)\delta + 6)y_0/\sigma_n\}}\} \tag{6.4.23}$$

The ratio $y_0/\sigma_n$ is related to the signal-to-noise ratio by

$$y_0/\sigma_n = \left(\eta\,\frac{2\,E_S}{N_0\sigma_a^2}\right)^{1/2} = \left(\eta\,\frac{3\log_2 M_I}{M_I^2 - 1}\,\frac{2\,E_S}{N_0}\right)^{1/2} \tag{6.4.24}$$

where

$$\eta = y_0^2/E_C E_{RD} \tag{6.4.24a}$$

and $\sigma_a^2 = (M_I^2 - 1)/3$. Using a Gray code, the bit error probability is related to the symbol error probability by

$$P_b(e) = P(e)/\log_2 M_I \tag{6.4.25}$$

**6.4.1.1 System with Nyquist function response** Here we assume that

$$g(t) = g_N(t) \tag{6.4.26}$$

where $g_N(t)$ is the Nyquist function as in (4.3.29) with amplitude $g_N(0) = 1$. Therefore

$$y_I(t) = A g_N(t) \cos \Delta\phi \tag{6.4.27}$$

$$y_Q(t) = Ag_N(t) \sin \Delta\phi \tag{6.4.28}$$

The normalized interference term is, from (6.4.2) and (6.4.10), assuming $A_A = 0$)

$$I' = \sum_i{}' a_{Ii} g_{N,k-i}/g_{N,0} + \sum_i a_{Qi} g_{N,k-i} \tan \Delta\phi/g_{N,0} \tag{6.4.29}$$

If the sampling times are ideal ($t_0 = 0$), then $g_{N,0} = 1, g_{N,i} = 0 \; (i \neq 0)$; hence the interference is a single term

$$I' = a_{Qk} \tan \Delta\phi \tag{6.4.30}$$

The factor, $\delta$, is here

$$\delta = g_{N,0} \cos \Delta\phi \tag{6.4.31}$$

and assuming a matched filter

$$G_C(f) = H_{RD}(f) = \sqrt{G_N(f)} = H_N(f) \tag{6.4.32}$$

we obtain in (6.4.24a) $\eta = 1$.

The results for QASK ($\varepsilon = 0$) with $M = 4 (M_I = 2)$ and $M = 16 \; (M_I = 4)$ is presented in Fig. 6.15 both for $t_0 = 0$ and $t_0 = 0.05T$. When $t_0 = 0$ the result is independent of excess bandwidth, $\beta$. When $t_0 \neq 0$, there is a strong dependence on $\beta$. Phase offset is more detrimental for $M = 16$ then for $M = 4$. For example, let $\Delta E_b/N_0$ be the additional energy require for $P_b(e) = 10^{-4}$ when the phase offset is increased from 0 to 5°. The results are 0.6 dB for $M = 4$ and 2.1 dB for $M = 16$ both for $\beta = 0.25$ and $\beta = 0.5$.

**6.4.1.2 System with Butterworth filters** Here we assume that the system has identical Butterworth filters in receiver and transmitter of order $N = 2, 3, 4$ and the same normalized, 3-dB bandwidth $B_0 = 2f_0T$. The detector is a simple, sample detector; hence in fact we discuss systems NS and HS of Table 4.3. The shaping functions are NRZ and HS; hence $g(t)$ is given in (4.5.17) and (4.5.30) with parameters as in (4.5.39) and (4.5.42). In Fig. 6.16 we show the results for quaternary OQASK with HS shaping function, also known as MSK. The sampling time, $t_0$, is optimal in the absence of offset. In Fig. 6.17 we show the effect of QCI and ISI for 16-ary QASK with NRZ shaping function (labeled QAM), 16-ary OQASK with NRZ shaping function (labeled NS), and 16-ary OQASK with HS shaping function (labeled HS). Here also phase offset is more detrimental for $M = 16$ than for $M = 4$. In these figures the phase offset is presented in radians rather then in degrees.

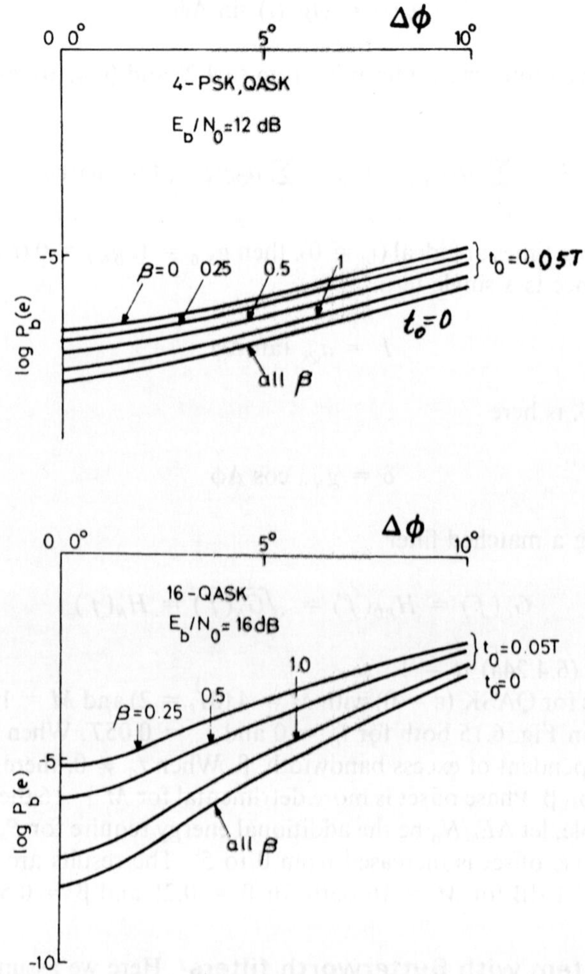


Fig. 6.15 Effect of phase offset on bit error probability of QASK and PSK with $M$ = 4, and 16 symbols for systems with Nyquist function reponse.

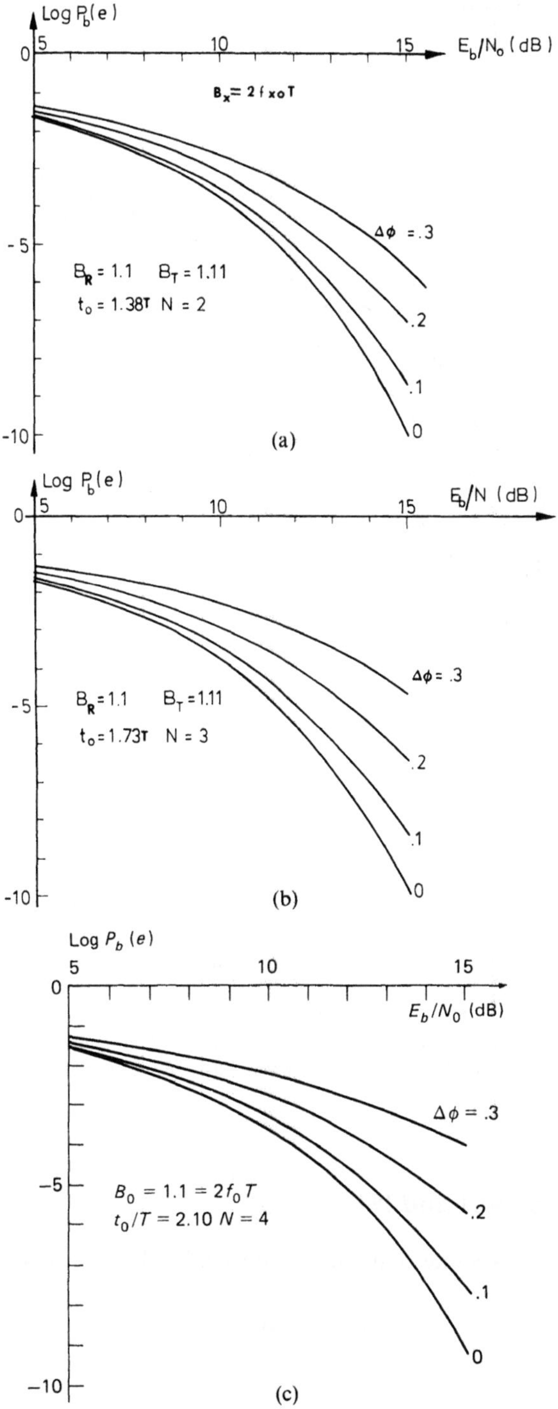


Fig. 6.16. Effect of phase offset on bit error probability of MSK with Butterworth filters in receiver and transmitter: (a) filter of order two, (b) filter of order three, (c) filter of order four (I. Korn, B. Seth, "Adjacent Channel and Quadrature Channel Interference in Minimum Shift Keying," *IEEE Tr. Sel. Ar. Comm.*, Vol. SAC-1, January 1983, pp. 21–28. Copyright © 1983 IEEE).

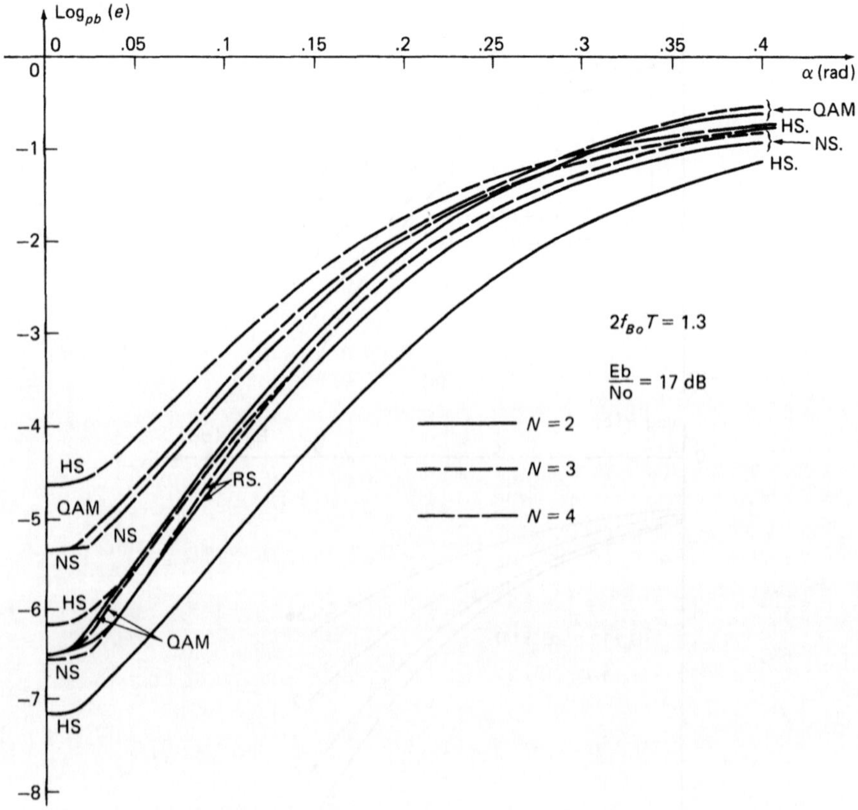


Fig. 6.17. Effect of phase offset on bit error probability of 16-ary OQASK with NRZ (NS) and HS (HS) shaping functions and 16-ary QASK with NRZ (QAM) shaping function. The system has identical Butterworth filters in received and transmitter with normalized bandwidth $B = 2f_0T = 1.3$. (I. Korn, Y. Tsang, "Effect of Intersymbol and Quadrature Channel Interference on Error Probability of 16-ary Offset Quadrature Amplitude Modulation with Sinusoidal and Rectangular Shaping." *IEEE Tr. Comm.*, Vol. COM-31, February 1983 pp. 264–269. Copyright © 1983 IEEE).

### 6.4.2 Effect of ACI and ISI

In this section we assume that there is no QCI, which means that

$$g_Q(t) = \Delta\phi = 0 \tag{6.4.33}$$

Hence

$$g_I(t) = g(t) \tag{6.4.34}$$

The interference contains now only three sums

$$I = \sum_i{}' a_{Ii} y_{K-i} + \sum_i b_{Ii} y_{I,k-i}(\tau, f_A) + \sum_i b_{Qi} y_{Q,k-i}(\varepsilon, \tau, f_A) \quad (6.4.35)$$

where the terms have been defined in (6.2.15) through (6.2.18). We thus have to compute $g(t, f_A)$, which can be written in two forms

$$\begin{aligned} g(t, f_A) &= h_S(t) \exp(j\omega_A t) * h_T(t) \exp(j\omega_A t) * h_{CD}(t) \\ &= g_T(t) \exp(j\omega_A t) * h_{CD}(t) \end{aligned} \quad (6.4.36)$$

where

$$g_T(t) = h_S(t) * h_T(t) \quad (6.4.37)$$

and

$$h_{CD}(t) = h_C(t) * h_R(t) * h_D(t) \quad (6.4.38)$$

We shall assume that both $g_T(t)$ and $h_{CD}(t)$ are real; hence

$$g(t, -f_A) = g^*(t, f_A) \quad ((6.4.39)$$

and it is sufficient to compute $g(t, f_A)$ for $f_A \geqq 0$ only.

**6.4.2.1 System with Nyquist function response** Here we assume that

$$G_T(f) = H_{CD}(f) = H_N(f) \quad (6.4.40)$$

where $H_N(f)$ is the square root of the Nyquist function, presented in eq. (4.3.36), so that

$$g(t) = g(t, 0) = g_N(t) \quad (6.4.41)$$

where $g_N(t)$ is the Nyquist function with excess bandwidth β. Using Fourier transforms, eq. (6.4.36) can also be written as

$$g(t, f_A) = \int_{-\infty}^{\infty} H_N(f - f_A) H_N(f) \exp(j\, 2\pi f t)\, df \quad (6.4.42)$$

Defining

$$F(f, f_A) = H_N(f - f_A/2) H_N(f + f_A/2) \quad (6.4.43)$$

which is a real function, symmetric both in $f$ and $f_A$, we obtain from (6.4.42)

$$g(t, f_A) = f(t, f_A) \exp(j\pi f_A t) \tag{6.4.44}$$

$$g(t) = g(t, 0) = f(t, 0) \tag{6.4.44a}$$

where $f(t, f_A)$ is a real function, symmetric both in $t$ and $f_A$, which depends on the numerical values of both $f_A$ and $\beta$ and their interrelation. The formula for $f(t, f_A)$ is rather lengthy; hence we shall not quote it here, but rather refer the reader to Ref. 6.8. However, a plot of $f(t, f_A)$ as a function of $t$ with $\beta$ and $f_A$ as parameters is shown in Fig. 6.18. This function is zero if $f_A \geqq (1 + \beta)/T$. From Fig. 6.18 we can obtain an intuitive feeling how the proximity in frequency of the adjacent channel signal, $f_A$, affects the system. We can see for example that when $\beta$ increases from 0.25 to 1, the number of significant interfering terms is reduced. We also see that when the ratio $f_A T/(1 + \beta)$ increases, $f(t, f_A)$ decreases.

When we substitute (6.4.43) into (6.2.17) and (6.2.18), we obtain

$$\begin{aligned} y_{I,k-i}(\tau, f_A) = \operatorname{Re} \{ & A_A f(t_0 + (k - i)T - \tau, f_A) \\ & \exp\{j(\Delta\phi_A + \pi f_A(t_0 + (k - i)T - \tau))\}\} \end{aligned} \tag{6.4.45}$$

$$\begin{aligned} y_{Q,k-i}(\varepsilon, \tau, f_A) = \operatorname{Im} \{ & A_A f(t_0 + (k - i - \varepsilon)T - \tau, f_A) \\ & \exp\{j(\Delta\phi_A + \pi f_A(t_0 + (k - i - \varepsilon)T - \tau))\}\} \end{aligned} \tag{6.4.46}$$

If $t_0 = 0$, there is no ISI, and the first sum in (6.4.15) is zero. We assume that $\tau$ is uniform distributed in $-T/2$—$T/2$ (or 0—$T$) and $\Delta\phi_A$ is uniformly distributed in $-\pi$—$\pi$ (or 0—$2\pi$). This assumption is reasonable because the signals in the main and adjacent channels are not synchronized in time or in phase. The conditional bit error probability, conditioned on specific values of $\tau$ and $\Delta\phi_A$, is as in (4.4.6)

$$P_b(e|\tau, \Delta\phi_A) = k_1 \overline{Q((k_2\, 2\, E_b/N_0)^{1/2}(1 + I'(\tau, \Delta\phi_A)))} \tag{6.4.47}$$

$$k_1 = 2(1 - M_I^{-1}) \log_2 M_I \tag{6.4.48}$$

$$k_2 = 3 \log_2 M_I/(M_I^2 - 1) \tag{6.4.49}$$

and

$$I' = I/(Af(0, 0)) = I/A \tag{6.4.50}$$

and we emphasize the fact that $I'$ is computed for specific values of $\tau$ and $\Delta\phi_A$. The average in (6.4.47) is only with respect to the rvs $\{b_{Ii}\}$ and $\{b_{Qi}\}$. The bit error probability is

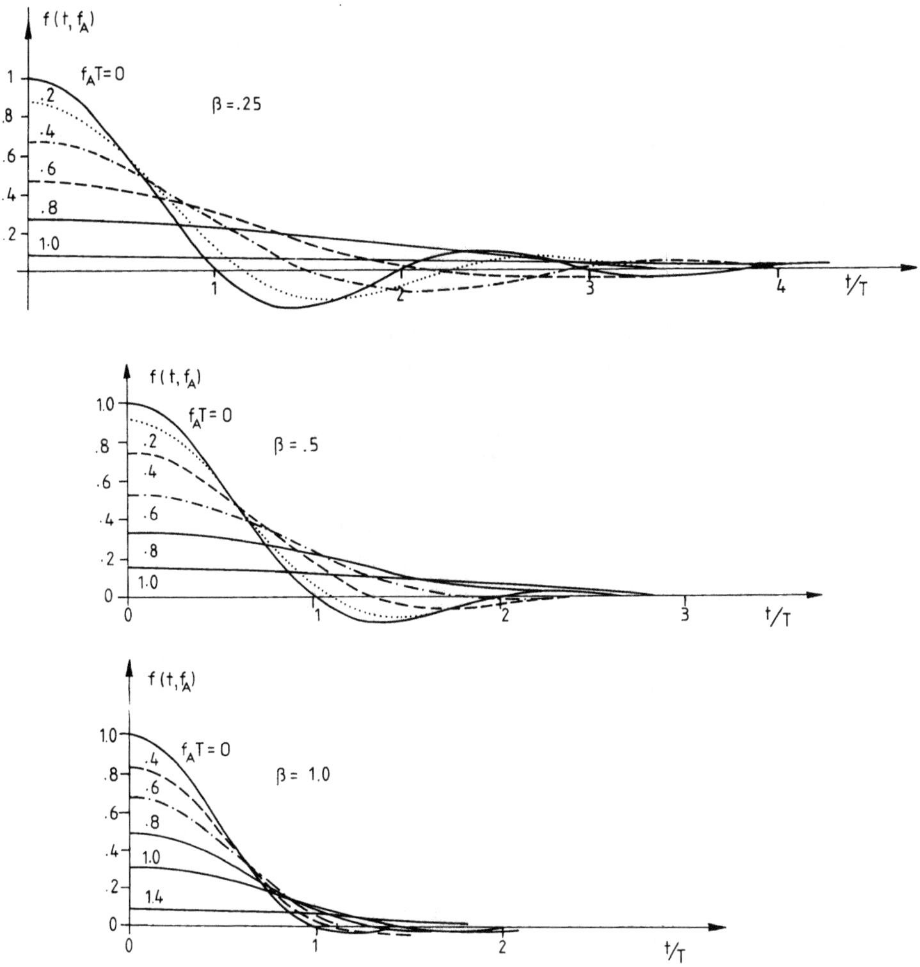


Fig. 6.18. The function $f(t, f_A)$ as a function of $t$ with β and $f_A$ as parameters.

$$P_b(e) = \int_0^T \int_0^{2\pi} P_b(e|\tau, \Delta\phi_A)\, d\tau\, d\Delta\phi_A (2\,\pi T)^{-1}$$

$$\simeq \sum_{i=0}^{N_\tau - 1} \sum_{k=0}^{N_\phi - 1} P_b(e|i\Delta\tau, k\Delta)(N_\tau N_\phi)^{-1} \tag{6.4.51}$$

where

$$\Delta\tau = T/N_\tau, \qquad \Delta = 2\,\pi/N_\phi \tag{6.4.52}$$

It was shown in Problem 1.6.3 that the modulo ($A$) sum of two independent rvs, one of which is uniformly distributed in 0—$A$, is also uniformly distributed in 0—$A$. This implies that

$$\Delta\phi_A + \pi f_A(t_0 + (k - i - \varepsilon)T - \tau) \tag{6.4.53}$$

is uniformly distributed in 0—2 $\pi$ and

$$\Delta\phi_A/(\pi f_A) + t_0 + (k - i - \varepsilon)T - \tau \tag{6.4.54}$$

is uniformly distributed in 0—$T$. Therefore, it is sufficient in (6.4.51) to compute the average with respect to $\tau$ only, i.e.

$$P_b(e) = \sum_{i=0}^{N_\tau - 1} P_b(e|i\Delta\tau, 0)/N_T \tag{6.4.55}$$

The resulting bit error probability for QASK with 4 and 16 symbols as a function of $E_b/N_0$ with $f_A T$ as a parameter is shown in Fig. 6.19. In the same figure we also include results for QASK with circular constellation under the label PSK, which we discuss in Section 6.5. In this figure it was assumed that the amplitude of the signal in the interfering channel is the same as in the main channel, i.e., $A_A = A$.

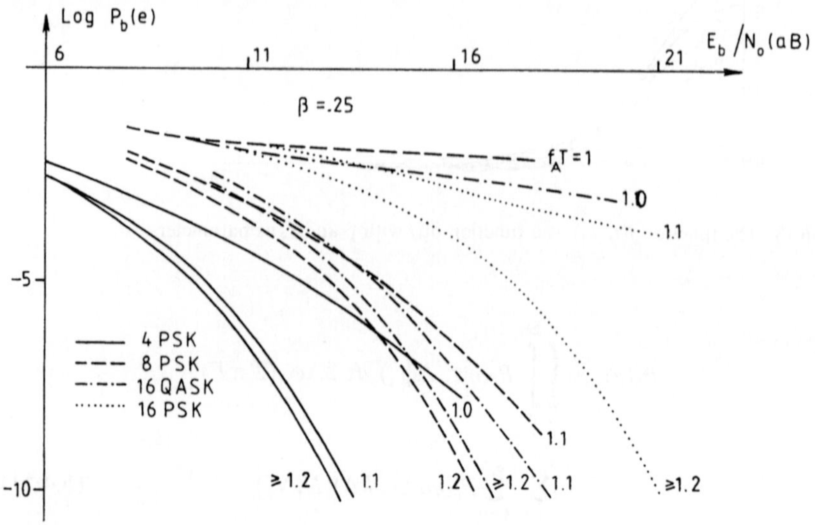


Fig. 6.19. Bit error probability as a function of signal-to-noise ratio per bit for PSK and QASK with 4, 8 and 16 symbols. The system has a Nyquist function response with excess bandwidth β.

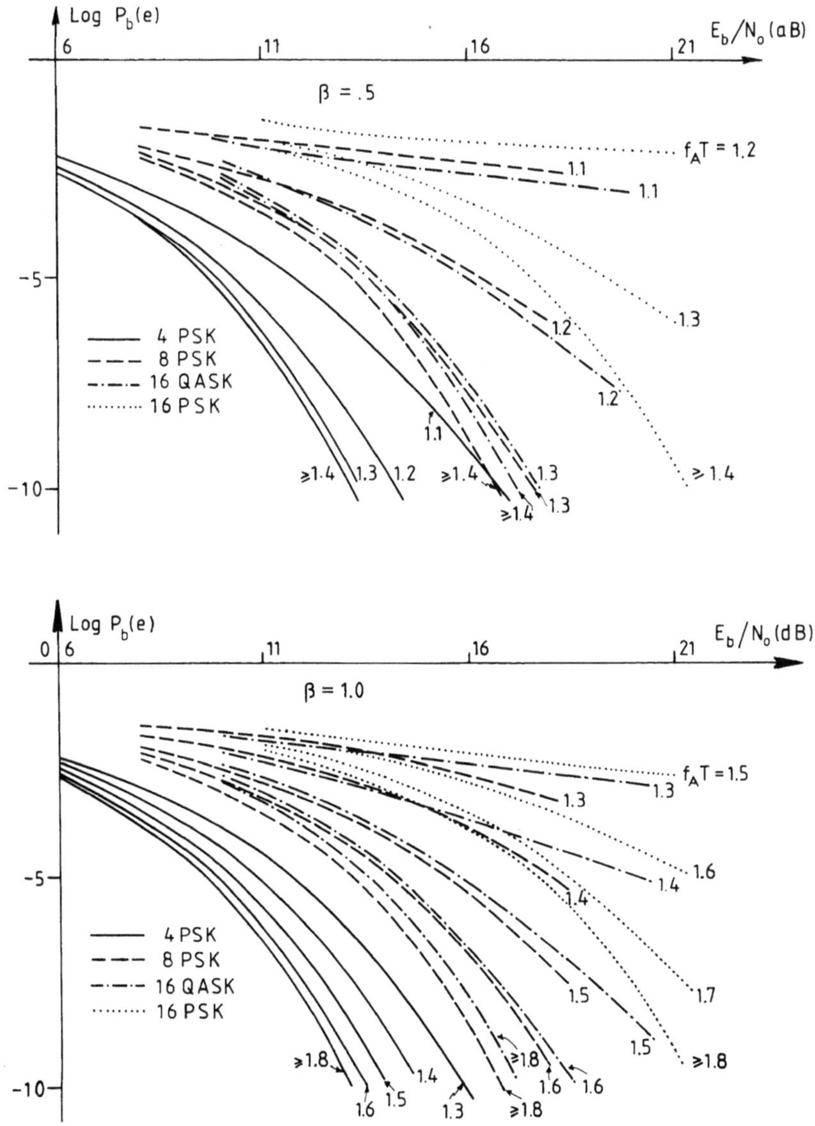

Log $P_b(e)$
6
11
16
21
$E_b/N_o$ (aB)
β = .5
$f_AT$ = 1.2
1.1
1.1
-5
1.3
1.2
4 PSK
8 PSK
16 QASK
16 PSK
1.2
1.1
≥1.4
1.3
1.2
≥1.4
1.3
≥ 1.4
-10
≥1.4
1.3
Log $P_b(e)$
0
6
11
16
21
$E_b/N_o$ (dB)
β = 1.0
$f_AT$ = 1.5
1.3
1.3
-5
1.6
1.4
1.4
4 PSK
8 PSK
16 QASK
16 PSK
1.5
1.7
1.5
≥1.8
≥1.8
≥1.8
1.4
1.6
1.6
-10
1.6
1.5
1.3
≥1.8


Fig. 6.19. (*con't.*)

*Example* 6.4.3
Assume that $\beta = 0.25$ or $\beta = 0.5$. The number of symbols is 4 or 16. Compute the signal-to-noise ratio per bit required to achieve a bit error probability of $10^{-5}$ if the frequency separation is $f_A T = 1.2$. Compute also the spectral efficiency of the system.

The first part can be solved using Fig. 6.19 by drawing a horizontal line through the point $\log P_b(e) = -5$ and then vertical lines through the intersections of the horizontal line with the curves for $f_A T = 1.2$. The result is

$$\begin{array}{lll} \beta = 0.25 & M = 4 & E_b/N_0 = 9.6 \text{ dB} \\ \beta = 0.25 & M = 16 & E_b/N_0 = 12.2 \text{ dB} \\ \beta = 0.5 & M = 4 & E_b/N_0 = 10.2 \text{ dB} \\ \beta = 0.5 & M = 16 & E_b/N_0 = 15.7 \text{ dB} \end{array}$$

The spectral efficiency is the ratio of bit rate, $R_b$, and bandwidth per signal, which is here $f_A$. Thus

$$\eta_B = R_b/f_A = (f_A T_b)^{-1} = \log_2 M(f_A T)^{-1} = \log_2 M/1.2$$

Thus for $M = 4$ $\eta_B = 1.66$ bps/Hz, and for $M = 16$ $\eta_B = 3.33$ bps/Hz.

**6.4.2.2 System with distinct poles filters**[6.6, 6.7] In this section we assume that the shaping function is either NRZ or HS

$$h_S(t) = \begin{cases} u_T(t) = u(t) - u(t - T) & \text{NRZ} \\ \sin(\pi t/T)u_T(t) = \sin(\pi t/T)u(t) + \sin(\pi(t - T)/T)u(t - T) & \text{HS} \end{cases} \tag{6.4.56}$$

Therefore for NRZ

$$h_S(t)\exp(j\omega_A t) = \exp(j\omega_A t)u(t) - \exp(j\omega_A T)\exp(j\omega_A(t - T))u_T(t - T) \tag{6.4.57}$$

and for HS

$$\begin{aligned} h_S(t)\exp(j\omega_A t) = {} & \sin(\pi t/T)\exp(j\omega_A t)u(t) \\ & + \exp(j\omega_A T)\sin(\pi(t-T)/T)\exp(j\omega_A(t-T))u_T(t-T) \end{aligned} \tag{6.4.58}$$

When we substitute (6.4.57) and (6.4.58) into (6.4.36), we obtain

$$g(t, f_A) = \begin{cases} g_N(t, f_A) - g_N(t - T, f_A)\exp(j\omega_A T) & \text{NRZ} \\ g_H(t, f_A) + g_H(t - T, f_A)\exp(j\omega_A T) & \text{HS} \end{cases} \tag{6.4.59}$$

where

$$g_N(t, f_A) = u(t) \exp(j\omega_A t) * h_{TD}(t, f_A) \tag{6.4.60}$$

$$g_H(t, f_A) = \sin(\pi t/T) \exp(j\omega_A t) u(t) * h_{TD}(t, f_A) \tag{6.4.61}$$

and

$$h_{TD}(t, f_A) = h_T(t) \exp(j\omega_A t) * h_{CD}(t) \tag{6.4.62}$$

The Laplace transform of (6.4.62) is

$$H'_{TD}(s; f_A) = H'_T(s - j\omega_A) H'_{CD}(s) \tag{6.4.63}$$

We assume that $H'_T(s)$ and $H'_{CD}(s)$ represent filters with simple poles

$$H'_T(s) = \sum_{i=1}^{N_T} \rho_{T,i}/(s + p_{T,i}) \tag{6.4.64}$$

$$H'_{CD}(s) = \sum_{i=1}^{N_R} \rho_{R,i}/(s + p_{R,i}) \tag{6.4.65}$$

where $\{\rho_{X,i}\}$ are the residua, $\{p_{X,i}\}$ are the poles, and $N_X$, $X = T, R$ is the number of poles. When we substitute (6.4.64) and (6.4.65) into (6.4.63), we obtain

$$H'_{TD}(s, f_A) = \sum_{i=1}^{N_{TR}} \rho_i/(s + p_i) \tag{6.4.66}$$

where

$$N_{TR} = N_T + N_R \tag{6.4.67}$$

$$\rho_i = \begin{cases} \rho_{R,i} H_T(-p_{R,i} - j\omega_A) & i = 1, \ldots, N_R \\ \rho_{T,i-N_R} H_R(j\omega_A - p_{T,i}) & i = N_R + 1, \ldots, N_{TR} \end{cases} \tag{6.4.68}$$

and

$$p_i = \begin{cases} p_{R,i} & i = 1, \ldots, N_R \\ p_{T,i-N_R} - j\omega_A & i = N_R + 1, \ldots, N_{TR} \end{cases} \tag{6.4.69}$$

Thus

$$h_{TD}(t, f_A) = \sum_{i=1}^{N_{TR}} \rho_i \exp(-p_i t) u(t) \tag{6.4.70}$$

and, after substitution into (6.4.60) and (6.4.61)

$$g_N(t, f_A) = \sum_{i=1}^{N_{TR}} \rho_i \frac{\exp(j\omega_A t) - \exp(-p_i t)}{p_i + j\omega_A} u(t) \tag{6.4.71}$$

$$g_H(t, f_A) = \sum_{i=1}^{N_{TR}} \rho_i \{(p_i + j\omega_A) \sin(\pi t/T) - (\pi/T) \cos(\pi t/T)\} \exp(j\omega_A T) + (\pi/T) \exp(-p_i t)\} u(t) / \{(p_i + j\omega_A)^2 + (\pi/T)^2\} \tag{6.4.72}$$

We have assumed for the numerical computation that $h_T(t)$ and $h_{CD}(t)$ are Butterworth filters of the same order $N$. This would apply to the case where the detector filter is a sample detector (i.e., $h_D'(s) = 1$), which, as we already know from Chapter 4, is better than the matched filter detector when the transmitter and receiver filters are narrowband, which they are in practice. Thus the systems we are discussing here are NS and HS as defined in Table 4.3. We have already stated in Section 6.4.2.1 that it is not necessary to compute (6.4.51); it is sufficient to compute either

$$P_b(e|\tau) = \sum_{k=0}^{N_\phi - 1} P_b(e|\tau, k\Delta)/N_\phi \tag{6.4.73}$$

or

$$P_b(e|\Delta\phi_A) = \sum_{i=0}^{N_\tau - 1} P_b(e|i\Delta\tau, \Delta\phi_A)/N_\tau \tag{6.4.74}$$

because

$$P_b(e) = P_b(e|\tau) = P_b(e|\Delta\phi_A) \tag{6.4.75}$$

This is in fact shown in Fig. 6.20 for quaternary QASK, system HS. In this figure the Butterworth filters have the same order $N$, a normalized 3-dB bandwidth $B_0 = 2f_0T$, and $B_A = f_AT$. In Figs. 6.21, 6.22, and 6.23, we show the bit error probability as a function of $B_0$, $B_A$ (here $B_R = 2f_{R0}T$, and $B_T = 2f_{T0}T$) or $E_b/N_0$, with the other variables as parameters for $N = 2, 3, 4$ and $A_A = A$. We can see from these figures that, given $B_A$, there is an optimal value of $B_0$. This is expected intuitively, because if $B_0$ is large we have more noise and ACI, and if $B_0$ is small we have more ISI. We also see that the optimal value of $B_0$ increases with $B_A$.

*Example* 6.4.4
Compute from Figs. 6.21, 6.22, and 6.23 the signal-to-noise ratio per bit required to achieve a bit error probability of $10^{-5}$, assuming $B_0 = 1.0$ and $B_A = 1.5$. Compute the spectral efficiency.

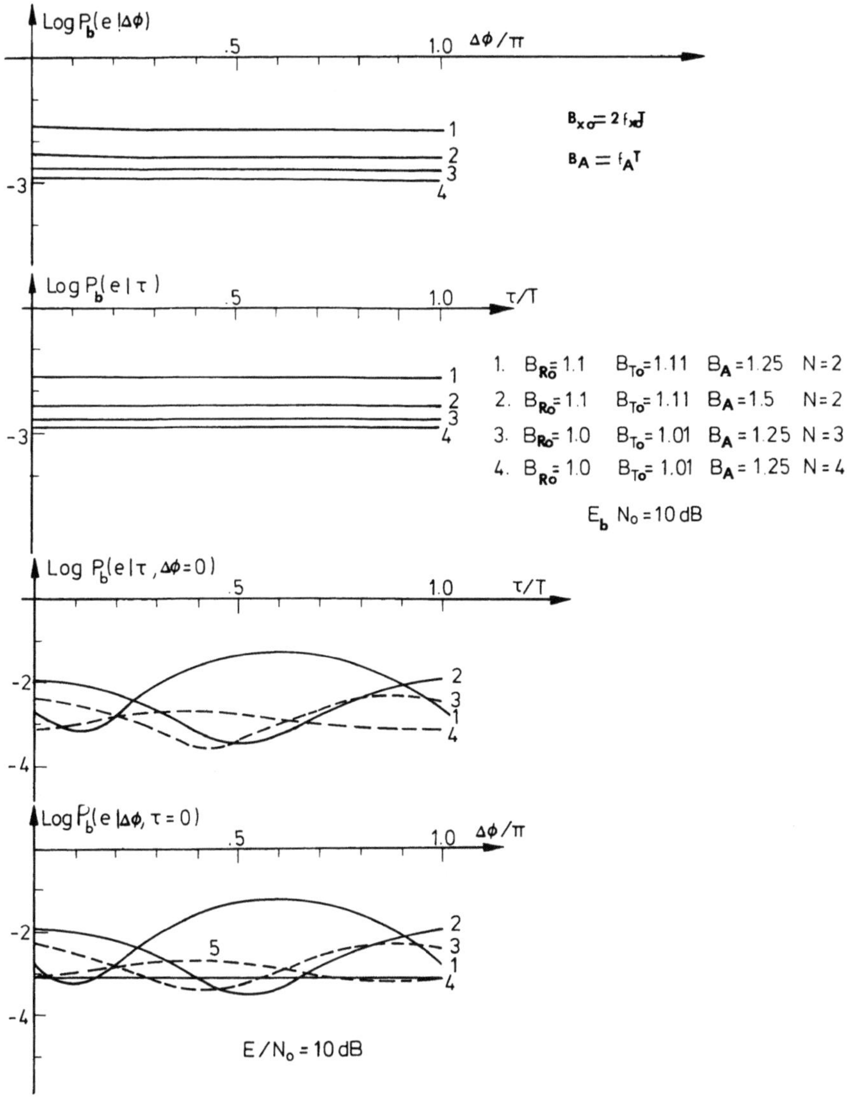


Fig. 6.20. Conditional and unconditional bit error probabilities for quaternary OQASK and MSK. The system has $N$th order Butterworth filters in receiver and transmitter (I. Korn, B. Seth, "Adjacent Channel and Quadrature Channel Interference in Minimum Shift Keying," *IEEE Tr. Sel. Ar. Comm.*, Vol. SAC-1, January 1983, pp. 21–28. Copyright © 1983 IEEE).

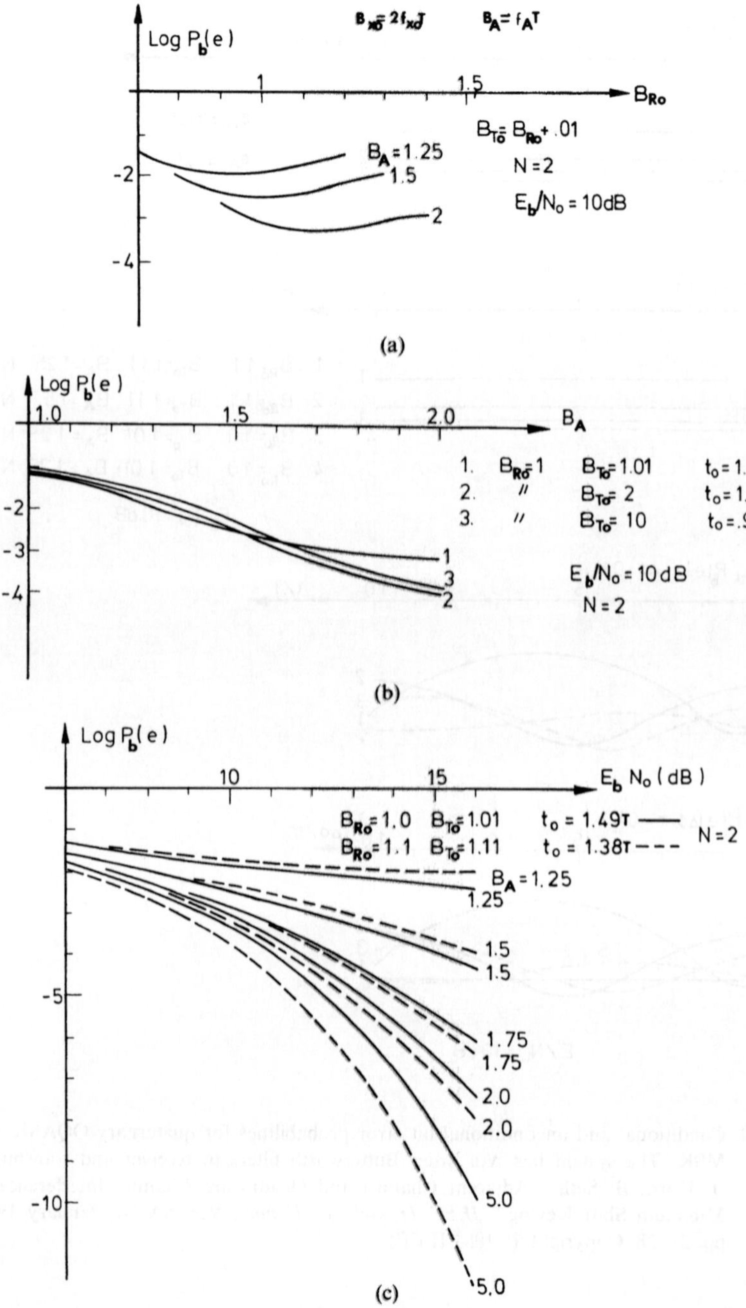


Fig. 6.21. Bit error probability as a function of (a) filter bandwidth, (b) frequency separation, (c) signal-to-noise ration per bit for MSK (quaternary OQASK with HS shaping function) with Butterworth filters of order $N = 2$ in transmitter and receiver.

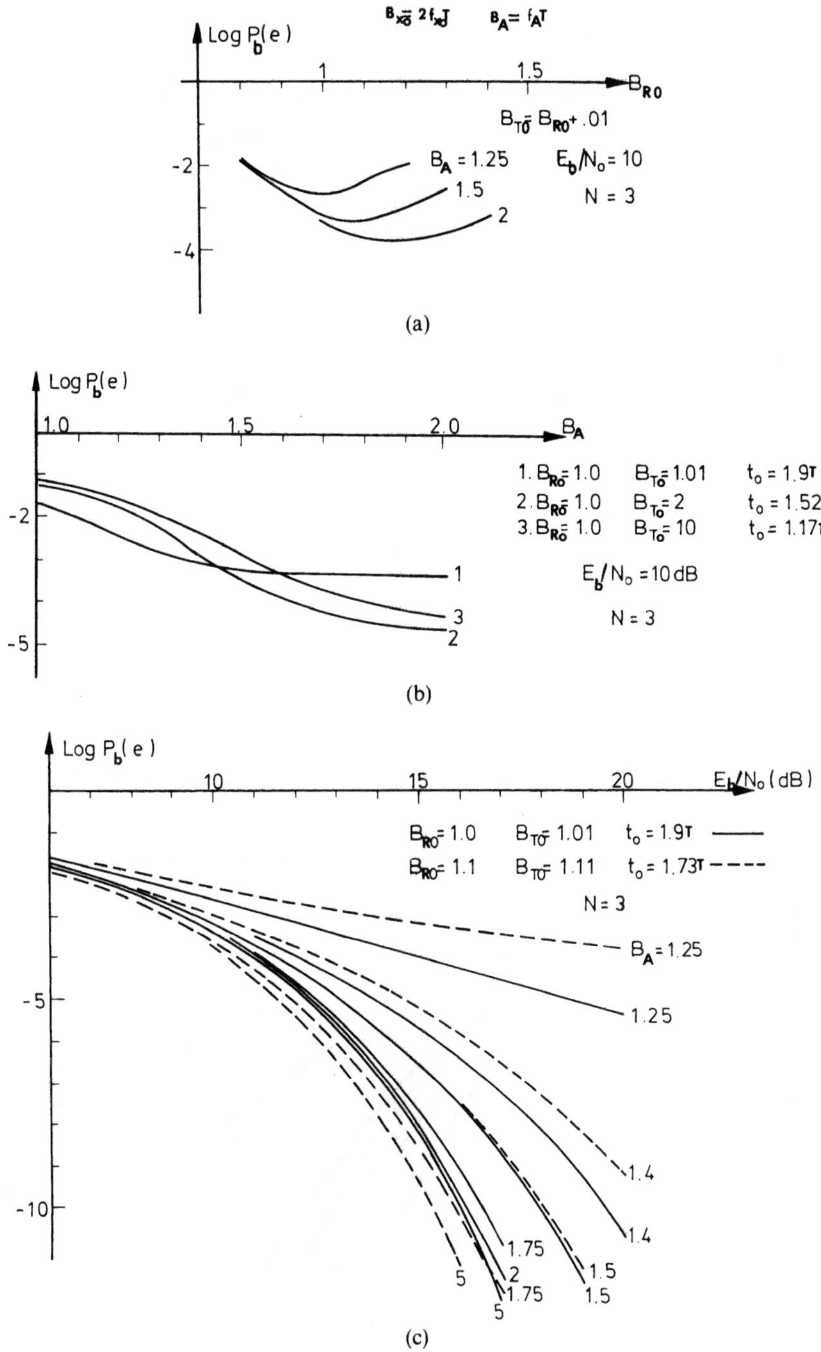


Fig. 6.22. The same as 6.21 but $N = 3$.

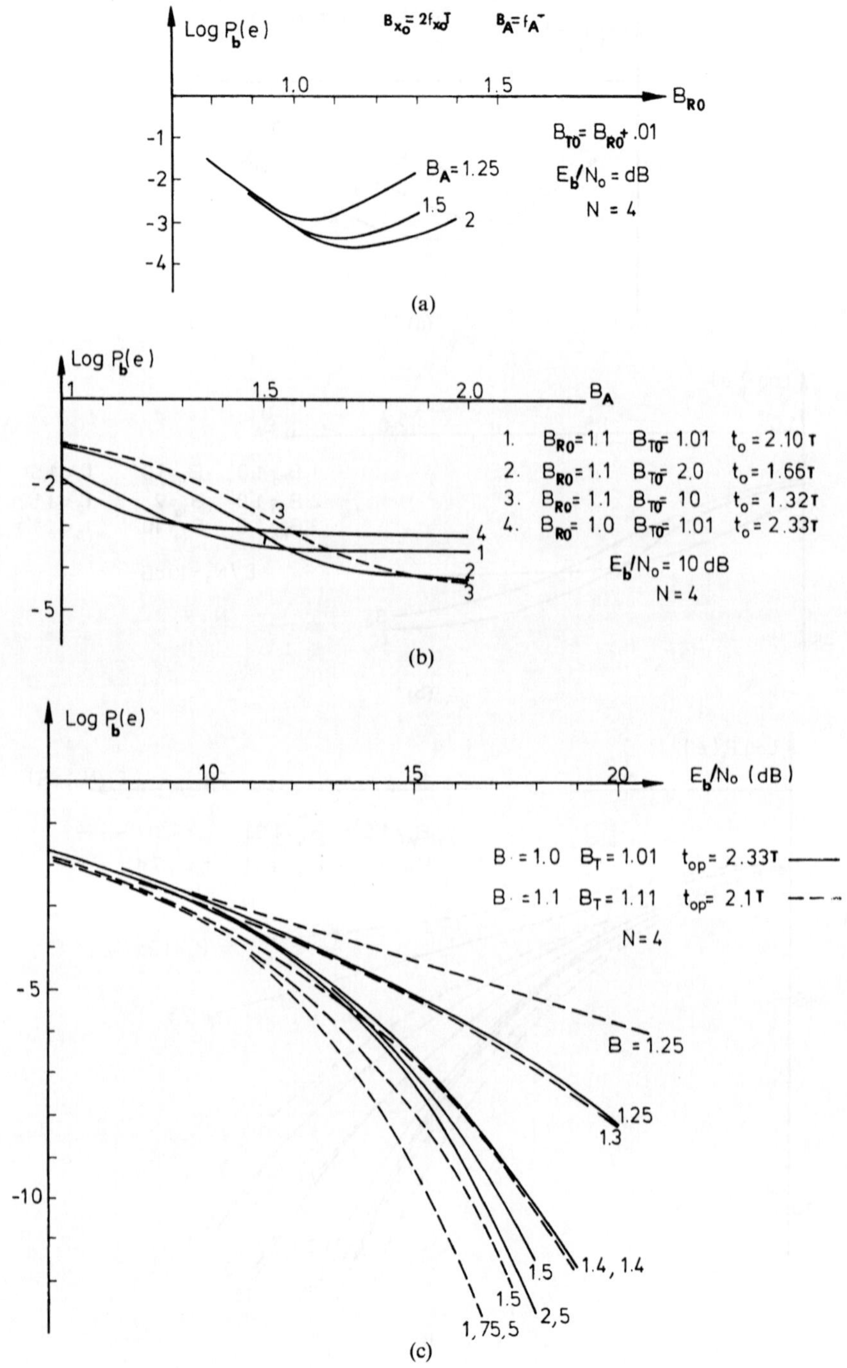


Fig. 6.23. The same as 6.21 but $N = 4$.

We find from these figures that $E_b/N_0 = 17.8$ dB for $N = 2$, 13.1 dB for $N = 3$, and 14.5 dB for $N = 4$.

The spectral efficiency is here

$$\eta_A = \frac{R_b}{f_A} = \frac{\log_2 4}{f_A T} = \frac{2}{1.5} = 1.33$$

When we compare these numbers with those of Example 6.4.3, we note that the spectral efficiency is reduced from 1.66 to 1.33 and the signal-to-noise ratio for the best filter ($N = 3$) is increased from 9.6 dB to 13.1 dB. This is the penalty we pay for using Butterworth filters instead of Nyquist, matched filters.

**6.4.2.3 MSK system with nonnegative impulse response filters**[6.9, 6.10] We have already mentioned the fact that, given the frequency separation, $f_A$, there is an optimal bandwidth for the transmitter and receiver filters, $f_0$. It would be of interest to find an analytic relation between $f_0$ and $f_A$. In general this is impossible due to the great complexity of the problem. However, if we make certain assumptions and approximations, such a formula can be found. The assumptions are:

a. The system is quaternary OQASK with HS shaping function and sampling detector, i.e., binary MSK.

b. The impulse responses of the filters $h_T(t)$ and $h_R(t)$ are nonnegative and the channel filter is ideal or is part of $h_R(t)$; hence

$$g(t) = \sin(\pi t/T)u_T(t) * h_T(t) * h_R(t) \geqq 0 \tag{6.4.76}$$

c. $g_0 \gg g_{\pm 1} \gg g_{\pm i}$, $i > 1$; therefore only two ISI symbols and one ACI symbol affect the system performance.

d. There is no QCI.

e. We shall compute a worst-case bound to the bit error probability, which will be, however, not remote from the true value.

Since MSK has two alternative formulations, it will be convenient to use the OQASK version for the main signal and the FSK version for the interfering signal

$$\begin{aligned} s(t) = {} & A \sum_i a_{Ii} \sin(\pi(t - iT)/T)u_T(t - iT) \\ & + jA \sum_i a_{Qi} \sin(\pi(t - iT - T/2)/T)u_T(t - iT - T/2) \end{aligned} \tag{6.4.77}$$

and

$$s_A(t) = A_A \exp\left\{ j\pi \int_{-\infty}^{t} \sum_i b_i u_T(t_1 - iT/2 - \tau)\, dt_1/T \right\} \tag{6.4.78}$$

where $a_{Ii}$, $a_{Qi}$, and $b_i$ are binary ($\pm 1$) independent equiprobable random variables, and $A$ is related to the energy per bit by

$$A = 2\sqrt{E_b/T} \tag{6.4.79}$$

Thus taking the real part of (6.1.16), we obtain

$$r_I(t) = x_I(t) + x_A(t) + n_I(t) \tag{6.4.80}$$

where

$$x_I(t) = A \sum_i a_{Ii} \sin(\pi(t - iT)/T) u_T(t - iT) * h_T(t) * h_R(t) \tag{6.4.81}$$

$$x_A(t) = \text{Re}\{s_A(t) \exp(j\omega_A t) * h_T(t) \exp(j\omega_A t) * h_R(t) \exp(j\Delta\phi_A)\} \tag{6.4.82}$$

and $n_I(t)$ is zero mean, Gaussian noise with variance

$$\sigma_n^2 = N_0 \int_{-\infty}^{\infty} |H_R(f)|^2 \, df \tag{6.4.83}$$

The decision about symbol $a_{I0}$ is taken at time $t_0$ (we lose nothing in generality if we consider symbol $k = 0$, because the error probability is independent of the index of the symbol); hence

$$\begin{aligned} r_{I,0} &= A a_{I0} g_0 + A \sum_i{}' a_{Ii} g_{-i} + x_{A,0} + n_{I,0} \\ &= A a_{I0} g_0 + I + n_{I,0} \end{aligned} \tag{6.4.84}$$

Because of our assumptions, $I$ contains only three terms that are significant

$$I = A a_{I1} g_{-1} + A a_{I,-1} g_1 + x_{A,0}(b_0) \tag{6.4.85}$$

where we emphasize the fact that in the ACI component only one symbol, say $b_0$, is dominant. Because this is a binary case, the bit error probability is

$$P_b(e) = \overline{Q((Ag_0 + I)/\sigma_n)} = \sum_{k=1}^{8} Q((Ag_0 + I_k)/\sigma_n)/8 \tag{6.4.86}$$

where $I_k$, $k = 1, 2, \ldots, 8$, are the eight different values of $I$ generated by the triple $(a_{I,1}, a_{I,-1}, b_0)$. Let the maximum value of $I$ be $I_M$

$$I_M = A(g_{-1} + g_1) + |x_{A,0}(b_0)| \tag{6.4.87}$$

Then

$$P_U(e)/8 \leqq P_b(e) \leqq P_U(e) \tag{6.4.88}$$

where

$$P_U(e) = Q((Ag_0 - I_M)/\sigma_n) \tag{6.4.89}$$

$P_U(e)$ is the worst case, caused when symbols $a_{I1} = a_{I,-1} = -1$, which is the opposite of $a_{I0} = 1$, and $b_0$ is such that $x_{A,0}$ is negative.

Since the symbols $a_{I,\pm 1}$, $i \geqq 2$, have no effect on the error probability, we can select them arbitrarily. For our convenience we shall assume that $a_{I,\pm 2} = 1$, $a_{I,\pm 3} = -1$, etc., so that the symbols are alternatively $\pm 1$. This implies that

$$\sum_i a_{Ii} \sin(\pi(t - iT)/T)u_T(t - iT) = \sin(\pi t/T) \tag{6.4.90}$$

Hence from (6.4.81)

$$x_I(t) = \text{Im}\{AH_T(f_N)H_R(f_N)\exp(j\omega_N t)\} \tag{6.4.91}$$

where

$$f_N = \omega_N/(2\,\pi) = (2\,T)^{-1} \tag{6.4.92}$$

is the Nyquist frequency.

Similarly, in the interfering signal we can select all symbols, except $b_0$, arbitrarily. For our convenience we shall assume that all symbols are $+1$ if $b_0 = +1$ and all symbols are $-1$ if $b_0 = -1$. Thus (6.4.78) and (6.4.82) are modified to

$$s_A(t) = A_A \exp(\pm j\omega_N t) \tag{6.4.93}$$

$$x_A(t) = \text{Re}\{A_A H_T(\pm f_N)H_R(f_A \pm f_N)\exp\{j(\Delta\phi_A + \omega_A t \pm \omega_N t)\} \tag{6.4.94}$$

The sampling time, $t_0$, is selected to maximize $x_I(t)$; thus

$$x_{I,0} = A|H_T(f_N)H_R(f_N)| \tag{6.4.95}$$

and the largest ACI value is

$$x_{A,0} = A_A|H_T(f_N)H_R(f_A - f_N)| \tag{6.4.96}$$

Thus

$$Ag_0 - I_M = A|H_T(f_N)H_R(f_N)|(1 - \rho_A|H_R(f_A - f_N)/H_R(f_N)|) \quad (6.4.97)$$

where

$$\rho_A = A_A/A \quad (6.4.98)$$

When we substitute (6.4.97), (6.4.79), and (6.4.83) into (6.4.89) we obtain

$$P_U(e) = Q\{(\eta\ 2\ E_b/N_0)^{1/2}\} \quad (6.4.99)$$

where

$$\eta = 2\frac{|H_T(f_N)H_R(f_N)|^2(1 - \rho_A|H_R(f_A - f_N)/H_R(f_N)|)^2}{T\int_{-\infty}^{\infty}|H_R(f)|^2\,df} \quad (6.4.100)$$

If we assume that $|H_T(f)| = |H_R(f)|$, we obtain a simpler formula.

*Example* 6.4.5 Gaussian filters

We assume that

$$H_T(f) = H_R(f) = \exp\{-(\alpha T_b f)^2\} \quad (6.4.101)$$

where $\alpha$ is related to the 3-dB bandwidth $B_0 = 2f_0T_b$ by

$$B_0 = (2\ln 2)^{1/2}\alpha \quad (6.4.102)$$

and $T_b = T/2$. When we substitute (6.4.101) into (6.4.100), we obtain

$$\eta = (2/\pi)^{1/2}\alpha\exp(-\alpha^2/4)\{1 - \rho_A\exp(-\alpha^2 B_A(B_A - 1)/4)\}^2 \quad (6.4.103)$$

where

$$B_A = 2f_AT_b \quad (6.4.104)$$

By taking the derivative of $\eta$ with respect to $\alpha$ and equating the result to zero, we find an equation for the optimal $\alpha$, $\alpha_{op}$, hence also $B_{op}$ as a function of $B_A$. The result is

$$\alpha_2\exp(\alpha_2 z)(\alpha_2 + 8\,\alpha_2 z + 16\,z)^{-1} = \rho_a\exp(-2\,z) \quad (6.4.105)$$

where

$$\alpha_2 = \alpha_{op}^2 - 2, \qquad z = B_A(B_A - 1)/4 \tag{6.4.106}$$

and thus

$$B_{op} = \{2 \ln 2/(2 + \alpha_2)\}^{1/2} \tag{6.4.107}$$

The relation between $B_{op}$ and $f_A T_b$ is shown in Fig. 6.24, and the degradation in signal-to-noise ratio when the filters with optimum bandwidth are used is

$$\frac{\Delta E_b}{N_0} = -10 \log \eta \text{ (dB)} \tag{6.4.108}$$

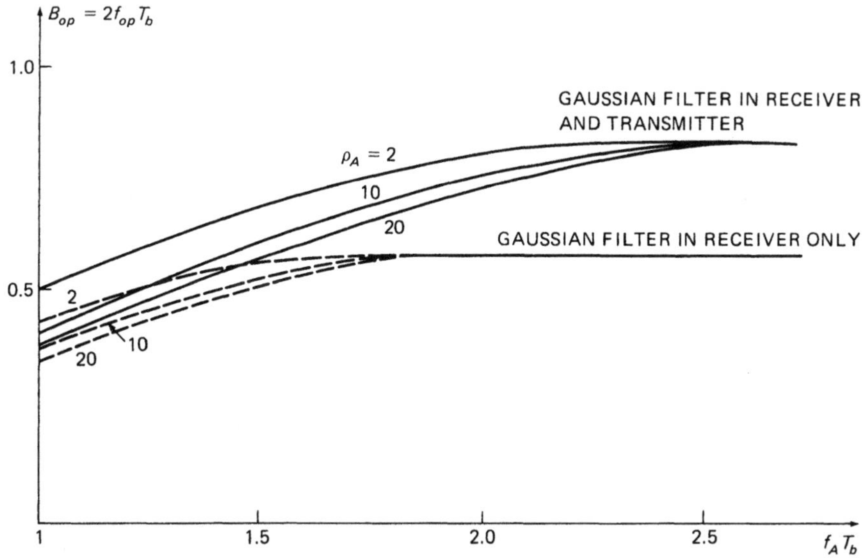


Fig. 6.24. Relation between optimal 3-dB filter bandwidth ($B_{op} = 2 f_0 T_b$) and frequency separation between signals in main and interfering channels.

is shown in Fig. 6.25. The case of filter in receiver only is obtained by substituting $H_T(f) = 1$.

We see from Fig. 6.24 that the filter bandwidth increases with frequency separation, because we have less adjacent channel interference. The filter bandwidth is reduced when the energy in the adjacent channel is increased. From Fig. 6.25 we can learn that the degradation is more severe when there are two filters (one in transmitter and one in receiver) rather than a single filter in receiver only. When $f_A T_b$ is large, the degradation is caused by ISI

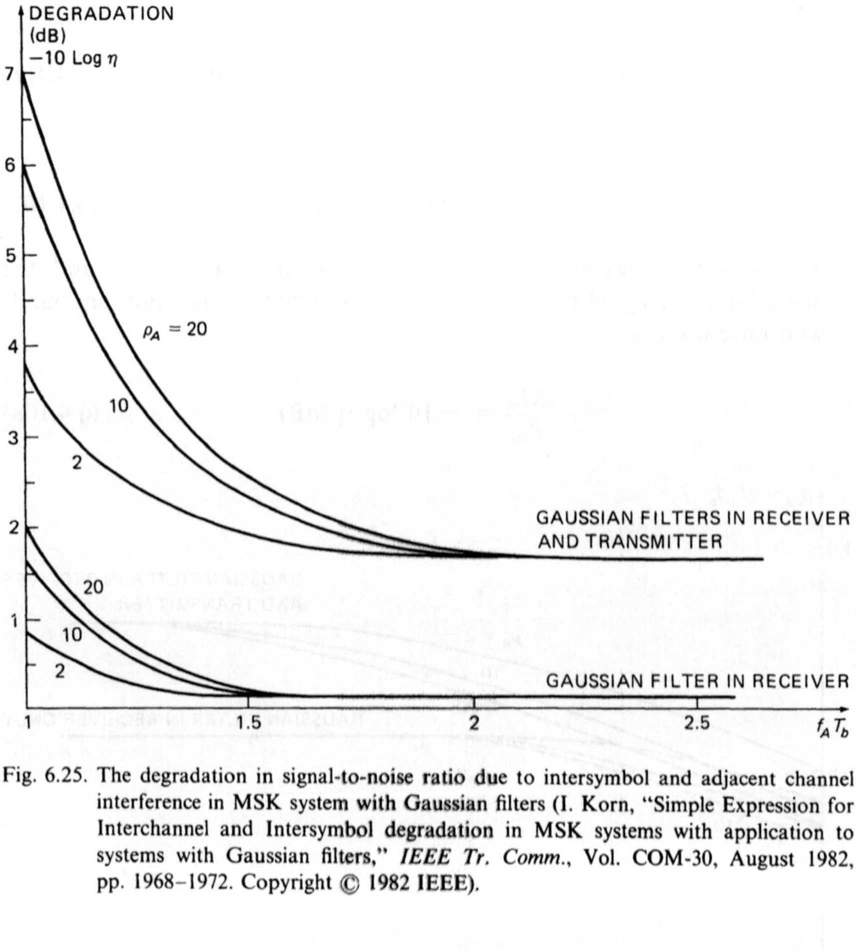


Fig. 6.25. The degradation in signal-to-noise ratio due to intersymbol and adjacent channel interference in MSK system with Gaussian filters (I. Korn, "Simple Expression for Interchannel and Intersymbol degradation in MSK systems with application to systems with Gaussian filters," *IEEE Tr. Comm.*, Vol. COM-30, August 1982, pp. 1968–1972. Copyright © 1982 IEEE).

only. Subtracting this value from the degradation, we obtain the degradation caused by ACI only. For example, in the case of two filters and frequency separation of $f_A T_b = 1$, the degradation is about 6 dB when the amplitude in the adjacent channel signal is 10 times the amplitude in the main channel. Out of this about 1.8 dB is caused by ISI and the rest by ACI.

## 6.5 EFFECT OF INTERFERENCE IN CIRCULAR CONSTELLATIONS (PSK)[6.11-6.18]

In a system with a circular symbol constellation, the main and interfering signals are

$$s(t) = A \sum_i \exp(j\pi a_i/M) u_T(t - iT) \tag{6.5.1}$$

$$s_A(t) = A_A \sum_i \exp(j\pi b_i/M)u_T(t - iT - \tau) \tag{6.5.2}$$

where $a_i \in \{\pm 1, \pm 3, \ldots, \pm(M - 1)\}$ or $a_i \in \{0, 2, 4, \ldots, 2M - 2\}$. With these equations (6.1.11) is simplified to

$$r(t) = A \sum_i \exp(j(\pi a_i/M + \Delta\phi)g(t - iT)$$
$$+ A_A \sum_i \exp(j(\pi b_i/M + \Delta\phi_A)g(t - iT - \tau, f_A) + n(t) \tag{6.5.3}$$

where $g(t)$ and $g(t, f_A)$ are given in (6.2.1) and (6.2.2) with $h_S(t) = u_T(t)$. Thus at the sampling time, $t_k$, we obtain

$$r_k = Ag_0 \exp(j(\pi a_k/M + \Delta\phi)) + I + n_k \tag{6.5.4}$$

where

$$I = A \sum_i{}' g_{k-i} \exp(j(\pi a_i/M + \Delta\phi))$$
$$+ A_A \sum_i g_{k-i}(\tau, f_A) \exp(j(\Delta\phi_A + \pi b_i/M) \tag{6.5.5}$$

Because the symbols are uniformly located on the circle and $I$ and $n_k$ are zero-mean symmetric random variables, the error probability is the same for all symbols. It is thus sufficient to compute the error probability under the assumption or condition that $a_k = 1$, as shown in Fig. 6.26. There will be an error when $a_k = 1$ if the tip of the noise lies in $B_1 \cup B_2$, which can be bounded as in (6.3.47)

$$\text{Max}\{P(r_k \in B_1), P(r_k \leqq B_2)\} \leqq P(e) \leqq P(r_k \in B_1) + P(r_k \in B_2) \tag{6.5.6}$$

and

$$r_k = Ag_0 \exp(j(\pi/M + \Delta\phi)) + I + n_k \tag{6.5.7}$$

We can assume, without any loss of generality, that $g(t)$ is real, because, if not, the phase of $g(t)$ can be part of $\Delta\phi$. If $\Delta\phi = 0$, because $I$ and $n_k$ are symmetric rvs

$$P(r_k \in B_1) = P(r_k \in B_2) \tag{6.5.8}$$

Hence, as in (6.3.50)

$$P_L(e) \leqq P(e) \leqq 2\,P_L(e) \tag{6.5.9}$$

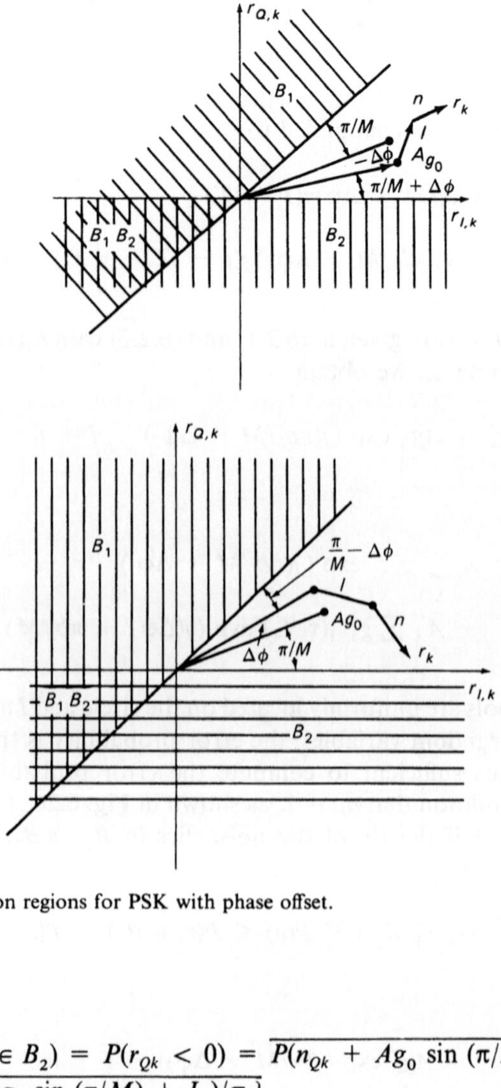


Fig. 6.26. Decision regions for PSK with phase offset.

where

$$P_L(e) = P(r_k \in B_2) = P(r_{Qk} < 0) = P(n_{Qk} + Ag_0 \sin(\pi/M) + I_Q < 0)$$
$$= Q\{(Ag_0 \sin(\pi/M) + I_Q)/\sigma_n\} \tag{6.5.10}$$

and

$$I_Q = \text{Im}\{I\} \tag{6.5.11}$$

If $\Delta\phi \neq 0$, (6.5.8) is no longer true. For $\Delta\phi > 0$, $r_k$ is on the average closer to the boundary of $B_1$ than to $B_2$. Hence

$$P(r_k \in B_1) > P(r_k \in B_2) \tag{6.5.12}$$

and vice versa for $\Delta\phi < 0$. In any case

$$\begin{aligned} P(r_k \in B_2) &= \overline{P(n_{Qk} + Ag_0 \sin(\pi/M + \Delta\phi) + I_Q < 0)} \\ &= \overline{Q\{(Ag_0 \sin(\pi/M + \Delta\phi) + I_Q)/\sigma_n\}} \end{aligned} \tag{6.5.13}$$

It seems that to compute $P(r_k \in B_1)$ is a more difficult job, but if we rotate Fig. 6.26 so that the boundary of $B_1$ is in the same position as the boundary of $B_2$ prior to the rotation, we have an identical situation. Hence

$$P(r_k \in B_1) = \overline{Q\{(Ag_0 \sin(\pi/M - \Delta\phi) + I_Q/\sigma_n\}} \tag{6.5.14}$$

We shall assume from now on that $|\Delta\phi| < \pi/M$, because otherwise there are errors without noise and interference. The error probability is thus bounded by

$$P_- \leqq P(e) \leqq P_- + P_+ \tag{6.5.15}$$

where

$$\begin{aligned} P_\pm &= Q\{Ag_0 \sin(\pi/M \pm |\Delta\phi|) - I_Q)/\sigma_n\} \\ &= Q\{(\eta\mu\, 2\, E_b/N_0)^{1/2}(\sin(\pi/M \pm \Delta\phi) + I')\} \end{aligned} \tag{6.5.16}$$

In the last expression

$$\mu = \log_2 M \tag{6.5.17}$$

$$\begin{aligned} I' = I_Q/(Ag_0) &= \sum_i{}' (g_{k-i}/g_0) \sin(\pi a_i/M + \Delta\phi) \\ &+ \sum_i \rho_A |g_{k-i}(\tau, f_A)/g_0| \sin(\pi b_i/M + \Delta\phi_A \\ &+ \arg(g_{k-i}(\tau, f_A))) \end{aligned} \tag{6.5.18}$$

$$\rho_A = A_A/A \tag{6.5.19}$$

and

$$g_{k-i}(\tau, f_A) = g(t_0 + (k - i)T - \tau, f_A) \tag{6.5.20}$$

Because $P_- > P_+$, the ratio between the upper and lower bound in (6.5.15) is even better than in (6.5.9). To compute the numerical values of $P_\pm$, we can use some of the methods presented in Section 4.4.3. Not all bounds and approximations are applicable here, because in (6.5.18) the interference is not a linear function of the symbols, though this is essential in some of the methods of Chapter 4 (for example, the method of Jenq et al.).

Let us rank $\{|g_k/g_0|\}$ $k \neq 0$, and $\{\rho_A g_k(\tau, f_A)|/g_0\}$ according to decreasing order, so that we obtain the sequence $\{h_i\}$, $i = 1, 2, 3$, $h_i \geq h_{i+1}$. Thus (6.5.11) can be replaced by

$$I' = \sum_{i=1}^{\infty} v_i h_i \tag{6.5.21}$$

where $v_i$ is either

$$v_i = \sin(\pi a_j/M + \Delta\phi) \tag{6.5.22}$$

or

$$v_i = \sin(\pi b_j/M + \Delta\phi_A + \arg(g_j(\tau, f_A))) \tag{6.5.23}$$

for some $j$.

Note that $\{v_i\}$ are independent, but not identically distributed rvs, each having $M$ values. If we take into account $N$ most significant terms, which we always do in practice, we obtain

$$I'_N = \sum_{i=1}^{N} v_i h_i \tag{6.5.24}$$

Now we can use, for example, eq. (4.4.26) with (4.4.29) replaced by

$$I'_N(j) = \sum_{i=1}^{N} v_i(j) h_i \tag{6.5.25}$$

where

$$\mathbf{v}(j) = \{v_1(j), v_2(j), \ldots, v_N(j)\} \tag{6.5.26}$$

is the $j$th realization of the vector

$$\mathbf{v} = \{v_1, v_2, \ldots, v_N\} \tag{6.5.27}$$

The Taylor and Legendre expansion methods, the Chernoff bound, and the quadrature formulas can and have been used to compute the error probability. The reader is referred to Refs. 6.11–6.16 for more details on the matter. In these references examples are given for systems with $M = 2, 4, 8$, and 16 symbols, NRZ shaping function, sample detector and mainly Butterworth filters. Since, for $M = 2$, PSK is identical to binary ASK and, for $M = 4$, the symbol constellation is rectangular, which is identical to parallel binary ASK systems, these cases are better treated within the ASK frame.

### 6.5.1 Extension of the method of Jenq et al. to circular constellation[4.25]

Because the method of Jenq et al. was so successful in application to ASK systems (hence also to systems with rectangular symbol constellations), it will be of great convenience if the method is extended to PSK. The difference is that, though in ASK

$$I = \sum_{i=1}^{N} a_i h_i \tag{6.5.28}$$

in PSK

$$I = \sum_{i=1}^{N} v_i h_i \tag{6.5.29}$$

where $v_i$ is a nonlinear function of the symbols $a_i \in \{\pm 1, \pm 3, \ldots, \pm(M-1)\}$. In general because $a_i$ has $M$ different equiprobable values, $v_i$ will also have $M$ equiprobable values (not all may be different). We have to consider only $M > 4$, because, as already stated, $M = 2, 4$ can be treated by methods used in ASK. We shall consider only $M = 8$ and $M = 16$, because systems with other numbers have not found application in practice. We see from (6.5.21) and (6.5.22) that

$$v_i = \sin(\pi a_i/M + \psi) \tag{6.5.30}$$

where $\psi$ is either $\Delta\phi$ or

$$\psi = \Delta\phi_A + \arg(g_j(\tau, f_A)) \tag{6.5.31}$$

and we have renamed $a_j$ and $b_j$ as $a_i$. When $\psi = 0$, we investigate the effect of ISI only; when $\psi = \Delta\phi$ we take also into account a phase offset; if $\psi$ is as in (6.5.31) we also take into account ACI.

$\underline{M = 8}$ First we assume that $\psi = 0$; thus

$$v_i = \sin(\pi a_i/M), \qquad a_i = \pm 1, 3 \tag{6.5.32}$$

and the values of $v_i$ are $\pm V_1$, $\pm V_2$, where

$$V_1 = \sin(3\pi/M), \qquad V_2 = \sin(\pi/M) \tag{6.5.33}$$

The rv $v_i$ can be represented as

$$v_i = a_{1i}x_i + a_{2i}x_2 \tag{6.5.34}$$

where $a_{1i}$, $a_{2i}$ are independent, binary ($\pm 1$), rvs and

$$x_i = 0.5\,(V_1 + V_2), \qquad x_2 = 0.5\,(V_1 - V_2) \tag{6.5.35}$$

Note, indeed, that taking all four values of the pair ($a_{1i}$, $a_{2i}$) in (6.5.34), we obtain all values of $v_i$ in (6.5.32). When we substitute (6.5.34) into (6.5.29), we obtain

$$I = \sum_{i=1}^{N} a_{1i}(x_1 h_i) + \sum_{i=1}^{N} a_{2i}(x_2 h_i) \tag{6.5.36}$$

which again can be reordered according to rank into a single summation with 2 $N$ terms.

If $\psi \neq 0$, $v_i$ has in general eight values; $\pm V_1$, $\pm V_2$, $\pm V_3$, $\pm V_4$, where $V_i$ is the $i$th largest value of $v_i$.

$$\begin{aligned} V_1 &= \sin\,(3\,\pi/8 + \psi), & V_2 &= \sin\,(5\,\pi/8 + \psi) \\ V_3 &= \sin\,(\pi/8 + \psi), & V_4 &= \sin\,(7\,\pi/8 + \psi) \end{aligned} \tag{6.5.37}$$

where we assumed that $0 \leq \psi \leq \pi/8$. This assumption does not impose any restriction on the generality of the discussion; any other value simply means a rotation of the symbols, without changing the values of $V_i$, $i = 1, 2, 3, 4$. This is illustrated in Fig. 6.27. Our intention is to approximate $v_i$ by a linear combination of nonnegative number $x_1 \geqq x_2 \geqq x_3 \geqq 0$

$$w_i = a_{1i}x_1 + a_{2i}x_2 + a_{3i}x_3 \tag{6.5.38}$$

where $a_{1i}$, $a_{2i}$, $a_{3i}$ are independent, binary ($\pm 1$) rvs. If we select

$$\begin{aligned} W_1 &= V_1 = x_1 + x_2 + x_3 \\ W_2 &= V_2 = x_1 + x_2 - x_3 \\ W_3 &= V_3 = x_1 - x_2 + x_3 \end{aligned} \tag{6.5.39}$$

i.e.

$$x_1 = 0.5\,(V_2 + V_3),\ x_2 = 0.5\,(V_1 - V_3),\ x_3 = 0.5\,(V_1 - V_2) \tag{6.5.40}$$

then

$$W_4 = x_1 - x_2 - x_3 = V_2 + V_3 - V_1 \tag{6.5.41}$$

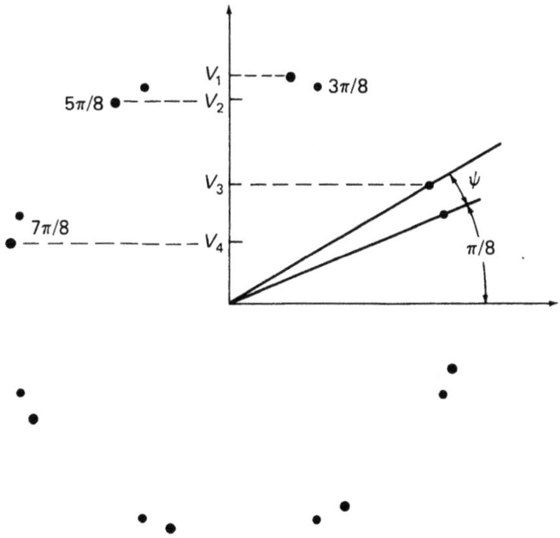


Fig. 6.27. Generation of variable $V_i$ in PSK.

is a linear combination of $V_1$, $V_2$, $V_3$, while $V_4$ is not linearly related to these values. Thus $W_4 \neq V_4$, and the difference is

$$
\begin{aligned}
W_4 - V_4 &= V_2 + V_3 - V_1 - V_4 = 2\,\{\cos(\pi/8) - \cos(3\,\pi/8)\}\,\sin\psi \\
&= 1.082 \sin\psi \leqq 0.414 \qquad (6.5.42)
\end{aligned}
$$

Thus when we approximate $v_i$ *by* $w_i$, we overestimate the interference. This implies that when we substitute (6.5.38), (6.5.40) into (6.5.29) instead of $v_i$, we obtain

$$
I_+ = \sum_{i=1}^{N} a_{1i}(h_i x_1) + \sum_{i=1}^{N} a_{2i}(h_i x_2) + \sum_{i=1}^{N} a_{3i}(h_i x_3) \qquad (6.5.43)
$$

which will give an upper bound to the error probability if this is substituted into (6.5.16)

If however, we select

$$
\begin{aligned}
W_1 &= V_1 = x_1 + x_2 + x_3 \\
W_2 &= V_2 = x_1 + x_2 - x_3 \\
W_4 &= V_4 = x_1 - x_2 - x_3
\end{aligned} \qquad (6.5.44)
$$

i.e.

$$
x_1 = 0.5\,(V_1 + V_4),\ x_2 = 0.5\,(V_2 - V_4),\ x_3 = 0.5\,(V_1 + V_2) \qquad (6.5.45)
$$

then

$$W_3 = x_1 - x_2 + x_3 = V_1 + V_4 - V_2 \tag{6.5.46}$$

The difference between $W_3$ and the correct value, $V_3$, is

$$\begin{aligned} W_3 - V_3 &= V_1 + V_4 + V_2 - V_3 = 2\,(\cos(3\,\pi/8) - \cos(\pi/8))\sin\psi \\ &= -1.082 \sin\psi \geqq -0.414 \end{aligned} \tag{6.5.47}$$

Thus when we approximate $v_i$ by $w_i$ with $x_1, x_2, x_3$, as given in (6.5.45), we underestimate the interference. This implies that when we substitute (6.5.38) and (6.5.45) into (6.5.29), instead of $v_i$ we obtain

$$I_- = \sum_{i=1}^{N} a_{1i}(h_i x_1) + \sum_{i=1}^{N} a_{2i}(h_i x_2) + \sum_{i=1}^{N} a_{3i}(h_i x_3) \tag{6.5.48}$$

which will give a lower bound to the error probability if (6.5.48) is substituted into (6.5.16). Equations (6.5.43) and (6.5.48) have the same form, but the values of $x_1$, $x_2$, $x_3$ are different, namely, (6.5.40) and (6.5.45).

The two bounds are close to each other because $w_i$ differs from $v_i$ only in the third or fourth significant term ($V_1$ and $V_2$ are not affected by the approximation), and the significant terms are dominant in ISI and ACI, particularly after the reordering (6.5.48) according to rank.

Another, simpler approximation, which is also an upper bound, is to use

$$w_i = a_{1i}x_1 + a_{2i}x_2 \tag{6.5.49}$$

$$x_1 = 0.5\,(V_1 + V_2), \qquad x_2 = 0.5\,(V_1 - V_2) \tag{6.5.50}$$

with $V_1$ and $V_2$ given in (6.5.37). In this approximation we have in fact replaced $V_3$ by $V_1$, which is an overestimate of the interference.

<u>$M = 16$</u> In this case when $\psi = 0$, $v_i$ has only eight values: $\pm V_1$, $\pm V_2$, $\pm V_3$, $\pm V_4$, where

$$V_i = \sin((2\,i - 1)\pi/16), \qquad i = 1, 2, 3, 4 \tag{6.5.51}$$

The error probability can be bounded using the method for $M = 8$, $\psi \neq 0$.

When $\psi \neq 0$, $v_i$ has 16 values: $\pm V_i$, $i = 1, 2, \ldots, 8$, where $V_i$ is the $i$th largest term from the set $\{\sin((2\,i - 1)\pi/16 + \psi)\}$. We may assume $0 \leqq \psi \leqq \pi/16$; hence

$$\begin{aligned} V_1 &= \sin(7\,\pi/16 + \psi), & V_2 &= \sin(9\,\pi/16 + \psi) \\ V_3 &= \sin(5\,\pi/16 + \psi), & V_4 &= \sin(11\,\pi/16 + \psi) \\ V_5 &= \sin(3\,\pi/16 + \psi), & V_6 &= \sin(13\,\pi/16 + \psi) \\ V_7 &= \sin(\pi/16 + \psi), & V_8 &= \sin(15\,\pi/16 + \psi) \end{aligned} \tag{6.5.52}$$

We will approximate $V_i$ by $W_i$

$$W_i = a_{1i}x_1 + a_{2i}x_2 + a_{3i}x_3 + a_{4i}x_4 \qquad (6.5.53)$$

where $a_{1i}$, $a_{2i}$, $a_{3i}$, $a_{4i}$ are independent, binary ($\pm 1$), equiprobable rvs. If we select

$$\begin{aligned} W_1 &= V_1 = x_1 + x_2 + x_3 + x_4 \\ W_2 &= V_2 = x_1 + x_2 - x_3 - x_4 \\ W_3 &= V_3 = x_1 + x_2 + x_3 + x_4 \\ W_5 &= V_5 = x_1 - x_2 + x_3 + x_4 \end{aligned} \qquad (6.5.54)$$

i.e.

$$\begin{aligned} x_1 &= 0.5\,(V_2 + V_3 + V_5 - V_1), \quad x_2 = 0.5\,(V_1 - V_5) \\ x_3 &= 0.5\,(V_1 - V_3), \quad x_4 = 0.5\,(V_1 - V_2) \end{aligned} \qquad (6.5.55)$$

then $W_4$, $W_6$, $W_7$, $W_8$ are determined by

$$\begin{aligned} W_4 &= x_1 + x_2 - x_3 - x_4 = V_2 + V_3 - V_1 > V_4 \\ W_6 &= x_1 - x_2 + x_3 - x_4 = V_2 + V_5 - V_1 > V_6 \\ W_7 &= x_1 - x_2 - x_3 + x_4 = V_3 + V_5 - V_1 > V_7 \\ W_8 &= x_1 - x_2 - x_3 - x_4 = V_2 + V_3 + V_5 - 2\,V_1 > V_8 \end{aligned} \qquad (6.5.56)$$

In fact the differences are

$$\begin{aligned} 0.00 &\leqq W_4 - V_4 \leqq 0.14 \\ 0.00 &\leqq W_6 - V_6 \leqq 0.25 \\ 0.21 &\leqq W_7 - V_7 \leqq 0.25 \\ 0.21 &\leqq W_8 - V_8 \leqq 0.56 \end{aligned} \qquad (6.5.57)$$

Therefore (6.5.53) and (6.5.54) overestimate the interference; hence after substitution of

$$I_+ = \sum_{i=1}^{N} a_{1i}(h_i x_1) + \sum_{i=1}^{N} a_{2i}(h_i x_2) + \sum_{i=1}^{N} a_{3i}(h_i x_3) + \sum_{i=1}^{N} a_{4i}(h_i x_4) \qquad (6.5.58)$$

into (6.5.16), we shall obtain an upper bound on the error probability. To obtain a lower bound, instead of using (6.5.54), we shall use

$$\begin{aligned} W_1 &= V_1 = x_1 + x_2 + x_3 + x_4 \\ W_2 &= V_2 = x_1 + x_2 + x_3 - x_4 \\ W_4 &= V_4 = x_1 + x_2 - x_3 - x_4 \\ W_8 &= V_8 = x_1 - x_2 - x_3 - x_4 \end{aligned} \qquad (6.5.59)$$

so that

$$x_1 = 0.5\,(V_1 + V_8),\ x_2 = 0.5\,(V_4 - V_8)$$
$$x_3 = 0.5\,(V_2 - V_4),\ x_4 = 0.5\,(V_1 - V_2) \tag{6.5.60}$$

Now $W_3$, $W_5$, $W_6$, and $W_7$ are fixed by

$$\begin{aligned} W_3 &= x_1 + x_2 - x_3 + x_4 = V_1 - V_2 + V_4 \\ W_5 &= x_1 - x_2 + x_3 + x_4 = V_1 - V_4 + V_8 \\ W_6 &= x_1 - x_2 + x_3 - x_4 = V_2 - V_4 + V_8 \\ W_7 &= x_1 - x_2 - x_3 + x_4 = V_1 - V_2 + V_8 \end{aligned} \tag{6.5.61}$$

The difference between $W_i - V_i$, $i = 3, 5, 6, 7$, when we vary $\psi$ from 0 to $\pi/16$, is

$$\begin{aligned} -0.14 &\leqq W_3 - V_3 \leqq 0.00 \\ -0.42 &\leqq W_5 - V_5 \leqq -0.21 \\ -0.21 &\leqq W_6 - V_6 \leqq -0.16 \\ -0.31 &\leqq W_7 - V_7 \leqq -0.00 \end{aligned} \tag{6.5.62}$$

thus $W_i \leqq V_i$, which means that we underestimate the interference. When we substitute (6.5.44) with the values of (6.5.60) into (6.5.16), we obtain a lower bound to the error probability. Because the dominant terms are similar in value when we use (6.5.54) or (6.5.59), the bounds are quite close to each other.

A simpler upper bound is obtained if, instead of (6.5.53), we use

$$W_i = a_{1i}x_1 + a_{2i}x_2 + a_{3i}x_3 \tag{6.5.63}$$

where $x_i$ are computed as in (6.5.40) with values of $V_1$, $V_2$, $V_3$, as given in (6.5.52). This is equivalent to leaving $V_i$, $i = 1, 2, 3$ intact and replacing $V_i$, $i = 4, 5, 6, 7, 8$ by $W_i > V_i$.

### 6.5.2 System with Nyquist function response

For this system $g(t)$ and $g(t, f_A)$ are given in (6.4.41) and (6.4.43). Using the bounds of Section 6.5.1 and the method of Jenq et al., we have computed the bit error probability as a function of signal-to-noise ratio per bit with sampling time $t_0$ and phase offset $\Delta\phi$ as parameters. This is shown in Fig. 6.28 for $M = 8$ and in Fig. 6.29 for $M = 16$. In these figures we have assumed that there is no ACI ($A_A = 0$). In Fig. 6.30 we have fixed the signal-to-noise ratio per bit, and the horizontal axis is the phase offset. The effect of adjacent channel interference was already presented in Fig. 6.19. We can see from

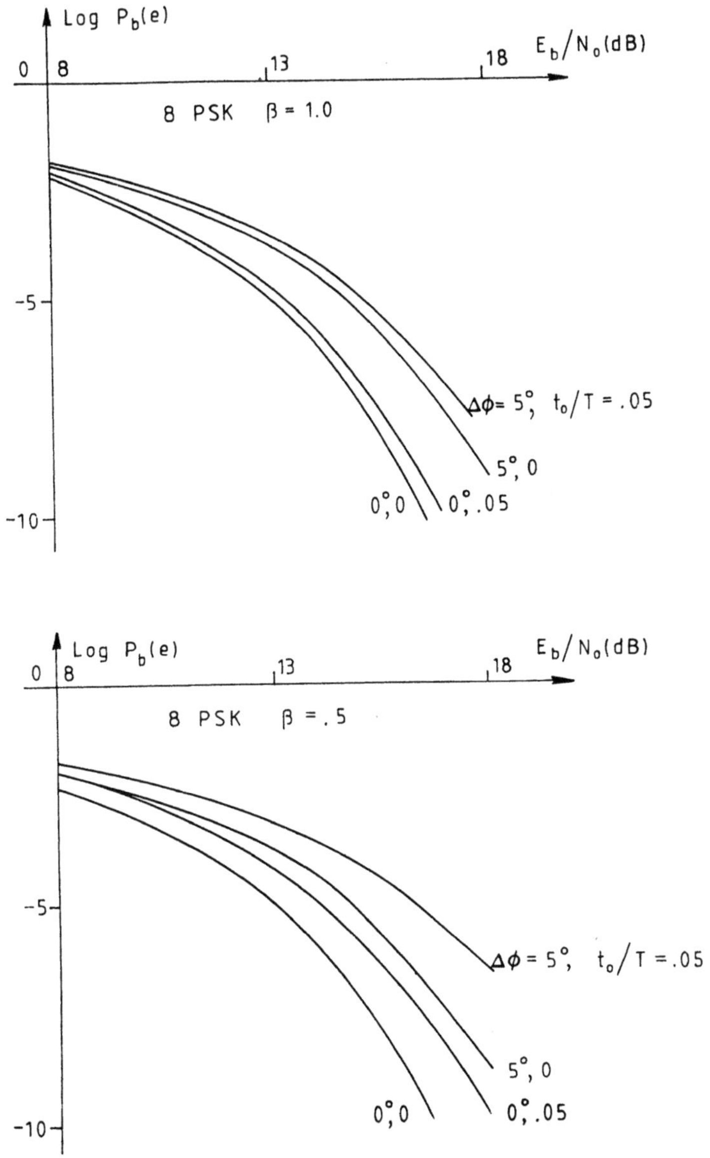


Fig. 6.28. Bit error probability as a function of signal-to-noise ratio per bit for QASK with circular constellation (PSK) with $M = 8$ symbols. The system has a Nyquist function response with excess bandwidth β; $t_0$ is the sampling time offset.

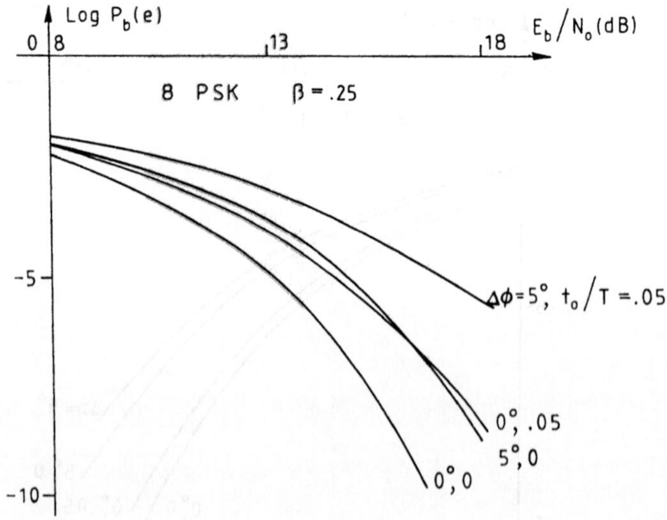


Fig. 6.28. (*con't.*)

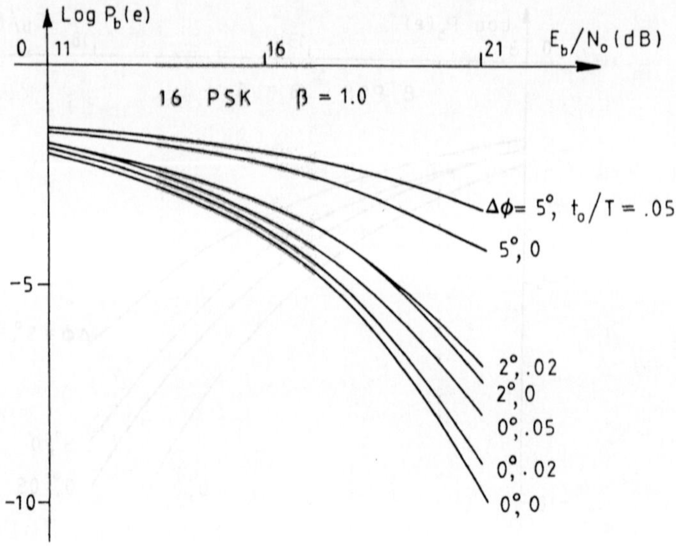


Fig. 6.29. The same as 6.28 but $M = 16$.

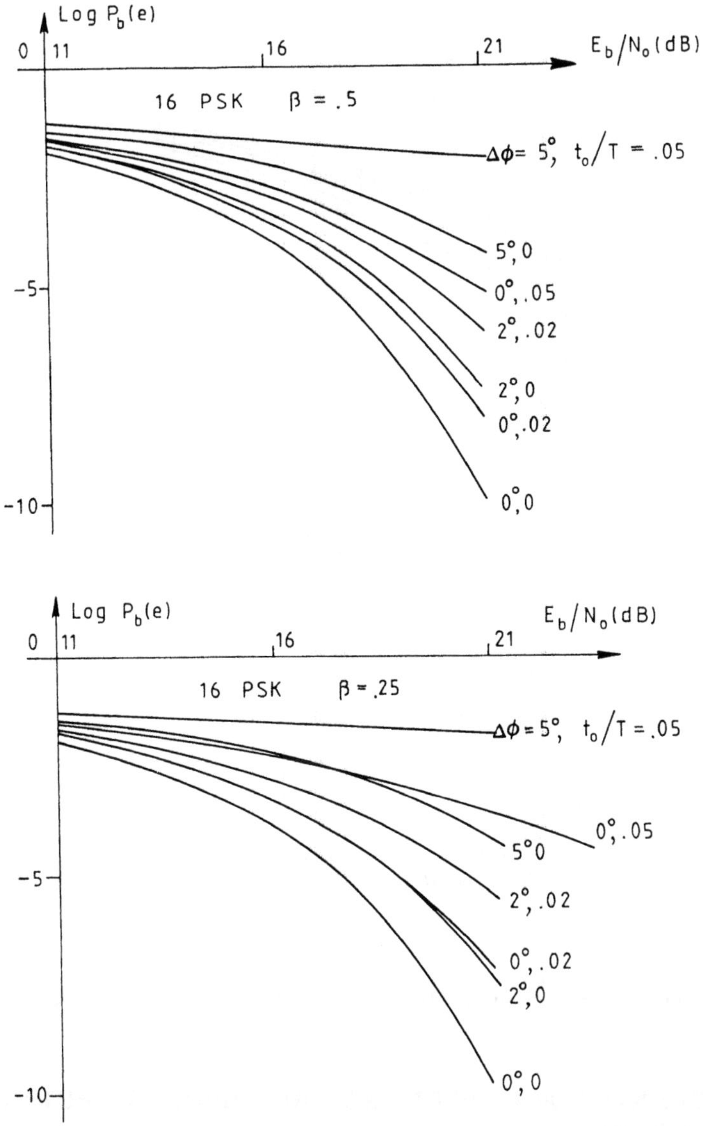
Log $P_b(e)$
0
11
16
21
$E_b/N_0$(dB)
16 PSK β = .5
Δφ= 5°, $t_0/T$ = .05
5°, 0
0°, .05
2°, .02
2°, 0
0°, .02
0°, 0
-5
-10
Log $P_b(e)$
0
11
16
21
$E_b/N_0$(dB)
16 PSK β = .25
Δφ = 5°, $t_0/T$ = .05
0°, .05
5° 0
2°, .02
0°, .02
2°, 0
0°, 0
-5
-10

Fig. 6.29. (*con't.*)

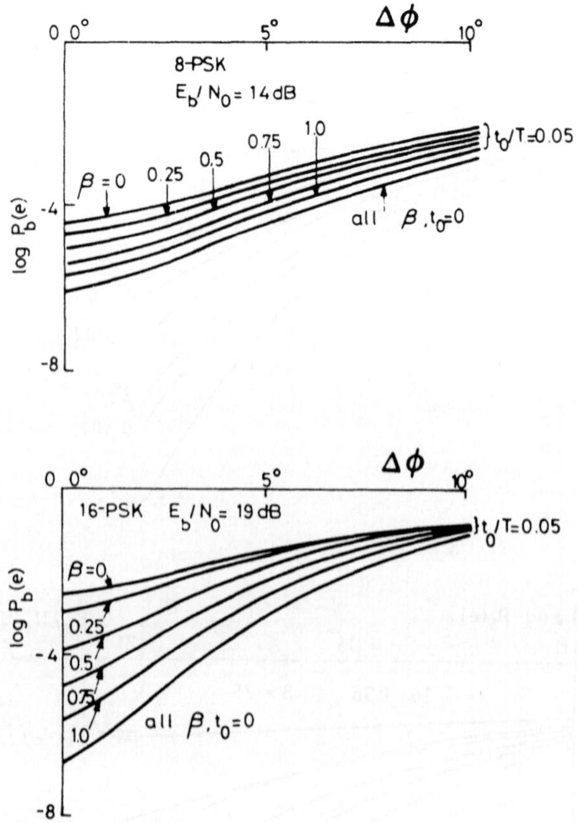


Fig. 6.30. Bit error probability as a function of phase offset for QASK with circular constellation (PSK) and $M = 8$ or 16 symbols. The system has a Nyquist function response.

these figures that even a phase offset of 2° greatly increases the error probability.

## 6.6 CHANNEL WITH FLAT AND FREQUENCY SELECTIVE FADING

Until now it was assumed that the channel can be modelled by a fixed, linear time-invariant filter that, for convenience, we may consider to be part of the transmitter filter or receiver filter. This model is sufficient when the channel is a coaxial cable, a waveguide, or a pair of copper wires. For a radio channel, the properties of which depend on reflections of electromagnetic waves from the ionosphere and other layers, this model is not good any more. A simple model of a radio channel is shown in Fig. 6.31. If the transmitter signal is

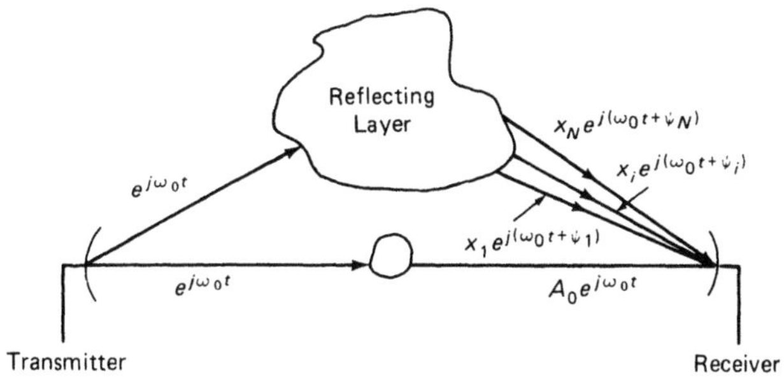


Fig. 6.31. Model of fading radio channel.

Re {exp ($j\omega_C t$)}, the received signal is

$$x(t) = \text{Re}\,\{\{A_0 + \sum_{i=1}^{N} x_i \exp(j\psi_i)\} \exp(j\omega_C t)\} \tag{6.6.1}$$

where $\{x_i\}$ are random amplitudes and $\{\psi_i\}$ random phases (which are related to time delays) associated with a particular path of the signal. $A_0$ may be a constant that represents the gain (in fact it will be an attenuation) of the specular component of the incoming signal. There is a certain delay for the specular component and in (6.6.1) we normalized the signal with respect to this delay.

Letting

$$x = \sum_{i=1}^{N} x_i \cos \psi_i \tag{6.6.2}$$

$$y = \sum_{i=1}^{N} x_i \sin \psi_i \tag{6.6.3}$$

the amplitude in (6.6.1) is

$$A_F = ((A_0 + x)^2 + y^2)^{1/2} \tag{6.6.4}$$

If there is no dominant value of $x_i$ and if $N$ is sufficiently large, it can be shown that $x$ and $y$ are independent, zero mean, Gaussian random variables. The pdf of $A_F$ is either Rayleigh (when $A_0 = 0$)

$$p_{A_F}(y) = y \exp(-0.5\, y^2/b)/b u(y) \tag{6.6.5}$$

or Rician

$$p_{A_F}(y) = y \exp(-0.5\,(y^2 + A_0^2)/b) I_0(yA_0/b)/b u(y) \tag{6.6.6}$$

where $b$ is a constant such that

$$\int_0^\infty p_{A_F}(y)\,dy = 1 \qquad (6.6.7)$$

and $I_0(.)$ is the modified Bessel function of the first kind and zero order. For large values of argument

$$I_0(z) = (2\,\pi z)^{-1/2} \exp(z) \qquad (6.6.8)$$

Hence for large values of $yA_0/b$, (6.6.6) is simplified to

$$p_{A_F}(y) = y(2\,\pi y A_0 b)^{-1/2} \exp(-0.5\,(y - A_0)^2/b) \qquad (6.6.9)$$

For small values of the argument

$$I_0(z) = \exp(z^2/4) \qquad (6.6.10)$$

Thus for $A_0 = 0$, (6.6.6) is reduced to (6.6.5).

With this model, the channel transfer function is

$$H_C(f) = A_F,\ h_C(t) = A_F\delta(t) \qquad (6.6.11)$$

which is independent of frequency..In reality $\{x_i\}$ and $\{\psi_i\}$ vary with time, so that $A_F$ fluctuates with time and is in fact a random process. However, if the fluctuations are slow in time in comparison with the symbol rate, we may assume that for a short sequence of symbols the channel gain, $A_F$, is constant. There are times when $A_F(t)$ is well below its average or nominal value; this is the time when the signal fades. Because the received signal energy is proportional to $A_F^2$, the signal-to-noise ratio, $E_b/N_0$, will drop during the fades below an acceptable level, and the result will be an increase in the bit error probability. The duration of the fades and their depth (how far below the nominal value $A_F$ is reduced) are determined experimentally for any given radio channel. The reader is referred to Refs. 6.18 and 6.19 and the references within for additional information on this matter.

We note that in (6.6.11) the channel transfer function is constant for all frequencies. Such fading is called flat fading.

Let $E_{b0}$ be the bit energy when $A_F = 1$, i.e., $E_{b0}$ is the nominal bit energy, and let

$$E_b = A_F^2 E_{b0} \qquad (6.6.12)$$

be the actual energy per bit. Let

$$P_b(e|E_b/N_0) = f(E_b/N_0) \tag{6.6.13}$$

be the error probability of a system when $E_b/N_0$ is fixed. To compute the average error probability in the presence of fading, we calculate

$$P_b(e) = \int_{-\infty}^{\infty} f(y^2 E_{b0}/N_0) p_{A_F}(y)\, dy \tag{6.6.14}$$

Alternatively, let

$$\rho = E_b/N_0$$

with an average of $\bar{\rho}$. Since $A_F^2$ is proportional to $\rho$, we obtain for Rayleigh fading a pdf for $\rho$ from (6.6.5)

$$p_\rho(\rho) = (\bar{\rho})^{-1} \exp(-\rho/\bar{\rho}) u(\rho) \tag{6.6.15}$$

and thus

$$P_b(e) = \int_0^{\infty} P_b(e|\rho) p_\rho(\rho)\, d\rho \tag{6.6.16}$$

*Example* 6.6.1 Rayleigh fading
Let

$$P_b(e|\rho) = k_1 Q(\sqrt{2\alpha\rho}) \tag{6.6.17}$$

as for example in (6.3.31) with

$$\alpha = \eta k_2 \tag{6.6.18}$$

and $k_1$, $k_2$ presented in Table 6.1. When we substitute (6.6.17) and (6.6.15) into (6.6.16), we obtain a closed form solution (after changing the order of integration)

$$P_b(e) = 0.5\, k_1 \left(1 - \frac{1}{\sqrt{1 + (\alpha\bar{\rho})^{-1}}}\right) \tag{6.6.19}$$

For example if $M = 4$ ($k_1 = k_2 = 1$) and matched filter ($\eta = 1$), we obtain

$$P_b(e) = 0.5\,(1 - (1 + 1/\bar{\rho})^{-1/2}) \tag{6.6.20}$$

which is shown in Fig. 6.32.

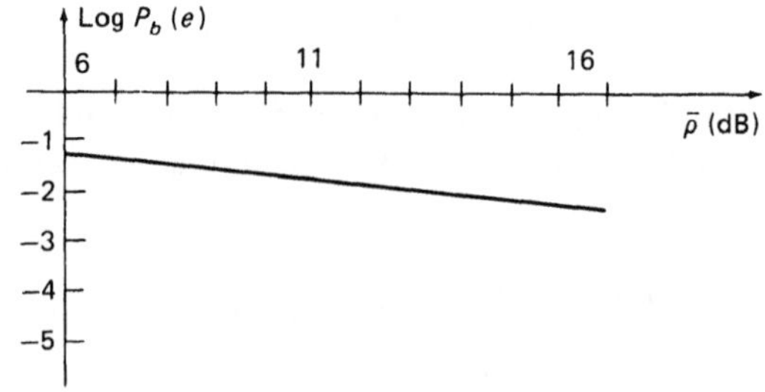


Fig. 6.32. Bit error probability of quaternary QASK in optimal system with Rayleigh fading as a function of average signal-to-noise ratio per bit.

As is obvious from Fig. 6.32, an increase in the average signal-to-noise ratio does not achieve a significant reduction in the average bit error probability. This can be achieved by *diversity*, i.e., several independent transmissions of the signal. The main methods of diversity are:

a. space diversity
b. frequency diversity
c. time diversity

In space diversity the signal is transmitted using several transmitter antennas or receiver antennas or both, situated several wavelengths apart, so that the fading in each such created diversity channel is independent.

In frequency diversity, the signal is modulated simultaneously on several carrier frequencies that fade independently.

In time diversity the signal is repeated.

The signals from the diversity channels are combined before a decision is made. There are various methods of combining the signals. In the method called *selection combining*, the decision is based on the largest signal only. In another method we simply add all signals with or without weightings. In the *maximal ratio combining* method, the weighting is proportional to the signal-to-noise ratio in each diversity channel. When the signal-to-noise ratio is the same, no weighting is required.

*Example* 6.6.2 Diversity

Let there be $K$ independent diversity channels. Let $\rho_k$ be the signal-to-noise ratio in channel $1 \leqq k \leqq K$. We assumed that the pdf of all $\rho_k$ is identical and as in (6.6.15). In maximal ratio combining

$$\rho = \sum_{k=1}^{K} \rho_k \tag{6.6.21}$$

with a pdf of

$$p_\rho(\rho) = (\bar{\rho})^{-1}(\rho/\bar{\rho})^{K-1} \exp(-\rho/\bar{\rho})/(K-1)!u(\rho) \tag{6.6.22}$$

with an average value of $K\bar{\rho}$. In selection combining

$$p_\rho(\rho) = (K/\bar{\rho}) \exp(-\rho/\bar{\rho})(1 - \exp(-\rho/\bar{\rho}))^{K-1}u(\rho) \qquad (6.6.23)$$

with an average value of $\bar{\rho} \sum_{k=1}^{K} k^{-1}$

When the fluctuation rate of $A_F$ is of the same order as the symbol rate, the fading is frequency dependent, or, in other words, frequency selective. Such fading will also cause distortion of the transmitted signal. A simple model of frequency selective fading is obtained if we take in (6.6.1) only two paths

$$x(t) = \text{Re}\,\{\{A_0 + x_1 \exp(j\psi_1)\} \exp(j\omega_C t)\} \qquad (6.6.24)$$

The baseband equivalent transfer function of the channel is thus

$$H_C(f) = A_0\{1 + b \exp(j\psi_1)\} \qquad (6.6.25)$$

where

$$b = x_1/A_0 \qquad (6.6.26)$$

and the phase, $\psi_1$, is related to the delay, $\tau_F$, by

$$\psi_1 = -2\,\pi f \tau_F + \psi_F \qquad (6.6.27)$$

The minimum value of $H_C(f)$ is obtained when

$$\psi_1 = \pi \qquad (\text{modulo } 2\,\pi) \qquad (6.6.28)$$

i.e., for $f = f_n$ (a notch frequency) such that

$$\psi_F = \pi + 2\,\pi f_n \tau_F \qquad (6.6.29)$$

When we substitute (6.6.29) into (6.6.27), we obtain

$$\psi_1 = -2\,\pi(f - f_n)\tau_F + \pi \qquad (6.6.30)$$

The transfer function of the channel is shown in Fig. 6.33.

Taking the inverse Fourier transform of (6.6.25), using (6.6.27), we obtain the impulse response

$$h_C(t) = A_0\{\delta(t) + b\delta(t - \tau_F) \exp(j\psi_F)\} \qquad (6.6.31)$$

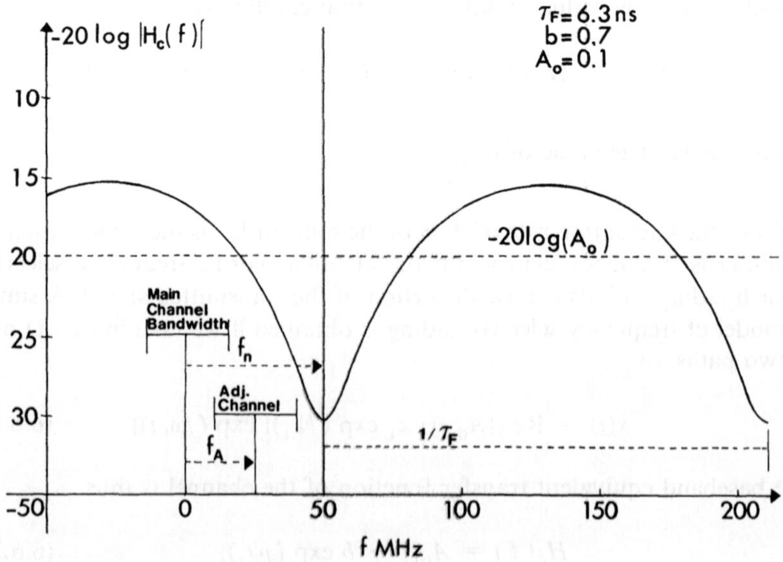


Fig. 6.33. Transfer function of channel with frequency selective fading.

The two-ray, frequency selective model was thoroughly investigated in Refs. 6.20–6.24 and applied to 4-PSK and 8-PSK systems in Ref. 6.22. In these references either $\tau_F$ or $f_n$ is a rv. In Refs. 6.20–6.24 the pdfs of $A_0$, $b$, and $f_n$ are presented, based on actual measurements in a system with a carrier frequency of 6 GHz and bandwidth of 30 MHz. With a fixed delay of $\tau_F = 6.3$ ns, the results are

$$P(1 - b < X) = X^{2.3} \tag{6.6.32}$$

$$P(-20 \log A_0 < Y) = Q(0.2\,(Y - \overline{A(b)})) \tag{6.6.33}$$

$$p_{fn}(f_n) = \begin{cases} 5\,\tau_F/3 & |f_n| \leq (4\,\tau_F)^{-1} \\ \tau_F/3 & (4\,\tau_F)^{-1} < |f_n| \leq (2\,\tau_F)^{-1} \end{cases} \tag{6.6.34}$$

and $\overline{A(b)}$ is the mean value of $-20 \log A_0$, which depends on $b$, and the graph of which can be found in Ref. 6.20. In Ref. 6.22 the model is simplified by assuming that $\tau_F$ and $b$ are independent with pdfs

$$p_{\tau_F}(\tau) = (\bar{\tau}_F)^{-1} \exp\,(-\tau/\bar{\tau}_F)u(\tau) \tag{6.6.35}$$

$$p_b(b) = \alpha_1(\exp\,(\alpha_1) - 1)^{-1} \exp\,(\alpha_1 b)u_1(b) \tag{6.6.36}$$

where $\tau_F$ is the average value of the delay, and $\alpha_1$ was selected as $\alpha_1 = 10$. This value was selected so that maximum fade depth exceeds 13 dB with a probability of 0.9, i.e.

$$\text{Prob}\{-20\log(1-b) \geqq 13\} = 0.9 \tag{6.6.37}$$

The average delay, $\tau_F$, depends on the distance between transmitter and receiver, $L$, by

$$\bar{\tau}_F = 0.296\,(L/20)^3 \tag{6.6.38}$$

where $L$ is in kilometers. In fact the exact form of $p_b(b)$ is not important, so long as it is continuous and nonzero in the vicinity of $b = 1$.

We found, in the beginning of this chapter, that the system impulse response in the absence of fading ($H_C(f) = 1$) is $g(t, f_A)$. In the presence of frequency selective fading, the system function is changed to $g_F(t, f_A)$, where, using (6.6.31)

$$g_F(t, f_A) = A_0\{g(t, f_A) + bg(t - \tau_F, f_A)\exp(j\psi_F)\} \tag{6.6.39}$$

Fixing the value of $A_0$, $b$, and $\tau_F$, we can compute the conditional bit error probability $P_b(e|A_0, \tau_F, b)$. In digital radio at microwave frequencies (carrier frequencies in the 6- 11-GHz band) most of the fading occurs during calm summer nights. So long as the error probability stays below a nominal value, say $P_{bn}(e) = 10^{-3}$, the system performance is acceptable, and the actual bit error probability is of no importance. The system fails if the error probability exceeds this value. The probability of failure is thus

$$P_F = \int_0^{\infty}\int_0^{\infty}\int_0^{1}\int_{P_{bn}(e)}^{1} dP_b(e|A_0, \tau_F, b)\,p_{A_0,\tau_F,b}(A_0, \tau_F, b)\,dA_0\,d\tau_F\,db \tag{6.6.40}$$

To find the fraction of time of a year during which failure occurs, eq. (6.6.40) must be multiplied by a time factor that, in Ref. 6.22, is given as $f_C(L/10)^3/p_b(1)$.

Let $b_c$ be the largest value of $b$ for which the bit probability is less than a nominal value, say $10^{-3}$. A system signature[6.24] is a curve of $1 - b_c$ as a function of the notch frequency, $f_n$. System A is better than system B if the signature of A is under the signature of B. Using a mean square error criterion (equivalent to a bit error probability of $10^{-3}$) and the following probabilities for the channel parameters

$$p_b(b) = u_1(b) \tag{6.6.41}$$

$$p_{\psi_F}(\alpha) = (2\,\alpha)^{-1}u_{2\pi}(\alpha + \pi) \tag{6.6.42}$$

$$p_{f_n|\tau_F}(f\,|\tau_F) = \tau_F u_{1/\tau_F}(f + 0.5/\tau_F) \tag{6.6.43}$$

we have computed[6.25] the signatures for QASK with 4, 16 and 64 symbols and PSK with 4, 8 and 16 symbols. It was assumed that the response of the system, excluding the channel is a raised cosine with excess bandwidth $\beta$ and the receiver is matched to the transmitter. One adjacent channel is present with relative amplitude $\rho_A$ ($\rho_A = A_A/A$). In Fig. 6.34 we show the signature for QASK with 16 symbols, $\beta = 0.5$, a bit rate of 140 Mbps and frequency separation between main and adjacent channel of 40 MHz. The bit error probability is proportional to the area under the signature. The area for the various systems is shown in Fig. 6.35 as a function of $\rho_A$. The system with a lower area is better. We conclude from this figure that (a) 16 QASK is better than 8 PSK for all values of $\rho_A$ (b) for small values of $\rho_A$ 4 QASK in the best system (c) for large values of $\rho_A$, 64 QASK is the best system and (d) for intermediate values of $\rho_A$ 16 QASK is the best modulation.

## 6.7 SUMMARY

In this chapter we have presented the conditions for the presence and absence of ISI, QCI, and ACI. Assuming no interference, we have computed the bit error probability as a function of signal-to-noise ratio for QASK and OQASK with general symbol constellations and concluded that the rectan-

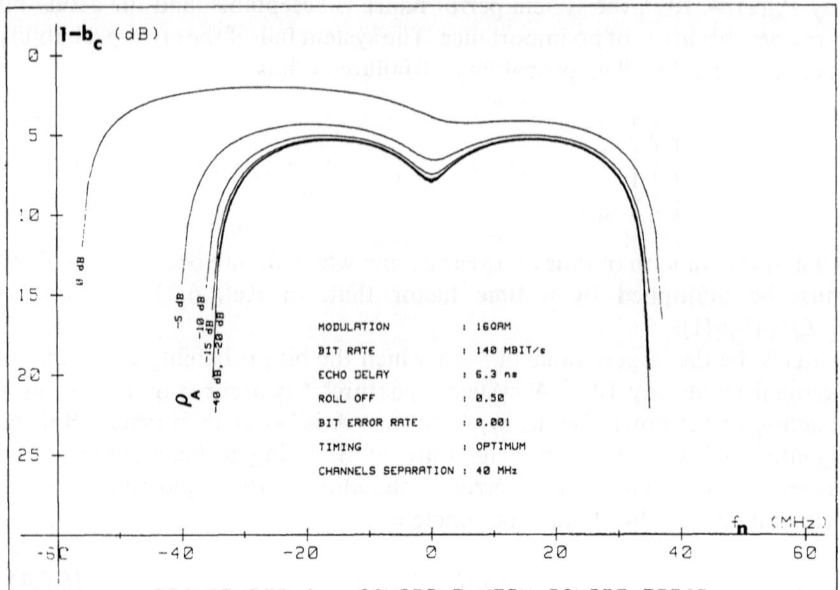


Fig. 6.34. Signature of 16 QASK in the presence of adjacent channel interference with relative amplitude $\rho_A$.

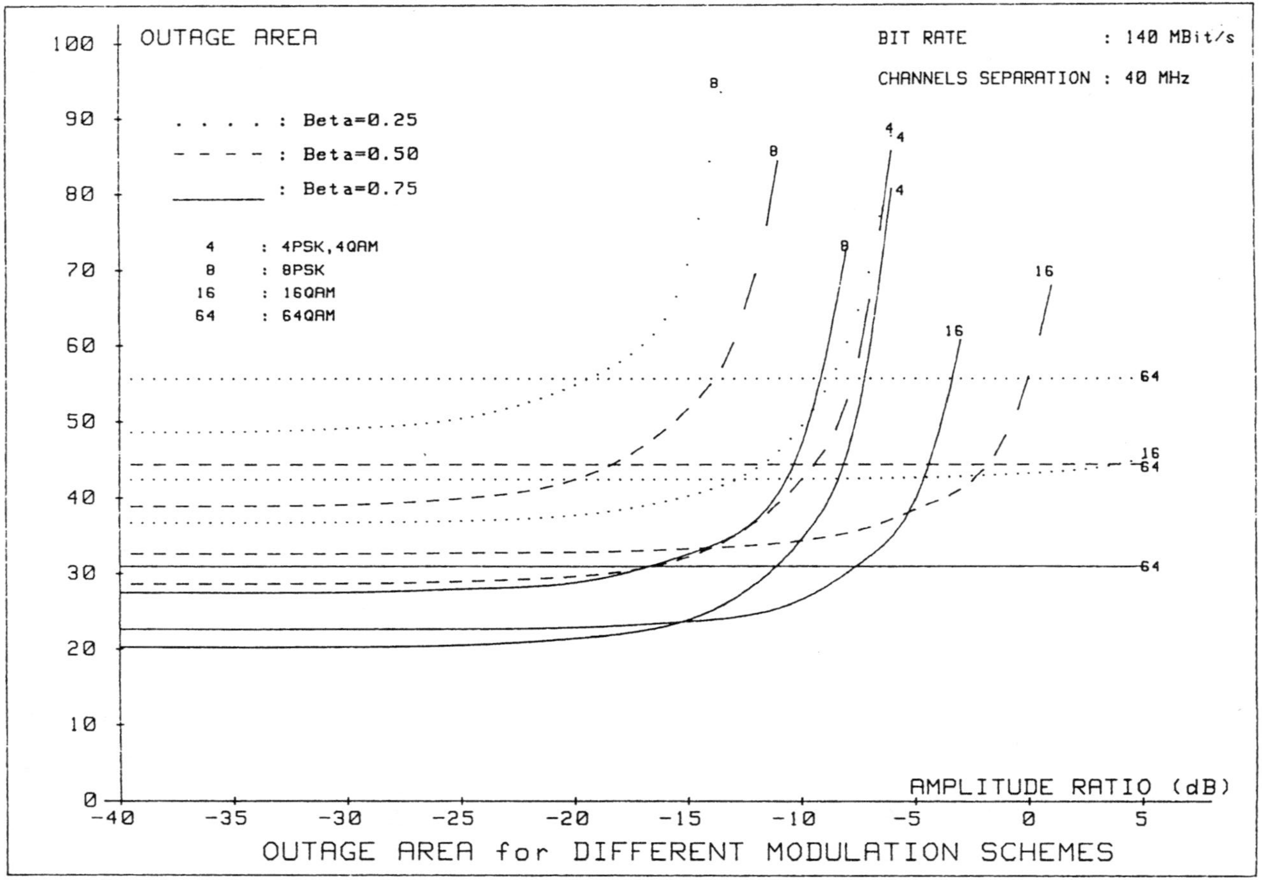


Fig. 6.35. Area under signature for QASK with 4, 16 and 64 symbols and 8 PSK as a function of $\rho_A$. $\beta$ is the excess bandwidth of the raised cosine signal. The bit rate is 140 Mbps and frequency separation is 40 MHz.

gular constellation is optimal for $M = 4$ and very close to optimal for other symbol numbers. When constant envelope signals are a necessity, QASK with a circular constellation, i.e., PSK, is a proper candidate. For QASK and OQASK with rectangular and circular constellations, we computed the bit error probability in the presence of ISI, ACI, and QCI. We considered three kinds of systems: (a) a system with receiver matched to the transmitter and overall Nyquist function system response; (b) a system with Butterworth filters in receiver and transmitter, sampling detector, and RZ and HS shaping functions; and (c) an MSK system with Gaussian filters in receiver and transmitter. For the system with Nyquist function response and bit error probability of $P_b(e) = 10^{-4}$, the signal-to-noise ratio per bit is 8.4 dB (4-QASK), 11.7 dB (8-PSK), 12.2 dB (16-QASK), and 16.3 dB (16-PSK) when there is no interference. In the presence of ISI, ACI, and QCI, additional energy is required to keep the error probability fixed at $10^{-4}$. This is stated in Table 6.3 for ACI and Table 6.4 for ISI and QCI. ISI is caused by nonideal sampling time ($t_0 \neq 0$) and QCI by phase offset ($\Delta\phi \neq 0$)

**Table 6.3 Additional energy (in dB) required for a bit error probability of $10^{-4}$ in the presence of ACI**

| $\beta$ | $f_A T$ | 4 QASK | 8 PSK | 16 QASK | 16 PSK |
|---|---|---|---|---|---|
| 0.25 | 1.1 | 0.2 | 0.9 | 0.6 | 5.8 |
| 0.5 | 1.2 | 0.4 | 2.5 | 1.7 | >10 |
| 0.75 | 1.3 | 1.8 | 3.6 | 3.4 | >10 |
| 1.00 | 1.5 | 0.6 | 2.0 | 1.8 | 9.3 |

**Table 6.4 Additional energy (in dB) required for a bit error probability of $10^{-4}$ in the presence of ISI and QCI**

| $\beta$ | $t_0/T$ | $\Delta\phi$ | 4-QASK | 8-PSK | 16-QASK | 16-PSK |
|---|---|---|---|---|---|---|
| 0.25 | 0.05 | 0 | 0.6 | 1.3 | 1.7 | 5.2 |
| 0.25 | 0 | 5° | 0.6 | 1.7 | 2.1 | 4.6 |
| 0.25 | 0.05 | 5° | 1.0 | 3.6 | 4.6 | >10 |
| 0.5 | 0.05 | 0 | 0.4 | 1.0 | 1.2 | 2.9 |
| 0.5 | 0 | 5° | 0.6 | 1.7 | 2.1 | 4.6 |
| 0.5 | 0.05 | 5° | 1.0 | 3.1 | 3.6 | >10 |

We see from Tables 6.3 and 6.4 that the ranking of the systems according to performance is: 4-QASK, 8-PSK, 16-QASK, 16-PSK, if only Gaussian noise, ISI, and QCI are taken into account. The positions of 8-PSK and 16-QASK are interchanged if only Gaussian noise and ACI are taken into account.

To compute the error probability of PSK, we extended the method of Jenq et al., which originally was applicable to ASK only.

We discussed the various channel models: with and without fading. We presented general formulas that can be used for the computation of error probability in the presence of flat and frequency selective fading.

In this chapter we have assumed that the ratio of bandwidth to carrier frequency is small, so that the baseband equivalents of the bandpass filters are symmetric filters. The case when this ratio is not small is discussed in Ref. 6.26.

The spectral efficiency of QASK and OQASK is the same as the efficiency of ASK with $\sqrt{M}$ symbols.

## 6.8 PROBLEMS

6.3.1 Determine the decision regions, and compute the bit error probability as a function of signal-to-noise ratio per bit in a QASK system with no interference, matched filter, and signal constellation with eight symbols, as in Fig. P6.3.1.

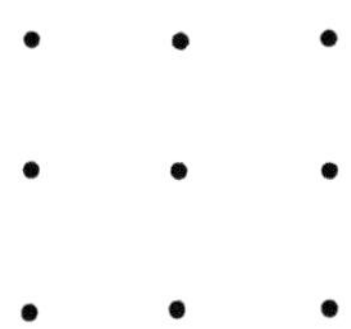

6.3.2 Determine the decision regions, and compute the bit error probability as a function of signal-to-noise ratio per bit in a PSK system with no interference, matched filter, and signal constellation with three symbols, as in Fig. P6.3.2.

6.3.3 In a QASK system with no interference, matched filter, and symbols $\{a_{Ii}\}, \{a_{Qi}\}$ from the set $\mathring{A}_{\pm} = \{\pm 1, \pm 3, \ldots, \pm(M_I - 1)\}$, the decision regions have been made under the assumption that the signal-to-noise ratio per bit, $E_b/N_0$ is 10 dB, though this ratio is actually 11 dB because of a greater energy.

a. Compute the bit error probability if $M_I = 2$.
b. Repeat (a) if $M_I = 4$.
c. Repeat (a) if the energy is reduced so that actually $E_b/N_0 = 9$ dB.
d. Repeat (c) with $M_I = 4$.

6.4.1 Compute the results presented in Fig. 6.15 for $t_0/T = 0.05$, $\beta = 0.5$ and four symbols.

6.4.2 Compute the function $g(t, f_A)$ in eq. (6.4.42) for $\beta = 0.5$. Sketch the function $f(t, f_A)$ as a function of $t/T$ for $f_A = 1/T$.

6.4.3 Compute the results presented in Fig. 6.19 for $\beta = 0.5, f_A = 1.2$, and four symbols.

6.4.4 Compute the spectral efficiency, and comment on the bit error probability (using Fig. 6.19) of the following systems.

| SYSTEM | BIT RATE $R_b$ (Mbps) | CHANNEL SPACING $f_A$ (MHz) |
|---|---|---|
| 4 QASK | 34 | 29 |
| | 68 | 30, 40 |
| 8 PSK | 68 | 30, 40 |
| | 140 | 30, 40 |
| 16 QASK | 140 | 30, 40 |
| 64 QASK | 140 | 30, 40 |
| | 210 | 30, 40 |

6.4.5 Assume that $H_C(f) = H_D(f) = 1$ and that $H_T(f)$, $H_R(f)$ are single-pole Butterworth filters with 3-dB frequencies, $f_{T0}$ and $f_{R0}$, respectively. Compute $g_N(t, f_A)$ and $g_H(t, f_A)$ in eqs. (6.4.71) and (6.4.72).

6.4.6

a. Show that for Gaussian filters

$$T_b \int_{-\infty}^{\infty} |H(f)|^2 \, df = (0.5\,\pi)^{1/2}/\alpha$$

where $\alpha$ is given in (6.4.102).

b. Show that for Gaussian filters and no adjacent channel interference, eq. (6.4.100) is simplified to

$$\eta = (2/\pi)^{1/2}\alpha \exp(-\alpha^2/4)$$

c. Show that $\eta$ in (b) is maximized if the 3-dB filter bandwidth is $B_{\text{op}} = \sqrt{\ln 2}$ and the maximal value is $\eta_{\max} = 2(e\pi)^{-1/2}$.

d. Compute $\eta$ in (6.4.100) assuming that $H_T(f) = 1$ and $H_R(f)$ is a Gaussian filter.

e. Compute for (d) the optimal 3-dB bandwidth and the resulting $\eta$ for $\rho_A = 0$ and $\rho_A = 10$.

6.5.1

a. Prove the inequalities in eq. (6.5.62).

b. Compute the range of $W_i - V_i$, $i = 1, 2, 3, 4$, if instead of (6.5.60), we use $x_i' = x_i/1.47$.

6.5.2 Compute the results presented in Fig. 6.2.8 for $\beta = 0.5$, $\Delta\phi = 5°$, $t_0/T = 0.05$.

6.6.1 Prove eqs. (6.6.19) and (6.6.20).

6.6.2 Let $\{\rho_k\}$ be independent rvs with identical Rayleigh pdf, as in eq. (6.6.15)

a. Show that the pdf of the sum $\rho = \sum_{k=1}^{K} \rho_k$ is as in (6.6.22).

b. Show that the pdf of $\rho = \max_{k=1,\ldots,K} \rho_k$ is as in (6.6.23).

6.6.3 Compute the bit error probability of eq. (6.6.16) with $P_b(e|\rho)$ as in (6.6.17) and $p_\rho(\rho)$ as in (6.6.22). Plot the result as a function of $\bar{\rho}$ for $K = 2, 3, 4$, and compare with Fig. 6.32.

6.6.4 Assume a system with two diversity channels. The outputs of the detector filters in the two channels are

$$r_1 = a_0 g_0 + n_1$$
$$r_2 = a_0 g_0 + n_2$$

where $n_1$ and $n_2$ are independent, zero mean, Gaussian noises with variances $\sigma_1^2$ and $\sigma_2^2$, respectively. The outputs are combined into

$$r = w_1 r_1 + w_2 r_2$$

where $w_1$, $w_2$ are weights. The decision about the symbols $a_0 = \pm 1$ is made by

$$\hat{a}_0 = \text{sign } r$$

a. Compute the bit error probability for given $w_1$ and $w_2$.

b. Specify the optimal weights, i.e., $w_1$, $w_2$, that minimize the bit error probability.

c. Repeat (a), assuming $w_1 = w_2 = 1$.
d. Compare (b) and (c) if $\sigma_1^2 = 2\,\sigma_2^2$.

6.6.4 Compute and sketch $|H_C(f)|$ of eqs. (6.6.25) and (6.6.30), assuming $A_0 = 1$, $b = 0.5$, and $\tau_F = 6.3$ nsec.

## 6.9 REFERENCES


6.1 E. Arthurs and H. Dym, "On the Optimum Detection of Digital Signals in the Presence of White, Gaussian, Noise—A Geometric Interpretation and a Study of Three Basic Data Transmission Systems," *IRE Tr. Comm. Syst.*, Vol. CS-10, December 1962, pp. 336–372.

6.2 G. J. Foschini, R. D. Gitlin, and S. B. Weinstein, "Optimisation of the Two-Dimensional Signal Constellations in the Presence of Gaussian Noise," *IEEE Tr. Comm.*, Vol. COM-22, January 1974, pp. 28–38.

6.3 C. M. Thomas, M. Y. Weidner, and S. H. Durrani, "Digital Amplitude-Phase Keying with *M*-ary alphabets," *IEEE Tr. Comm.*, Vol. COM-22, February 1974, pp. 168–180.

6.4 R. D. Gitlin and E. Y. Ho, "The Performance of Staggered Quadrature Amplitude Modulation in the Pressence of Phase Jitter," *IEEE Tr. Comm.*, Vol. COM-23, March 1975, pp. 398–352.

6.5 Y. C. Jenq, B. Liu, and J. B. Thomas, "Threshold Effect on Error Probability in QAM Systems," *IEEE Tr. Comm.*, Vol. COM-28, July 1980, pp. 1047–1051.

6.6 I. Korn and B. Seth, "Adjacent Channel and Quadrature Channel Interference in Minimum Shift Keying," *IEEE Tr. Sel. Ar. Comm.*, Vol. SAC-1, January 1983, pp. 21–28.

6.7 I. Korn and Y. Tsang, "Effect of Intersymbol and Quadrature Channel Interference on Error Probability of 16-ary Offset Quadrature Amplitude Modulation with sinusoidal and rectangular shaiping," *IEEE Tr. Comm.*, Vol. COM-31, February 1983, pp. 264–269.

6.8 I. Korn, "Error Probability of QASK with Rectangular and Circular Symbol Constellations in the Presence of Intersymbol, Quadrature Channel and Adjacent Channel Interference," *Proc. IEE*, Part F, CRSP, Vol. 131, April 1984, pp. 194–202.

6.9 M. Ishizuka and K. Hirade, "Optimum Gaussian Filter and Deviated Frequency Locking Scheme for Coherent Detection of MSK," *IEEE Tr. Comm.*, Vol. COM-28, June 1980, pp. 850–857.

6.10 I. Korn, "Simple Expression for Interchannel and Intersymbol Interference Degradation in MSK Systems with Application to Systems with Gaussian Filters," *IEEE Tr. Comm.*, Vol. COM-30, August 1982, pp. 1968–1972.

6.11 V. K. Prabhu, "Performance of Coherent Phase Shift Keyed Systems with Intersymbol Interference," *IEEE Tr. Inf. Theory*, Vol. IT-17, July 1971, pp. 418–431.

6.12 V. K. Prabhu, "Error Rate Considerations for Coherent Phase Shift Keyed Systems with Co-channel Interference," *BSTJ*, Vol. 48, March 1969, pp. 743–767.

6.13 S. Benedetto and E. Biglieri, "Performance of *M*-ary PSK systems in the Presence of Intersymbol Interference and Additive Noise," *Alta Frequenza*, Vol. 41, April 1972, pp. 225–239.

6.14 O. Shimbo, R. J. Fang, and M. Celebiler, "Performance of *M*-ary PSK Systems in Gaussian Noise and Intersymbol Interference", *IEEE Tr. Inf. Theory*, Vol. IT-19, January 1973, pp. 44–58.

6.15 V. K. Prabhu, "Error Probability Performance of *M*-ary CPSK Systems with Intersymbol Interference," *IEEE Tr. Comm.*, Vol. COM-21, February 1973, pp. 98–109.

6.16 S. Benedetto, E. Biglieri, and V. Castellani, "Combined Effects of Intersymbol, Interchannel and Co-channel Interference in *M*-ary CPSK Systems," *IEEE Tr. Comm.*, Vol. COM-21, September 1973, pp. 997–1008.

6.17 R. Fang and O. Shimbo, "Unifield Analysis of a Class of Digital Systems in Additive Noise and Interference," *IEEE Tr. Comm.*, Vol. COM-21, October 1973, pp. 1075–1091.

6.18 M. Schwartz, W. R. Bennett, and S. Stein, *Communication Systems and Techniques*, McGraw-Hill, Inc., New York, N.Y., 1966.

6.19 K. Feher, *Digital Communications: Microwave Applications*, Prentice-Hall, Inc., Englewood Cliffs, N.J., 1981.

6.20 W. D. Rummler, "A New Selective Fading Model: Application to Propagation Data," *BSTJ*, Vol. 58, May–June 1979, pp. 1037–1071.

6.21 C. W. Lundgren and D. W. Rummler, "Digital Radio Outage due to Selective Fading Observation vs Prediction from Laboratory Simulation," *BSTJ*, Vol. 58, May–June 1979, pp. 1073–1100.

6.22 L. J. Greenstein and V. K. Prabhu, "Analysis of Multipath Outage with Application to 90 Mbit/s Systems in 6 and 11 GHz," *IEEE Tr. Comm.*, Vol. COM-27, January 1979, pp. 68–75.

6.23 W. D. Rummler, "A Statistical Model of Multipath Fading on a Space-diversity Radio Channel", *BSTJ*, Vol. 61, Nov. 82, pp. 2805–2219.

6.24 A. J. Giger, W. T. Barnett, "Effects of Multipath Propagation of Digital Radio", *IEEE Tr. Comm.*, Vol. COM-29, Sept. 81, pp. 1345–1352.

6.25 I. Korn, "Effect of Adjacent Channel Interference and Frequency Selective Fading on Outage of Digital Radio". Submitted for publication.

6.26 I. Korn, "Probability of Error in a Bandlimited Quadriphase Communication System," *IEEE Tr. AES*, Vol. AES-9, July 1973, pp. 535–543.

# 7 PSK AND DPSK

## 7.1 INTRODUCTION

In Chapter 6 we analyzed phase shift keying (PSK) with a rectangular shaping function, because this is essentially the same as QASK with a circular constellation. When the shaping function is not rectangular, especially when it is overlapping, PSK deviates from QASK. This is discussed in Section 7.2. In that section we also derive the joint probability density function (pdf) of the phase and amplitude of a complex, Gaussian random variable (rv), as well as their individual pdfs. This leads to an exact expression for the error probability, although in most cases upper and lower bounds that are very tight are more useful, especially when we have to compute the effect of intersymbol interference (ISI). In Section 7.3 we analyze differential PSK (DPSK) with or without ISI. The analysis is fundamentally different and significantly more difficult than the analysis of LSK or PSK. The reason for that is the inherently nonlinear detection process of DPSK, which leads to a product of Gaussian rvs. Except for binary DPSK without ISI, the formulas for the error probability are very complicated. In PSK the transmitted power is constant: hence nonlinear amplifiers can be used. DPSK is an improvement upon PSK because the absolute phase is not required at the receiver.

In Section 7.4 we present a summary, followed by problems in Section 7.5 and a list of references in Section 7.6.

## 7.2 PSK

A PSK system is shown in Fig. 7.1a. The phase of the carrier depends on the symbols $\{a_i\}$, which are assumed to be independent and equiprobable from the $M$-ary set $\mathring{A} = \{2k - 1, k = 1, 2, \ldots, M\}$. A baseband equivalent model is shown in Fig. 7.1b. In this model all bandpass filters have been replaced by their lowpass equivalent form, and we have assumed that the phase of the local oscillator is the same as the phase of the carrier, i.e., $\phi_R = \phi_T$. It was shown in Chapter 2 that in the general case, when the shaping function, $h_s(t)$, has duration $KT$ (where $K$ is an integer and $R = 1/T$ is the symbol rate), the complex envelope of the PSK signal is

$$\begin{aligned} s_1(t) &= A \exp\left(jK_p \sum_i a_i h_s(t - iT)\right) \\ &= A \sum_i b(t - iT, \mathbf{a}_i) \end{aligned} \tag{7.2.1}$$

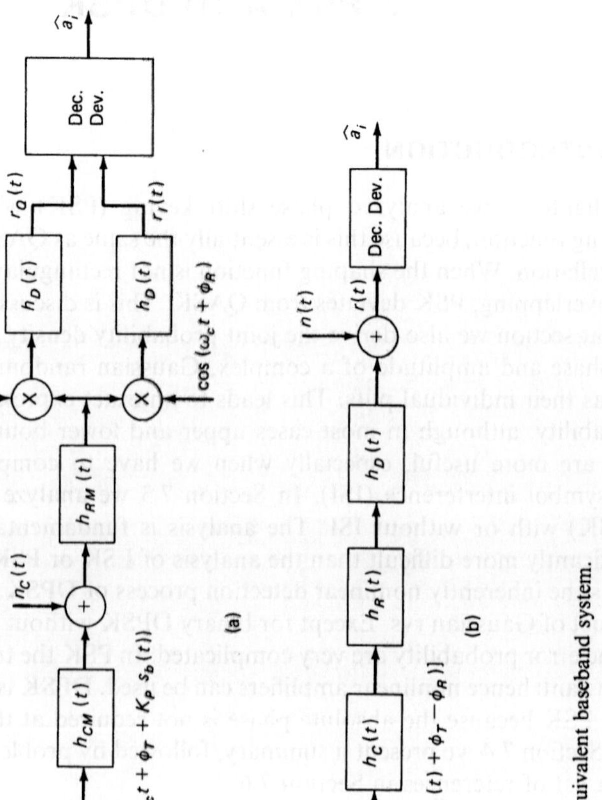


Fig. 7.1. Model of PSK system: (a) bandpss system, (b) equivalent baseband system.

where

$$b(t, \mathbf{a}_i) = \exp\left\{jK_p \sum_{k=0}^{K-1} a_{i-k} h_{sk}(t)\right\} u_T(t) \tag{7.2.2}$$

$$h_{sk}(t) = h_s(t + kT)u_T(t) \tag{7.2.3}$$

$$u_T(t) = \begin{cases} 1 & 0 \leqq t \leqq T \\ 0 & \text{otherwise} \end{cases} \tag{7.2.4}$$

and

$$K_p = \pi/M \tag{7.2.5}$$

if the maximal value of $h_s(t)$ is 1.

Equation (7.2.1) can be slightly generalized if $u_T(t)$ in equation (7.2.2) is replaced by an arbitrary function of duration $T, f(t)$. This is equivalent to the introduction of amplitude modulation in addition to phase modulation.

The case when the shaping function is an NRZ pulse

$$h_s(t) = u_T(t) \tag{7.2.6}$$

was already discussed within the frame of LSK in Chapter 6. This case is in fact the most commonly used PSK.[7.1–7.4]

The case of nonoverlapping shaping functions (i.e., $K = 1$)

$$h_s(t) = h_s(t)u_T(t) \tag{7.2.7}$$

was presented in Refs. 7.5–7.8. The only paper that analyzes PSK with overlapping shaping function is Ref. 7.8. The reason for attempting to use other then NRZ shaping functions is the improvement in spectral efficiency, as explained in Chapter 3.

The input to the decision device is the complex signal

$$r(t) = s_I(t) + n_I(t) + j(s_Q(t) + n_Q(t)) \tag{7.2.8}$$

where $n_I(t)$, $n_Q(t)$ are zero-mean, Gaussian, independent rvs with the same variance

$$\sigma_n^2 = N_0 \int_{-\infty}^{\infty} |H_R(f)H_D(f)|^2 \, df = N_0 E_{RD} \tag{7.2.9}$$

and $s_I(t)$ ($s_Q(t)$) is the real (imaginary) part of

$$s(t) = \sum_i y(t - iT, \mathbf{a}_i) \tag{7.2.10}$$

and

$$y(t, \mathbf{a}_i) = Ag(t, \mathbf{a}_i) \tag{7.2.11}$$

$$g(t, \mathbf{a}_i) = b(t, \mathbf{a}_i) * h(t) \tag{7.2.12}$$

$$h(t) = h_T(t) * h_C(t) * h_R(t) * h_D(t) \tag{7.2.13}$$

In (7.2.9) $N_0/2$ is the power spectral density of the white noise, $n_C(t)$ of Fig. 7.1a. A is related to the energy per symbol at the input of the transmitter filter by $E_s = A^2T/2$; hence the signal-to-noise ratio is defined here by

$$\rho_s = 0.5\ A^2/\sigma_n^2 = (E_s/N_0)(TE_{RD})^{-1} \tag{7.2.14}$$

The phase of $r(t)$ at time $t_k = t_0 + kT$ is

$$\phi_{r,k} = \phi_r(t_k) \tag{7.2.15}$$

where

$$\tan \phi_r(t) = \frac{s_Q(t) + n_Q(t)}{s_I(t) + n_I(t)} \tag{7.2.16}$$

The decision about the value of symbol $a_k$ is based on $\phi_{r,k}$, so that if

$$|\phi_{r,k} - \pi a_k/M| \leq \pi/M \tag{7.2.17}$$

there is no error. Because of stationarity, we may assume that $k = 0$. Because of symmetry of the symbol constellation, the error probability is the same for all symbols; hence we may assume that $a_0 = 1$. Thus the error probability is

$$P(e) = P(|\phi_{r,0} - \pi/M| > \pi/M) = P(2\ \pi/M < \phi_{r,0} < 2\ \pi) \tag{7.2.18}$$

where $\phi_{r,0}$ is computed under the condition that $a_0 = 1$. In order to compute this error probability, we need the probability density function (pdf) of $\phi_{r,0}$. This can be avoided, if we are satisfied with tight bounds on $P(e)$. It was shown in Section 6.5 that the error probability can be bounded by

$$P_L \leq P(e) \leq 2\ P_L \tag{7.2.19}$$

where

$$\begin{aligned} P_L &= P(r_Q(t_0) < 0) = P(s_Q(t_0) + n_Q(t_0) < 0) \\ &= \overline{Q(s_Q(t_0)/\sigma_n)} \end{aligned} \tag{7.2.20}$$

In (7.2.20) $s_Q(t_0)$ is computed under the assumption that $a_0 = 1$, the average is over all symbols $\{a_k, k \neq 0\}$, and

$$Q(x) = \int_x^\infty (2\pi)^{-0.5} \exp(-y^2/2)\, dy \tag{7.2.21}$$

is the tail of a Gaussian curve.

For $M = 2$ the error probability is $P_L$, and for $M \geqq 4$ the error probability is closer to 2 $P_L$ then to $P_L$. The average in (7.2.20) can be computed or bounded by the methods presented in Chapters 4 and 6. Usually $s_Q(t_0)$ can be approximated by only $N$ significant terms in (7.2.10). When $M$ and $N$ are small the exhaustive method is the best suitable.

*Example* 7.2.1
In this example it is assumed that

$$h_S(t) = \sin^2(\pi t/T) u_T(t)$$

which is a raised cosine (RC) of duration $T$. It is assumed that

$$h(t) = h_R(t) = \omega_0 \exp(-\omega_0 t) u(t)$$

where $u(t)$ is the step function and $\omega_0 = 2\pi f_0$, with $f_0$ the 3-dB bandwidth of the filter. The filter introduces intersymbol interference; therefore the optimal sampling time is not $t_0 = 0.5\ T$, but is optimized. The error probability as a function of signal-to-noise ratio, $\rho_S$ is shown in Fig. 7.2 for binary symbols and in Fig. 7.3 for quaternary symbols, the parameter is the normalized bandwidth $2 f_0 T$. In Fig. 7.4 we compare the values of $\rho_S$ of PSK with raised cosine and NRZ ($h_S(t) = u_T(t)$) shaping functions, which give the same error probability of $P(e)\ 10^{-6}$. It can be seen from this figure that the performance of PSK with NRZ shaping function is better than the one with the RC shaping function.

*Example* 7.2.2
In this example the symbols are binary and the shaping functions are: NRZ, cosine, triangle, and raised cosine of duration $T$ and a raised cosine of duration 2 $T$

$$h_S(t) = \sin^2(0.5\ \pi t/T) u_{2T}(t)$$

It is assumed that

$$h(t) = h_R(t)$$

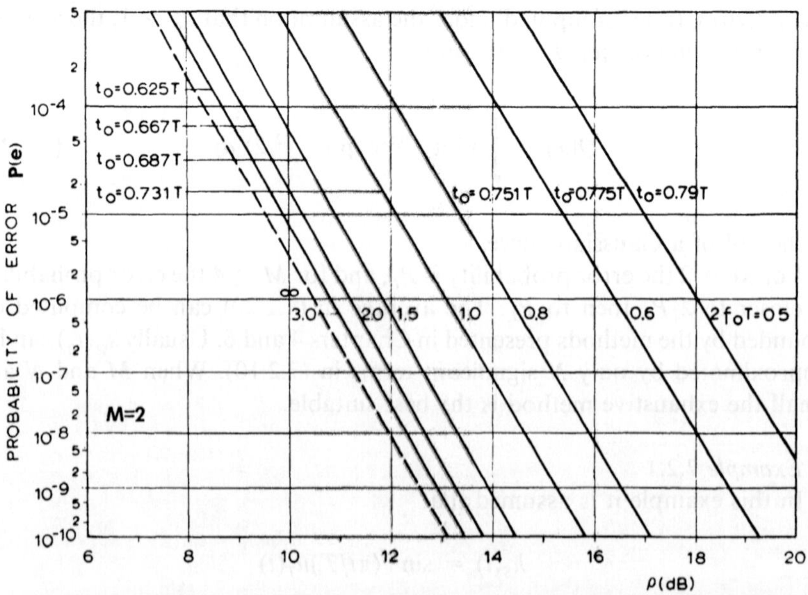


Fig. 7.2. Error probability of binary PSK with raised cosine shaping function of duration $T$ as a function of SNR (reprinted from S. Benedetto, E. Biglieri, "Performance of $M$-ary PSK Systems in the Presence of Intersymbol Interference and Additive Noise," *Alta Frequenza*, Vol. XLI, 1972, pp. 225–239).

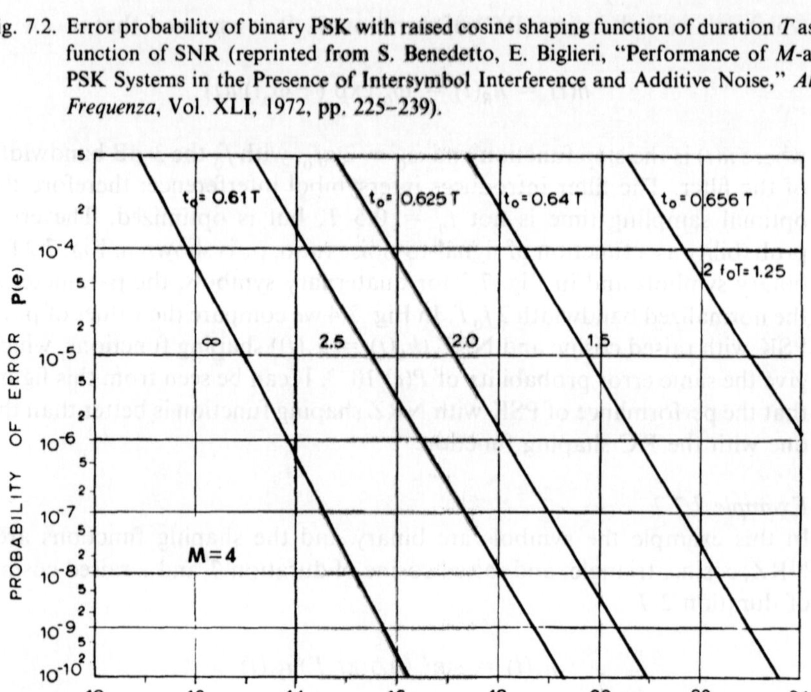


Fig. 7.3. The same as 7.2 but quaternary symbols (S. Benedetto, E. Biglieri, "Performance of $M$-ary PSK Systems in the Presence of Intersymbol Interference and Additive Noise," *Alta Frequenza*, Vol. XLI, 1972, pp. 225–239).

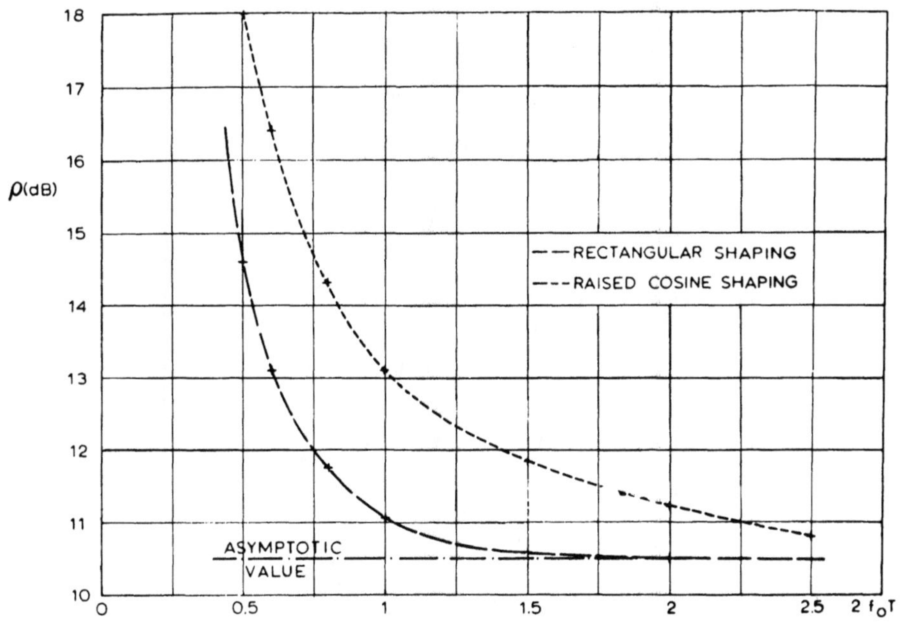


Fig. 7.4. SNR as a function of filter bandwidth for binary PSK with rectangular and raised cosine shaping functions for an error probability of $10^{-6}$ (S. Benedetto, E. Biglieri, "Performance of $M$-ary PSK Systems in the Presence of Intersymbol Interference and Additive Noise," *Alta Frequenza*, Vol. XLI, 1972, pp. 225–239).

is a Butterworth filter of order $N = 4$ and bandwidth

$$B_R = \int_{-\infty}^{\infty} |H_R(f)|^2\, df = 2 f_0/\text{sinc}\ (0.5/N) = 2.052 f_0$$

The error probability as a function of a signal-to-noise ratio $E_S/N_0$ is presented in Fig. 7.5, where in each case the optimal $B_R T$ was selected and $t_0$ was optimized.

The curve labeled *ideal* corresponds to an NRZ shaping function with matched filter detection, i.e.

$$h(t) = u_T(t)$$

It can be seen from this figure that PSK with NRZ shaping function is superior.

*Example* 7.2.3

In this example the symbols are binary, the shaping function is a raised

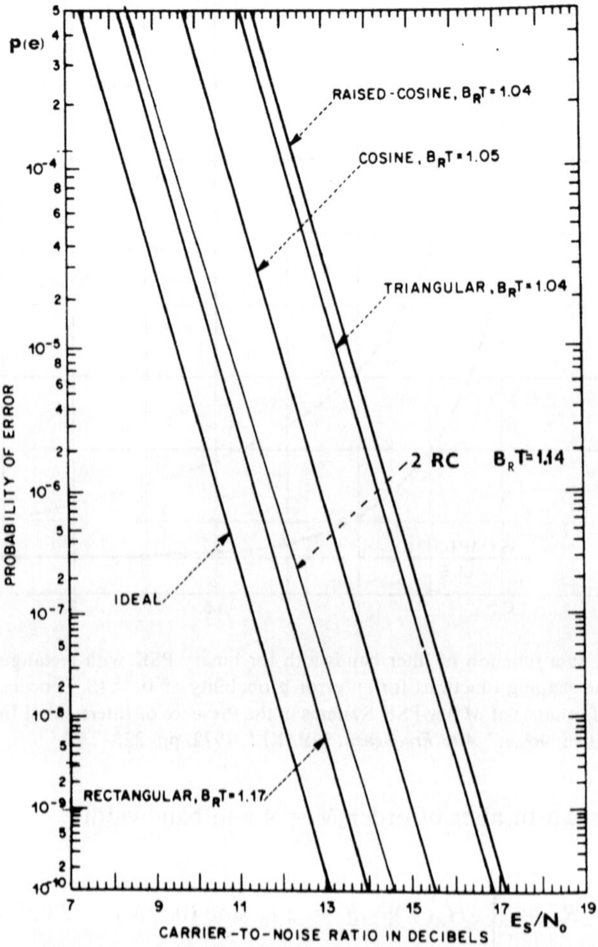


Fig. 7.5. Error probability of binary PSK with rectangular, raised cosine, and triangular shaping functions of duration $T$ and raised cosine shaping function of duration $2T$ as a function of energy-to-noise ratio $E/N_0$ (V. K. Prabhu, "PSK Type Modulation with Nonoverlapping Baseband Pulses," *IEEE Tr. Comm.*, Vol. COM-25, September 1977, pp. 980–990. Copyright © 1977 IEEE).

cosine of duration 2 $T$, and

$$h(t) = h_T(f) * h_R(t)$$

where both $h_T(f)$ and $h_R(t)$ are Butterworth filters of order 4. The bandwidth $B_R$ is optimized as in Example 7.3. The bandwidth of the transmitter filter is selected so that the signal at its output contains 99% of the power of its input. This bandwidth is denoted by $f_{99}$ and will be

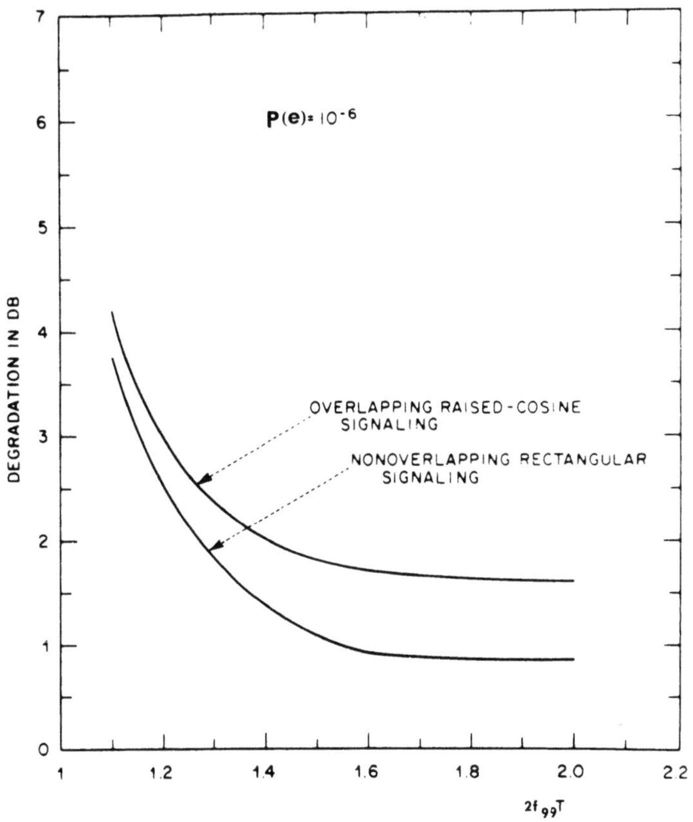


Fig. 7.6. Degradation in signal-to-noise ratio for binary PSK with rectangular shaping function of duration $T$ and raised cosine shaping the duration 2 $T$ as a function of normalized 99% bandwidth of transmitter filter for an error probability of $10^{-6}$ (S. Benedetto, E. Biglieri, C. Castelani, "Combined Effects of intersymbol, Interchannel and Co-channel Interferences in $M$-ary CPSK Systems," *IEEE Tr. Comm.*, Vol. COM-21, September 1973 pp. 997–1008. Copyright © 1973 IEEE).

different for different shaping functions. Figure 7.6 shows the additional $E_s/N_0$ relative to ideal NRZ and a function of $2 f_{99}T$ for an error probability of $10^{-6}$ for PSK with RC shaping. The conclusion is again clear: NRZ shaping is better than the 2 $T$, RC shaping.

### 7.2.1 The pdf of phase and amplitude of a complex, Gaussian random variable

Before leaving this section we shall derive the pdf of the phase of a complex Gaussian rv as well as its amplitude, which are useful in computing the exact value of error probability both here and in the next section.

Let

$$r = r_I + jr_Q = A_r \exp(j\phi_r) = s + n = s_I + js_Q + n_I + jn_Q$$
$$= A_S \exp(j\phi_S) + n \qquad (7.2.22)$$

be a complex, Gaussian rv with average

$$\bar{r} = s \qquad (7.2.23)$$

variance

$$\sigma^2 = 0.5\,\overline{(r - s)(r - s)^*} = 0.5\,(\overline{n_I^2} + \overline{n_Q^2}) = \sigma_n^2 \qquad (7.2.24)$$

and $A_r(A_S)$, $\phi_r(\phi_S)$ represent the noisy (noiseless) amplitude and phase, as shown in Fig. 7.7.

We assume that $n_I$ and $n_Q$ are independent, zero-mean, Gaussian rv with variance $\sigma_n^2$ and joint pdf

$$p_{n_I,n_Q}(n_I, n_Q) = (2\,\pi\sigma_n^2)^{-1} \exp\{-0.5\,(n_I^2 + n_Q^2)/\sigma_n^2\} \qquad (7.2.25)$$

Applying the method presented in Section 1.6.3 and already used in Section 6.3, the joint pdf of $A_r$, $\phi_r$ is for $0 \leq A_r$ and any $2\,\pi$ section of $\phi_r$

$$p_{Ar,\phi r}(A_{r,\phi r}) = A_r p_{nI,nQ}(r_I - s_I, r_Q - s_Q)$$
$$= (2\,\pi\sigma^2)^{-1} A_r \exp\{-0.5\,(A_r^2 + A_S^2 - 2\,A_S A_r \cos(\phi_r - \phi_S)/\sigma^2\} \qquad (7.2.26)$$

When we integerate with respect to $A_r$, we obtain the pdf of $\phi_r$

$$p_{\phi r}(\phi_r) = \int_{-\infty}^{\infty} p_{Ar,\phi r}(A_r, \phi_r)\,dA_r$$
$$= \int_0^{\infty} (x/\pi) \exp\{-(x^2 + \rho_S - 2\,x(\rho_S)^{0.5} \cos(\phi_r - \phi_S))\}\,dx$$
$$= \exp(-\rho_S)/(2\,\pi) + (\rho_S/\pi)^{0.5} \exp(-\rho_S \sin^2(\phi_r - \phi_S))$$
$$\cos(\phi_r - \phi_S)\{1 - Q((2\,\rho_S)^{0.5} \cos(\phi_r - \phi_S))\} \qquad (7.2.27)$$

where

$$\rho_S = 0.5\,A_S^2/\sigma^2 \qquad (7.2.28)$$

is the signal-to-noise ratio, $E_S/N_0$, in the ideal case (no intersymbol interference, matched filter), and $E_S$ is the energy per symbol.

Note that $\phi_r$ is a symmetric random variable around $\phi_S$ and $\phi_S$ is its average value.

$$\overline{\phi_r} = \phi_S \tag{7.2.29}$$

We can define the phase error as

$$\theta = \phi_r - \phi_S \tag{7.2.30}$$

with a pdf

$$p_\theta(\theta) = \exp(-\rho_S)/(2\pi) + (\rho_S/\pi)^{0.5} \exp\{-\rho_S \sin^2\theta\} \cos\theta\,\{1 - Q((2\rho_S)^{0.5}\cos\theta)\} \tag{7.2.31}$$

for $|\theta| \leqq \pi$ or $0 \leqq \theta \leqq 2\pi$. For large values of $\rho_S$ and small values of $\theta$, eq. (7.2.31) can be approximated by

$$p_\theta(\theta) \simeq (\rho_S/\pi)^{0.5} \exp(-\rho_S \sin^2\theta) \tag{7.2.32}$$

When we integerate (7.2.26) with respect to $\phi_r$ (or $\theta$), we obtain the pdf of $A_r$

$$\begin{aligned} p_{A_r}(A_r) &= \int_0^{2\pi} p_{A_r,\phi_r}(A_r, \phi_r)\, d\phi_r \\ &= \exp(-\rho_S)(A_r/\sigma^2)\exp(-0.5\,A_r^2/\sigma^2) I_0((2\rho_S)^{0.5}A_r/\sigma) \end{aligned} \tag{7.2.33}$$

where

$$I_0(z) = \int_0^{2\pi} \exp(z\cos\theta)\, d\theta/(2\pi) \tag{7.2.34}$$

The pdf in (7.2.33) is called Rician while if $\rho_S = 0$ it is called Rayleigh.

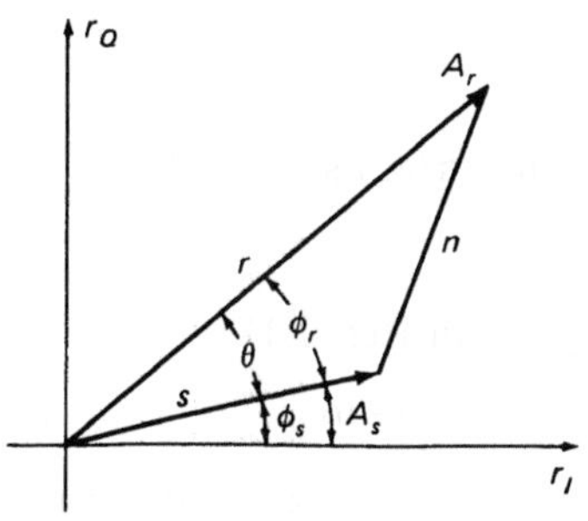


Fig. 7.7. Gaussian, complex random variable.

### 7.2.2 Exact error probability

The error probability is, from (7.2.18) (we replace $\phi_{r,0}$ by $\phi_r$)

$$P(e) = \int_{2\pi/M}^{2\pi} p_{\phi r}(\phi_r)\, d\phi_r = \int_{2\pi/M-\phi_S}^{2\pi-\phi_S} p_\theta(\theta)\, d\theta \tag{7.2.35}$$

For each sequence of symbols $\{a_i, a_0 = 1\}$, we obtain a certain value of $\phi_S$ and $\rho_S$ from eq. (7.2.10); hence (7.2.35) must be averaged with respect to all these sequences. In the ideal case where

$$b(t, a_i) = \exp(j\pi a_i/M) \tag{7.2.36}$$

a receiver matched to transmitter and no intersymbol interference

$$s = s(t_0) = A \exp(j\pi/M) \tag{7.2.37}$$

Hence

$$\phi_S = \pi/M \tag{7.2.38}$$

Thus from the symmetry of $p_\theta(\theta)$

$$P(e) = 2\int_{\pi/M}^{\pi} p_\theta(\theta)\, d\theta \tag{7.2.39}$$

The probability distribution function of $p_\theta(\theta)$ was tabulated in Ref. 7.9. Various simplifications can be obtained when we substitute (7.2.27) or (7.2.31) into (7.2.39). For example Ref. 7.10 shows that

$$P(e) = (2\pi)^{-1}\int_{-\infty}^{\cot(\pi/M)} (1 + x)^2 \exp\{-\rho_S(1 + x^2)\} \sin^2(\pi/M)\, dx$$

$$= \int_{-\pi/2}^{\pi/2-\pi/M} \exp\{-\rho_S \sin^2(\pi/M) \sec^2\theta\}\, d\theta \tag{7.2.40}$$

Another expression is given in Ref. 7.11

$$P(e) = (2/\pi)^{0.5} \tan(\pi/M) \int_0^{(2\rho_S)^{0.5}\cos(\pi/M)} \exp\{-0.5\, z^2 \tan^2(\pi/M)\} Q(z)\, dz - 1/M \tag{7.2.41}$$

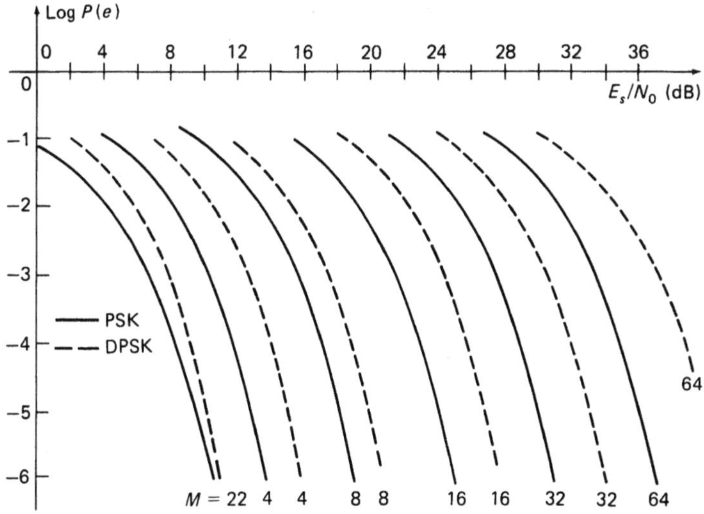


Fig. 7.8. Symbol error probability as a function of signal-to-noise ratio, $E_s/N_0$ for ideal $M$-ary PSK and DPSK.

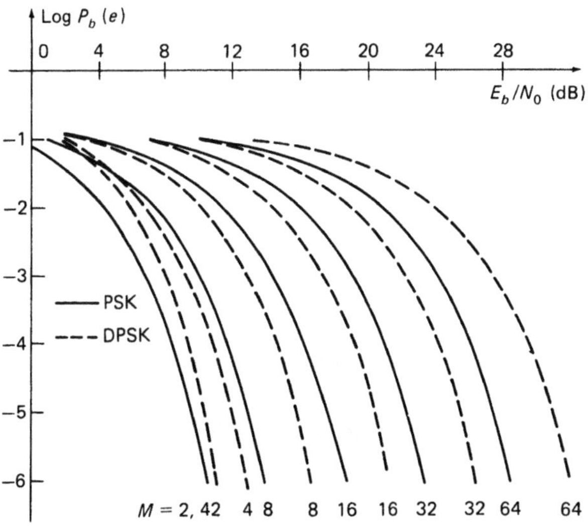


Fig. 7.9. Bit error probability as a function at signal-to-noise ratio per bit, $E_b/N_0$ for ideal $M$-ary PSK and DPSK.

For large signal-to-noise ratio (such that $P(e) \leq 10^{-3}$) and $M > 2$, we can approximate

$$P(e) = 2\,Q((2\,\rho_S)^{0.5} \sin(\pi/M)) \tag{7.2.42}$$

The error probability as a function of signal to noise is shown in Fig. 7.8. The bit error probability as a function of signal-to-noise ratio per bit is shown in Fig. 7.9. In doing so we assume that a Gray code is used; thus $E_b = E_S/\log_2 M$ and $P_b(e) = P(e)/\log_2 M$.

## 7.3 DPSK

A model of a differential PSK (DPSK) system is shown in Fig. 7.10, where (a) is the bandpass system and (b) is the equivalent baseband system. DPSK is an improvement upon PSK, because the receiver is not required to generate the phase of the transmitter carrier in order to detect the transmitted symbols. Instead the receiver computes the phase difference at consecutive time instants $t_{k-1}$ and $t_k = t_{k-1} + T$. The information symbols, $\{a_i\}$, are respresented as phase differences at the transmitter rather then absolute phase, so that the phase transmitted during the interval $iT \leq t \leq (i+1)T$ is

$$a_i'\pi/M = (a_{i-1}' + a_i)\pi/M \tag{7.3.1}$$

Because the phase is taken modulo 2 $\pi$, both $a_i$ and $a_i'$ are taken from the set $\{2\,m - 1, m = 1, 2, \ldots, M)$. The modulated signal is

$$\begin{aligned} s_M(t) &= \mathrm{Re}\,(A \exp\{j(\omega_C t + K_p \sum_i a_i' u(t - iT) + \phi_T)\} \\ &= \mathrm{Re}\,\{A \exp\{j(\omega_C t + \phi_T)\} \sum_i \exp(jK_p a_i') u(t - iT))\} \end{aligned} \tag{7.3.2}$$

where $K_p = \pi/M$. The output of the receiver filter is

$$r_M(t) = \mathrm{Re}\,\{r(t) \exp\{j(\omega_C t + \phi_T)\}\} \tag{7.3.3}$$

where

$$r(t) = A \sum_i \exp(jK_p a_i') g(t - iT) + n(t) \tag{7.3.4}$$

$$g(t) = u_T(t) * h_T(t) * h_C(t) * h_R(t) \tag{7.3.5}$$

$$n(t) = n_I(t) + jn_Q(t) \tag{7.3.6}$$

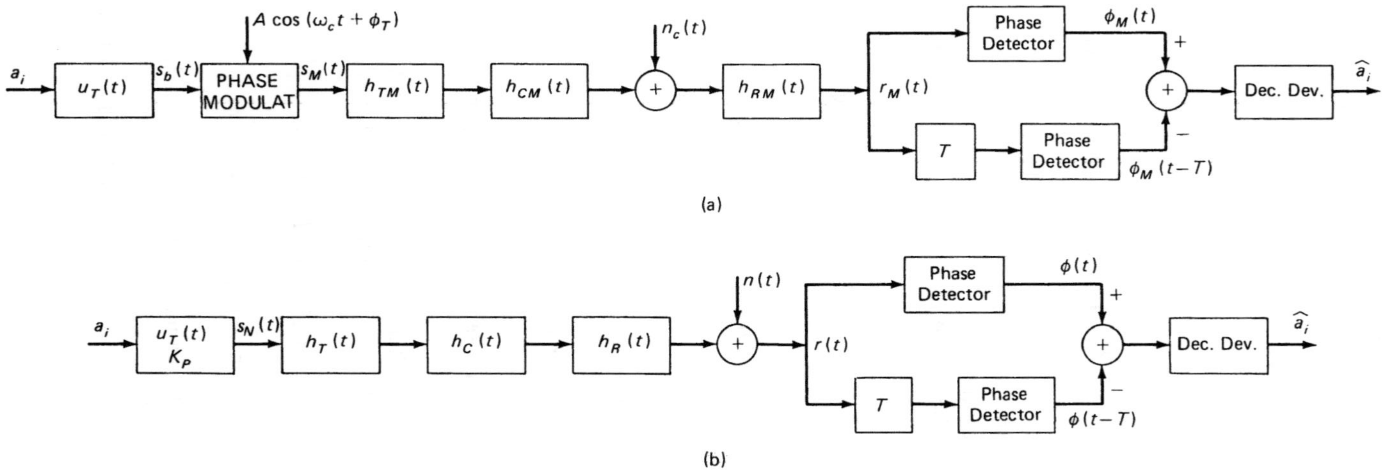


Fig. 7.10 Model of DPSK system: (a) bandpass system, (b) equivalent baseband system.

$n_I(t)$, $n_Q(t)$ are zero-mean, independent random variables with identical variance

$$\sigma_n^2 = N_0 \int_{-\infty}^{\infty} |H_R(f)|^2 \, df \tag{7.3.7}$$

and autocorrelation

$$R_n(\tau) = N_0 \int_{-\infty}^{\infty} |H_R(f)|^2 \cos (2\pi f\tau) \, df \tag{7.3.8}$$

Section 1.8 showed that $n_I(t)$, $n_Q(t)$ are independent random processes if $H_R(f)$ is a symmetric function.

Let $\phi_M(t)$ and $\phi_r(t)$ be the phase of $r_M(t)$ and $r(t)$, respectively. The phase differences are

$$\Delta\phi_M = \phi_M(t_k) - \phi_M(t_{k-1}) = \omega_C T + \phi_r(t_k) - \phi_r(t_{k-1}) = \omega_C T + \Delta\phi \tag{7.3.9}$$

If we assume that $\omega_C T$ is an integer multiple of $2\pi$, we obtain

$$\Delta\phi_M = \Delta\phi \qquad (\text{modulo } 2\pi) \tag{7.3.10}$$

Thus it is sufficient to compute the phase of $r_k$ and $r_{k-1}$, which from (7.3.4) is

$$r_k = A \sum_i \exp (jK_p a_i') g_{k-i} + n_k = s_k + n_k \tag{7.3.11}$$

$$r_{k-1} = A \sum_i \exp (jK_p a_i') g_{k-1-i} + n_{k-1} = s_{k-1} + n_{k-1} \tag{7.3.12}$$

and we denote $x_k = x(t_k)$ where $x$ stands for $r$, $g$, and $n$. If $g(t)$ is a Nyquist function ($g_0 = 1$, $g_i = 0$, $i \neq 0$), there is no ISI, and

$$r_k = A \exp (jK_p a_k') + n_k \tag{7.3.13}$$

$$r_{k-1} = A \exp (jK_p a_{k-1}') + n_{k-1} \tag{7.3.14}$$

Without loss in generality we may assume that $k = 1$. Thus

$$\Delta\phi = \arg r_1 - \arg r_0 = \arg (r_1 r_0^*) = \arg (v) \tag{7.3.15}$$

where

$$v = r_1 r_0^* \tag{7.3.16}$$

The decision rule is the same as in PSK, namely, (7.2.17) with $\phi_{r,k}$ replaced by $\Delta\phi$; hence the error probability can be computed as in (7.2.18) with $\phi_{r,0}$ replaced by $\Delta\phi$ or can be bounded as in (7.2.19), provided $r_Q = \text{Im}\,(r(t_0))$ is replaced by

$$v_Q = \text{Im}\,(v) \tag{7.3.17}$$

i.e.

$$P_L = P(\text{Im}\,(v) < 0) = P(\text{Re}\,(-jv) < 0) \tag{7.3.18}$$

Since

$$\text{Re}\,(-jv) = \text{Re}\,(-jr_1 r_0^*) = (|r_1 + jr_0|^2 - |r_1 - jr_0|^2)/4 \tag{7.3.19}$$

we also obtain

$$P_L = P(R_+ < R_-) \tag{7.3.20}$$

where $R_\pm$ is the amplitude of

$$r_\pm = (r_1 \pm jr_0)/2 \tag{7.3.21}$$

For $M = 2$, the error probability is $P_L$, and for $M \geqq 4$ the error probability is closer to 2 $P_L$ then to $P_L$.

### 7.3.1 Ideal DPSK

By *ideal* we mean that (7.3.13) and (7.3.14) hold. The difference between the phases is, from (7.3.15) and (7.3.1)

$$\Delta\phi = \phi_{r1} - \phi_{r0} = \phi_{s1} - \phi_{s0} + \theta_1 - \theta_0 = \pi a_1/M + \Delta\theta \tag{7.3.22}$$

where

$$\Delta\theta = \theta_1 - \theta_0 \tag{7.3.23}$$

and

$$\theta_i = \phi_{ri} - \phi_{si} \qquad i = 1, 0 \tag{7.3.24}$$

are the phase errors. The error probability is as in (7.2.35) or (7.2.39), provided $\theta$ is replaced by

$$\psi = \Delta\theta \qquad (\text{mod } 2\,\pi) \tag{7.3.25}$$

The pdf of $\Delta\theta$ can be computed from

$$p_{\Delta\theta}(\Delta\theta) = \int_{-\infty}^{\pi} p_{\theta 1}(\Delta\theta + \theta_0) p_{\theta 0}(\theta_0)\, d\theta_0 \tag{7.3.26}$$

where the pdfs of $\theta_1$ and $\theta_0$ are given in eq. (7.2.31) provided $\rho_0$ is replaced by $\rho_1 = \rho_{s1}$ and $\rho_0 = \rho_{s0}$, respectively. In our particular case, in view of (7.3.13) and (7.3.14)

$$\rho_1 = \rho_0 = \rho_s \tag{7.3.27}$$

but in general they may differ. In writing (7.3.27) we assume that $\theta_0$ and $\theta_1$ are independent rvs, which is true if $n_k$ and $n_{k-1}$ are uncorrelated. This is certainly true when the receiver filter is the square root of a Nyquist function and also true whenever the autocorrelation of noise at the receiver output $R_n(T)$ is close to zero. For Butterworth filters of order $N$ and 3-dB bandwidth, $f_0$, $R_n(T)/R_n(0)$ is shown in Fig. 7.11.

To compute (7.3.26), we expand (7.2.31) in a Fourier series

$$p_{\theta i}(\theta_i) = \sum_{k=0}^{\infty} \varepsilon_k C_k(\rho_i) \cos (k\theta_i)/(2\pi), \qquad i = 0, 1 \tag{7.3.28}$$

where

$$\varepsilon_0 = 1, \qquad \varepsilon_k = 2 \qquad k > 0 \tag{7.3.29}$$

$$C_k(\rho_i) = \int_{-\pi}^{\pi} p_{\theta i}(\theta_i) \cos (k\theta_i)\, d\theta_i = (\pi\rho_i/4)^{0.5} \exp(-\rho_i/2)\{I_{(k-1)/2}(\rho_i/2) + I_{(k+1)/2}(\rho_i/2)\} \tag{7.3.30}$$

where

$$I_k(z) = \int_0^{2\pi} \exp(z \cos\theta) \cos(k\theta)\, d\theta/(2\pi) \tag{7.3.31}$$

is the modified Bessel function of order $k$. When we substitute (7.3.28) into (7.3.26) and apply the orthogonality of the cosine function $\{\cos (k\theta)\}$, we obtain

$$p_{\Delta\theta}(\Delta\theta) = 0.5 \sum_{k=0}^{\infty} \varepsilon_k C_k(\rho_1) C_k(\rho_0) \cos (k\Delta\theta)/(2\pi) \tag{7.3.32}$$

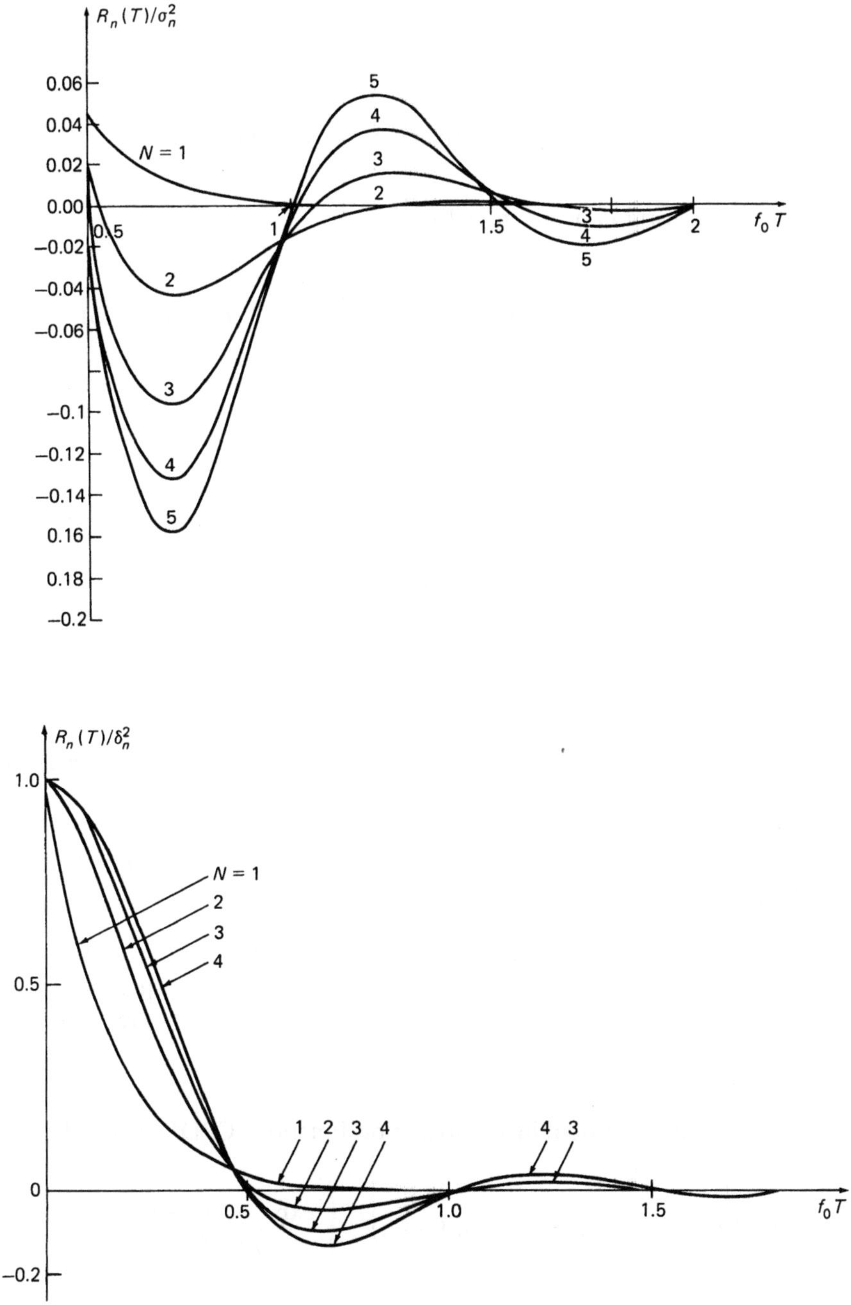


Fig. 7.11. Correlation at time $T$ of noise at output of Butterworth filter of order $N$ and 3-dB bandwidth $f_0T$.

The pdf of $\psi$ is

$$p_\psi(\beta) = p_{\Delta\theta}(\beta) + p_{\Delta\theta}(\beta + 2\pi)$$
$$= \sum_{k=0}^{\infty} \varepsilon_k C_k(\rho_1) C_k(\rho_0) \cos(k\beta)/(2\pi) \tag{7.3.33}$$

A closed form formula is given in Ref. 7.11

$$p_\psi(\beta) = (2\pi)^{-1} \exp(-\rho_m)\{\cosh(\rho_d) + 0.5 \int_0^\pi (\rho_m \sin\alpha + \rho_g \cos\beta)$$
$$\cosh(\rho_d \cos\alpha) \exp(\rho_g \sin\alpha \sin\beta)\, d\alpha\} \tag{7.3.34}$$

where

$$\rho_m = 0.5(\rho_1 + \rho_0),\ \rho_d = 0.5(\rho_1 - \rho_0),\ \rho_g = (\rho_0\rho_1)^{0.5} \tag{7.3.35}$$

When $\rho_0 = \rho_1 = \rho_s$, this is simplified to

$$p_\psi(\beta) = (2\pi)^{-1} \exp(-\rho_s)\{1 + 0.5 \int_0^\pi \rho_s(\sin\alpha + \cos\beta)$$
$$\exp(\rho_s \sin\alpha \sin\beta)\, d\alpha\} \tag{7.3.36}$$

This pdf is shown in Fig. 7.12.

For large values of $\rho_s$, this is approximated by (for $\beta = \pi/2$ there is equality)

$$p_\psi(\beta) \simeq \begin{cases} (\rho_s/(2\pi\cos\beta))^{0.5} \cos^2(\beta/2) \exp(-2\rho_s \sin^2(\beta/2)) & 0 \leqq \beta \leqq \pi/2 \\ (1 + \rho_s)\exp(-\rho_s)/(2\pi) & \beta = \pi/2 \\ \sec^2\beta/(2\pi\rho_s)\exp(-\rho_s) & \pi/2 < \beta \leqq \pi \end{cases} \tag{7.3.37}$$

The complementary probability distribution function (CPDF) is for $\beta \geqq 0$

$$Q_\psi(\beta) = P(\psi \geqq \beta) = \rho_g \sin\beta\, (4\pi)^{-1} \int_0^\pi \frac{\exp(-f(\alpha, \beta))}{f(\alpha, \beta)}\, d\alpha \tag{7.3.38}$$

where

$$f(\alpha, \beta) = \rho_m - \rho_d \cos\alpha - \rho_g \sin\alpha \cos\beta \tag{7.3.39}$$

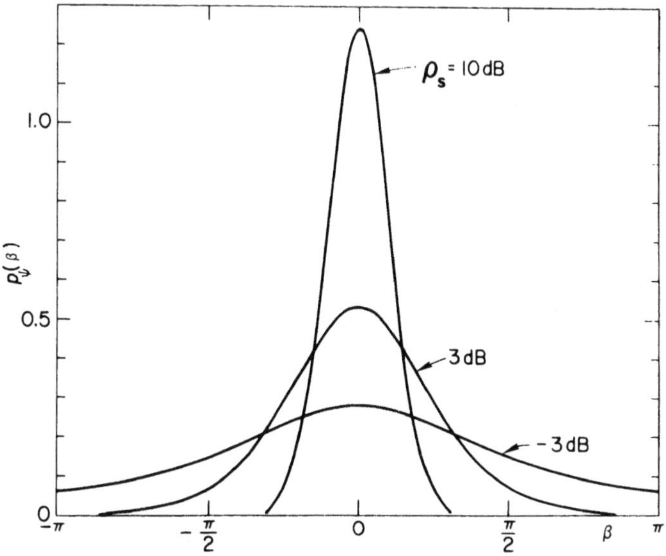


Fig. 7.12. The pdf of the modulo 2π difference of two phases (R. F. Pawula, "On the Theory of Error Rates for Narrow Band Digital FM," *IEEE Tr. Comm.*, Vol. COM-29, November 1981 pp. 1634–1643. Copyright © 1981 IEEE).

which for $\rho_0 = \rho_1 = \rho_s$ is simplified to

$$f(\alpha, \beta) = \rho_s(1 - \sin\alpha\cos\beta) \tag{7.3.40}$$

The CPDF is shown in Fig. 7.13. For large signal-to-noise ratios we have the approximation (for $\beta = \pi/2$ there is equality)

$$Q_\psi(\beta) \simeq \begin{cases} \cot(\beta/2)(8\,\pi\rho_s\cos\beta)^{-0.5}\exp(-2\,\rho_s\sin^2(\beta/2)) & 0 \leqq \beta \leqq \pi/2 \\ 0.25\exp(-\rho_s) & \beta = \pi/2 \\ -\tan\beta\exp(-\rho_s)/(2\,\pi\rho_s) & \pi/2 < \beta \leqq \pi \end{cases} \tag{7.3.41}$$

The error probability is

$$P(e) = 2\int_{\pi/M}^{\pi} p_\psi(\beta)\,d\psi = 2\,Q_\psi(\pi/M) \tag{7.3.42}$$

which for the binary case is simply

$$P(e) = 0.5\exp(-\rho_s) \tag{7.3.43}$$

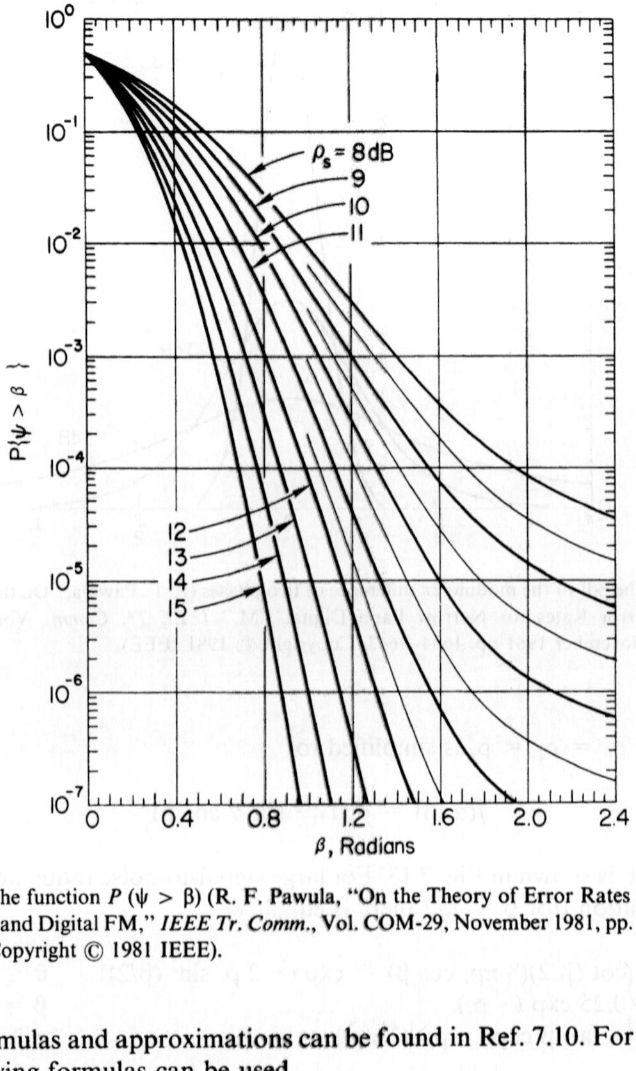


Fig. 7.13. The function $P(\psi > \beta)$ (R. F. Pawula, "On the Theory of Error Rates for Narrow Band Digital FM," *IEEE Tr. Comm.*, Vol. COM-29, November 1981, pp. 1634–1643. Copyright © 1981 IEEE).

Other formulas and approximations can be found in Ref. 7.10. For example, the following formulas can be used

$$P(e) \simeq 2\, Q((2\,\rho_s)^{0.5} \sin(\pi\, 2^{-0.5}/M)) \tag{7.3.44}$$

$$P(e) \lesssim 2\, Q\left\{\rho_s\left(\frac{2}{1+2\,\rho_s}\right)^{0.5} \sin(\pi/M)\right\} \tag{7.3.45}$$

$$P(e) \simeq 2 \cos(0.5\,\pi/M)(\cos(\pi/M))^{-0.5}\, Q((\rho_s)^{0.5}\, 2 \sin(0.5\,\pi/M)) \tag{7.3.46}$$

The error probability as a function of signal-to-noise ratio is shown in Fig. 7.8, where we assumed that the receiver is matched to the transmitter. The bit error probability, as a function of signal-to-noise ratio per bit, is presented in Fig. 7.9.

### 7.3.2 Bounds to error probability

Here we are computing eq. (7.3.20). If we assume that $R_+$ and $R_-$ are independent rvs, then

$$P_L = P(R_- > R_+) = \int_0^\infty \left\{ \int_{R+}^\infty p_{R-}(R_-)\, dR_- \right\} p_{R+}(R_+)\, dR_+ \quad (7.3.47)$$

where the pdf of $R_\pm$ is given in (7.2.33) after replacement of $A_r$, $\rho_s$ by $R_\pm$, $\rho_\pm$, respectively, where

$$\rho_\pm = 0.5\ R_{s\pm}^2/\sigma_\pm^2 \quad (7.3.48)$$

$\sigma_\pm^2$ is the variance of $r_\pm$ in (7.3.21), and $R_{s\pm}$ is the amplitude of the signal component of $r_\pm$.
Letting

$$r_\pm = s_\pm + n_\pm = R_{s\pm} \exp(j\phi_{s\pm}) + n_\pm \quad (7.3.49)$$

we obtain from (7.3.11) and (7.3.12)

$$s_\pm = (s_1 \pm js_0)/2 \quad (7.3.50)$$

$$n_+ = n_{I+} + jn_{Q+} = (n_1 + jn_0)/2 = 0.5\ \{n_{I,1} - n_{Q,0} + j(n_{Q,1} + n_{I,0})\} \quad (7.3.51)$$

$$n_- = n_{I-} + jn_{Q-} = (n_1 - jn_0)/2 = 0.5\ \{n_{I,1} + n_{Q,0} + j(n_{Q,1} - n_{I,0})\} \quad (7.3.52)$$

$n_\pm$ are complex, zero-mean, Gaussian rvs with variance and correlation

$$\overline{n_{I\pm}^2} = 0.5\ (\sigma_n^2 \mp R_{nI,nQ}(T)) \quad (7.3.53)$$

$$\overline{n_{Q\pm}^2} = 0.5\ (\sigma_n^2 \pm R_{nI,nQ}(-T)) \quad (7.3.54)$$

$$\overline{n_{I+}n_{I-}} = \overline{n_{I+}n_{Q+}} = \overline{n_{Q+}n_{Q-}} = \overline{n_{Q-}n_{I-}} = 0 \quad (7.3.55)$$

$$\overline{n_{I+}n_{Q-}} = -\overline{n_{I-}n_{Q+}} = R_n(T) \quad (7.3.56)$$

In most cases $H_R(f)$ is a symmetric function; hence $n_I$ and $n_Q$ are uncorrelated. Thus

$$\overline{n_{I\pm}^2} = \overline{n_{Q\pm}^2} = 0.5\,\sigma_n^2 \tag{7.3.57}$$

We shall also assume that $R_n(T) = 0$, which is certainly true when $H_R(f)$ is the square root of a Nyquist function and approximately true for Butterworth filters. This implies that $r_+(r_-)$ are independent Gaussian rvs with average $s_+(s_-)$ and the same variance

$$\sigma_\pm^2 = 0.5\,\overline{n_+ n_+^*} = 0.5\,\overline{n_I n_I^*} = 0.5\,\sigma_n^2 = \sigma^2 \tag{7.3.58}$$

Thus

$$\rho_\pm = R_{s\pm}^2/\sigma_n^2 \tag{7.3.59}$$

and we can indeed use (7.3.47). When we substitute (7.2.33) into (7.3.47), we obtain

$$P_L = \int_0^\infty Q(R_{s-}/\sigma,\ R_+/\sigma)\,p_{R+}(R_+)\,dR_+ \tag{7.3.60}$$

where

$$Q(a, b) = \int_b^\infty x \exp\{-0.5\,(a^2 + x^2)\} I_0(ax)\,dx \tag{7.3.61}$$

is the Marcum function[7.12] with the properties (note that $I_0(0) = 1$)

$$Q(a, 0) = 1 \tag{7.3.62}$$

$$Q(0, b) = \exp(-b^2/2) \tag{7.3.63}$$

It was shown in Ref. 7.13 that

$$\begin{aligned} P_L &= 0.5\,\{1 - Q(\rho_+^{0.5}, \rho_-^{0.5}) + Q(\rho_-^{0.5}, \rho_+^{0.5})\} \\ &= 0.5\,(\rho_+ - \rho_-)(\rho_+ + \rho_-)^{-1} \int_{0.5(\rho_+ + \rho_-)}^\infty \exp(-y) \\ &\quad I_0(2\,(\rho_+\rho_-)^{0.5}(\rho_+ + \rho_-)^{-1}y)\,dy \end{aligned} \tag{7.3.64}$$

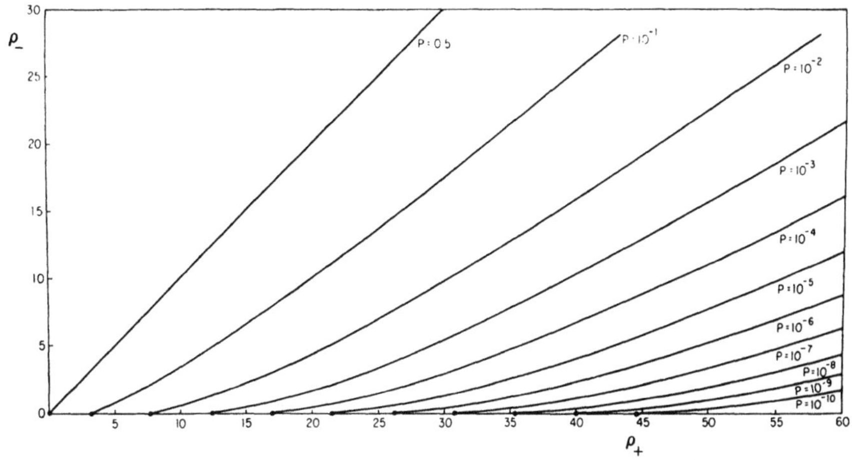


Fig. 7.14. The function $P = 0.5\{1 - Q(\rho_+^{0.5}, \rho_-^{0.5}) + Q(\rho_-^{0.5}, \rho_b^{0.5})\}$ (S. Stein, "Unified Analysis of Certain Coherent and Noncoherent Binary Communication Systems," *IRE Tr. Inf. Th.*, Vol. IT-10, January 1964, pp. 43–51. Copyright © 1964 IEEE).

The function is illustrated in Fig. 7.14

*No intersymbol interference (ISI)*[7.13–7.16] If we assume that (7.3.13) and (7.3.14) are valid and substitute these equations into (7.3.50), we obtain

$$s_{\pm} = 0.5\, A\{\exp(j\pi a_1'/M) \pm \exp(j\pi a_0'/M)\} \tag{7.3.65}$$

with amplitudes

$$R_{s\pm} = A\{0.5\,\{1 \pm \sin(\pi a_1/M)\}\}^{0.5} \tag{7.3.66}$$

where $a_1 = 1$. Substitution into (7.3.59) gives

$$\rho_{\pm} = \rho_s(1 \pm \sin(\pi/M)) \tag{7.3.67}$$

where $\rho_s$ is defined in (7.2.28) because in this case $A_s = A$. We substitute (7.3.67) into (7.3.64), resulting in

$$P_L = 0.5 \sin(\pi/M) \int_{\rho_s}^{\infty} \exp(-y) I_0(y \cos(\pi/M))\, dy \tag{7.3.68}$$

It is shown in Ref. 7.14 that $P_L$ can be bounded by

$$KP_+ \leqq P_L \leqq P_+ \tag{7.3.69}$$

where

$$P_+ = 0.5\,\pi \cos(0.5\,\pi/M)\cos^{-0.5}(\pi/M)Q(2\,\rho_s^{0.5}\sin(\pi/M)) \quad (7.3.70)$$

and

$$K = (2/\pi)\{1 - 2\,Q(\rho^{0.5}\pi\cos^{0.5}(\pi/M))\} \quad (7.3.71)$$

Because the error probability is as in (7.2.19), we obtain bounds on $P(e)$

$$KP_+ \leqq P(e) \leqq 2\,P_+ \quad (7.3.72)$$

and the ratio between the upper and lower bound is $2/K$, which for $M > 4$ $\rho > 1$ is bounded by

$$\pi \leqq 2/K \leqq 1.035\,\pi \quad (7.3.73)$$

These are the tightest available bounds for DPSK.

*Effect of ISI*[7.4, 7.17–7.18] Here we obtain from (7.3.11), (7.3.12), and (7.3.50)

$$s_\pm = 0.5\,A\sum_k\{\exp(j\pi a'_{1-k}/M) \pm \exp(j\pi a'_{-k}/M)\}g_k \quad (7.3.74)$$

Although generally $\{g_k\}$ may be complex if the transfer function, $G(f)$, is symmetric, they are real. We shall assume that indeed this is the case; thus the amplitudes are

$$R_{s\pm} = (A/2^{0.5})\left\{\sum_k g_k^2(1 \pm \sin(\pi a_{1-k}/M))\right\}^{0.5} \quad (7.3.75)$$

Because $a_1 = 1$, we obtain after substitution into (7.3.59)

$$\rho_\pm = \rho\left\{g_0^2(1 \pm \sin(\pi/M)) + \sum_{k\neq 0} g_k^2(1 \pm \sin(a_{1-k}\pi/M))\right\} \quad (7.3.76)$$

When there is no interference ($g_0 = 1$, $g_k = 0$, $k \neq 0$) this is reduced to (7.3.67). We substitute (7.3.76) into (7.3.64), the result being

$$P_L = 0.5\,K_1\int_{\rho E_g}^{\infty}\exp(-y)I_0(K_2 y)\,dy \quad (7.3.77)$$

where

$$E_g = \sum_k g_k^2 \quad (7.3.78)$$

$$K_1 = \sum_k g_k^2 \sin(\pi a_{1-k}/M)/E_g \tag{7.3.79}$$

$$K_2 = \left\{ \sum_k g_k^2 (1 + \sin(\pi a_{1-k}/M)) \sum_k g_k^2 (1 - \sin(\pi a_{1-k}/M)) \right\}^{0.5} \Big/ E_g \tag{7.3.80}$$

and $a_1 = 1$. In the actual computation we assume that only $N + 1$ terms in (7.3.78) are significant. The same terms are used in calculation of $K_1$ and $K_2$. Thus $K_1$ and $K_2$ depend on a set of $N$ symbols, say $\mathbf{a} = \{a_1, a_2, \ldots, a_N\}$, and similarly $P_L$ is in fact $P_L(\mathbf{a})$. There are $L = M^N$ realizations of $\mathbf{a}$. Thus the error probability is in fact

$$\overline{P_L} \leqq P(e) \leqq 2\,\overline{P_L} \tag{7.3.81}$$

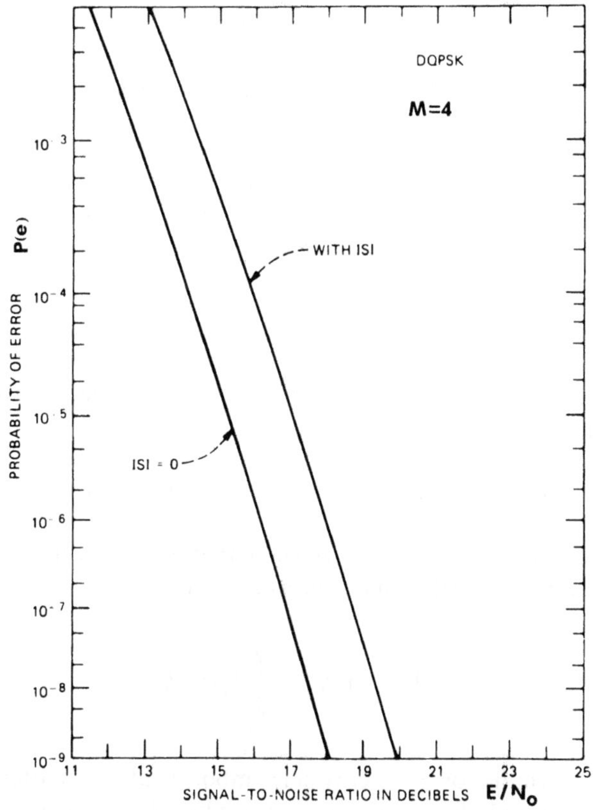


Fig. 7.15. Error probability as a function of $E/N_0$ for quaternary DPSK with and without ISI (reprinted with permission from *The Bell System Technical Journal*. Copyright © 1981, AT&T).

*Example* 7.3.1 Quaternary DPSK
We assume here that

$$g(t) = u_T(t) * h_T(t) * h_R(t)$$

where $h_T(t)$ and $h_R(t)$ are Butterworth filters of order 4 and 3-dB bandwidth $f_{T0}T = 1$ and $f_{R0}T = 0.52$, respectively. The error probability as a function of signal-to-noise ratio is shown in Fig. 7.15. In the same figure, taken from Ref. 7.4, the case of no ISI is also shown.

The effect of cochannel interference and impulsive noise can be found in Refs. 7.20–7.21.

## 7.4 SUMMARY

In this chapter we have derived the error probability of PSK and DPSK. In PSK the shaping function may be rectangular (this was discussed at length in Chapter 6), nonooverlapping, and overlapping. It was found that the usage of the latter shaping function does not improve the error probability performance with respect to the former. In dealing with DPSK, a rectangular shaping function has been assumed throughout. Exact values and bounds on the error probability have been presented with or without intersymbol interference.

## 7.5 PROBLEMS

7.2.1 A PSK signal has amplitude $A$. The signal is applied to a system with total response

$$g(t) = b(t) * h_T(t) * h_R(t) = g_T(t) * h_R(t)$$

The white noise has a psd of $N_0/2$. Assume that $b(t)$ is a rectangular pulse of duration $T$ and that $h_R(t)$ is matched to $g_T(t)$. Let

$$\int_{-\infty}^{\infty} g_T^2(t)\, dt = \int_{-\infty}^{\infty} h_R^2(t)\, dt$$

a. Write a formula for the energy per symbol, $E$, at transmitter filter input.
b. Write a formula for the energy per symbol, $E_s$, at receiver filter input.
c. Write a formula for the noise power, $\sigma_n^2$, at receiver filter output.
d. Compare the ratios $E/\sigma_n^2$, $E_s/\sigma_n^2$, and $\rho = 0.5\, A^2/\sigma_n^2$. When are they identical?

7.2.2 In a PSK system, the shaping function is a raised cosine of duration $T$. Assume a system such that

$$h(t) = h_R(t) = \omega_0 \exp(-\omega_0 t)u(t)$$

$\omega_0 = 2\pi f_0$, and $f_0 T = 1, 1.2, 1.4$.

a. Compute

$$g(t, a_0) = \exp(j\pi a_0/Mh_s(t))u_T(t) * h(t)$$

assuming that $a_0 \in \{1, 3, \ldots, 2M - 1)\}$ with $M = 2, 4, 8$.

b. Determine in each case the value of $t$ for which $|g(t, a_0)|$ is maximum. Denote that value by $t_{op}$.

c. Assume that only two past symbols and one future symbol contribute to the intersymbol interference. Compute the error probability as a function of signal-to-noise ratio $E/N_0$ for the various values of $f_0 T$.

7.2.3 The same as problem 7.2.2, but the shaping functions are

a. triangular of duration $T$

b. cosine of duration $T$

c. raised cosine of duration $2T$.

7.2.4 In a PSK system the shaping function is a raised cosine of duration $T$ or $2T$; the symbols are binary, quaternary, or octal; and the system is such that

$$h(t) = h_R(t) * h_T(t)$$

where $h_R(t)$ and $h_T(t)$ are Butterworth filters of the same order $N = 1, 2, 3, 4$. Compute the error probability as a function of signal-to-noise ratio assuming that the 3-dB bandwidths of the filters are $f_{T0}T = 1.5 f_{R0}T$, $f_{0R}T = 1$. Optimize the sampling time. Assume only three or four interfering symbols.

7.2.5 Derive eqs. (7.2.26), (7.2.27), and (7.2.33).

7.2.6 Derive eq. (7.2.40).

7.2.7 Derive eq. (7.2.41).

7.3.1 Show that eq. (7.2.19) can be used to bound the error probability of DPSK, provided $P_L$ is as given in eq. (7.3.18).

7.3.2 Show that eq. (7.3.33) is the pdf of

$$\psi = \theta_1 - \theta_0 \bmod (2\pi)$$

7.3.3 Prove eq. (7.3.34).

7.3.4 Prove eq. (7.3.37).

7.3.5 Derive the approximation in (7.3.46), (7.3.44), and (7.3.45).

7.3.6 Prove eqs. (7.3.53)–(7.3.56).

7.3.7 Prove eq. (7.3.64).

7.3.8 Derive eqs. (7.3.66) and (7.3.68).

7.3.9 Derive eq. (7.3.70).

7.3.10 In a DPSK system the symbols are binary. Assume that

$$h(t) = h_T(t) * h_R(t)$$

where $h_T(t)$ and $h_R(t)$ are Butterworth filters of order $N = 1$ and 3-dB bandwidth $f_{T0}T = f_{R0}T = 1.1$. Assume only three interfering terms in intersymbol interference.

a. Compute the error probability as a function of signal-to-noise ratio $E/N_0$.
b. Repeat (a) assuming quaternary symbols.
c. Repeat (a) assuming $N = 2, 3, 4$.
d. Repeat (b) assuming $N = 2, 3, 4$.
e. Repeat (a) assuming $M = 8$ symbols.
f. Repeat (a) assuming $N = 2, 3, 4$.

## 7.6 REFERENCES


7.1 C. R. Cahn, "performance of Digital Phase Modulation Communication Systems," *IRE Tr. Comm. Sys.*, Vo. CS-7, May 1959, pp. 3–6.

7.2 O. Shimbo, R. J. Fang, and M. Celebiler, "Performance of *M*-ary PSK Systems in Gaussian Noise and Intersymbol Interference," *IEEE Tr. Inf. Theory*, Vol. IT-19, January 1973, pp. 44–58.

7.3 S. Kabasawa, N. Morinaga, and T. Namekawa, "*M*-ary CPSK Detection with Noisy Reference and Interference," *IEEE Tr. Aer. Elect. Sys.*, Vol. AES-16, September 1980, pp. 712–719.

7.4 V. K. Prabhu and J. Salz, "On the Performance of Phase Shift Keying Systems," *BSTJ*, Vol. 60, December 1981, pp. 2307–2343.

7.5 S. Benedetto and E. Biglieri, "Performance of *M*-ary PSK Systems in the Presence of Intersymbol Interference and Additive Noise," *Alta Frequenza*, Vol. XLI, 1972, pp. 225–239.

7.6 V. K. Prabhu, "Error Probability Performance of *M*-ary CPSK systems with Intersymbol Interference," *IEEE Tr. Comm.*, Vol. COM-21, February 1973, pp. 97–108.

7.7 S. Benedetto, E. Biglieri, and C. Castelani, "Combined Effects of Intersymbol, Interchannel and Co-channel Interferences in $M$-ary CPSK Systems," *IEEE Tr. Comm.*, Vol. COM-21, September 1973, pp. 997–1008,

7.8 V. K. Prabhu, "PSK Type Modulation with Overlapping Baseband Pulses," *IEEE Tr. Comm.*, Vol. COM-25, September 1977, pp. 980–990.

7.9 F. S. Weinstein, "A Table of the Cumulative Probability Distribution of the Phase of a Sine Wave in Narrow-Band Normal Noise," *IEEE Tr. Inf. Theory*, Vol. IT-23, September 1977, pp. 640–643.

7.10 R. F. Pawula, S. O. Rice, and J. H. Roberts, "Distribution of the Phase Angle between Two Vectors Perturbed by Gaussian Noise," *IEEE Tr. Comm.*, Vol. COM-30, August 1982, pp. 1828–1841.

7.11 R. F. Pawula, "On the Theory of Error Rates of Narrow Band Digital FM," *IEEE Tr. Comm.*, Vol. COM-29, November 1981, pp. 1634–1643.

7.12 Y. I. Marcum, "A Statistical Theory of Target Detection by Pulsed Radar," *IEEE Tr. Inf. Theory*, Vol. IT-6, April 1960, pp. 145–267.

7.13 S. Stein, "Unified Analysis of Certain Coherent and Noncoherent Binary Communication Systems," *IRE Tr. Inf. Theory*, Vol. IT-10, January 1964, pp. 43–51.

7.14 V. K. Prabhu "Error Rate for Differential PSK," *IEEE Tr. Comm.*, Vol. COM-30, December 1982, pp. 2547–2550.

7.15 A. Arthurs and H. Dym, "On the Optimum Detection of Digital Signals in the Presence of White Gaussian Noise—A Geometric Interpolation and a Study of Three Basic Data Transmission Systems," *IRE Tr. Comm. Sys.*, Vol. CS-10, December 1962, pp. 336–372.

7.16 J. J. Busgang and M. Leiter, "Error Rate Approximation for Differential Phase Shift Keying," *IRE Tr. Comm. Sys.*, Vol. CS-12, March 1964, pp. 18–27.

7.17 W. M. Hubbard, "The Effect of Intersymbol Interference on Error Rate in Binary Differentially Coherent Phase Shift Keyed Systems," *BSTJ*, Vol. 46, July–August 1967, pp. 1149–1172.

7.18 L. Calandrino, G. Crippa, and G. Immovilli, "Intersymbol Interference in Binary and Quaternary PSK and DPSK System," *Alta Frequenza*, Vol. XXXVIII, May 1969, pp. 87–94 (Part 1), pp. 156–163 (Part 2).

7.19 O. Shimbo, M. J. Celebiler, and R. J. Fang, "Performance Analysis of DPSK Systems in Both the Thermal Noise and Intersymbol Interferences," *IEEE Tr. Comm. Techn.*, Vol. COM-19, December 1971, pp. 1179–1188.

7.20 A. S. Rosenbaum, "Binary PSK Error Probabilities with Multiple Cochannel Interferences," *IEEE Tr. Comm. Techn.*, Vol. COM-18, June 1970, pp. 241–253.

7.21 A. S. Rosenbaum, "Error Performance of Multiphase DPSK with Noise and Interference," *IEEE Tr. Comm. Techn.*, Vol. COM-18, December 1970, pp. 821–824.

7.22 S. Oshita and K. Feher, "Performance of PSK and DPSK Systems in an Impulsive and Gaussian Noise Environment," *IEEE Tr. Comm.*, Vol. COM-30, December 1982, pp. 2540–2546.

# 8 FSK

## 8.1 INTRODUCTION

In frequency shift keying (FSK) the instantaneous frequency is a linear function of the transmitted symbols. A model of an FSK system is shown in Fig. 8.1, and various detectors are shown in Figs. 8.2–8.4. We assume that the symbols $\{a_i\}$ are independent, equiprobable, are transmitted at the rate of $R = 1/T$ symbols per second, and take values from the $M$-ary set $\mathring{A}_\pm = \{\pm 1, \pm 3, \ldots, \pm(M - 1)\} = \{a(1), \ldots, a(M)\}$, so that

$$a(m) = 2m - 1 - M \tag{8.1.1}$$

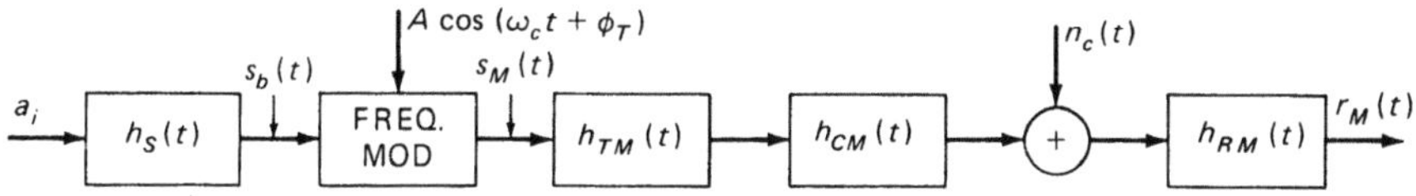


Fig. 8.1. Model of FSK transmitter and channel.

Prior to modulation the symbols are converted into a baseband signal

$$s_b(t) = \sum_i a_i h_S(t - iT) \tag{8.1.2}$$

where the shaping function $h_S(t)$ is arbitrary and may have a duration exceeding $T$. The majority of the results in the literature are for systems with binary symbols ($\pm 1$) and NRZ shaping function

$$h_S(t) = u_T(t) = u(t) - u(t - T) \tag{8.1.3}$$

where $u(t)$ is a unit step function.

The modulated signal is

$$s_M(t) = A \cos(\omega_C t + \phi_T + \phi(t)) = \mathrm{Re}\,\{A \exp(j\phi(t)) \exp(j(\omega_C t + \phi_T))\} \tag{8.1.4}$$

where $A$, $f_C = \omega_C/(2\pi)$, and $\phi_T$ are the amplitude, carrier frequency, and phase of unmodulated carrier signal and

$$\phi(t) = \omega_d \int_{-\infty}^{t} s_b(t')\, dt' \tag{8.1.5}$$

where $f_d = \omega_d/(2\pi)$ is a frequency deviation. The instantaneous frequency deviation is

$$f_{\text{dev}}(t) = (2\pi)^{-1}\, d\phi(t)/dt = f_d \sum_i a_i h_S(t - iT) \tag{8.1.6}$$

We showed in Chapter 2 that

$$A \exp(j\phi(t)) = A \sum_i b(t - iT, a_i) \tag{8.1.7}$$

where

$$b(t, a_i) = \exp\{j(a_i\beta(t) + \phi_i)\}u_T(t) \tag{8.1.8}$$

$$\beta(t) = \omega_d \int_0^t h_S(\tau)\, d\tau u(t) \tag{8.1.9}$$

and if the phase is continuous

$$\phi_i = \beta(T) \sum_{-\infty}^{i-1} a_k \tag{8.1.10}$$

or if the phase is not continuous

$$\phi_i = \phi(a_i) \tag{8.1.11}$$

Particularly for an NRZ pulse

$$b(t, a_i) = \exp(j(a_i\omega_d t + \phi_i))u_T(t) \tag{8.1.12}$$

the instantaneous frequency deviation is a constant

$$f_{\text{dev}}(t) = a_i f_d \tag{8.1.13}$$

and the instantaneous frequency is

$$f(t) = f_C + a_i f_d \tag{8.1.14}$$

There are $M$ such frequencies $\{f_1, f_2, \ldots, f_M\}$ corresponding to the $M$ symbols

$$f_m = f_C + a(m)f_d \tag{8.1.15}$$

The maximum frequency deviation is $f_d(M - 1)$. In narrowband FSK $f_d$ is small, so that $f_d(M - 1)T$ is close to 1. In wide band FSK $f_dT$ is an integer, so that $f_d(M - 1)T$ is proportional to $M$. In wideband FSK we also assume that $f_CT$ is an integer so that $f_mT$ is an integer, and we can write

$$s_M(t) = \sum_i b_M(t - iT, a_i) \tag{8.1.16}$$

where when $a_i = a(m)$

$$b_M(t, a(m)) = A \cos(\omega_m t + \phi_T)u_T(t), \; m = 1, \ldots, M \tag{8.1.17}$$

Wideband FSK can be detected using a bank of matched filters, matched to the signals (8.1.17), as shown in Fig. 8.2. This implies the knowledge of phase $\phi_T$, and such detection is called *coherent*. In noncoherent detection, shown in Fig. 8.3, we use a bank of $M$ identical (except for center frequency) filters $\{H(f, m)\}$ followed by envelope detectors (or squares) and detector filters. The filters $\{H(f, m)\}$ have nonoverlapping spectra and are usually wideband. A binary version of a noncoherent receiver is shown in Fig. 8.4.

Narrowband FSK is detected using a frequency detector, which is a frequency-to-voltage converter called a *discriminator*, followed sometimes by a detector filter, which is usually a matched filter to the shaping function. This is shown in Fig. 8.5. In Fig. 8.1, $h_{TM}(t)$, $h_{CM}(t)$ and $h_{RM}(t)$ are bandpass filters with center frequency $f_C$, their baseband equivalent filters denoted by $h_T(t)$, $h_C(t)$, and $h_R(t)$, respectively. $n_C(t)$ is white Gaussian noise with power spectral density $N_0/2$. The output of the receiver filter is

$$\begin{aligned} r_M(t) &= A_r(t) \cos(\omega_C t + \phi_T + \phi_r(t)) \\ &= \text{Re}\,\{r(t) \exp(j(\omega_C t + \phi_T)\} \end{aligned} \tag{8.1.18}$$

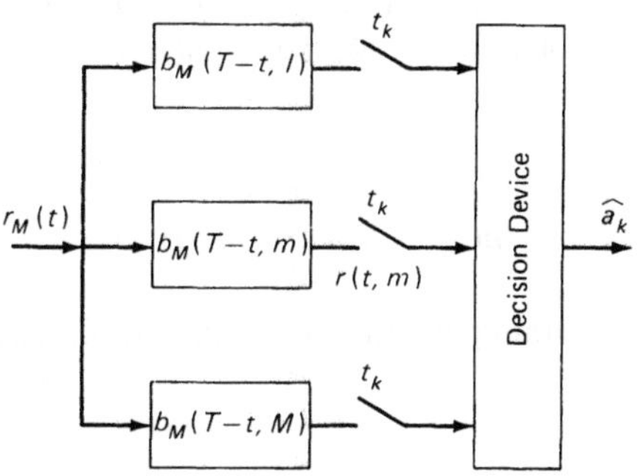


Fig. 8.2 Coherent receiver of wideband FSK.

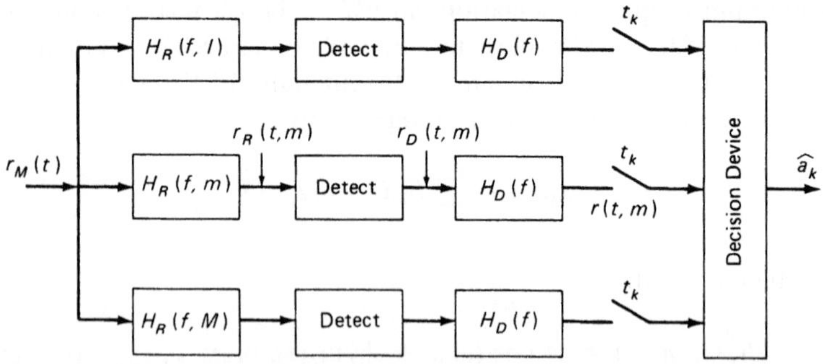


Fig. 8.3. Noncoherent receiver of wideband FSK.

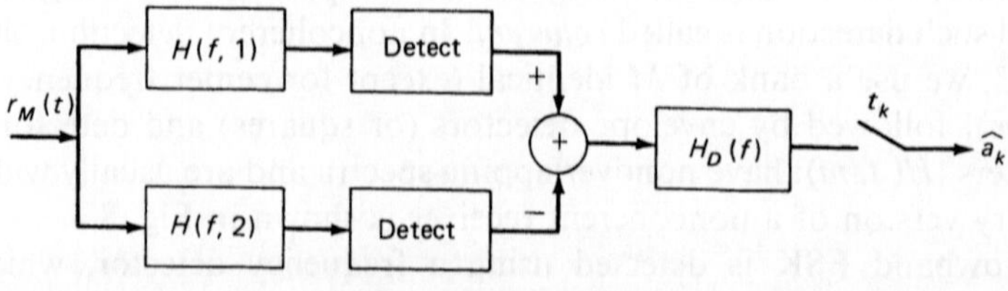


Fig. 8.4. Noncoherent receiver of wideband binary FSK.

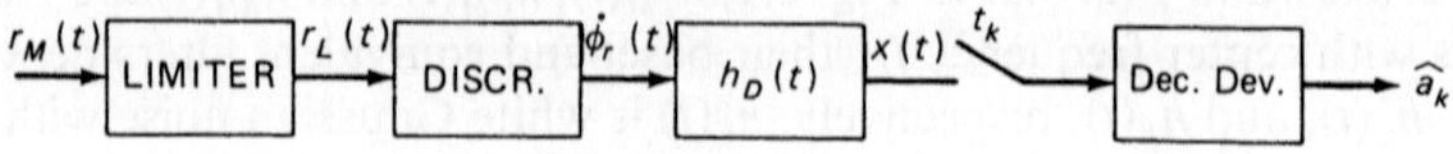


Fig. 8.5. Discriminator receiver of narrowband FSK.

where

$$r(t) = s(t) + n(t) = A_r(t) \exp(j\phi_r(t)) = r_I(t) + jr_Q(t) \tag{8.1.19}$$

$$\begin{aligned} s(t) &= A \exp(j\phi(t)) * h_T(t) * h_C(t) * h_R(t) \\ &= A_S(t) \exp(j\phi_S(t)) = s_I(t) + js_Q(t) \end{aligned} \tag{8.1.20}$$

and

$$n(t) = n_I(t) + jn_Q(t) \tag{8.1.21}$$

where $n_I(t)$, $n_Q(t)$ are independent, zero mean, Gaussian rvs (random variables) with variance

$$\sigma_n^2 = N_0 \int_{-\infty}^{\infty} |H_R(f)|^2 \, df = N_0 B_R \tag{8.1.22}$$

where $B_R$ is the noise equivalent filter bandwidth. Note that the transmitted signal may be distorted by filters (if they are narrowband) so that the amplitude has changed from a constant $A$ to $A_S(t)$, and the phase has changed from $\phi(t)$ to $\phi_S(t)$. In addition the amplitude and phase are corrupted by the noise. Because the information, about the symbols is retained in the frequency, the amplitude variations can be eliminated. This is done by the limiter (shown in Fig. 8.5, which can also be present in the other models), which produces the signal

$$r_L(t) = K \cos (\omega_C t + \phi_T + \phi_r(t)) \tag{8.1.23}$$

where $K$ may be 1. The discriminator has an output

$$\hat{\omega}(t) = \dot{\phi}_r(t) \tag{8.1.24}$$

which may be further processed by the detector filter so that

$$x(t) = \hat{\omega}(t) * h_D(t) = \int_{-\infty}^{t} h_D(t - \tau)\hat{\omega}(\tau)\, d\tau \tag{8.1.25}$$

Usually $h_D(t)$ is eliminated ($h_D(t) = \delta(t)$, the impulse function); hence

$$x(t) = \hat{\omega}(t) \tag{8.1.26}$$

or $h_D(t)$ is an ideal integrate and dump circuit, which is a matched filter to the NRZ pulse, hence

$$x(t) = \int_{t-T}^{t} \hat{\omega}(\tau)\, d\tau = \phi_r(t) - \phi_r(t - T) \tag{8.1.27}$$

Samples are taken at times $\{t_k = t_0 + kT\}$, from which the decisions are made about the values of the symbols. The decisions are $\hat{a}_k$. The decision rule for each detector will be specified later.

In this chapter we are computing the error probability of FSK with the various detectors as a function of signal-to-noise ratio $E_S/N_0$, where

$$E_S = A^2T/2 \tag{8.1.28}$$

is the energy per symbol at transmitter filter input. This energy is related to the energy per bit by

$$E_S = E_b \log_2 M \tag{8.1.29}$$

We shall also use another definition of signal-to-noise ratio

$$\rho_S = 0.5\, A^2/\sigma_n^2 = (E_S/N_0)(B_R T)^{-1} \tag{8.1.30}$$

which differs from $E_S/N_0$ by the constant $B_R T$. Note that if $h_R(t)$ is an ideal Nyquist filter, this constant is 1.

This chapter has the following outline. In Section 2 we discuss FSK with a coherent detector. In Section 3 the object is FSK with noncoherent detector. In Section 4 we present the performance of FSK with discriminator detector. In Section 5 we analyze FSK with discriminator detector and detector filter. In Section 6 we discuss briefly the detection of FSK signals using an observations interval that is larger then a single-symbol interval. In Section 7 we have a summary, which is followed by problems in Section 8 and a list of references in Section 9.

## 8.2 COHERENT FSK

Here we assume that

$$h_M(t) = h_{TM}(t) * h_{CM}(t) * h_{RM}(t) \tag{8.2.1}$$

is wideband (theoretically $h_M(t) = \delta(t)$), so that in Fig. 8.2

$$r_M(t) = s_M(t) + n_C(t) \tag{8.2.2}$$

In any time interval $iT \leq t \leq (i + 1)T$, $s_M(t)$ is one of the $M$ signals

$$b_M(t, a(m)) = A \cos(2\,\pi f_m t + \phi_T)u_T(t) \tag{8.2.3}$$

Without any loss in generality we may assume that $i = 0$.

### 8.2.1 Orthogonal FSK

We select the frequencies $\{f_m\}$ so that the signals $\{b_M(t, a(m))\}$ are orthogonal. Letting

$$b_M(t, a(m)) = (E_S)^{0.5}\phi_m(t) \tag{8.2.4}$$

$$\phi_m(t) = (2/T)^{0.5} \cos(2\,\pi f_m t + \phi_T)u_T(t) \tag{8.2.5}$$

the signals $\{\phi_m(t)\}$ are orthogonal, i.e.

$$\int_0^T \phi_m(t)\phi_k(t)\,dt = \begin{cases} 1 & k = m \\ 0 & k \neq m \end{cases} \tag{8.2.6}$$

The optimal receiver is composed of a bank of matched filters, matched to $\{\phi_m(t)\}$; hence the output of the $m$th filter is

$$r(t, m) = r_M(t) * \phi_m(T - t) = s(t, m) + n(t, m) \tag{8.2.7}$$

At time $t = T$

$$s_m = s(T, m) = \int_0^T \phi_m(\tau) s_M(\tau)\, d\tau = \begin{cases} (E_S)^{0.5} & \text{if } s_M(t) = b_M(t, a(m)) \\ 0 & \text{otherwise} \end{cases} \tag{8.2.8}$$

and

$$n_m = n(T, m) = \int_0^T \phi_m(\tau) n_C(\tau)\, d\tau \tag{8.2.9}$$

is zero mean, Gaussian noise, independent of $n_k$, with variance

$$\sigma_n^2 = 0.5\, N_0 \tag{8.2.10}$$

because

$$\overline{n_m n_k} = \int_0^T \int_0^T \phi_m(\tau)\phi_k(\tau')\overline{n_C(\tau) n_C(\tau')}\, d\tau\, d\tau'$$

$$= 0.5\, N_0 \int_0^T \phi_m(\tau)\phi_k(\tau)\, d\tau = \begin{cases} 0.5\, N_0 & m = k \\ 0 & m \neq k \end{cases} \tag{8.2.11}$$

The decision rule is

$$\hat{a}_0 = a(m) = 2m - 1 - M \text{ if } r_m \geqq r_k \text{ for all } k \tag{8.2.12}$$

where $r_m = r(T, m)$. Because of symmetry we may assume without loss in generality that the transmitted symbol is $a_0 = 1 - M$, which corresponds to $m = 1$. We shall make a correct decision if

$$r_1 = (E_S)^{0.5} + n_1 \tag{8.2.13}$$

is larger than $r_k = n_k$ $k = 2, 3, \ldots, M$. Because $\{n_k\}$ are identically distributed, independent Gaussian rvs, we obtain the probability of a correct decision

$$P(c) = P(c|m = 1) = \int_{-\infty}^{\infty} p(r_1 = y, r_2 < y, \ldots, r_M < y)\, dy$$

$$= \int_{-\infty}^{\infty} p_{n1}(y - (E_S)^{0.5})) \prod_{k=2}^{M} P(n_k < y)\, dy$$

$$= (2\,\pi)^{-0.5} \int_{-\infty}^{\infty} \exp\,(-0.5y^2)\{1 - Q(y + (2\,E_S/N_0)^{0.5})\}^{M-1}\, dy \qquad (8.2.14)$$

where

$$Q(y) = \int_{y}^{\infty} (2\,\pi)^{-0.5} \exp\,(-0.5\,x^2)\, dx \qquad (8.2.15)$$

The error probability is simply

$$P(e) = 1 - P(c) \qquad (8.2.16)$$

This is illustrated as a function of $E_S/N_0$ in Fig. 8.6. The bit error probability

$$P_b(e) = \frac{0.5\,M}{M - 1} P(e) \simeq 0.5\,P(e) \qquad (8.2.17)$$

as a function of signal-to-noise ratio per bit $E_b/N_0$ is shown in Fig. 8.7. When we substitute (8.1.29) into (8.2.16) and take the limit with $M \to \infty$, we obtain

$$P(e) = \begin{cases} 0 & E_b/N_0 \geqq 0.69\ (-1.6\text{ dB}) \\ 1 & E_b/N_0 < 0.69 \end{cases} \qquad (8.2.18)$$

*Example* 8.2.1

Compute the required signal-to-noise ratio per bit if the bit error probability is $10^{-4}$ and $M = 2, 4, 8, 16, 32$, and 64. Compare the result with the corresponding values for PSK. Give a possible reason for the difference.

The solution is given in Fig. 8.7. The result is: $E_b/N_0 = 11.3, 8.7, 7.4, 6.5, 5.8$, and 5.3 dB. The corresponding results for PSK are: $E_b/N_0 = 8.4, 8.4, 11.7, 16.3, 21$, and 25 dB, taken from Fig. 7.8. We see that for $M = 2$ and 4, PSK requires less energy than FSK. This is reversed for $M \geqq 8$.

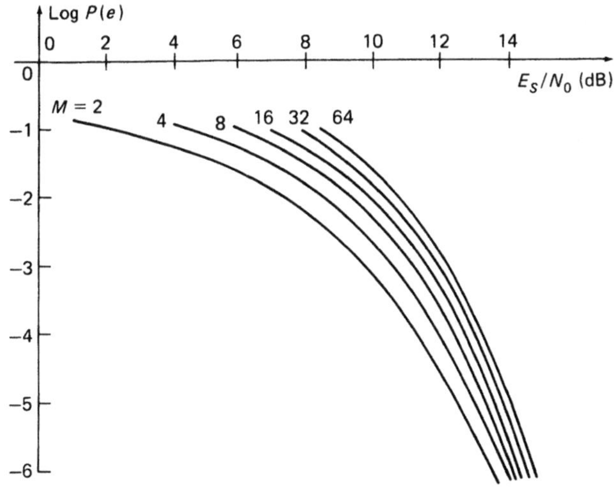


Fig. 8.6. Error probability as a function of signal-to-noise ratio for $M$-ary orthogonal FSK with coherent detection.

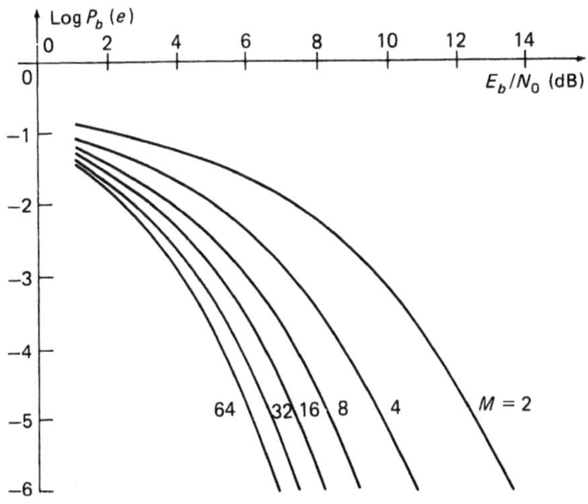


Fig. 8.7. Bit error probability as a function of signal-to-noise ratio per bit for $M$-ary orthogonal FSK with coherent detection.

Orthogonal FSK requires a much larger bandwidth than PSK. The bandwidth is proportional to the number of dimensions in the orthogonal signal set.

To obtain the orthogonal signal set of (8.2.6) we selected the frequencies so that $f_m T$ is an integer; however a sufficient condition is that $2(f_m - f_k)T$ is an integer.

### 8.2.2 An upper bound to error probability

A simple upper bound to error probability can be derived if we view the $M$ orthogonal signals as $M$ vectors in an $M$-dimensional space. From this point of view, $s(T, m)$ is actually the vector

$$\mathbf{s}_m = (0, 0, \ldots \underset{\uparrow m}{(E_S)^{0.5}}, 0, 0) \tag{8.2.19}$$

which has only one nonzero component at its $m$th position. The received signal is

$$\mathbf{r} = \mathbf{s} + \mathbf{n} \tag{8.2.20}$$

when $\mathbf{s} \in \{\mathbf{s}_1, \mathbf{s}_2, \ldots, \mathbf{s}_M\}$ and $\mathbf{n}$ is a noise vector, whose components are zero mean, independent, Gaussian rvs with variance as in (8.2.10). The optimal decision rule is a partitioning of the space into nonoverlapping regions so that if $\mathbf{r}$ belongs to region

$$DR_m = \{\mathbf{r}: |\mathbf{r} - \mathbf{s}_m| \leq |\mathbf{r} - \mathbf{s}_k|, \textit{all } k \neq m\} \tag{8.2.21}$$

the decision is $a_0 = a(m)$. The error probability is

$$P(e) = P(e|m = 1) = \sum_{k=2}^{M} P(\mathbf{r} \in DR_k|m = 1) \tag{8.2.22}$$

We may simplify the decision rule into a binary one by the following argument. Let

$$DR_{m,k} = \{\mathbf{r}: |\mathbf{r} - \mathbf{s}_m| \leqq |\mathbf{r} - \mathbf{s}_k|\} \tag{8.2.23}$$

which certainly implies

$$DR_m \subset DR_{m,k} \tag{8.2.24}$$

Hence

$$P(e) \leqq \sum_{k=2}^{M} P(\mathbf{r} \in DR_{k,1}|m = 1) = (M - 1)P(\mathbf{r} \in DR_{2,1}|m = 1) \tag{8.2.25}$$

where the last equality follows from the symmetry of the problem in all dimensions. The binary decision rule is illustrated in Fig. 8.8. From this figure, there will be an error if the noise in the specified direction will exceed

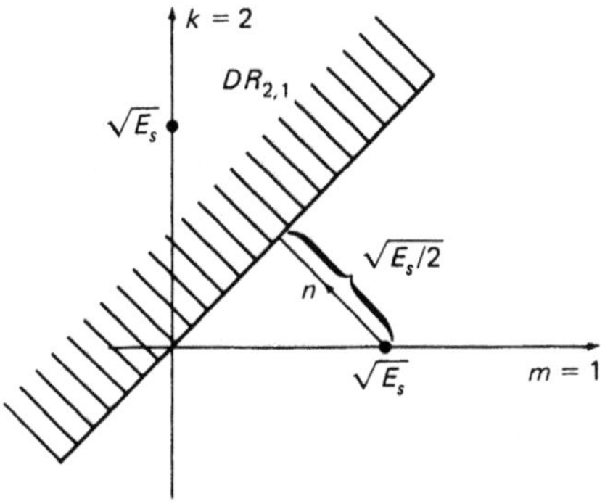


Fig. 8.8. Two-dimensional decision regions for orthogonal FSK.

half the distance between the signal vectors. The distance is simply

$$d = \left( \int_0^T \{s(t, 1) - s(t, 2)\}^2 \, dt \right)^{0.5} = (2 \, E_S)^{0.5} \tag{8.2.26}$$

and, because the noise is circularly symmetric (the same variance in all directions)

$$P(\mathbf{r} \in DR_{2,1} | m = 1) = P(n > d/2) = Q(0.5 \, d/\sigma_n) = Q((E_S/N_0)^{0.5}) \tag{8.2.27}$$

Thus

$$P(e) \leqq (M - 1) Q((E_S/N_0)^{0.5}) \tag{8.2.28}$$

For binary symbols the error probability is always

$$P_b(e) = Q(0.5 \, d/\sigma_n) \tag{8.2.29}$$

Hence the upper bound is the exact value. For $M > 2$ and $P(e) \leqq 10^{-3}$ the upper bound is an excellent approximation to the true value.

### 8.2.3 Binary coherent FSK

Here we assume that the signals are

$$b_M(t, \pm) = A \cos (2 \pi \, (f_C \pm f_d) t + \phi_T) u_T(t) \tag{8.2.30}$$

with arbitrary $f_d$, which means that they are not necessarily orthogonal. This is illustrated in Fig. 8.9. The error probability is as in (8.2.29) with (here $E_S = E_b$ because the symbols are binary)

$$d^2 = 2\, E_b\, (1 - \mathrm{sinc}\, (2\, h)) \tag{8.2.31}$$

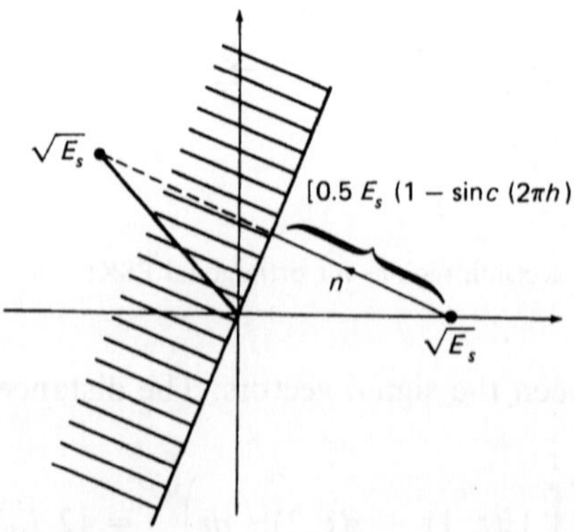


Fig. 8.9. Decision regions for binary FSK.

where

$$h = 2\, f_d T \tag{8.2.32}$$

is the normalized frequency deviation and

$$\mathrm{sinc}\, x = \sin\, (\pi x)/(\pi x) \tag{8.2.33}$$

The error probability is thus

$$P_b(e) = Q\{\sqrt{(E_b/N_0)(1 - \mathrm{sinc}(2\, h))}\} \tag{8.2.34}$$

which can be minimized by maximizing the distance $d$, which depends on $h$. The optimal $h$ and the minimal error probability is

$$h = h_{op} = 0.715 \tag{8.2.35}$$

$$P_b(e) = Q(\sqrt{1.217\, E_b/N_0}) \tag{8.2.36}$$

In orthogonal FSK the result is $Q((E_b/N_0)^{1/2})$ and in PSK and antipodal ASK the result is $Q((2\, E_b/N_0)^{1/2})$. Relative to PSK the penalty in signal-to-noise ratio is 3 dB for orthogonal FSK and 2.15 dB for optimal FSK. The bit error probability for the three cases is shown in Fig. 8.10.

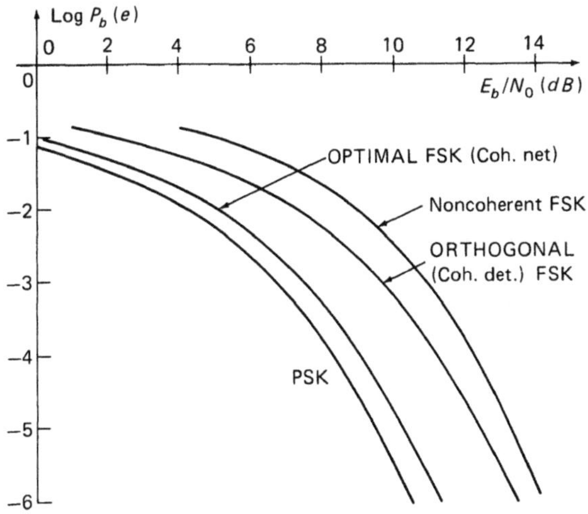


Fig. 8.10. Error probabilities comparison of binary FSK systems.

## 8.3 NONCOHERENT FSK

The receiver is shown in Fig. 8.3. The input signal is as in (8.2.2) and (8.2.3). The filters $\{H_R(f, m)\}$ have the form

$$H_R(f, m) = H_R(f - f_m) \tag{8.3.1}$$

i.e., they are identical except for their center frequencies. The spectra of these filters do not overlap, so that when $a_0 = a(1)$, only filter $H(f, 1)$ has a nonzero output in the absence of noise. The noise at the output of the $m$th filter is

$$n_m(t) = n_{Im}(t) \cos(\omega_m t + \phi_T) + n_{Qm}(t) \sin(\omega_m t + \phi_T) \tag{8.3.2}$$

where $\{n_{Im}(t), n_{Qm}(t)\}$ are independent, zero mean, Gaussian rvs with variance $\sigma_n^2$. The output of filter $H(f, 1)$ is thus

$$r_R(t, 1) = (A + n_{I1}(t)) \cos(\omega_1 t + \phi_T) + n_{Q1}(t) \sin(\omega_1 t + \phi_T) \tag{8.3.3}$$

while of the other filters, $m = 2, 3, \ldots, M$

$$r_R(t, m) = n_m(t) \tag{8.3.4}$$

The output of the envelope detectors is

$$r_D(t, m) = \begin{cases} \{(A + n_{I1}(t))^2 + n_{Q1}^2(t)\}^{0.5} & m = 1 \\ \{n_{Im}^2(t) + n_{Qm}^2(t)\}^{0.5} & m = 2, \ldots, M \end{cases} \tag{8.3.5}$$

The output of the square law detectors, after we eliminate the high-frequency terms (frequencies $2 f_m$), is

$$r_D(t, m) = \begin{cases} (A + n_{I1}(t))^2 + n_{Q1}^2(t) & m = 1 \\ n_{Im}^2(t) + n_{Qm}^2(t) & m = 2, \ldots, M \end{cases} \tag{8.3.6}$$

### 8.3.1 No detector filters

If there is no detector filter, then

$$r(T, m) = r_D(T, m) = \begin{cases} A_m & \text{Env. Det.} \\ A_m^2 & \text{Sq. Law Det.} \end{cases} \tag{8.3.7}$$

where we denoted

$$A_m = \begin{cases} ((A + n_{I1}(T))^2 + n_{Q1}^2(T))^{0.5} & m = 1 \\ (n_{I1}^2(T) + n_{Q1}^2(T))^{0.5} & m = 2, \ldots, M \end{cases} \tag{8.3.8}$$

In either case the decision rule is that if

$$A_m \geqq A_k \qquad k = 1, 2, \ldots, M \tag{8.3.9}$$

then $a_0 = a(m)$. Thus there is no error if $A_1 \geqq A_m$, $m = 2, \ldots, M$. Because of independence and the identical distribution of $A_2, \ldots, A_M$, we obtain

$$P(c) = \int_{-\infty}^{\infty} p_{A1}(y)\{P(A_2 \leqq y)\}^{M-1}\, dy \tag{8.3.10}$$

It was shown in section 7.2 that the pdf of $A_1$ is Rician

$$p_{A1}(y) = \exp(-\rho_S)(y/\sigma_n^2) \exp(-0.5\, y^2/\sigma_n^2) I_0((2\rho_S)^{0.5} y/\sigma_n) u(y) \tag{8.3.11}$$

and the pdf of $A_2$ is obtained from (8.3.11) by setting $\rho_S = 0$

$$p_{A2}(y) = (y/\sigma_n^2) \exp(-0.5\, y^2/\sigma_n^2) u(y) \tag{8.3.12}$$

It is easy to compute

$$P(A_2 \leqq y) = 1 - \exp(-0.5\, y^2/\sigma_n^2) \tag{8.3.13}$$

and since

$$(1 - x)^n = \sum_{k=0}^{n} C_k^n (-x)^k \tag{8.3.14}$$

$$C_k^n = \frac{n!}{k!(n-k)!} \tag{8.3.15}$$

we obtain after substitution of (8.3.11), (8.3.13), and (8.3.14) into (8.3.10)

$$P(c) = \exp(-\rho_S) \sum_{k=0}^{M-1} \int_{-\infty}^{\infty} (-1)^k C_k^{M-1} (y/\sigma_n^2) I_0((2\rho_S)^{0.5} y/\sigma_n) \exp(-0.5(1+k)y^2/\sigma_n^2)\, dy \tag{8.3.16}$$

Changing variables

$$z = y(1+k)^{0.5} \tag{8.3.17}$$

and noting that

$$\int_0^{\infty} p_{A1}(y)\, \mathrm{d}y = 1 \tag{8.3.18}$$

independent of the value of $\rho_S$, we obtain

$$P(c) = \sum_{k=0}^{M-1} (-1)^k C_k^{M-1} \exp(-k\rho_S/(1+k))/(1+k) \tag{8.3.19}$$

The error probability is

$$P(e) = 1 - P(c) = \sum_{k=1}^{M-1} (-1)^{k+1} C_k^{M-1} \exp(-k\rho_S/(1+k))/(1+k) \tag{8.3.20}$$

The error probability as a function of $\rho_S$ is shown in Fig. 8.11, and the bit error probability as a function of

$$\rho_b = \rho_S/\log_2 M \tag{8.3.21}$$

is shown in Fig. 8.12.

*Example* 8.3.1
Compute the error probability for binary and quaternary symbols.
We obtain from (8.3.20) for $M = 2$

$$P(e) = P_b(e) = 0.5 \exp(-0.5\,\rho_S) = 0.5 \exp(-0.5\,\rho_b) \tag{8.3.22}$$

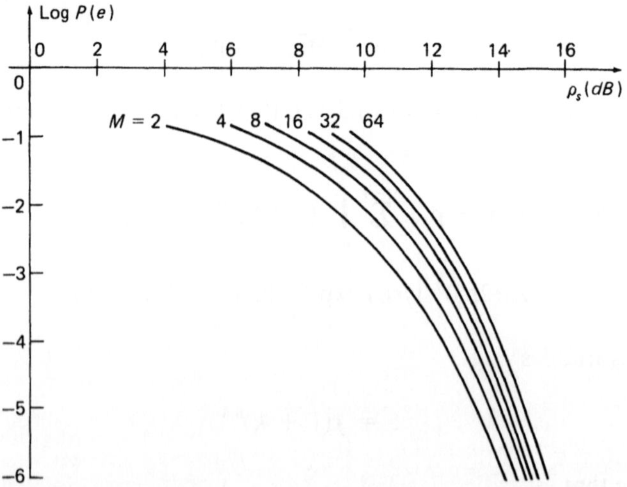


Fig. 8.11. Error probability as a function of signal-to-noise ratio for orthogonal $M$-ary FSK with noncoherent detection.

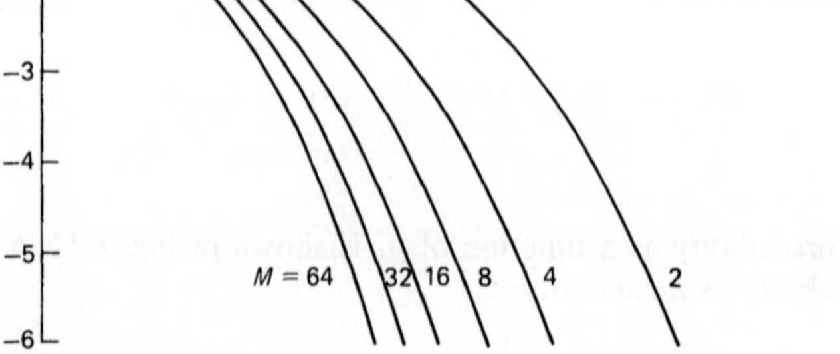


Fig. 8.12. Bit error probability as a function of signal-to-noise ratio per bit of orthogonal $M$-ary FSK with noncoherent detection.

If we interpret $\rho_b$ as $E_b/N_0$, this equation is also shown in Fig. 8.10. For $M = 4$ we obtain

$$P(e) = 1.5 \exp(-0.5\,\rho_S) - \exp(-2\,\rho_S/3) + 0.25 \exp(-0.75\,\rho_S)$$

### 8.3.2 With detector filters

The reason for introducing a narrowband detector filter is the excessive noise caused by the wideband receiver filters $H_R(f, m)$, which may have a bandwidth $N = B_R T \geqq 10$. Such a system would be required if the frequencies $\{f_m\}$ are widely separated and have an uncertainty about their exact value caused, for example, by the Doppler effect. In this system

$$r(T, m) = \int_0^T h_D(T - \tau) r_D(\tau, m)\, d\tau \simeq \frac{T}{N} \sum_{k=0}^{N-1} h_D(T - \tau_k) r_D(\tau_k, m) \quad (8.3.23)$$

where

$$\tau_k = kT/N \quad (8.3.24)$$

Specifically, when $h_D(t)$ is a matched filter to the NRZ pulse, i.e.

$$h_D(t) = \frac{1}{T} u_T(t) \quad (8.3.25)$$

the output is

$$r(T, m) = \frac{1}{T} \int_0^T r_D(\tau, m)\, d\tau \simeq \frac{1}{N} \sum_{k=0}^{N-1} r_D(\tau_k, m) \quad (8.3.26)$$

It is assumed that the rvs $\{r_D(\tau_k, m)\}$ are independent, which would be true if $H_R(f)$ is a brick wall filter. They are identically distributed with average value and variance

$$m_D(m) = \overline{r_D(\tau_k, m)} = \begin{cases} \overline{A_m} \\ \overline{A_m^2} \end{cases}$$

$$\sigma_D^2(m) = \overline{\{r_D(\tau_k, m) - \overline{r_D(\tau_k, m)}\}^2} = \begin{cases} \overline{A_m^2} - (\overline{A_m})^2 \\ \overline{A_m^4} - (\overline{A_m^2})^2 \end{cases} \quad (8.3.27)$$

It was shown in Ref. 8.7 that taking these moments with respect to the pdf of (8.3.11) for $m = 1$ and with respect to the pdf in (8.3.12) for $m = 2, \ldots, M$, we obtain

$$m_D(1) = \begin{cases} (0.5\, N_0 N \pi)^{0.5}\, {}_1F_1(-0.5; 1; -\rho_S) \\ 2\, N_0 N(1 + \rho_S) \end{cases} \quad (8.3.28)$$

$$m_D(2) = \begin{cases} 0.5\,(N_0 N\pi)^{0.5} \\ 2\,N_0 N \end{cases} \tag{8.3.29}$$

$$\sigma_D^2(1) = \begin{cases} 2\,E_S + 2\,N_0 N - 0.5\,N_0 N\pi\,{}_1F_1^2(-0.5;\,1;\,-\rho_S) \\ (2\,N_0)^2 N(1 + 2\,\rho_S) \end{cases} \tag{8.3.30}$$

$$\sigma_D^2(2) = \begin{cases} 2\,N_0 N(1 - 0.25\,\pi) \\ (2\,N_0)^2 N \end{cases} \tag{8.3.31}$$

where the hypergeometric function[8.13]

$$\begin{aligned} {}_1F_1(-0.5;\,1;\,-\rho_S) = \exp\,(-0.5\,\rho_S)\{(1 + \rho_S)I_0(0.5\,\rho_S) \\ + \rho_S I_1(0.5\,\rho_S)\} \end{aligned} \tag{8.3.32}$$

is expressed in terms of modified Bessel functions.

Gaussian approximation (large $N$) For large values of $N$, the summation in (8.3.23), being a large sum of independent rvs, is approximately Gaussian with average and variance

$$\overline{r_m} = \overline{r(T,\,m)} = \overline{r_D(m)} \int_0^T h_D(\tau)\,d\tau \tag{8.3.33}$$

$$\sigma_m^2 = \sigma_D^2(m) \int_0^T h_D^2(\tau)\,d\tau \tag{8.3.34}$$

The error probability is

$$\begin{aligned} P(e) &= 1 - \int_{-\infty}^{\infty} p_{r(T,1)}(y)\{P(r(T,\,2) \leqq y)\}^{M-1}\,dy \\ &= 1 - (2\,\pi)^{-0.5} \int_{-\infty}^{\infty} \exp\,(-0.5\,y^2)\{1 - Q((y\sigma_1 + \overline{r_1} - \overline{r_2})/\sigma_2)\}^{M-1}\,dy \\ &= \sum_{k=1}^{M-1} (-1)^{k+1} C_k^{M-1} \int_{-\infty}^{\infty} Q^k\{(y\sigma_1 + \overline{r_1} - \overline{r_2})/\sigma_2\}(2\pi)^{-0.5} \\ &\quad \exp\,(-0.5\,y^2)\,dy \end{aligned} \tag{8.3.35}$$

Assuming an NRZ detector filter, the error probability as a function of signal-to-noise ratio per bit is shown for a square law detector in Fig. 8.13.

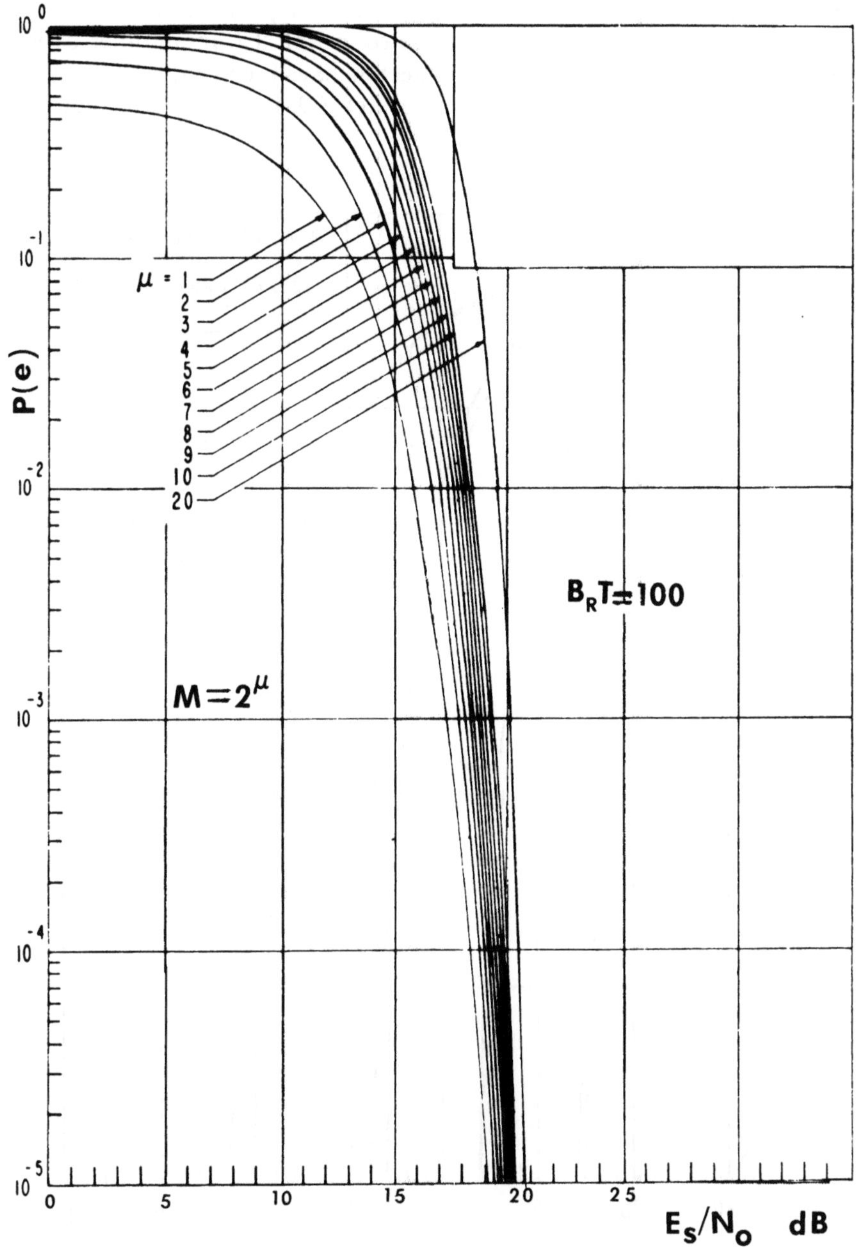


Fig. 8.13. Error probability of wideband FSK with square law detector ($B_R T = 100$) and NRZ detector filter as a function of signal-to-noise ratio (A. B. Glenn, *RCA Review*, Vol. 27, pp. 272–319, June 1966).

The binary case for both the square law and envelope detectors is shown in Fig. 8.14. These figures were first presented in Ref. 8.7. In all other papers only the binary case and square law detectors have been analyzed. Thus the effect of a bandpass limiter is analyzed in Ref. 8.9. In Ref. 8.10 the detector

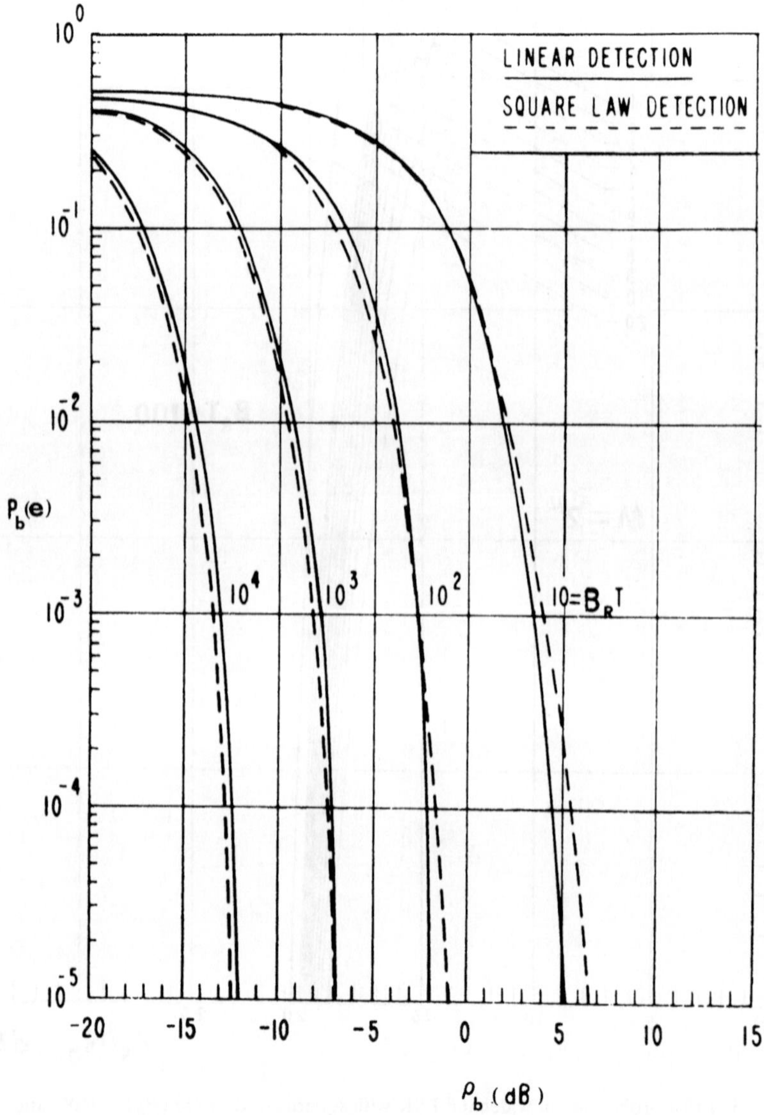


Fig. 8.14. Bit error probability of wideband binary FSK with square law and envelope detectors and NRZ detector filters as a function of signal-to-noise ratio (A. B. Glenn, *RCA Review*, Vol. 27, pp. 272–319, June 1966).

filter is NRZ or Butterworth of order 1 or 2. In Ref. 8.10 the effect of intersymbol interference is taken into account by replacing in (8.3.23) the lower limit of the integral to $-kT$, so that $k$ preceding symbols affect the system. It was found there that the optimal 3-dB bandwidth of the Butterworth filters of order 1 and 2 is $f_0T = 0.37$ and 0.52, respectively. The resulting error probability is shown in Fig. 8.15.

*No approximation* (small $N$) In Refs. 8.8 and 8.11, $B_RT$ is not necessarily large; hence the probability density of $r(T, m)$ is computed using the characteristic function method. In Ref. 8.8 the detector filter is NRZ, and the

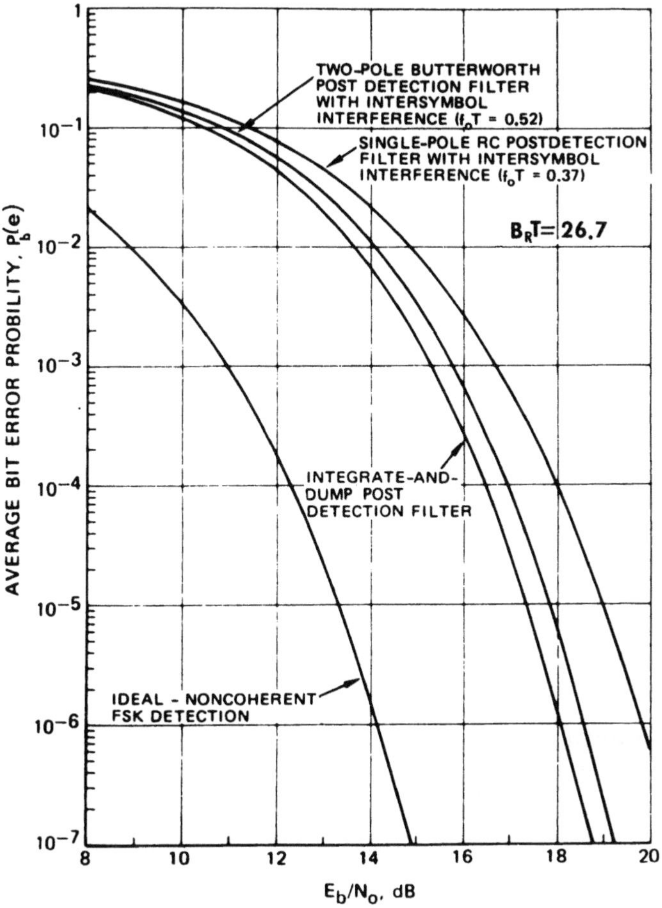


Fig. 8.15. Bit error probability of wideband binary FSK with square law detector and various detector filters ($B_RT = 26.7$) (M. C. Austin, "Wide Band Frequency Shift Keyed Receiver Performance in the Presence of Intersymbol Interference," *IEEE Tr. Comm.*, Vol. COM-23, April 1975, pp. 453–458. Copyright © 1975 IEEE).

effect of multipath fading is analyzed. In Ref. 8.11 the detector filter is either NRZ or Butterworth. The amplitude of the signals may also be shaped, so that the signals are, instead of (8.2.3)

$$b_M(t, a(m)) = A(t) \cos (2 \pi f_m t + \phi_T) \tag{8.3.36}$$

where $A(t)$ is an arbitrary positive function of duration $T$. In the binary case the probability of error is the probability that $x(T) \leqq 0$ where

$$x(T) = r(T, 1) - r(T, 2) = \int_0^T \{(A(\tau) + n_{I1}(\tau))^2 + n_{Q1}^2(\tau)$$

$$- n_{I2}^2(\tau) - n_{Q2}^2(\tau)\}h(T - \tau)\, d\tau$$

$$\simeq \sum_0^{N-1} \{(A_k + n_{I1k})^2 + n_{Q1k}^2 + n_{I2k}^2 - n_{Q2k}^2\}h_k T/N \tag{8.3.37}$$

where we denoted

$$A_k = A(\tau_k),\ n_{yik} = n_{yi}(\tau_k),\ y = Q, I,\ i = 1, 2$$

$$h_k = h(T - \tau_k)$$

The characteristic function of $x = x(T)$ is

$$C_x(v) = \sum_{k=0}^{N-1} \exp \{j\, 2\, \pi h_k A_k^2 (v/\sigma_n)(1 - j\, 4\, \pi v h_k \sigma_n)^{-1}\}/(1 + (4\, \pi v h_k \sigma_n)^2) \tag{8.3.38}$$

which for constant $h_k = 1$ and $A_k = A$ is simplified to

$$C_x(v) = \exp \{j\, 2\, \pi A^2 (v/\sigma_n)(1 - j\, 4\, \pi v \sigma_n)^{-1}\}\{1 + (4\, \pi v \sigma_n)^2\}^{-1} \tag{8.3.39}$$

The error probability is

$$P_b(e) = \int_{-\infty}^{0} \left\{ \int_{-\infty}^{\infty} C_x(v) \exp (-j\, 2\, \pi v x)\, dv \right\} dx \tag{8.3.40}$$

For an NRZ filter and constant amplitude, the result is

$$P_b(e) = 2^{-(2N-1)} \exp (-0.5\, E_b/N_0) \sum_{k=0}^{N-1} \left( C_k^{2N-1} \sum_{n=0}^{N-1-k} (0.5\, E_b/N_0)^n/n! \right) \tag{8.3.41}$$

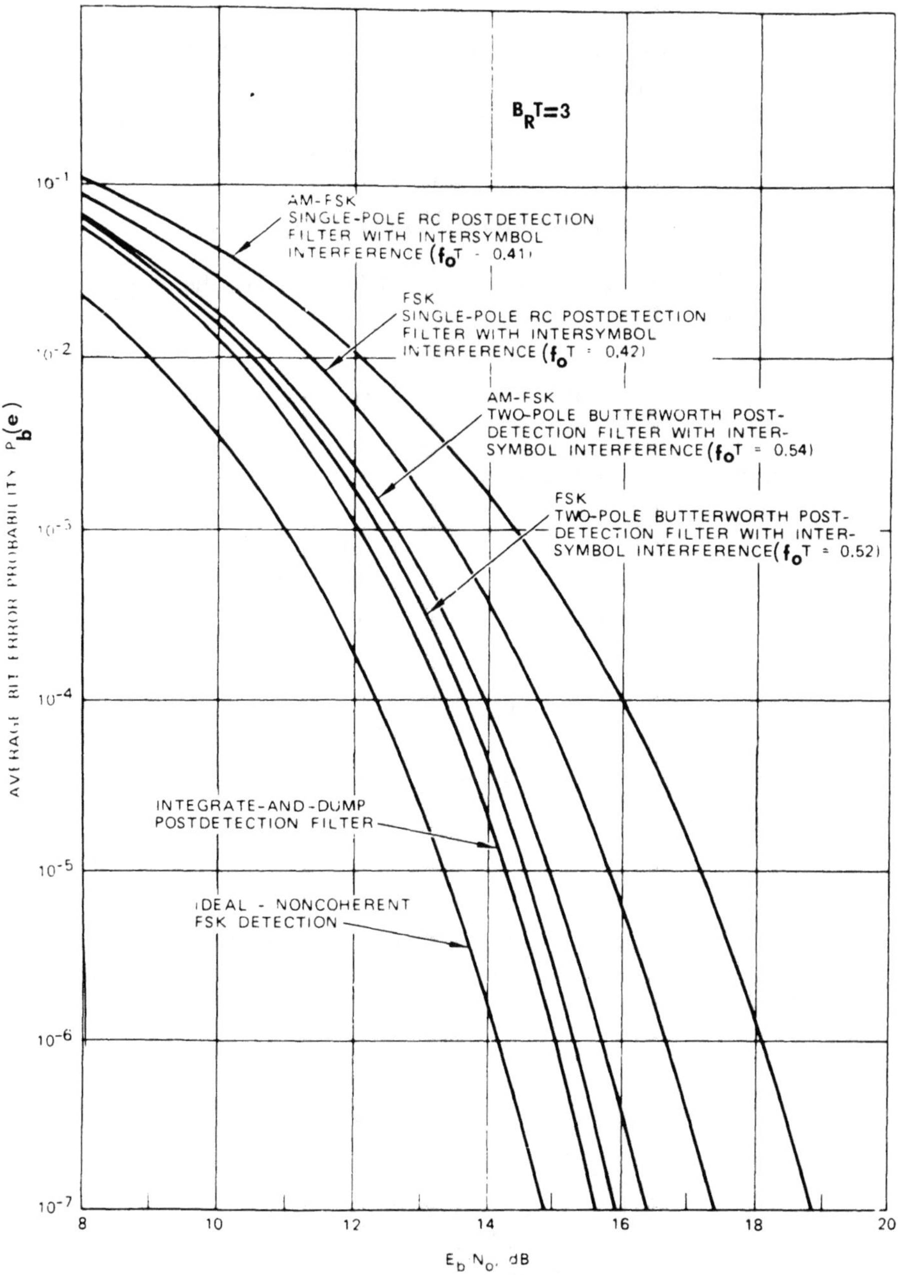


Fig. 8.16. Bit error probability of wideband binary FSK with square law detector and various detector filters ($B_RT = 3$) (L. B. Milstein and M. C. Austin, "Performance of Noncoherent FSK and AM-FSK Systems with Postdetection Filtering," *IEEE Tr. Comm.*, Vol. COM-23, November 1975, pp. 1300–1305. Copyright © 1975 IEEE).

ISI can be accounted for by extending the lower limit in (8.3.37) to $-kT$. The error probability is shown in Fig. 8.16, taken from Ref. 8.11. The variable amplitude is assumed to be a triangle with a peak at $T/2$. In Ref. 8.12, using a different approach, it is claimed that $H_R(f)$ may also be narrowband, and the contribution of this filter to the ISI can also be computed.

## 8.4 FSK WITH DISCRIMINATOR DETECTOR

Referring to Figs. 8.1 and 8.5 and eqs. (8.1.13)–(8.1.21), the output of the discriminator is

$$\hat{\omega}(t) = \dot{\phi}_r(t) = \frac{d}{dt}\arg r(t) \tag{8.4.1}$$

In the absence of distortion and noise

$$\hat{\omega}(t) = \dot{\phi}_S(t) = \omega_d \sum_i a_i h_S(t - iT) \tag{8.4.2}$$

Thus at the sampling time, $t = t_k$, we obtain ideally (the assumption is that $h_S(t_k) = 1$)

$$\dot{\phi}_r(t) = a_k \omega_d \tag{8.4.3}$$

As can be seen from Fig. 8.17, the phase noise

$$\phi_n(t) = \tan^{-1}\frac{n'_Q(t)}{A_S(t) + n'_I(t)} \tag{8.4.4}$$

is symmetric around zero, because $n'_Q(t)$, $n'_I(t)$ are zero mean, Gaussian rvs with variance $\sigma_n^2$. This was shown in 1.8. The decision rule is thus the same as for ASK, namely

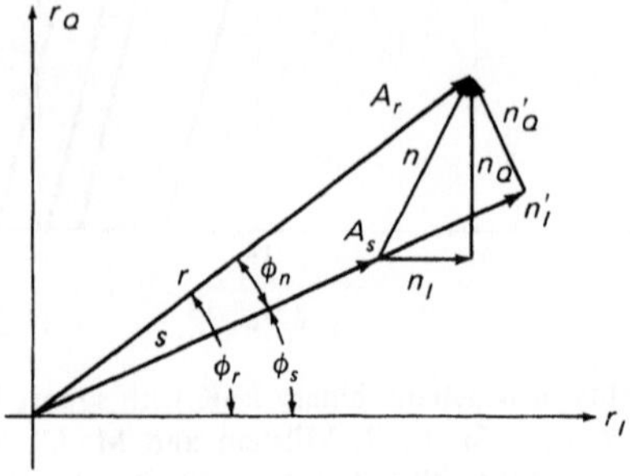


Fig. 8.17. Phase error of signal and Gaussian noise.

$$|\hat{\omega} - a(m)\omega_d| < \omega_d \rightarrow \hat{a}_k = a(m), m = 2, 3, \ldots, M - 1$$
$$\hat{\omega} < -(M - 2)\omega_d \rightarrow \hat{a}_k = -M + 1 \quad (8.4.5)$$
$$\hat{\omega} > (M - 2)\omega_d \rightarrow \hat{a}_k = M - 1$$

where, to simplify notation, we dropped the dependence on $t_k$. The error probability is

$$P(e) = M^{-1} \sum_{m=1}^{M} P(e|m) \quad (8.4.6)$$

$$P(e|m) = \begin{cases} P(|\hat{\omega} - a(m)\omega_d| > \omega_d | a_k = a(m)), m = 2, 3, \ldots, M - 1 \\ P(\hat{\omega} > -(M - 2)\omega_d | a_k = -M + 1) \\ P(\hat{\omega} < (M - 2)\omega_d | a_k = M - 1) \end{cases} \quad (8.4.7)$$

Because of symmetry around the zero frequency

$$P(e|m) = P(e|M - m) \quad (8.4.8)$$

Hence for an even $M$

$$P(e) = (2/M) \sum_{m=1}^{M/2} P(e|m) \quad (8.4.9)$$

and for the binary case

$$P_b(e) = P(e|a_k = +1) = P(\hat{\omega} < 0|a_k = +1) \quad (8.4.10)$$

When there is no distortion, (8.4.7) is simplified to

$$P(e|m) = \begin{cases} P(|\dot{\phi}_n| > \omega_d) & m = 2, 3, \ldots, M - 1 \\ P(\dot{\phi}_n > \omega_d) & m = 1 \\ P(\dot{\phi}_n < -\omega_d) & m = M \end{cases} \quad (8.4.11)$$

Hence

$$P(e) = 2(1 - M^{-1})P(\dot{\phi}_n > \omega_d) \quad (8.4.12)$$

We thus see that in order to compute the error probability we need the pdf of $\hat{\omega} = \dot{\phi}_r$.

### 8.4.1 The PDF of instantaneous frequency

The PDF (probability distribution function) of the instantaneous frequency was derived using various methods in Refs. 8.14–8.19. We shall follow here

Refs. 8.15 and 8.19. It follows from (8.4.1) that

$$\hat{\omega}(t) = \frac{d}{dt}\text{Im}\,\{\ln r(t)\} = \text{Im}\left[\frac{\dot{r}(t)}{r(t)}\right] = \text{Im}\left[\frac{r^*(t)\dot{r}(t)}{|r(t)|^2}\right]$$
$$= \text{Re}\,\{-jr^*(t)\dot{r}(t)\}/|r(t)|^2 \tag{8.4.13}$$

The PDF of $\hat{\omega}(t)$ is thus (we drop for convenience the dependence on $t = t_k$)

$$P(\hat{\omega} < x) = P\left(\frac{\text{Re}\{-jr^*\dot{r}\}}{|r|^2} < x\right) = P(\text{Re}\{-jr^*\dot{r} - x|r|^2 < 0\})$$
$$= P(Re\{r_1^* r_2\} < 0) \tag{8.4.14}$$

where

$$r_1 = r = s_1 + n_1 = s + n \tag{8.4.15}$$

and

$$r_2 = -j\dot{r} - xr = s_2 + n_2 = -j\dot{s} - xs - j\dot{n} - xn \tag{8.4.16}$$

The averages, variances, and correlation of $r_1$, $r_2$ are

$$\overline{r}_1 = s_1 = A_S(t)\exp(j\phi_S(t)) \tag{8.4.17}$$

$$\overline{r}_2 = s_2 = -jA_S(t)\exp(j\phi_S(t))\{\dot{A}_S/A_S + j\dot{\phi}_S\} - xA_S\exp(j\phi_S) \tag{8.4.18}$$

$$\sigma_1^2 = \sigma_n^2 \tag{8.4.19}$$

$$\sigma_2^2 = \sigma_n^2(x^2 + \omega_{\text{ef}}^2 - 2\,x\omega_{\text{av}}) \tag{8.4.20}$$

where

$$\omega_{\text{ef}} = 2\,\pi f_{\text{ef}},\ \omega_{\text{av}} = 2\,\pi f_{\text{av}} \tag{8.4.21}$$

$$f_{\text{ef}}^2 = \int_{-\infty}^{\infty} f^2|H_R(f)|^2\,df/B_R \tag{8.4.22}$$

$$f_{\text{av}} = \int_{-\infty}^{\infty} f|H_R(f)|^2\,df/B_R \tag{8.4.23}$$

$$\lambda = 0.5\,\overline{n_2^* n_1}/(\sigma_1\sigma_2) = (\omega_{\text{av}} - x)(x^2 + \omega_{\text{eq}}^2 - 2\,\omega_{\text{av}}x)^{-0.5}$$

In deriving these equations we have used the results from Section 1.8.3 with $x_1 = n_I, x_2 = n_Q$.

It is not difficult to show that

$$P(\text{Re}\{r_1^* r_2\} < 0) = P(|r_1 + r_2|^2 < |r_1 - r_2|^2) \\ = P(|z_1|^2 < |z_2|^2) \tag{8.4.24}$$

where

$$z_1 = 0.5\,\{(1 + K)r_1 + (1 - K)r_2\} \tag{8.4.25}$$

$$z_2 = 0.5\,\{(1 - K)r_1 + (1 + K)r_2\} \tag{8.4.26}$$

If we select

$$K = \left(\frac{\sigma_1^2 + \sigma_2^2 + 2\,\sigma_1\sigma_2\lambda}{\sigma_1^2 + \sigma_2^2 - 2\,\sigma_1\sigma_2\lambda}\right)^{0.5} \tag{8.4.27}$$

$z_1$ and $z_2$ are independent rvs. In Section 7.3 we have already presented a formula for (8.4.24) (there $z_1, z_2$ are called $r_+, r_-$), assuming that $\sigma_1 = \sigma_2 = \sigma$. Using the same method, it is shown in Refs. 8.15 and 8.19 that

$$P(\hat{\omega} < x) = 0.5\,(1 + \lambda)(1 - Q(b^{0.5}, a^{0.5})) + 0.5\,(1 - \lambda)Q(a^{0.5}, b^{0.5}) \tag{8.4.28}$$

where

$$a = A_{s2}^2/(\sigma_1^2 + \sigma_2^2) = 0.5\,\rho_s\{(\dot{A}_s\delta(x)/A_s)^2 + (1 - (\dot{\phi}_s - x)\delta(x))^2\} \tag{8.4.29}$$

$$b = A_{s1}^2/(\sigma_1^2 + \sigma_2^2) = 0.5\,\rho_s\{\dot{A}_s\delta(x)/A_s)^2 + (1 + (\dot{\phi}_s - x)\delta(x))^2\} \tag{8.4.30}$$

$$\delta(x) = (x^2 + \omega_{\text{ef}}^2 - 2\,\omega_{\text{av}}x)^{-0.5} \tag{8.4.31}$$

and $Q(\ ,\ )$ is the Marcum function.

*Example* 8.4.1 No distortion and Butterworth filter
If there is no distortion

$$A_s(t) = A \rightarrow \dot{A}_s = 0 \tag{8.4.32}$$

$$\dot{\phi}_s(t) = a_k\omega_d \tag{8.4.33}$$

The first statement is always correct when a bandpass limiter is used. There will be no distortion if

$$H_R(f) = (H_T(f)H_C(f))^{-1} \tag{8.4.34}$$

Since $H_R(f)$ is a Butterworth filter

$$\omega_{\text{av}} = 0 \tag{8.4.35}$$

and for a Butterworth filter of order $N$

$$f_{\text{ef}}^2 = \int_{-\infty}^{\infty} f^2(1 + (f/f_0)^{2N})^{-1}\, df \Big/ \int_{-\infty}^{\infty} (1 + (f/f_0)^{2N})^{-1}\, df$$

$$= f_0^2 \sin(0.5\,\pi/N)\sin(1.5\,\pi/N) \tag{8.4.36}$$

where we have used the formula

$$\int_{-\infty}^{\infty} x^{\lambda_1 - 1}(1 + x^{\lambda_2})^{-1}\, dx = 2\,\pi/\{\lambda_2 \sin(\lambda_1\pi/\lambda_2)\} \qquad 0 < \lambda_1 < \lambda_2 \tag{8.4.37}$$

Thus

$$\lambda = -x(x^2 + \omega_{\text{ef}}^2)^{-0.5} = -x\,\delta(x) \tag{8.4.38}$$

$$\delta(x) = (x^2 + \omega_{\text{ef}}^2)^{-0.5} \tag{8.4.39}$$

### 8.4.2 Binary FSK

The error probability is, from (8.4.10)

$$P(\hat{\omega} < 0) = 0.5\,\{1 - Q(b^{0.5}, a^{0.5}) + Q(a^{0.5}, b^{0.5})\} \tag{8.4.40}$$

where, since

$$\delta(x) = 1/\omega_{\text{ef}} \tag{8.4.41}$$

$$a = 0.5\,\rho_s\{(\dot{A}_s/(A_s\omega_{\text{ef}}))^2 + (1 - \dot{\phi}_s/\omega_{\text{ef}})^2\} \tag{8.4.42}$$

$$b = 0.5\,\rho_s\{(\dot{A}_s/(A_s\omega_{\text{ef}}))^2 + (1 + \dot{\phi}_s/\omega_{\text{ef}})^2\} \tag{8.4.43}$$

When there is no distortion ($\dot{A}_s = 0, \dot{\phi}_s = \omega_d$)

$$a = 0.5\ \rho_s(1 - f_d/f_{\text{ef}})^2 \tag{8.4.44}$$

$$b = 0.5\ \rho_s(1 + f_d/f_{\text{ef}})^2 \tag{8.4.45}$$

$$\rho_s = 0.5A^2/\sigma_n^2 \tag{8.4.46}$$

Particularly if we select

$$f_d = f_{\text{cf}} \tag{8.4.47}$$

we obtain

$$a = 0,\ b = 2\ \rho_s \tag{8.4.48}$$

Since

$$Q(b^{0.5}, 0) = 1,\ Q(0, b^{0.5}) = \exp\,(-0.5\ b) \tag{8.4.49}$$

the result is

$$P_b(e) = P(\hat{\omega} < 0) = 0.5\ \exp\,(-\rho_s) \tag{8.4.50}$$

When we compare this result with eq. (8.3.22) for noncoherent FSK with separate receiver filters for the two signals, there seems to be an improvement in the error probability, because of the factor 0.5 in the exponential. This is only an illusion, however, because the factor $B_RT$ in the definition of $\rho_s$ in (8.4.50) is about twice the corresponding value in (8.3.22). The reason for that is simple: the receiver filter with a discriminator detector must be wide enough to accommodate the two signals, though the individual filters in Section 8.3 accommodate only one of these signals. Other formulas for the error probability of binary FSK can be found in Refs. 8.14, 8.16, 8.21, and 8.22. For example, in Ref. 8.14 the bit error probability is presented as

$$P_b(e) = Q((2\ \rho_s)^{0.5}) + (\rho_s/\pi)^{0.5} \int_{-1}^{1} \exp\,(-\rho_s x^2)$$

$$Q\{a(2\ \rho_s(1 - x^2))^{0.5} - bx\}\ dx \tag{8.4.51}$$

where

$$a = (B_R)^{0.5}\dot{\phi}_s/\omega_{\text{ef}} \tag{8.4.52}$$

$$b = (0.5)^{0.5}\dot{A}_s/\omega_{\text{ef}} \tag{8.4.53}$$

with a minimum value when $b = 0$. The minimum value is

$$P_b(e) = \pi^{-1} \int_0^{\pi/2} \exp\{-a^2 \rho_s (1 + (a^2 - 1)\cos^2\theta)^{-1}\}\, d\theta \quad (8.4.54)$$

which is shown in Fig. 8.18 with $a$ as a parameter. It can be seen from this figure that if $a \geqq 1$ there is no great change in the error probability. $P_b(e)$ can be well approximated by

$$P_b(e) = \begin{cases} V_1 \exp(-\rho_s) & a > 1 \\ 0.5 \exp(-\rho_s) & a = 1 \\ V_2 \exp(-a^2 \rho_s) & a < 1 \end{cases} \quad (8.4.55)$$

where

$$V_1 = \frac{f_{ef}}{A_s \dot{\phi}_s (a^2 - 1)^{0.5}} \quad (8.4.56)$$

$$V_2 = \frac{f_{ef}}{A_s \dot{\phi}_s (1 - a^2)^{0.5}} \quad (8.4.57)$$

*Example* 8.4.2
Let the receiver filter be an ideal filter with bandwidth $B_R$ wide enough so that the signal is not distorted. Thus here with $a_o = 1$

$$b = 0, \dot{\phi}_s = \omega_d$$

$$\omega_{ef}^2 = \int_{-0.5B_R}^{0.5B_R} (2\pi f)^2 \, df = (\pi B_R)^2 B_R / 3$$

and

$$a = (3)^{0.5} 2 f_d / B_R = (3)^{0.5} h/(B_R T)$$

where $h$ is the normalized frequency deviation. If we select $a = 1$ and $h = 0.7$, we obtain $B_R T = 1.21$. The error probability can be computed from Fig. 8.18.

### 8.4.3 Condition of no ISI

We have seen that the error probability depends on $A_s$, $\dot{A}_s$, and $\dot{\phi}_s$ at $t = t_0$. In Section 4.3 we derived the conditions of no ISI (intersymbol interference)

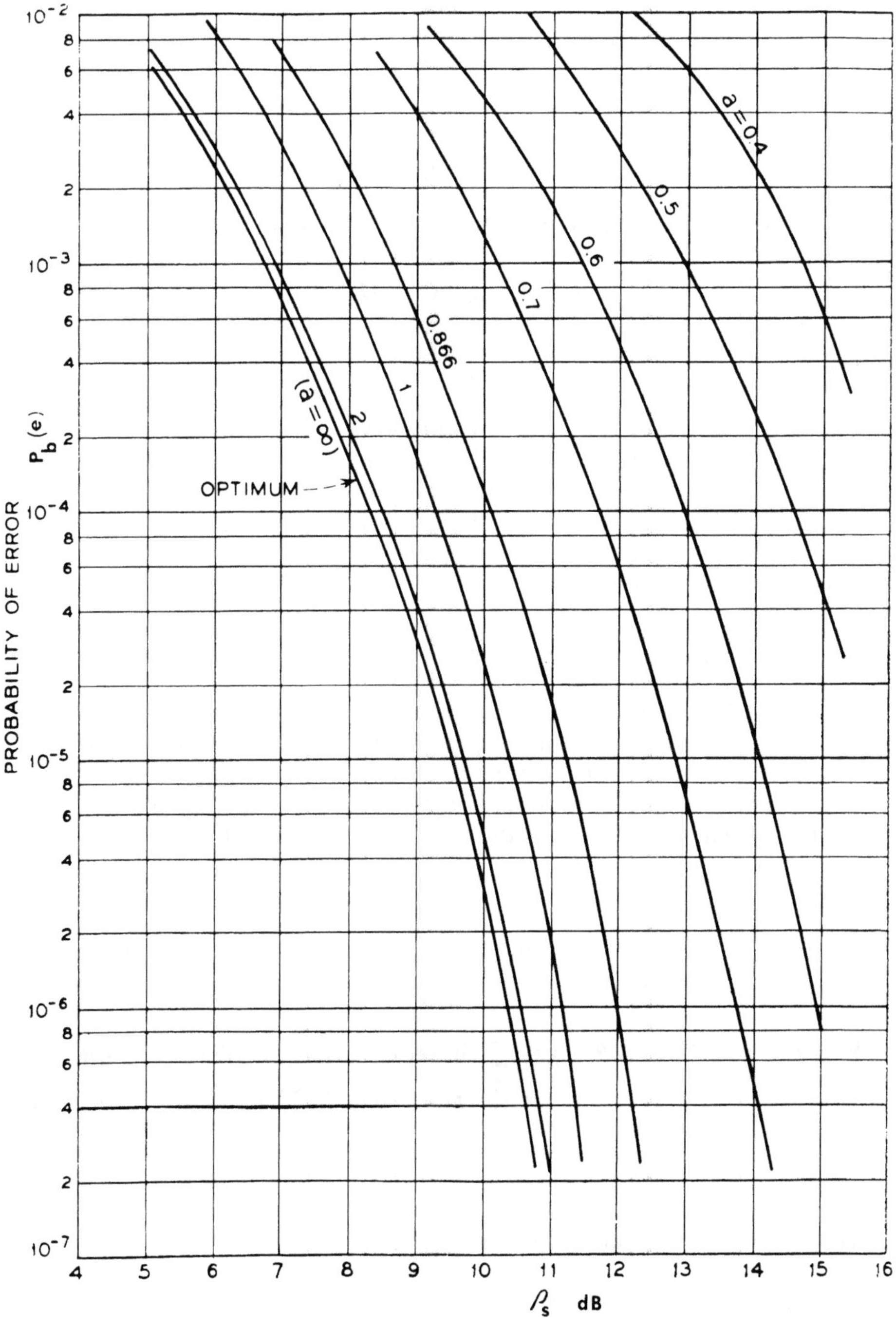


Fig. 8.18. Error probability as a function of signal-to-noise ratio for binary FSK with discriminator detector (Reprinted with permission from *The Bell System Technical Journal*. Copyright © 1963, AT&T).

for ASK and QASK signals. Here we derive similar conditions for an FSK signal. This was derived earlier in Refs. 8.23–8.25.

Let

$$h(t) = h_T(t) * h_C(t) * h_R(t) \tag{8.4.58}$$

When we substitute (8.1.7), (8.1.12) into (8.1.20), we obtain

$$s(t) = A \sum_i g(t - iT, a_i) \tag{8.4.59}$$

where

$$\begin{aligned} g(t, a_i) &= b(t, a_i) * h(t) = \exp\{j(a_i\omega_d t + \phi_i)\}u_T(t) * h(t) \\ &= \exp\{j(a_i\omega_d t + \phi_i)\}z(t - 0.5\,T, a_i) \end{aligned} \tag{8.4.60}$$

$$z(t, a_i) = u_T(t + 0.5\,T) * h(t)\exp(-ja_i\omega_d t) \tag{8.4.61}$$

with Fourier transform

$$Z(f, a_i) = T\,\text{sinc}(fT)H(f + a_i f_d) \tag{8.4.62}$$

There is no ISI if at the sampling time, $t_0$, $g(t_0, a_i) \neq 0$, while $g(t_0 - kT, a_i) = 0$ for all $k \neq 0$ and the derivative $\dot{g}(t_0 - kT, a_i) = 0$ for all $k$. This is achieved if $z(t_0, a_i) = T$, $z(t_0 - kT, a_i) = 0$, $k \neq 0$, and $\dot{z}(t_0 - kT, a_i) = 0$ all $k$. We may assume that $t_0 = 0$, because, if not, the same would apply to $z(t - t_0, a_i)$. This infinite number of equations can be reduced to the two equations

$$\begin{aligned} \sum_k Z(f - kR, a_i) &= T \sum_k \text{sinc}\{(f - kR)T\}H(f - kR + a_i f_d) \\ &= T \sum_k \text{sinc}\{(f - kR - a_i f_d)T\}H(f - kR) = T \end{aligned} \tag{8.4.63}$$

$$\begin{aligned} \sum_k \pi(f - kR)Z(f - kR, a_i) &= \sum_k \sin\{\pi(f - kR - a_i f_d)T\}H(f - kR) \\ &= \sin\{\pi(f - a_i f_d)T\} \sum_k (-1)^k H(f - kR) = 0 \end{aligned} \tag{8.4.64}$$

where $R = 1/T$. We thus have to solve the $M + 1$ equations

$$\sum_k \text{sinc}\{(f - kR - a_i f_d)T\}H(f - kR) = 1, \; a_i \in \{\pm 1, \ldots, \pm(M - 1)\} \tag{8.4.65}$$

$$\sum_k (-1)^k H(f - kR) = 0 \qquad (8.4.66)$$

There is an infinite number of functions $H(f)$ that satisfy (8.4.65) and (8.4.66). The one with the least bandwidth will be nonzero in a bandwidth of $(M + 1)R$.

*Example* 8.4.3
Find $H(f)$ that will cause no ISI in FSK for binary symbols and has a minimum bandwidth.
We assume that

$$H(f) \neq 0 \quad \text{for} \quad |f| \leqq 1.5\ R$$

The equations are

$$b_{-1,+}H(f + R) + b_{0,+}H(f) + b_{1,+}H(f - R) = 1$$

$$b_{-1,-}H(f + R) + b_{0,-}H(f) + b_{1,-}H(f - R) = 1$$

$$-H(f + R) + H(f) - H(f - R) = 0$$

where

$$b_{k,\pm} = \text{sinc}\{(f - kR \pm f_d)T\}$$

The particular solution can be found in Ref. 8.25.

Although it is possible to obtain an FSK signal without ISI, the large resulting bandwidths of the filters are prohibitive, because they will introduce excessive noise. In practice, binary FSK with a bandwidth of $R$ only (instead of 3 $R$) is achievable with only a moderate amount of ISI.

### 8.4.4 Effect of filter on FSK signal

We assume that $h_T(t)$, $h_C(t)$, and $h_R(t)$ are causal, real filters with a finite number of distinct poles. It was shown in Section 4.5 that the composite filter $h(t)$ has also a finite number of poles. Thus we can write

$$h(t) = \sum_{n=1}^{K} \rho_n \exp(-p_n t)u(t) \qquad (8.4.67)$$

where $\{p_n\}$ are the poles (either real or complex conjugate pairs) and $\{\rho_n\}$ are the residua (also real or in conjugate pairs), so that $h(t)$ is real. Because

$$b(t, a_i) = \exp\{j(\phi_i + a_i\omega_d t)\}u_T(t) = \exp(j\phi_i)$$
$$\{\exp(ja_i\omega_d t)u(t) - \exp(ja_i\omega_d T)\exp\{ja_i\omega_d(t - T)\}u(t - T)\} \tag{8.4.68}$$

we obtain in (8.4.60)

$$g(t, a_i) = \exp(j\phi_i)\{g_u(t, a_i) - \exp(ja_i\omega_d T)g_u(t - T, a_i)\} \tag{8.4.69}$$

where

$$g_u(t, a_i) = \exp(ja_i\omega_d t)u(t) * h(t)$$
$$= \sum_{n=1}^{K} \rho_n(p_n + ja_i\omega_d)^{-1}\{\exp(ja_i\omega_d t) - \exp(-p_n t)\}u(t) \tag{8.4.70}$$

We shall also need the derivative

$$\dot{g}_u(t, a_i) = \sum_{n=1}^{K} \rho_n(p_n + ja_i\omega_d)^{-1}\{ja_i\omega_d \exp(ja_i\omega_d t) + p_n \exp(-p_n t)\}u(t) \tag{8.4.71}$$

At sampling time $t = t_0$, we obtain

$$A_s = (s_I^2(t_0) + s_Q^2(t_0))^{0.5} \tag{8.4.72}$$

$$\dot{A}_s = (s_I(t_0)\dot{s}_I(t_0) + s_Q(t_0)\dot{s}_Q(t_0))/A_s \tag{8.4.73}$$

$$\dot{\phi}_s = \{s_I(t_0)\dot{s}_Q(t_0) - s_Q(t_0)\dot{s}_I(t_0)\}/A_s^2 \tag{8.4.74}$$

where

$$s_I(t_0) = A\sum_i g_I(t_0 - iT, a_i) \tag{8.4.75}$$

$$s_Q(t_0) = A\sum_i g_Q(t_0 - iT, a_i) \tag{8.4.76}$$

and $g_I(t, a_i)$, $g_Q(t, a_i)$ is the real and imaginary part of $g(t, a_i)$ and can be computed from (8.4.69). In practice when we compute (8.4.75) and (8.4.76), only a finite number of terms, adjacent to $a_0$, will be significant, say $N_1 + N_2$ terms, so that

$$s_I(t_0) = A\sum_{i=-N_1}^{N_2} g_I(t_0 - iT, a_i) \tag{8.4.77}$$

$$s_Q(t_0) = A\sum_{i=-N_1}^{N_2} g_Q(t_0 - iT, a_i) \tag{8.4.78}$$

$N_2$ is less than $K$ where $KT < t_0 \leqq (K + 1)T$. For a given value of $a_0$, there are $L = M^{(N_1+N_2)}$ such terms. When we apply the formulas of error probability (for example, (8.4.8)), we in fact compute the conditional error probability, conditioned on a certain sequence $\mathbf{a}(m) = (a_{-N_1}, \ldots a_{-1}, a(m), a_1, \ldots a_{N_2})$, and

$$P(e|m) = \sum_{i=1}^{L} P(e|\mathbf{a}_\iota(m))/L \tag{8.4.79}$$

where $a_\iota(m)$ is the ιth realization of $\mathbf{a}(m)$.

## 8.5 FSK WITH DISCRIMINATOR AND DETECTOR FILTER

It can be seen from Fig. 8.17 that

$$\dot{\phi}_r(t) = \dot{\phi}_s(t) + \dot{\phi}_n(t) \tag{8.5.1}$$

where $\phi_n(t)$ is given in (8.4.4). Because $n_Q'(t)$ and $n_I'(t)$ have the same properties as $n_Q(t)$ and $n_I(t)$, we shall drop the prime; hence here

$$\phi_n(t) = \tan^{-1} \{n_Q(t)/(A_s(t) + n_I(t)\} \tag{8.5.2}$$

The pdf of this phase is given in eq. (7.2.31), where it is called $\theta$, with $\rho_s$ replaced by

$$\rho_s(t) = 0.5\, A_s^2(t)/\sigma^2{}_n \tag{8.5.3}$$

The detector filter is a filter matched to the shaping function. An analysis of the system is available only when the shaping function is an NRZ pulse or split phase. For an NRZ pulse the detector filter is an integrate and dump circuit, the output of which is

$$x(t) = \int_{t-T}^{t} \dot{\phi}_r(\tau)\, d\tau = \phi_s(t) - \phi_s(t - T) + \int_{t-T}^{t} \dot{\phi}_n(\tau)\, d\tau \tag{8.5.4}$$

The phase noise $\phi_n(t)$ is determined by the relative values of the Gaussian processes $n_Q(t)$, $n_I(t)$. If we do not reduce $\phi_n(t)$ to its modulo $2\pi$ value, it has several branches with a range of $2\pi$ each, and the principal branch is defined as $|\phi_n(t)| \leqq \pi$.

In Fig. 8.19 we show several paths for the signal

$$v(t) = A_s + n_I(t) + jn_Q(t) \tag{8.5.5}$$

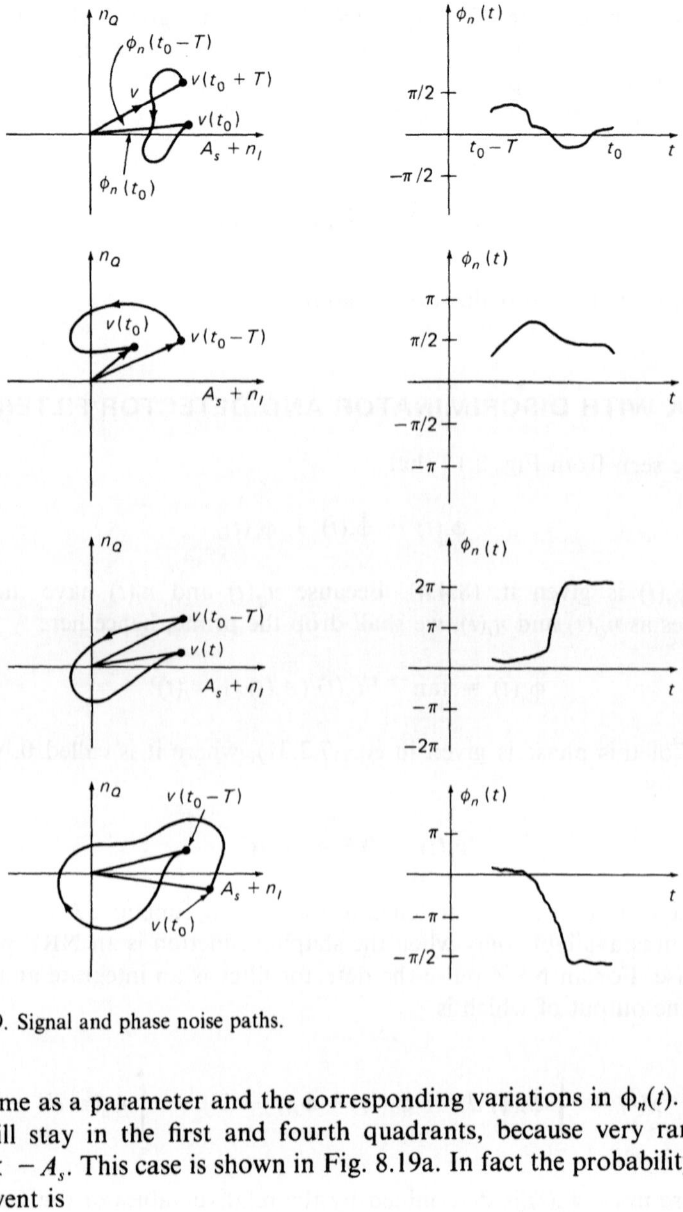


Fig. 8.19. Signal and phase noise paths.

with time as a parameter and the corresponding variations in $\phi_n(t)$. Usually $v(t)$ will stay in the first and fourth quadrants, because very rarely will $n_I(t) < -A_s$. This case is shown in Fig. 8.19a. In fact the probability of this rare event is

$$P(n_I(t) < -A_s) = Q(A_s/\sigma_n) = Q((2\,\rho_s)^{0.5}) \qquad (8.5.6)$$

and depends on the signal-to-noise ratio. Even if $v(t)$ crosses the vertical axis, it will be for a short moment only and will return immediately to the right-hand plane. The crossing into the left-hand plane may result in a sudden change of phase by $2\pi$, or equivalently $\phi_n(t)$ will climb to its next branch. This depends on the behavior of $n_Q(t)$. If $n_Q(t)$ does not change sign as shown in Fig. 8.19b, the phase stays within its principal branch. If $n_Q(t)$ does change sign as shown in Fig. 8.19c, there is a change of $2\pi$, and $\phi_n(t)$ will take values on the branch $\pi \leqq \phi_n(t) \leqq 3\pi$. In Fig. 8.19d we show a similar change of $-2\pi$. When we take the derivative of the phase, there will be a positive or negative narrow pulse of area $2\pi$ whenever there is a change of phase of $\pm 2\pi$. This is illustrated in Fig. 8.20. Because the pulses are narrow (compared with $1/B_d$, where $B_d$ is the bandwidth of the detector filter), they may be replaced by impulses of area $2\pi$. The occurrence of the impulses may be assumed to be a Poisson process.

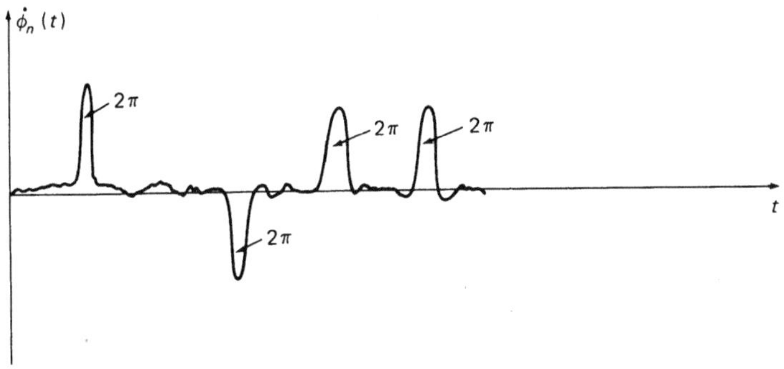


Fig. 8.20. The derivative of phase noise.

Therefore when we integrate $\dot{\phi}_n(t)$, the result is

$$\Delta\phi_n = \{\phi_n(t) - \phi_n(t - T)\} \bmod 2\pi + 2\pi N \tag{8.5.7}$$

where $\phi_n(t)$, $\phi_n(t - T)$ are phases confined to the principal branch of $-\pi$—$\pi$, and $N$ is a discrete random variable that represents the number of encirclements of the origin by $\phi_n(t)$ during the time interval $t - T$—$t$.

This theory of the behavior of a frequency modulated (FM) signal with noise was first presented in Refs. 8.26 and 8.27. Because in FM radio the occurrence of a pulse causes a "click" in the loudspeaker, the theory is sometimes called Rice's "click" theory. The theory was adapted to FSK in Refs. 8.28–8.32.

Let us denote

$$\theta_1 = \phi_n(t), \; \theta_0 = \phi_n(t - T) \tag{8.5.8}$$

and

$$\Delta\theta = \theta_1 - \theta_0, \; \psi = \Delta\theta \text{ (modulo } 2\pi) \tag{8.5.9}$$

The pdf of $\theta_0$ and $\theta_1$ is given in eq. (7.2.31), the pdf of $\Delta\theta$ (assuming that $\theta_0$ and $\theta_1$ are independent) in eq. (7.3.32), and that of $\psi$ in eq. (7.3.34)). The CPDF of $\psi$ is presented in eq. (7.3.38). In these equations

$$\rho_1 = \rho_s(t) = 0.5\ A_s^2(t)/\sigma_n^2 \tag{8.5.10}$$

$$\rho_0 = \rho_s(t - T) = 0.5\ A_s^2(t - T)/\sigma_n^2 \tag{8.5.11}$$

are the signal to noise ratios. For large values of $\rho_s$ (the definition of $\rho_m$, $\rho_d$, and $\rho_g$ are given in eq. (7.3.35)), the following approximations are given in refs. 8.18 and 8.32

$$Q_\psi(\beta) = \begin{cases} (\rho_m + u)\exp(u - \rho_m)\{8\ \pi u(\rho_m^2 - u^2)\}^{-0.5} & 0 < \beta < \pi/2 \\ 0.25\ \{1 - (\rho_g/\rho_m)\mathrm{Ie}(\rho_d/\rho_m, \rho_m)\} & \beta = \pi/2 \\ -\tan\beta\exp(-\rho_m)\{(\rho_m - 1)\cosh\rho_d + \rho_d\sinh\rho_d\}/(2\ \pi\rho_g^2) & \pi/2 < \beta < \pi \end{cases} \tag{8.5.12}$$

where

$$u^2 = \rho_m^2\cos^2\beta + \rho_d^2\sin^2\beta \tag{8.5.13}$$

and

$$\mathrm{Ie}(y, x) = \int_0^x I_0(yt)\exp(-t)\,dt$$

$$= (1 - y^2)^{-0.5} - \int_0^x \frac{\exp\{-x(1 - y\cos\theta)\}}{\pi(1 - y\cos\theta)}\,d\theta \tag{8.5.14}$$

The pdf of $\Delta\phi_n$ in (8.5.7) is thus the convolution of the pdfs of $\psi$ and of $N$. The random variable $N$ is the difference between the number of positive and negative going "clicks"

$$N = N_+ - N_- \tag{8.5.15}$$

with averages $\bar{N}_+$ and $\bar{N}_-$, respectively, in a time interval of duration $T$. $\bar{N}_+$ and $\bar{N}_-$ are equal when the carrier is unmodulated ($\phi_s(t) = 0$). When the carrier is modulated and $\phi_s(t) > 0$, we can ignore the positive going clicks, and if $\phi_s(t) < 0$, we can ignore the negative going clicks. Because of symmetry it is sufficient to discuss the first case only. The probability that we obtain exactly $N = k$ clicks, assuming $\phi_s > 0$, is given by the Poisson probability

$$P(N = -k) = \exp(-\bar{N})(\bar{N})^k/k! \qquad k = 0, 1, 2, \ldots \tag{8.5.16}$$

with the average $\bar{N}$ given by

$$\bar{N} = \int_{t-T}^{t} \dot{\phi}_s(\tau) \exp(-\rho_s(\tau))\, d\tau/(2\pi) \tag{8.5.17}$$

which for an undistorted signal, i.e., $\rho_s(\tau) = \rho_s$ and

$$\dot{\phi}_s(t) = a_0 \omega_d \qquad a_0 = 1, 3, \ldots, (M - 1) \tag{8.5.18}$$

is simply

$$\bar{N} = \bar{N}(a_0) = a_0 f_d T \exp(-\rho_s) \tag{8.5.19}$$

The joint pdf of $\Delta\phi_n$, assuming independence of $\psi$ and $N$, is

$$p_{\Delta\phi n}(\alpha) = \sum_{k=0}^{\infty} p_\psi(\alpha + 2\pi k) P(N = -k) \tag{8.5.20}$$

which is illustrated in Fig. 8.21. Since, for reasonable values of $\rho_s$, $\bar{N}$ is a small number, we may ignore in (8.5.20) all but the first two terms, and we can also approximate

$$P(N = 0) = \exp(-\bar{N}) \simeq 1 \tag{8.5.21}$$

$$P(N = -1) \simeq P(N < 0) = 1 - \exp(-\bar{N}) \simeq \bar{N} \tag{8.5.22}$$

Therefore

$$P_{\Delta\phi n}(\alpha) \simeq p_\psi(\alpha) + \bar{N} p_\psi(\alpha + 2\pi) \tag{8.5.23}$$

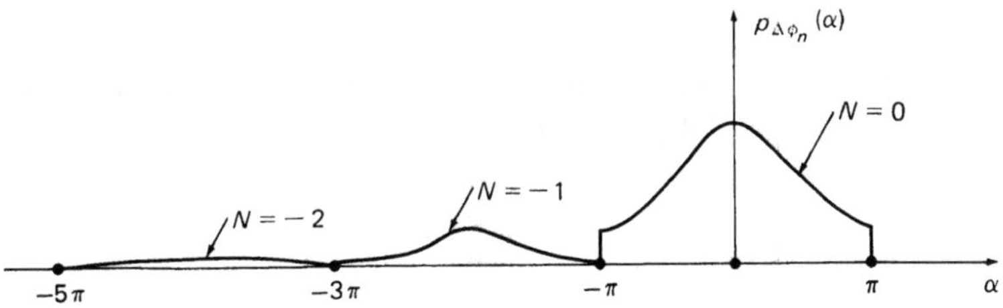


Fig. 8.21. The probability density function of the difference of two phases.

### 8.5.1 Error probability for NRZ shaping functions

If we assume that

$$h_D(t) = u_T(t) \tag{8.5.24}$$

the output of the detector filter is combining (8.5.4) and (8.5.7), for $t = t_0$

$$x(t) = \phi_s(t) - \phi_s(t - T) + \Delta\phi_n = \Delta\phi_s + \Delta\phi_n \tag{8.5.25}$$

In the absence of distortion

$$\Delta\phi_s = a_0\omega_d T \tag{8.5.26}$$

Hence

$$x(t) = a_0\omega_d T + \Delta\phi_n \tag{8.5.27}$$

The decision rule is the same as in eq. (8.4.5) with $\omega_d$ replaced by $\omega_d T$, and the error probability is as in eq. (8.4.7) with $\hat{\omega}$ replaced by $x(t_0)$ and $\omega_d$ by $\omega_d T$. Because of symmetry it is sufficient to compute the error probability for the positive symbols only; thus

$$P(e) = (2/M) \sum_{m=1}^{M/2} P(e|a_0 = 2\,m - 1) \tag{8.5.28}$$

where for $a_0 = 1, 3, \ldots, M - 3$

$$\begin{aligned} P(e|a_0 = 2\,m - 1) &= P(|x(t) - (2\,m - 1)\omega_d T| > \omega_d T|a_0 = 2\,m - 1) \\ &= P(|\Delta\phi_s + \Delta\phi_n - (2\,m - 1)\omega_d T| > \omega_d T|a_0 \\ &= 2\,m - 1) \\ &= P(\Delta\phi_n > 2\,m\omega_d T - \Delta\phi_s|a_0 = 2\,m - 1) \\ &\quad + P(\Delta\phi_n < 2(m - 1)\omega_d T - \Delta\phi_s|a_0 = 2\,m - 1) \end{aligned} \tag{8.5.29}$$

and for $a_0 = M - 1$

$$\begin{aligned} P(e|a_0 = M - 1) &= P(\Delta\phi_s + \Delta\phi_n - (M - 1)\omega_d T < -\omega_d T|a_0 = M - 1) \\ &= P(\Delta\phi_n < (M - 2)\omega_d T - \Delta\phi_s|a_0 = M - 1) \end{aligned} \tag{8.5.30}$$

In the binary case we obtain

$$P_b(e) = P(e|a_0 = 1) = P(\Delta\phi_n < -\Delta\phi_s|a_0 = 1) \tag{8.5.31}$$

**8.5.1.1 No intersymbol interference** When there is no distortion and $a_0 = 2m - 1$, we obtain

$$\Delta\phi_s = (2m - 1)\omega_d T \qquad (8.5.32)$$

Hence for $a_0 = 1, 3, \ldots, M - 3$

$$\begin{aligned} P(e|a_0 = 2m - 1) &= P(\Delta\phi_n > \omega_d T|a_0 = 2m - 1) \\ &\quad + P(\Delta\phi_n < -\omega_d T|a_0 = 2m - 1) \\ &= P(|\Delta\phi_n| > \omega_d T|a_0 = 2m - 1) \end{aligned} \qquad (8.5.33)$$

and

$$P(e|a_0 = M - 1) = P(\Delta\phi_n < -\omega_d T|a_0 = M - 1) \qquad (8.5.34)$$

We can see from Fig. 8.21 and eq. (8.5.23) that for $0 < \omega_d T \leqq \pi$

$$P(\Delta\phi_n > \omega_d T|a_0 = 2m - 1) = P(\psi > \omega_d T) \qquad (8.5.35)$$

while

$$\begin{aligned} P(\Delta\phi_n < -\omega_d T|a_0 = 2m - 1) &= P(\psi < -\omega_d \mathrm{T}) + \bar{N}(a_0) \\ &= P(\psi > \omega_d T) + \bar{N}(a_0) \end{aligned} \qquad (8.5.36)$$

We substitute (8.5.33)–(8.5.36) into (8.5.28) and, using (8.5.12) (or its simplified version eq. (7.3.37), because here $\rho_m = \rho_g = \rho_s$, $\rho_d = 0$) and (8.5.19), we obtain

$$P(e) = 2(1 - M^{-1})Q_\psi(\omega_d T) + 0.5\, M f_d T \exp(-\rho_s) \qquad (8.5.37)$$

For the binary case this is simply

$$P_b(e) = Q_\psi(\omega_d T) + f_d T \exp(-\rho_s) \qquad (8.5.38)$$

For $M$-ary FSK we select the frequency separation so that

$$\omega_d T = \pi/M \qquad (8.5.39)$$

Hence for $M > 2$ we are using the first equation in (7.3.37). The error probability as a function of signal-to-noise ratio for $M = 4, 8, 16, 32$ is shown in Fig. 8.22.

For binary FSK we select

$$\omega_d T = h\pi \qquad (8.5.40)$$

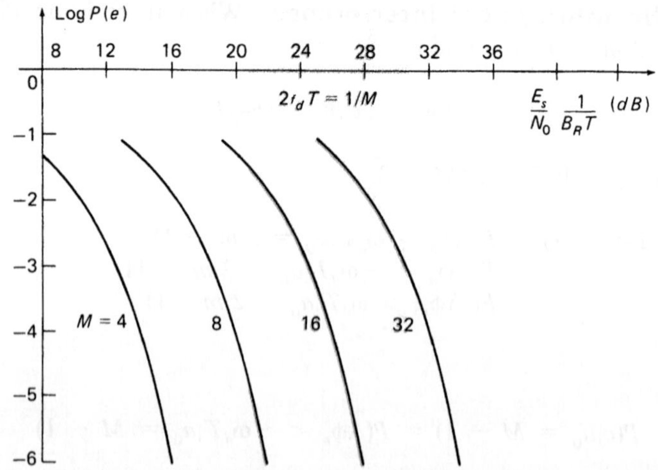


Fig. 8.22. Error probability as a function of signal-to-noise ratio for FSK with discriminator and NRZ detector filter for $h = 1/M$ and no distortion.

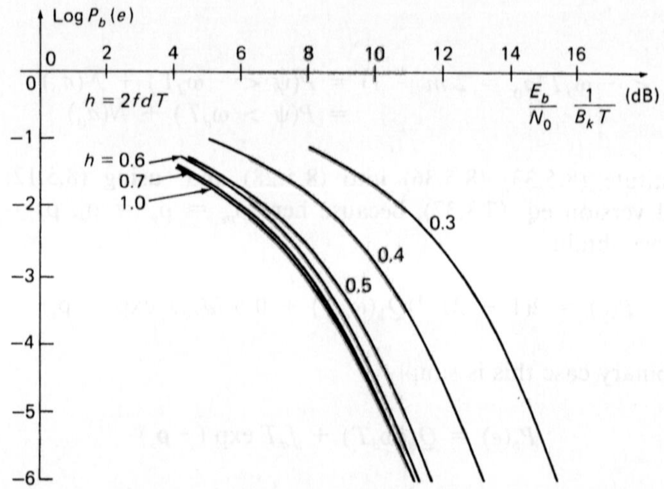


Fig. 8.23. Bit error probability as a function of signal-to-noise ratio of binary FSK with discriminator and NRZ detector filter for variable $h$.

where $h$ is arbitrary. The bit error probability as a function of signal-to-noise ratio with $h$ as a parameter is shown in Fig. 8.23. It was shown in Chapter 3 that the bandwidth of the modulated signal increases with $h$; hence a larger bandwidth will be required to pass the signal without distortion. Therefore a value of $h = 0.7$ is a reasonable selection.

### 8.5.1.2 With intersymbol interference

When there is signal distortion we have to return to eqs. (8.5.28)–(8.5.31). The difference in the signal phase is

$$\Delta\phi_s(t) = \phi_s(t) - \phi_s(t - T) \tag{8.5.41}$$

where

$$\phi_s(t) = \tan^{-1}(s_Q(t)/s_I(t)) \tag{8.5.42}$$

and $s_I(t)$, $s_Q(t)$ are given in eq. (8.4.75) and (8.4.76). In practice only a finite number of symbols, adjacent to $a_0$, must be taken into account; hence in fact eq. (8.4.75) and (8.4.78) will be used. Thus for a given value of $a_0 = 2m - 1$, $m = 1, 2, \ldots, M/2$, $\Delta\phi_s(t)$ will depend on the sequence

$$\mathbf{a}(m) = (a_{-N1}, \ldots a_{-1}, 2m - 1, a_1, \ldots, a_{N2}) \tag{8.5.43}$$

Hence in fact we should write

$$\Delta\phi_s(t) = \Delta\phi_s(t, \mathbf{a}(m)) \tag{8.5.44}$$

There are $L = M^{N1+N2}$ such sequences, all of which are equiprobable, $\mathbf{a}_\iota(m)$ being the $\iota$th sequence $1 \leqq \iota \leqq L$. The numbers $N_1$, $N_2$ will depend on the bandwidth, $B$, of the filter $h(t)$. For $BT > 1$, $N_1$ and $N_2$ must not be greater than 2.

Let the signal error caused by the $\iota$th sequence be

$$\varepsilon(\iota, m) = (2m - 1)\omega_d T - \Delta\phi_s(t, \mathbf{a}_\iota(m)) \tag{8.5.45}$$

We shall assume that this error is small enough so that

$$|\varepsilon(\iota, m)| \leqq \omega_d T \tag{8.5.46}$$

Thus we obtain from (8.5.29), (8.5.35), and (8.5.36), for $a_0 = 2m - 1$, $m = 1, 2, \ldots, 0.5M - 1$

$$\begin{aligned} P(e|\mathbf{a}_\iota(m)) &= P(\Delta\phi_n > \omega_d T + \varepsilon(\iota, m)) + P(\Delta\phi_n < -\omega_d T + \varepsilon(\iota, m)) \\ &= Q_\psi(\omega_d T + \varepsilon(\iota, m)) + Q_\psi(\omega_d T - \varepsilon(\iota, m)) + \bar{N}(\iota, m) \end{aligned} \tag{8.5.47}$$

and from (8.5.30) for $m = 0.5M$

$$P(e|\mathbf{a}_\iota(0.5M)) = Q_\psi(\omega_d T - \varepsilon(\iota, 0.5M)) + \overline{N(\iota, 0.5M)} \tag{8.5.48}$$

where $N(\iota, m)$ is computed using (8.5.17) for the sequence $\mathbf{a}_\iota(m)$.
After substitution into (8.5.28) we obtain

$$P(e) = 2(LM)^{-1}\left[\sum_{m=1}^{0.5M}\sum_{\iota=1}^{L}(Q_\psi(\omega_d T - \varepsilon(\iota, m)) + \overline{N(\iota, m)})\right.$$
$$\left.+ \sum_{m=1}^{0.5M-1}\sum_{\iota=1}^{L} Q_\psi(\omega_d T + \varepsilon(\iota, m))\right] \tag{8.5.49}$$

For the binary case this is simplified to

$$P_b(e) = L^{-1}\sum_{k}^{L} [Q_\psi(\Delta\phi_s(t_0, \mathbf{a}_\iota(1)) + \overline{N(\iota, 1)}] \tag{8.5.50}$$

In computing these equations we are using eq. (8.5.12) with $\rho_1$, $\rho_0$ as defined in (8.5.10) and (8.5.11), and $t = t_0$. In computing $\overline{N(\iota, m)}$ in (8.5.17) we have to use an approximation to the integral

$$\overline{N(\iota, m)} = T(2\pi K)^{-1}\sum_{k=0}^{K-1}\dot{\phi}_s(t_0 - T + kT/K)\exp(-\rho_s(t_0 - T + kT/K)) \tag{8.5.51}$$

and the sequence $\mathbf{a}_\iota(m)$ is assumed. If the filters in the system have a finite number of poles, the equations of Section 8.4.4 can be used to derive the numerical results.

The approach outlined here is in some aspects similar to the method presented in Ref. 8.33 however in this reference it was assumed that the sampling time, the "click" noise and decision levels are not affected by the filters and no examples are presented. Let us clarify how the decision levels are effected by the filters. In deriving (8.5.45) and (8.5.49) we have assumed that the decision levels are midway between the signal levels in the absence of distortion. When the signal is distorted by the filters the signal levels are changed hence the decision levels must be modified. This can be done simply by replacing in (8.5.45) and (8.5.49) $\omega_d T$ by $\omega_d T thr$ and the parameter $thr$ can be optimised. We have computed in ref. 8.48 and 8.49 the error probability of FSK with various filters. In Fig. 8.24 we show the bit error probability as a function of $E_b/N_0$ (signal to noise ratio per bit) for binary and quaternary symbols, assuming a wide band transmitter filter and a Butterworth filter in receiver with 2, 3, 4 poles. In the quaternary case we have either $thr = 1$ which corresponds to unmodified decision levels or the optimal value of $thr$. The sampling time was also optimised in each case.

In the binary case, three other methods have been published in Refs. 8.32–8.34 and 8.36.

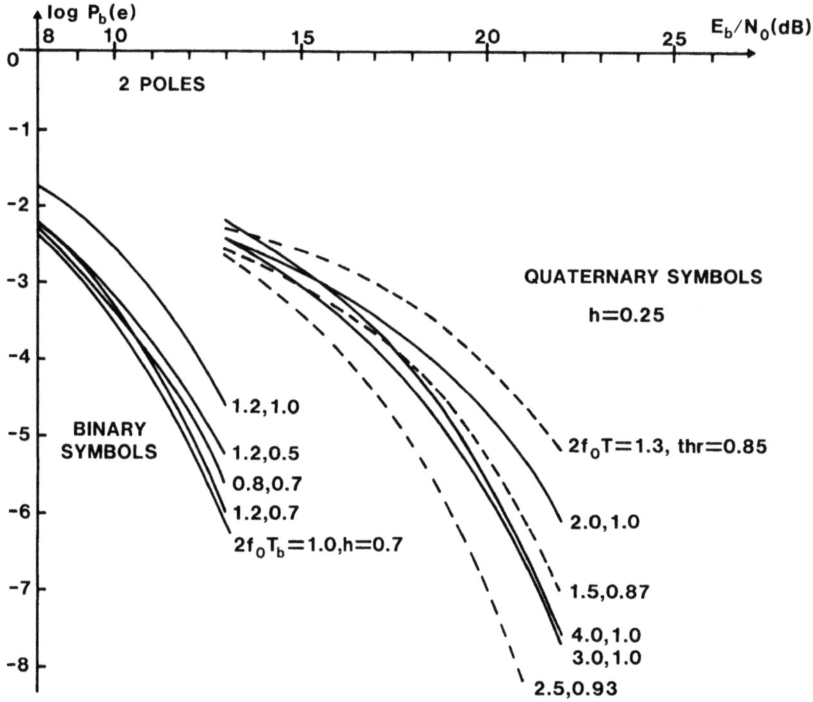


Fig. 8.24. Bit error probability as a function of signal-to-noise ratio per bit for binary and quaternary FSK with discriminator detector and NRZ detector filter. The transmitter filter is wide band, the receiver filter is a Butterworth filter with (a) 2, (b) 3 and (c) 4 poles. The decision levels are fixed (thr = 1) or are optimised. The sampling time is optimised. The parameters are normalised bandwidth ($2\,f_0T$) and frequency deviation ($h$).

In Ref. 8.34 the random modulating signal in (8.1.2) is replaced by a periodic signal with period

$$T_p = 30T \tag{8.5.52}$$

generated by a repetition of the pseudorandom sequence of 30 symbols

$$\{110\ 000\ 010\ 110\ 111\ 001\ 111\ 101\ 001\ 000\}$$

and an NRZ shaping function. In this case $\exp\{j\phi(t)\}$ is also periodic with a Fourier series

$$\exp\{j\phi(t)\} = \sum_n C_n \exp(j\,2\,\pi n f_p t) \tag{8.5.53}$$

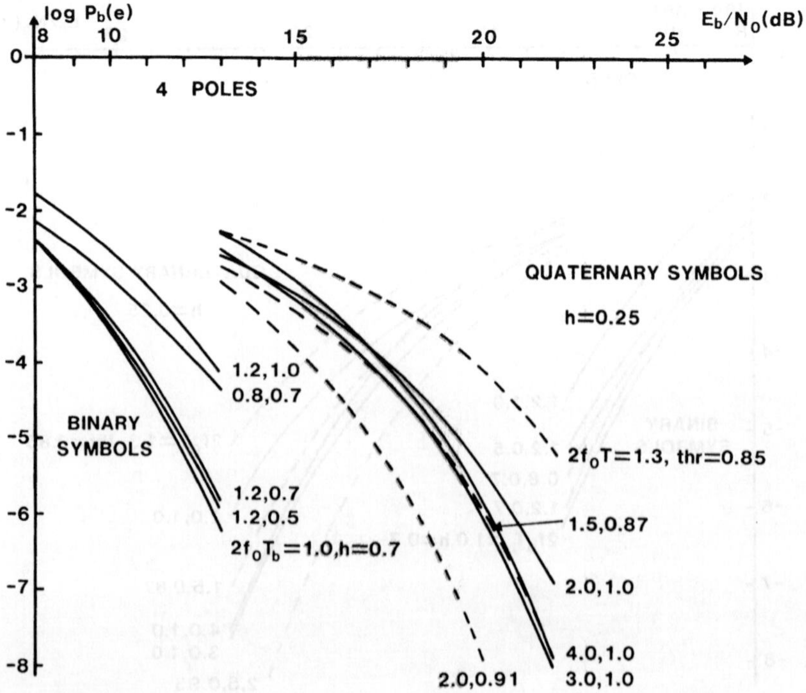

log Pb(e)
Eb/N0(dB)
8
10
15
20
25
0
-1
-2
-3
-4
-5
-6
-7
-8
4 POLES
QUATERNARY SYMBOLS
h=0.25
1.2,1.0
0.8,0.7
BINARY
SYMBOLS
2f0T=1.3, thr=0.85
1.2,0.7
1.2,0.5
1.5,0.87
2f0Tb=1.0,h=0.7
2.0,1.0
4.0,1.0
2.0,0.91
3.0,1.0


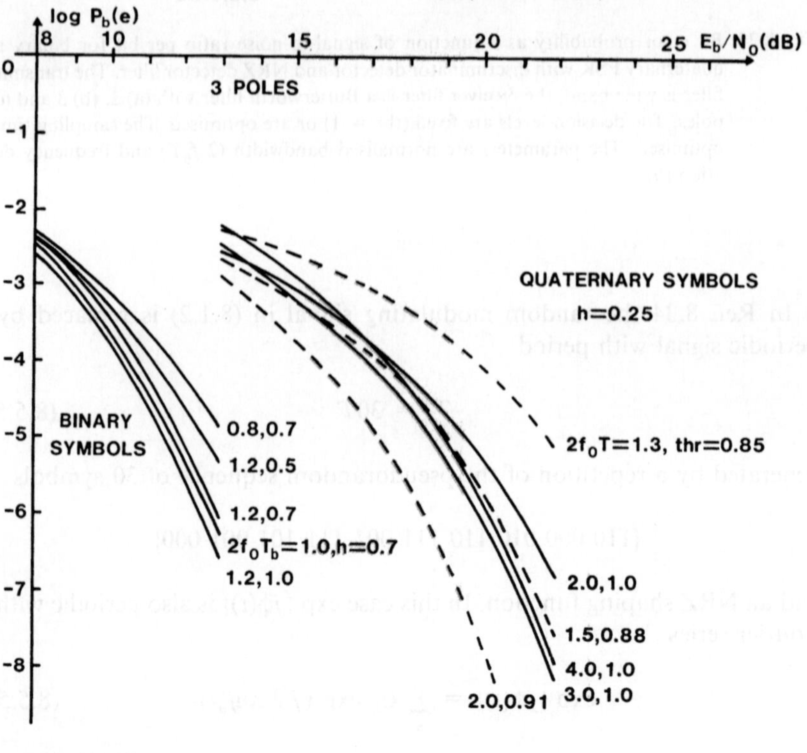

log Pb(e)
8
10
15
20
25
Eb/N0(dB)
0
3 POLES
-1
-2
-3
-4
-5
-6
-7
-8
QUATERNARY SYMBOLS
h=0.25
BINARY
SYMBOLS
0.8,0.7
2f0T=1.3, thr=0.85
1.2,0.5
1.2,0.7
2f0Tb=1.0,h=0.7
1.2,1.0
2.0,1.0
1.5,0.88
4.0,1.0
2.0,0.91
3.0,1.0


Fig. 8.24. (*con't.*)

where

$$f_p = 1/T_p \tag{8.5.54}$$

and $\{C_n\}$ are the Fourier coefficients

$$C_n = T_p^{-1} \int_{-0.5T_p}^{0.5T_p} \exp\{j(\phi(t) - 2\pi n f_p t)\}\, dt \tag{8.5.55}$$

At the output of the receiver filter we obtain

$$s(t) = A \sum_n C_n H(nf_p) \exp(j\, 2\pi n f_p t) \tag{8.5.56}$$

from which we can compute $\phi_s(t)$, $\dot{\phi}_s(t)$, and $A_s(t)$. When the product $BT$ is not too small ($B$ is the bandwidth of the filter $H(f)$), the ISI is caused mainly by two adjacent symbols on each side of $a_0$. The pseudorandom sequence contains almost all sequences of length five. Curves are presented in Ref. 8.34 under the assumption that all filtering is done in the receiver and the filter is either a brick wall or Gaussian filter. The conclusion there is that the optimal normalized frequency deviation, $h$, is about 0.7, and the optimal normalized bandwidth, $B_R T$ is about 1–1.2. Comparisons with coherent ASK and PSK favor binary FSK for $B_R T \leq 1$. The optimal $h$ is a compromise between the contribution of the clicks and the smooth portion of the phase noise to the error probability. The optimal value of $B_R T$ is a compromise between the contribution of ISI and noise to the error probability.

In Ref. 8.35 a modified version of (8.5.50) is used. The modifications are

a. Instead of $\rho_1$ and $\rho_2$, only one value, the average

$$\rho_{\text{av}} = \int_{t_0 - T}^{t_0} A_s^2(t, \mathbf{a}_\iota(1))\, dt/(2\, N_0 B_R T) \tag{8.5.57}$$

is used.

b. $\overline{N(\iota, 1)}$ is approximated by

$$\overline{N(\iota, 1)} = (f_d T)_{\text{av}} \exp(-\rho_{\text{av}}) \tag{8.5.58}$$

where

$$(f_d T)_{\text{av}} = \int_{t_0 - T}^{t_0} \Delta\phi_s(t, \mathbf{a}_\iota(1))\, dt/(2\pi) \tag{8.5.59}$$

In Ref. 8.31 are given numerical results assuming a Butterworth filter in the receiver. The optimal $h$ is 0.72, the optimal $B_R T$ is about 1 for second- and third-order filters. With the third-order filter the error probability is the same as with a coherent detector.

In Ref. 8.32 it is assumed that only one neighboring symbol, on each side of $a_0$ causes ISI. This assumption is justified for $3 \geqq BT \geqq 1$ and $h < 1.5$. Therefore, with $a_0 = 1$, we have to consider only the four sequences 111, 010, 011, and 110, which can be arbitrarily extended on both sides, because the additional symbols do not cause ISI. The sequence 111 is extended to an all "1" sequence leading to

$$A \exp(j\phi(t)) = A \exp(j\, 2\, \pi f_d t) \tag{8.5.60}$$

The sequence 010 is extended to an alternating sequence of "0" and "1", which is periodic with period $T_p = 2\,T$; hence $A \exp(j\phi(t))$ can be expanded into a Fourier series. The sequence 011 is extended on the left by an alternating sequence and to the right by an all "1" sequence. The opposite is done for the 110 sequence. Therefore it is assumed that the properties of the last two sequences are the average of the properties of the first two sequences, namely

$$\Delta\phi_s(t, 110) = \Delta\phi_s(t, 011) = 0.5\,\{\Delta\phi_s(t, 010) + \Delta\phi_s(t, 111)\} \tag{8.5.61}$$

$$\overline{N(110)} = \overline{N(011)} = 0.5\,\{\overline{N(010)} + \overline{N(111)}\} \tag{8.5.62}$$

Thus when we use (8.5.50) we have only four terms, which are reduced because of (8.5.61) and (8.5.62) to three terms only

$$\begin{aligned} P_b(e) = 0.25\,\{&Q_\psi(\Delta\phi_s(t_0, 111)) + Q_\psi(\Delta\phi_s(t_0, 010)) \\ &+ 2\,Q_\psi(\Delta\phi_s(t_0, 110)) + \bar{N}(111) + \bar{N}(010) + 2\,\bar{N}(110)\} \end{aligned} \tag{8.5.63}$$

The curves in Refs. 8.32 and 8.34 coincide. In Fig. 8.24 we show the error probability as a function of signal-to-noise ratio for a Gaussian filter in the receiver. Almost identical results have been obtained for a second-order Butterworth filter.

### 8.5.2 Error probability for split-phase shaping function

For a split-phase shaping function the detector filter has an impulse response

$$h_D(t) = u_{0.5T}(t) - u_{0.5T}(t - 0.5\,T) \tag{8.5.64}$$

Hence the output at $t = t_0$ is

$$x(t) = \int_{t-T}^{t-0.5T} \dot{\phi}_r(\tau)\, d\tau - \int_{t-0.5T}^{t} \dot{\phi}_r(\tau)\, d\tau = \Delta\phi_s(t) + \Delta\phi_n(t) + 2\,\pi(N_1 - N_2) \tag{8.5.65}$$

where

$$\Delta\phi_s(t) = 2\phi_s(t - 0.5\,T) - \phi_s(t) - \phi_s(t - T) \tag{8.5.66}$$

$$\Delta\phi_n(t) = 2\,\phi_n(t - 0.5\,T) - \phi_n(t) - \phi_n(t - T)\ (\text{modulo } 2\,\pi) \tag{8.5.67}$$

and $N_1$, $N_2$ is the number of clicks during the intervals $t - 0.5\,T$—$t - T$ and $t$—$t - 0.5\,T$, respectively. When there is no distortion

$$\Delta\phi_s(t) = a_0\omega_d T \tag{8.5.68}$$

If we assume that the three terms in (8.5.67) are independent, the pdf of $\Delta\phi_n(t)$ is the convolution of three pdfs, each of which has the form of eq. (7.3.32). A closed form expression for this pdf is not known yet, Hence numerical methods must be applied for its computation.

Assuming a high signal-to-noise ratio, $\phi_n(t)$ in (8.5.2) can be approximated by

$$\phi_n(t) = n_Q(t)/A_s \tag{8.5.69}$$

which is a zero-mean, Gaussian rv with variance

$$\sigma_{\phi n}^2 = \sigma_n^2/A_s^2 = 0.5/\rho_s \tag{8.5.70}$$

This can also be noted in Fig. 7.12. Therefore $\Delta\phi_n(t)$ is also zero-mean, Gaussian with variance

$$\sigma_{\Delta\phi}^2 = 6\,\sigma_{\phi n}^2 = 3/\rho_s \tag{8.5.71}$$

$N_1$ and $N_2$ have the same probability function given in (8.5.16) with

$$\bar{N}_1 = \int_{t-T}^{t-0.5T} \dot{\phi}_s(\tau) \exp(-\rho_s(\tau))\, d\tau/(2\,\pi) \tag{8.5.72}$$

$$\bar{N}_2 = -\int_{t-0.5T}^{t} \dot{\phi}_s(\tau) \exp(-\rho_s(\tau))\, d\tau/(2\,\pi) \tag{8.5.73}$$

which in the case of no distortion and $a_0 = 1$ is simplified to

$$\bar{N}_1 = \bar{N}_2 = 0.5 f_d T \exp(-\rho_s) \tag{8.5.74}$$

Since for large signal-to-noise ratio

$$P(N = 0) = \exp(-\bar{N}) \simeq 1,\ P(N = 1) \simeq P(N \geqq 1) = 1 - \exp(-\bar{N}) \simeq \bar{N} \tag{8.5.75}$$

we obtain, assuming independence between $N_1$ and $N_2$

$$P(N_1 - N_2 = 0) = 1 - 2\exp(\bar{N}_1) \simeq 1 \tag{8.5.76}$$

$$P(N_1 - N_2 = 1) = P(N_1 - N_2 = -1) = \bar{N}_1 \exp(-\bar{N}_1) \simeq \bar{N}_1 \tag{8.5.77}$$

In the binary case the error probability is thus

$$\begin{aligned} P_b(e) &= P(\Delta\phi_n + 2\pi(N_1 - N_2) > \omega_d T) \\ &\simeq Q(h\pi(\rho_s/3)^{0.5}) + 0.25\, h \exp(-\rho_s) \end{aligned} \tag{8.5.78}$$

This method, ignoring the clicks, was presented in Ref. 8.36. In Ref. 8.37 is applied the method of Ref. 8.34 (the psuedorandom sequence was increased to 32 symbols), and graphs of error probability are presented for Gaussian filter in receiver and various values of $h$ and $B_R T$. The optimal values are $B_R T = 1.8$ and $h = 1.3$.

## 8.6 OBSERVATION INTERVAL LONGER THAN $T$

Until now it was assumed that a decision about the value of a symbol was based on observation and processing of the receiver signal during an interval of duration $T$ seconds. In FSK with continuous phase the signal in any $T$ interval depends not only on the current signal, but also on all previous symbols. (This is illustrated in Fig. 8.25. See also Figs. 2.17, 2.19, and 2.20a). Therefore it makes sense to extend the observation and processing time to $NT$, $N > 1$. This indeed was done for binary symbols in Refs. 8.38–8.41 and for $M$-ary symbols in Ref. 8.42 for NRZ shaping functions of duration $T$. The analysis was extended to other shaping functions of duration $T$ and to various partial response (of duration larger than $T$, say, $KT$) shaping functions in Refs. 8.43–8.46. In all these papers it is assumed that the signal is not distorted by the filters. Thus the received signal is

$$r(t) = A\exp(j\phi(t)) + n(t) = s(t) + n(t) \tag{8.6.1}$$

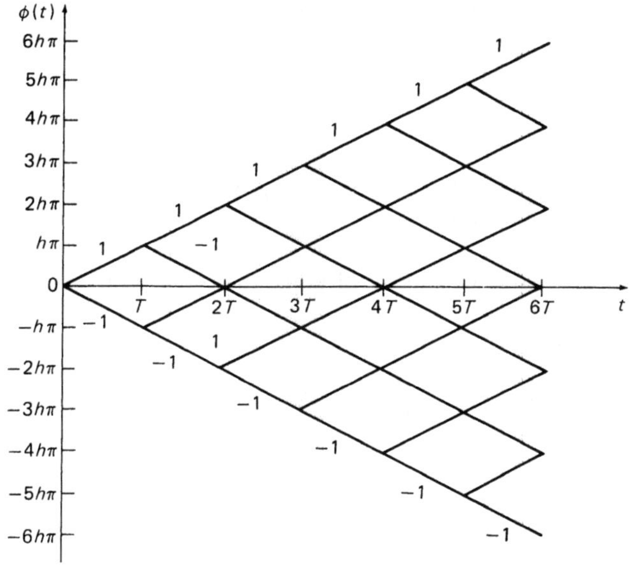


Fig. 8.25. Trajectories of the phase of an FSK signal with NRZ shaping function.

where

$$\phi(t) = 2\,\pi h \sum_i a_i \beta'(t - iT) \tag{8.6.2}$$

$$\beta'(t) = \int_0^t h_s(\tau)\, d\tau u(t)/(2\,\pi h) \tag{8.6.3}$$

and $h_s(t)$ is such that $\beta'(KT) = 0.5$. We observe $r(t)$ over the interval 0—$NT$, during which the sequence $\mathbf{a} = \{a_0, a_1, \ldots, a_{N-1}\}$ is transmitted and make a decision about the value of the first symbol, $a_0$, only. The optimal coherent receiver with a maximum likelihood decision rule (the derivation of this rule may be found in Ref. 8.47) is

$$\hat{a}_0 = a(m) \text{ if } \lambda_m = \max_k \{\lambda_k, k = 1, \ldots, M\} \tag{8.6.4}$$

where

$$a(m) = 2\,m - M - 1, m = 1, \ldots M \tag{8.6.5}$$

$$\lambda_m = \overline{\exp\left(2\,N_0^{-1} \int_0^{NT} r(t)s(t, \mathbf{a}(m))\, dt\right)} \tag{8.6.6}$$

$$\mathbf{a}(m) = \{a(m), a_1, \ldots, a_{N-1}\} \tag{8.6.7}$$

and the average is over the $N - 1$ independent rvs $a_1, \ldots, a_{N-1}$. When we perform the average we obtain

$$\lambda_m = \sum_{\iota=1}^{L} \exp\left(2 N_0^{-1} \int_0^{NT} r(t)s(t, \mathbf{a}_\iota(m))\, dt\right) \tag{8.6.8}$$

where $\mathbf{a}_\iota(m)$ is the $\iota$th realization of $\mathbf{a}(m)$, the total number of which is

$$L = M^{N-1} \tag{8.6.9}$$

When the signal-to-noise ratio is large, there is one term in (8.6.8) that is dominant; thus

$$\lambda_m \simeq \exp\left(2 N_0^{-1} \int_0^{NT} r(t)s(t, \mathbf{a}_\lambda(m))\, dt\right) \tag{8.6.10}$$

and $\mathbf{a}_\lambda(m)$ is the sequence that gives the largest term in (8.6.8). Thus instead of (8.6.4) the decision rule is equivalently

$$\hat{a}_0 = a(m) \text{ if } \Lambda_m = \max_k \{\Lambda_k, k = 1, \ldots, M\}$$

where

$$\Lambda_m = \int_0^{NT} r(t)s(t, \mathbf{a}_\lambda(m))\, dt \tag{8.6.11}$$

We can give the equation the following physical interpretation: we find the sequence that gives the largest correlation with the received signal; the first symbol of this sequence is $a_0$. The error probability can be upper-bounded using the union bound by

$$P(e) \leq L^{-1} \sum_{k \neq m} \sum_{m} Q(D(\mathbf{a}_\lambda(m), \mathbf{a}_\lambda(k))(2 N_0)^{-0.5}) \tag{8.6.12}$$

where $D$ is the Euclidian distance between the signals with the two sequences, i.e.

$$D^2(\mathbf{a}_\lambda(m), \mathbf{a}_\lambda(k)) = \int_0^{NT} \{s(t, \mathbf{a}_\lambda(m)) - s(t, \mathbf{a}_\lambda(k))\}^2\, dt$$

$$= \sum_{i=0}^{N-1} \int_{iT}^{(i+1)T} \{s(t, \mathbf{a}_\lambda(m)) - s(t, \mathbf{a}_\lambda(k))\}^2\, dt \tag{8.6.13}$$

When we substitute (8.6.1) into (8.6.13) we obtain

$$D^2(\mathbf{a}_\lambda(m), \mathbf{a}_\lambda(k)) = 2\,E\left(N - T^{-1}\int_0^{NT} \cos\phi(t, \mathbf{a}_\lambda(m) - \mathbf{a}_\lambda(k))\,dt\right) \quad (8.6.14)$$

For large signal-to-noise ratios, there is one dominant term, in (8.6.12); thus we approximate

$$P(e) = BQ\{D_{\min}(2\,N_0)^{-0.5}\} \quad (8.6.15)$$

where $B$ is a positive constant, and $D_{\min}$ is computed from

$$D_{\min}^2 = 2\,E \min_{\mathbf{b}} \{N - T^{-1}\int_0^{NT} \cos\phi(t, \mathbf{b})\,dt\} \quad (8.6.16)$$

where

$$\mathbf{b} = \{b_0, b_1, \ldots b_{N-1}\} = \mathbf{a}_\lambda(m) - \mathbf{a}_\lambda(k) \quad (8.6.17)$$

is a difference sequence, such that $b_0 \neq 0$ and

$$b_i = 0, \pm 2, \ldots, \pm 2(M - 1) \quad (8.6.18)$$

Therefore in (8.6.16)

$$\phi(t, \mathbf{b}) = 2\,\pi h \sum_{i=0}^{N} b_i \beta'(t - iT) \quad (8.6.19)$$

Since $E = E_b \log_2 M$, we can define the normalized distance by

$$d^2 = D^2/(2\,E_b) \quad (8.6.20)$$

thus

$$P(e) = BQ((2\,E_b/N_0)^{0.5} \log_2 M\, d_{\min}) \quad (8.6.21)$$

and

$$d^2(\mathbf{b}) = \log_2 M\left(N - T^{-1}\int_0^{NT} \cos\phi(t, \mathbf{b})\,dt\right) \quad (8.6.22)$$

The minimum value of $d$ will be obtained for a fixed $N$ by a sequence that maximizes the integral in (8.6.22). If the integral remains unchanged for $N \geqq$

$N_1$, there is no point in increasing $n$ beyond $N_1$. The complexity of the system increases with $N$.

*Example* 8.6.1
Assume binary symbols and a shaping function of duration $T$. The phase trajectories for an NRZ shaping function are shown in Fig. 8.25. The minimum distance will be obtained by the paths generated by the sequences

$$\mathbf{a}(1) = 1, -1, a_2, \ldots a_{N-1}$$

$$\mathbf{a}(-1) = -1, +1, a_2, \ldots a_{N-1}$$

which coincide for $t \geqq 2T$ independent of $\{a_2, \ldots a_{N-1}\}$. Thus here we select $N = 2$ and

$$d^2 = 2 - T^{-1} \int_0^{2T} \cos\{4\pi h(\beta'(t) - \beta'(t - T))\}\, dt = 2(1 - \mathrm{sinc}(2h))$$

It is shown in Refs. 8.40, 8.42, and 8.43 that for binary symbols the optimal $h$ is 0.715; for $M = 4$ the optimal $h$ is 1.75 if we select $N = 2$ and only 0.8 for $N \geqq 3$, and for $M = 8$ the optimal $h$ is 0.875.

In Fig. 8.26 we show the error probability as a function of $E_b/N_0$ in the case of NRZ shaping function of duration $T$, coherent detection, and $M = 2$, 4, 8. Similar results with noncoherent detection are shown in Fig. 8.27. These figures are reproduced from Ref. 8.43.

It can be seen from Fig. 8.26(a) that with $N = 5$ there is an improvement of about 1.1 dB over coherent PSK, which is the optimal for a single symbol processing interval. From Fig. 8.26(b) we conclude that with $N = 2$ we have an improvement of 2.5 dB, and for $N = 5$ an improvement of 3.5 dB over coherent QPSK. From Fig. 8.26(c) we see an improvement of 1.9 dB for $N = 2$ and of 2.6 dB for $N = 3$ over coherent orthogonal FSK. The results in Fig. 8.27 are even more remarkable. Here with noncoherent detection we have for low error probabilities an advantage of 0.5 dB over coherent PSK for $M = 2$. For $M = 4$ the advantage is 2.8 dB for a five-symbol observation interval.

## 8.7 SUMMARY

In this chapter we have presented the theory of FSK. We started with coherent FSK in which the phase of the transmitted signal is tracked by the receiver and presented formulas of error probability for orthogonal $M$-ary

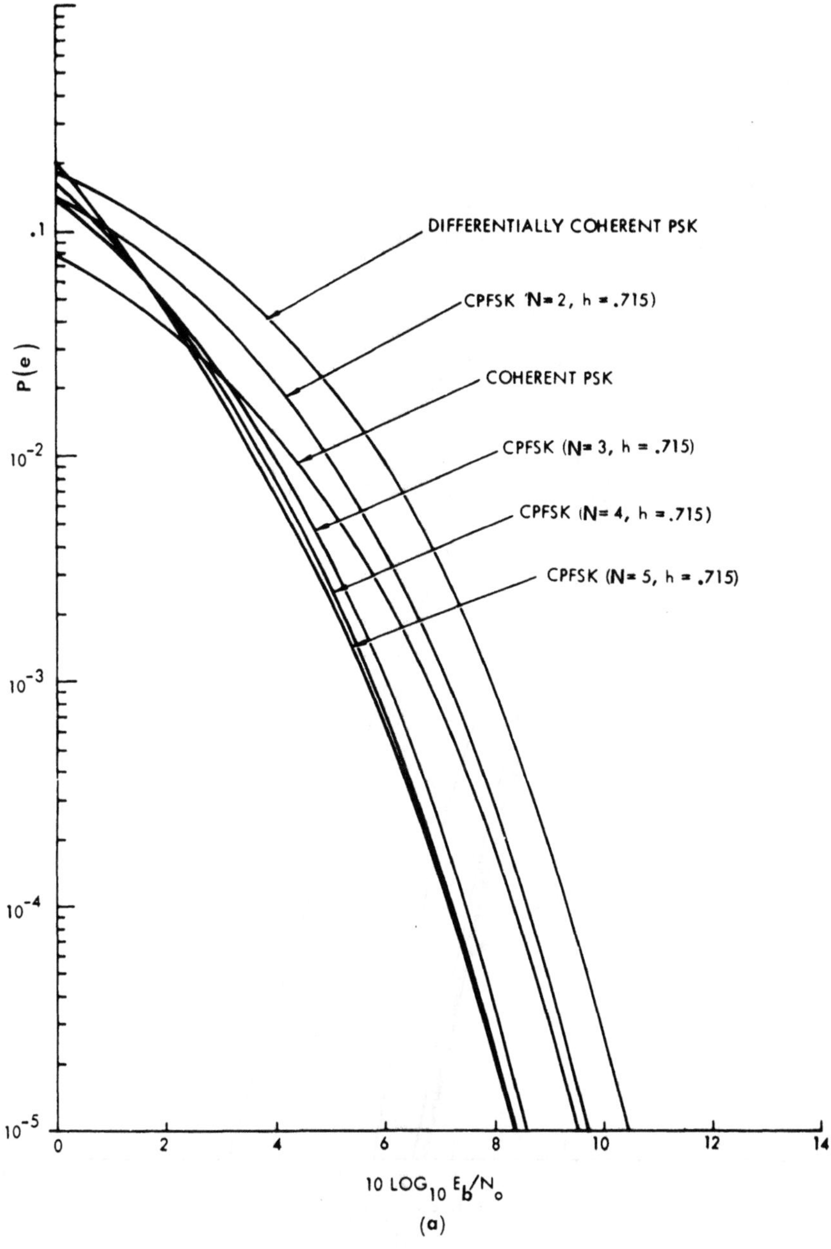


Fig. 8.26. Error probability as a function of $E_b/N_0$ for FSK with coherent detection and observation interval NT: (a) binary symbols, (b) quaternary symbols, (c) octal symbols (T. A. Schonoff, "Symbol Error Probabilities for $M$-ary CPFSK: Coherent and Noncoherent Detection," *IEEE Tr. Comm.*, Vol. COM-24, June 1976, pp. 699–652. Copyright © 1976 IEEE).

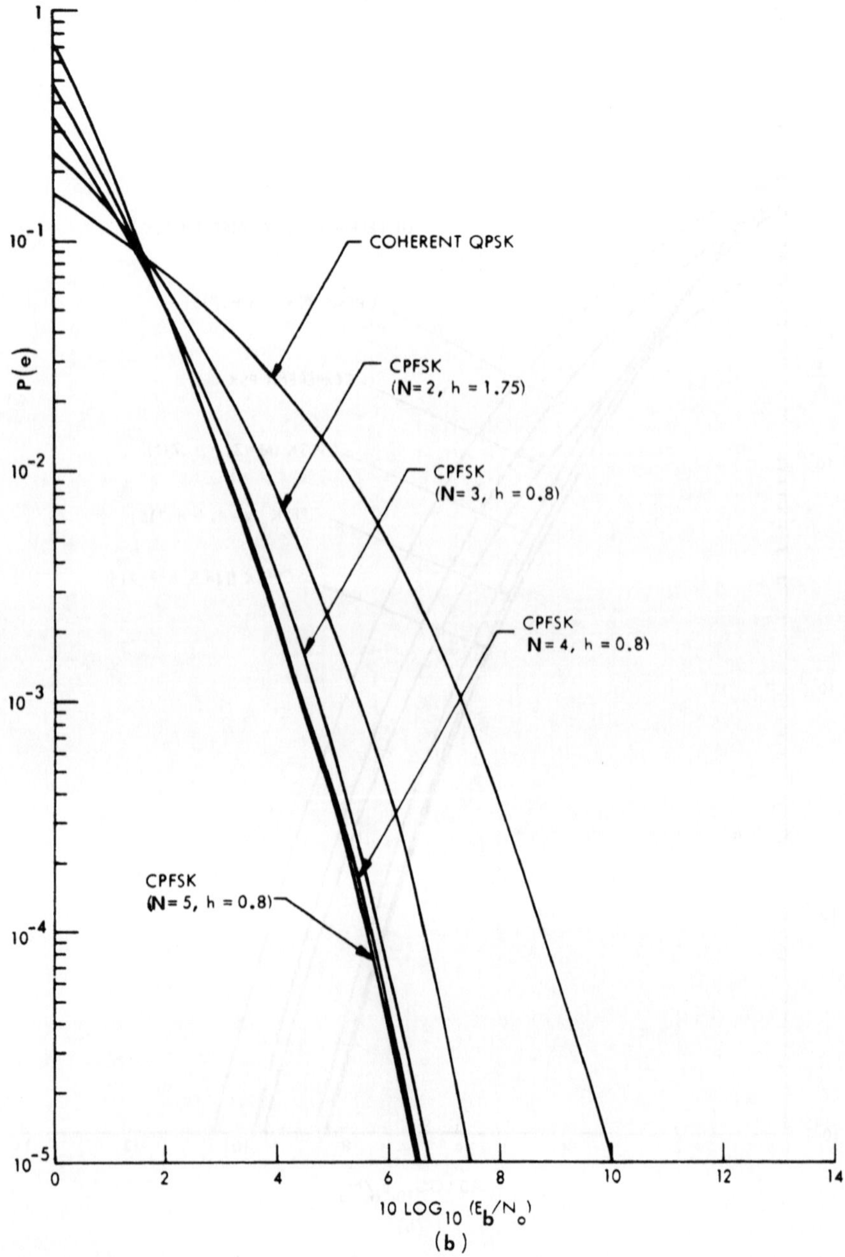
1
$10^{-1}$
$10^{-2}$
$10^{-3}$
$10^{-4}$
$10^{-5}$
P(e)
COHERENT QPSK
CPFSK
(N= 2, h = 1.75)
CPFSK
(N= 3, h = 0.8)
CPFSK
N= 4, h = 0.8)
CPFSK
(N= 5, h = 0.8)
0
2
4
6
8
10
12
14
10 LOG$_{10}$ ($E_b/N_o$)
(b)

Fig. 8.26. (*con't.*)

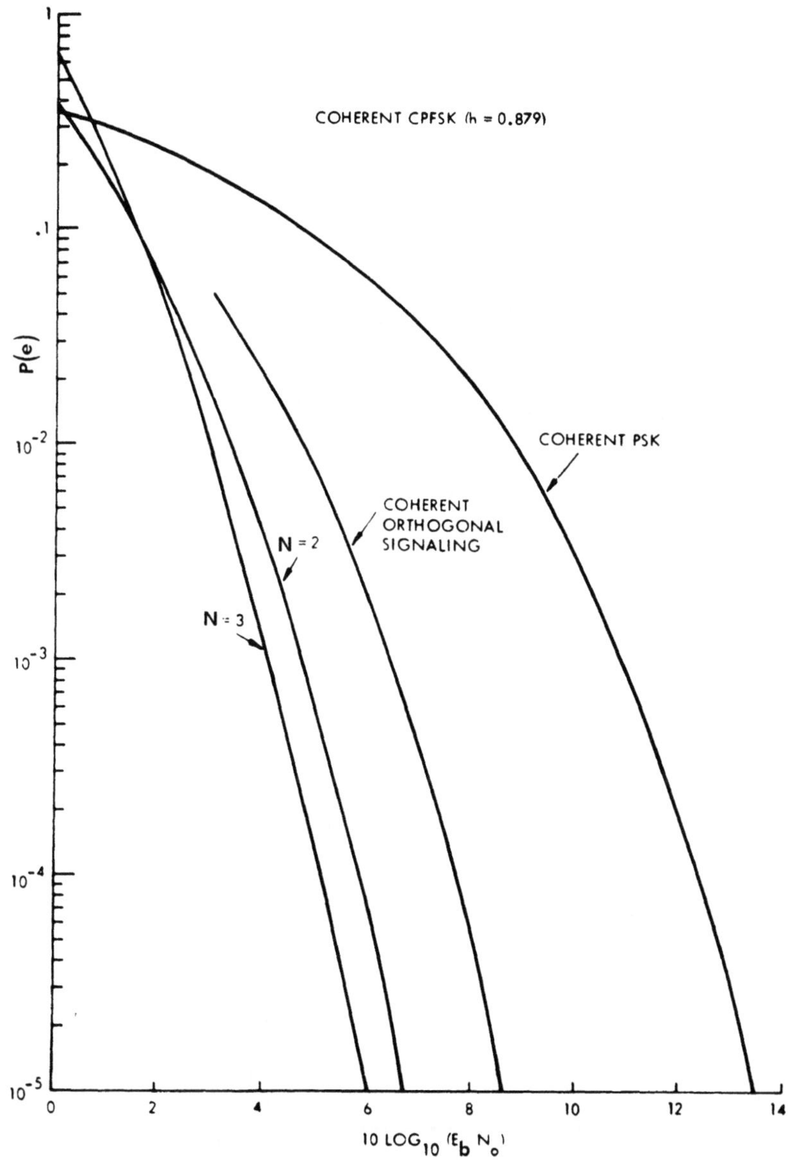


(c)

Fig. 8.26. (*con't.*)

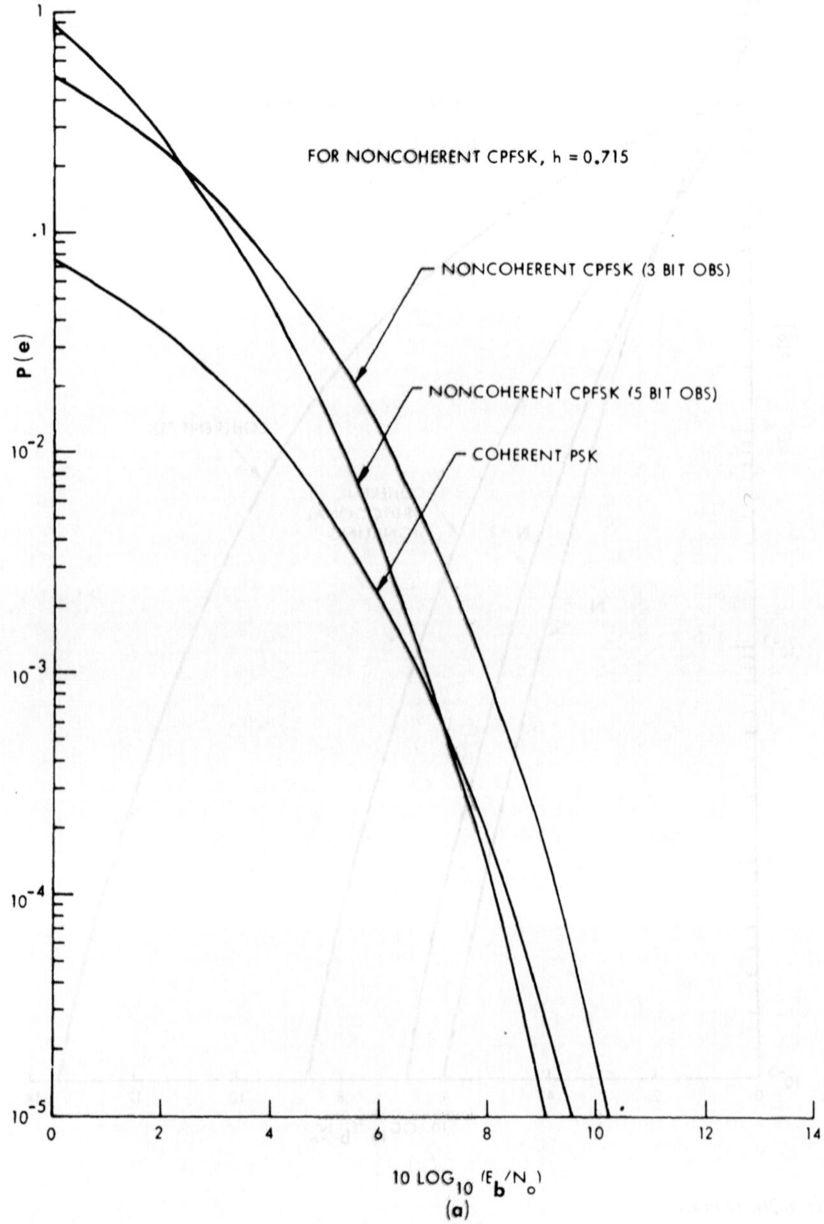


Fig. 8.27. The same as 8.26, but noncoherent detection.

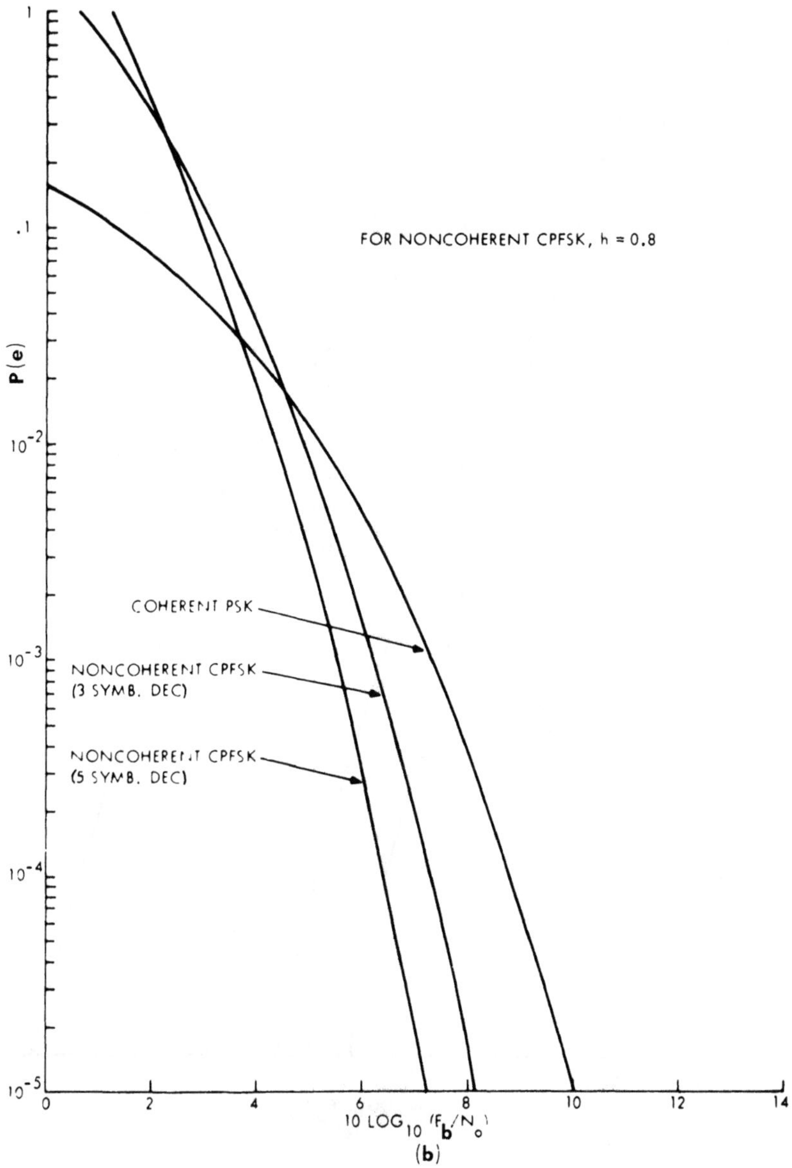

1
.1
P(e)
10^-2
10^-3
10^-4
10^-5
FOR NONCOHERENT CPFSK, h = 0.8
COHERENT PSK
NONCOHERENT CPFSK
(3 SYMB. DEC)
NONCOHERENT CPFSK
(5 SYMB. DEC)
0
2
4
6
8
10
12
14
10 LOG10 (Eb/No)
(b)


Fig. 8.27. (*con't.*)

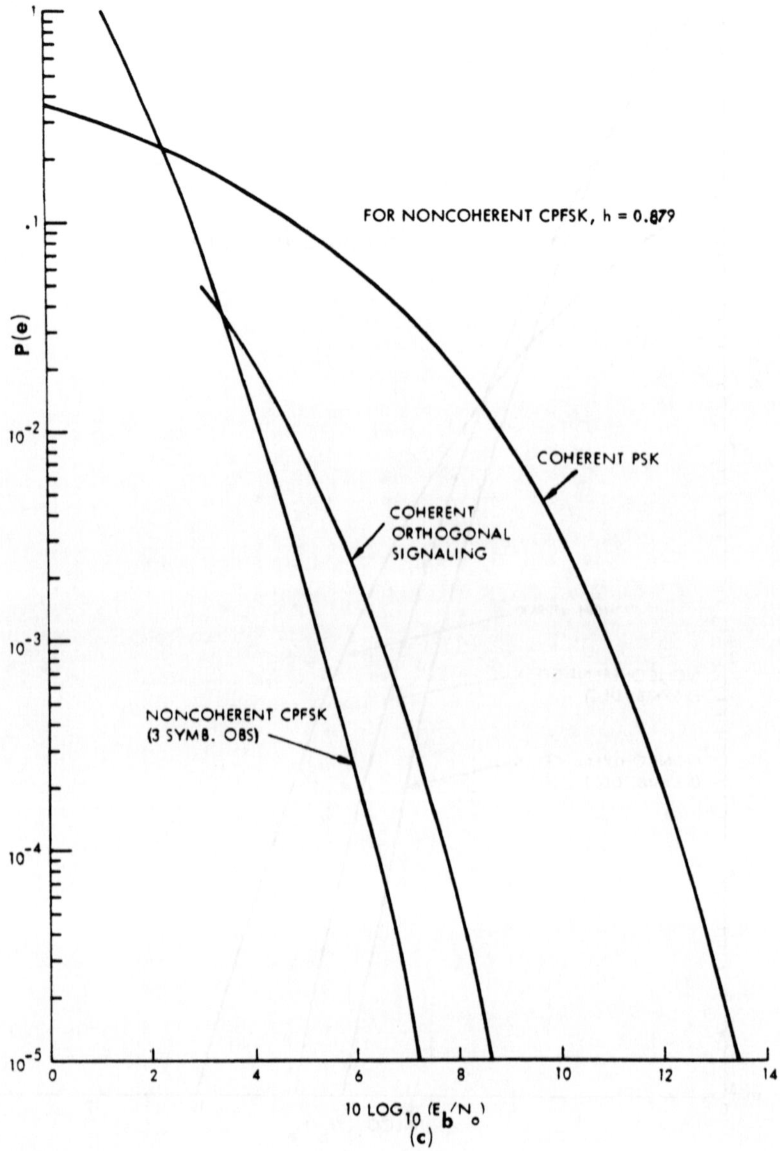

P(e)
1
.1
$10^{-2}$
$10^{-3}$
$10^{-4}$
$10^{-5}$
0
2
4
6
8
10
12
14
FOR NONCOHERENT CPFSK, h = 0.879
COHERENT PSK
COHERENT ORTHOGONAL SIGNALING
NONCOHERENT CPFSK (3 SYMB. OBS)
$10 \log_{10} (E_b/N_o)$
(c)


Fig. 8.27. (*con't.*)

signals and arbitrary FSK signals. We found that in the binary case the best results are obtained with normalized frequency deviation of $h = 0.715$. Next we discussed noncoherent detection of $M$-ary wideband FSK with or without a narrowband detector filters. This was followed by a section about detection of narrowband FSK using a discriminator. We have established conditions of no intersymbol interference, but these conditions lead to filters that cause excessive noise. We presented formulas for the effect of filters on an FSK signal. In 8.5 a detector filter followed the discriminator. We presented formulas for the computation of the error probability in the presence of ISI and described approximations from the literature. We showed that, using a receiver filter with an optimal bandwidth and an optimal frequency deviation, the error probability is almost the same as for optimal coherent FSK. Finally we briefly discussed the effect of extending the processing interval on the error probability.

## 8.8 PROBLEMS

8.2.1 Let a FSK signal set be defined by

$$s_m(t) = A \cos((\pi k/T + 2\,\pi m f_d t) \qquad m = \pm 1, \pm 3, \ldots, \pm(M-1)$$

where $k$ is a large integer.

a. Compute the minimal value of $f_d$ that will make the signals orthogonal.

b. Repeat (a) if the signals are

$$s_m(t) = A \sin((\pi k/T + 2\,\pi m f_d)t)$$

c. Repeat (a) for the set composed of the two sets. Note that the composite set has 2 $M$ signals.

d. Assume that the number of signals in cases (a), (b), and (c) is $M$ each. Compute the minimal required bandwidth in each case.

8.2.2 Show that for orthogonal signals the bit error probability is related to the symbol error probability by

$$P_b(e) = \frac{0.5\,M}{M-1} P(e)$$

8.2.3 Show that when $M \to \infty$ the error probability for orthogonal signals as a function of $E_b/N_0$ is given by

$$\lim_{M \to \infty} P(e) = 1 - u(E_b/N_0 - 0.69)$$

where $u(.)$ is the unit step function.

8.2.4 Given an $M$-ary orthogonal FSK system with $M = 2, 4, 8, 16, 32$ and 64 and coherent detection

a. Compute the bit error probability if $E_b/N_0 = 6$ dB.
b. Compute the values of $E_b/N_0$ if $P_b(e) = 10^{-5}$.

8.3.1 In a binary communication system the error probability is $10^{-5}$. Compute the required value of $E_b/N_0$ in the following cases

a. PSK
b. optimal coherent FSK
c. orthogonal coherent FSK
d. orthogonal noncoherent FSK

8.3.2 Given an $M$-ary orthogonal FSK system with $M = 2, 4, 8, 16, 32$ and 64 and noncoherent detection

a. Compute the bit error probability if $\rho_b = 6$ dB.
b. Compute the required signal-to-noise ratio per bit, $\rho_b$, if $P_b(e) = 10^{-5}$.
c. Compute in each case the value of $E_b/N_0$ if the bandwidth is $BT = M$.
d. Compare the results with those of Problem 8.2.4.

8.3.3 In a wideband FSK system with binary symbols and noncoherent detector, the detector filter is matched to the NRZ shaping function.

a. Assuming that in (8.3.23) $N$ is large ($N = 100$), compute the error probability for $\rho_b = 6$–$10$ dB.
b. Repeat (a) when $N = 2$.

8.4.1 Compute $f_{ef}$ and $f_{av}$ for

a. Butterworth filters of order $N = 1, 2, \ldots, 6$
b. Gaussian filter
c. Brick wall filter

8.4.2 Show that if we select $K$ as in eq. (8.4.27) the rvs $z_1$ and $z_2$ are independent.

8.4.3 In a binary FSK system with discriminator detector and wideband Gaussian filter in the receiver

a. Compute the parameter, $a$.
b. Compute the error probability as a function of $\rho_s$.

8.4.4 Continue Example 8.4.3 by specifying the filter with no intersymbol interference for FSK.

8.4.5 An FSK signal with NRZ shaping function is passing through a second-order Butterworth filter.

a. Sketch the amplitude and phase of $g(t, a_0)$, $a_0 = \pm 1$, $0 \leqq t \leqq 5\,T$, assuming that $2\,f_d T = 0.5$—$1.0$ and $f_0 T = 1$—$2$.

b. Repeat (a) for $\dot{g}(t, a_0)$.

c. Draw conclusions on the number of significant intersymbol intereference terms.

8.5.1 Derive eqs. (8.5.37) and (8.5.38).

8.5.2 Given an $M$-ary FSK system ($M = 2$, 4, 8, 16, 32 and 64) with discriminator detector and integrate and dump detector filter, and assuming that $B_R T = 2$ and $h = 1/M$, so that there is no signal distortion

a. Compute the error probability if $E_b/N_0 = 8$ dB.

b. Compute the values of $E_b/N_0$ if $P(e) = 10^{-5}$.

8.5.3 Compute the error probability of binary FSK with discriminator detector and integrate and dump detector filter if $B_R T = 2$, $h = 0.3$—$1.0$ and $E_b/N_0 = 13$ dB. Assume that the signal is not distorted.

8.5.4 Compute the error probability of binary FSK with discriminator detector and integrate and dump detector filter and a second-order Butterworth filter in the receiver with bandwidth $B_R T = 1$, using the method that led to eq. (8.5.50).

8.5.5 Repeat Problem 8.5.4 using the method of Ref. 8.32.

8.5.6 Repeat Problem 8.5.4 using the method of Ref. 8.34.

8.5.7 Repeat Problem 8.5.4 using the method of Ref. 8.35.

8.5.8 Derive a formula for the probability density of $\Delta\phi_n(t)$ in eq. (8.5.67).

8.5.9 Derive a formula for the probability of $N_1 - N_2$ if $N_1$, $N_2$ are independent discrete rvs with Poisson probability.

8.5.10 Derive eq. (8.5.78).

8.5.11 Apply the method of Refs. 8.34 and 8.37 to compute the error probability of binary FSK with split-phase shaping function and second-order Butterworth filter with bandwidth $B_R T = 2$ in the receiver. The detector filter is matched to the shaping function.

8.5.12 Show that eq. (8.6.4) is the maximum likelihood decision rule for a coherent receiver with observation time $NT$.

8.5.13 Derive eq. (8.6.8) from (8.6.6).

8.5.14 Prove the bound in eq. (8.6.12).

8.5.15 Assume binary FSK with NRZ shaping function and arbitrary normalized frequency deviation, $h$. Compute the distance $d^2(\mathbf{a}(1), \mathbf{a}(-1))$ for the various sequences of symbols of length $N = 1, 2, 3, 4$ and 5, which differ in the first symbol. For each $N$ select $h$ that maximizes the minimal distance.

8.5.16 In binary FSK systems with observation interval $NT$, the error probability is $10^{-5}$. Specify the required value of $E_b/N_0$ (in dB) for the following cases with $h = 0.715$

a. coherent detection and $N = 1, 2, 3, 4$ and 5
b. noncoherent detection and $N = 1, 3$ and 5
c. Compare (a) and (b) with binary PSK.

## 8.9 REFERENCES


8.1 E. Arthurs and H. Dym, "On the Optimum Detection of Digital Signals in the Presence of White Gaussian Noise—A geometric Interpretation and a Study of Three Basic Data Transmissions," *IRE Tr. Comm. Sys.*, Vol. CS-10, December 1962, pp. 336–372.

8.2 G. F. Montgomery, "A Comparison of Amplitude and Angle Modulation for Narrow-band Communication of Binary Coded Messages in Fluctuation Noise," *Proc. IRE*, Vol. 42, February 1954, pp. 447–454.

8.3 S. Stein, "Unified Analysis of Certain Coherent and Noncoherent Binary Communication Systems," *IEEE Tr. Inf. Theory*, Vol. IT-10, January 1964, pp. 43–51.

8.4 E. F. Smith, "Attainable Error Probabilities in Demodulation of Random Binary PCM/FM Waveforms," *IRE Tr. Space Elect. Tele.* Vol. SET-8, December 1962, pp. 290–297.

8.5 R. W. Lucky, J. Salz, and E. J. Weldon, *Principles of Data Communication*, McGraw-Hill Book Co., New York, N.Y., 1968, Chapter 8.

8.6 W. C. Lindsay and M. K. Simon, *Telecommunication System Engineering*, Prentice-Hall, Inc., Englewood Cliffs, N.J., 1973, Chapter 5.

8.7 A. B. Glenn, "Analysis of Noncoherent FSK System with Large Ratios of Frequency Uncertainties to Information Rates," *RCA Review*, Vol. 27, June 1966, pp. 272–314.

8.8 H. D. Chadwick, "The Error Probability of a Wide Band FSK Receiver in the Presence of Multipath Fading," *IEEE Tr. Comm. Tech.*, Vol. COM-19, October 1971, pp. 690–707.

8.9 M. K. Simon and J. C. Springett, "The Performance of a Noncoherent FSK Receiver Preceded by a Bandpass Limiter," *IEEE Tr. Comm.*, Vol. COM-20, December 1972, pp. 1128–1136.

8.10 M. C. Austin, "Wide Band Frequency Shift Keyed Receiver Performance in the Presence of Intersymbol Interference," *IEEE Tr. Comm.*, Vol. COM-23, April 1975, pp. 453–458.

8.11 L. B. Milstein and M. C. Austin, "Performance of Noncoherent FSK and AM-FSK Systems with Postdetection Filtering," *IEEE Tr. Comm.*, Vol. COM-23, November 1975, pp. 1300–1306.

8.12 S. Y. Kwon and N. M. Shehadeh, "Effects of Bandlimiting on the Noncoherent Detection of Frequency Shift Keyed (FSK) Signals," *Inter. Jour. Elect.*, Vol. 43, June 1977, pp. 537–553.

8.13 S. O. Rice, "Mathematical Analysis of Random Noise," *BSTJ*, Vol. 24, January 1945, pp. 95–157.
8.14 W. R. Bennett and J. Salz, "Binary Data Transmission by FM over a Real Channel," *BSTJ*, Vol. 42, September 1963, pp. 2387–2426.
8.15 J. Salz and S. Stein, "Distribution of Instantaneous Frequency for Signal plus Noise," *IEEE Tr. Inf. Theory*, Vol. IT-10, October 1964, pp. 272–274.
8.16 N. G. Gatkin, V. A. Geranin, M. I. Karnovsky, L. G. Krasnyy, and N. I. Cherney, "Probability Density of Phase Derivative of the Sum of a Modulated Signal and Gaussian Noise," *Radio Eng. Elect. Phys.* (USSR), 1965, pp. 1223–1229.
8.17 J. H. Roberts, *Angle Modulation*, Peter Peregrinus Ltd., England, 1977.
8.18 R. F. Pawula, S. O. Rice, and J. H. Roberts, "Distribution of the Phase Angle between the Two Vectors Perturbed by Gaussian Noise," *IEEE Tr. Comm.*, Vol. COM-30, August 1982, pp. 1828–1841.
8.19 M. Schwartz, W. R. Bennett, and S. Stein, *Communication Systems and Techniques*, McGraw-Hill Book Co., New York, N.Y., 1966, Chapter 8.
8.20 J. E. Mazo and J. Salz, "Probability of Error for Quadratic Detectors," *BSTJ*, Vol. 44, November 1965, pp. 2165–2186.
8.21 W. R. Bennett and J. R. Davey, *Data Transmission*, McGraw-Hill Book Co., New York, N.Y., 1965.
8.22 P. C. Jain, "Error Probabilities in Binary Modulation," *IEEE Tr. Inf. Theory*, Vol. IT-20, January 1974, pp. 36–42.
8.23 K. W. Cattermole, "Digital Transmission by Frequency Shift Keying with Zero Intersymbol Interference," *Elect. Letters*, Vol. 10, August 1974, pp. 349–350.
8.24 M. Tomlinson, "Realisable Filters which Give Zero Intersymbol Interference in an FSK System," *Circuit Th. and Appl.*, Vol. 2, 1974, pp. 291–297.
8.25 M. J. O'Mahony and K. W. Cattermole, "Distortionless Frequency Shift Keying: Further Results," *Elect. Letters*, Vol. 11, November 1975, pp. 605–606.
8.26 J. Cohn, "A New Approach to the Analysis of FM Threshold Extensions," *Proc. NEC*, Vol. 12, 1956, pp. 221–236.
8.27 S. O. Rice, "Noise in FM Receivers," Chapter 25, pp. 375–424, in *Proceedings, Symposium on Time Series Analysis*, M. Rosenblatt (ed.), John wiley & Sons, Inc., New Yor, 1963.
8.28 J. E. Mazo and J. Salz, "Theory of Error Rates for Digital FM," *BSTJ*, vol. 45, November 1966, pp. 1511–1535.
8.29 J. H. Roberts, "FM Click Rates," *Elect. Letters*, Vol. 10, 1974, pp. 16–17 and correction p. 208.
8.30 J. Klapper, "Demodulator Threshold Performance and Error Rates in Angle Modulated Digital Signals," *RCA Rev.*, June 1966, pp. 226–244.
8.31 D. L. Schilling, E. Hoffman, and E. A. Nelson, "Error Rates for Digital Signals Demodulated by an FM discriminator," *IEEE Tr. Comm. Tech.*, Vol. COM-15, August 1967, pp. 507–517.
8.32 R. F. Pawula, "On the Theory of Error Rates for Narrowband Digital FM," *IEEE Tr. Comm.*, Vol. COM-29, November 1981, pp. 1634–1643.
8.33 P. Papantoni-Kazakos and I. M. Paz, "The Performance of Digital FM Systems with Discriminator: Intersymbol Interference Effects," *IEEE Tr. Comm.*, Vol. COM-23, September 1975, pp. 867–877.
8.34 T. T. Tjhung and P. H. Wittke, "Carrier Transmission of Binary Data in a Restricted Band," *IEEE Tr. Comm. Tech.*, Vol. COM-18, August 1970, pp. 295–304.
8.35 R. T. Bobilin, "Distortion Analysis of Binary FSK," *IEEE Tr. Comm. Tech.*, Vol. COM-19, August 1971, pp. 478–486.
8.36 I. Korn, "Analysis of Manchester Coded FSK," *Austral. Tel. Res.* (ATR), Vol. 14, 1980, pp. 3–6.
8.37 C. H. Tan, T. T. Tjhung, and H. Singh, "Performance of Narrowband Manchester Coded

FSK with Discriminator Detector," *IEEE Tr. Comm.*, Vol. COM-31, May 1983, pp. 659–667.

8.38 M. G. Pelchat, R. C. Davies, and M. B. Luntz, "Coherent Demodulation of Continuous Phase FSK Signals," *Int. Telem. Conf. Conv. Rev.* (Washington D.C.), 1971, pp. 181–190.

8.39 R. DeBuda, "Coherent Demodulation of Frequency Shift Keying with Low Deviation Ratio," *IEEE Tr. Comm.*, Vol. COM-20, June 1972, pp. 429–435.

8.40 G. D. Forney, Jr., "The Viterbi Algorithm," *Proc. IEEE*, Vol. 61, March 1973, pp. 268–278.

8.41 W. P. Osborne and M. B. Luntz, "Coherent and Noncoherent Detection of CPFSK," *IEEE Tr. Comm.*, Vol. COM-22, August 1974, pp. 1023–1036.

8.42 T. A. Schonhoff, "Symbol Error Probabilities for *M*-ary CPFSK: Coherent and Noncoherent Detection," *IEEE Tr. Comm.*, Vol., COM-24, June 1976, pp. 644–652.

8.43 J. B. Anderson, C. E. W. Sundberg, T. Aulin, and N. Rydbeck, "Power Bandwidth Performance of Smoothed Phase Modulation Codes," *IEEE Tr. Comm.*, Vol. COM-29, March 1981, pp. 187–195.

8.44 T. Aulin and C. E. W. Sunberg, "Continuous Phase Modulation—part I: Full Response Signalling," *IEEE Tr. Comm.*, Vol. COM-29, March 1981, pp. 196–209.

8.45 T. Aulin and C. E. W. Sundberg, "Continuous Phase Modulation—part II: Partial Response Signalling," *IEEE Tr. Comm.*, Vol. COM-29, March 1981, pp. 210–225.

8.46 T. Aulin and C. E. W. Sundberg, "Partially Coherent Detection of Digital Full Response Continuous Phase Modulated Signals," *IEEE Tr. Comm.*, Vol. COM-30, May 1982, pp. 1096–1117.

8.47 J. M. Wozencraft and R. M. Jacobs, *Principles of Communication Engineering*, John Wiley & Sons, Inc., New York, 1966.

8.48 I. Korn, "Effect of bandlimiting filters on binary FSK with limiter—discriminator detector and integrator filter". Submitted for publication.

8.49 I. Korn, "Effect of narrowband filters on the error probability of M-ary FSK with limiter—discriminator—integrator detector", Submitted for publication.

# 9 PARTIAL RESPONSE SIGNALS

## 9.1 INTRODUCTION

We showed in Section 4.3 that to prevent intersymbol interference (ISI), the overall system response must be a Nyquist function with excess bandwidth $\beta$. The bandwidth of this function is $(1 + \beta)f_N$, where $f_N = 0.5/T$ is the Nyquist frequency, and $R = 1/T$ is the symbol rate. The function with minimum bandwidth is

$$G(f) = G_N(f) = g_0 T u_R(f + f_N) \tag{9.1.1}$$

and has zero excess bandwidth. This brick wall function cannot be realized; thus in practice an excess bandwidth of 0.25–0.5 is required with a reduced spectral efficiency. If we insist on having a function with minimum bandwidth, $f_N$, which is realizable, we introduce ISI. Because we can control the location and values of the ISI terms, however, it may be possible to reduce or even to eliminate the negative effects by a clever detector circuit. Signals with a controlled amount of ISI are called partial response signals (PRS), or correlative level signals.[9.1–9.10] The duration of these signals extends beyond a single symbol interval, $T$. Systems with PRS require usually a larger signal-to-noise ratio than full response signals or Nyquist function for the same error probability. In systems with a maximum likelihood or Viterbi decoder,[6.17–6.19] the penalty in signal-to-noise ratio is negligible.

In addition to being spectrally efficient, PRS have an intrinsic structure that can be used to monitor errors and for error detection and correction.[9.10,9.11,9.16,9.22,9.24]

This chapter has the following outline. In Section 9.2 we define quite broadly PRS systems. In Section 9.3 we show how error propagation can be eliminated using decision feedback. A precoding method for the same purpose is described in Section 9.4. In Section 9.5 we indicate how structural rules of PRS can be used to monitor, detect, and correct errors. A summary, problems, and references are presented in Sections 9.6, 9.7, and 9.8, respectively.

## 9.2 DEFINITION OF PRS

A signal $g(t)$ is called PRS of length $N + 1$ if its samples at times $t_i = t_0 + iT$ satisfy

$$g_i = \begin{cases} 0 & i < 0, i > N \\ \text{nonzero integer} & i = 0, i = N \\ \text{arbitrary integer} & 0 < i < N \end{cases} \tag{9.2.1}$$

Let $g_N(t)$ be a Nyquist function with $g_N(0) = 1$. We may generate a PRS function from the Nyquist function as a starting point by

$$g(t) = \sum_0^N g_i g_N(t - t_0 - iT) = \sum_0^N g_i \delta(t - iT) * g_N(t - t_0) \tag{9.2.2}$$

which in the frequency domain is

$$G(f) = \sum_0^N g_i \exp(-j\, 2\, \pi f i T) G_N(f) \exp(-j\, 2\, \pi f t_0) \tag{9.2.3}$$

Because the $\{g_i\}$, $i = 0, \ldots, N$ characterize the PRS we may call

$$G_p(f) = \sum_0^N g_i \exp(-j\, 2\, \pi f i T) \tag{9.2.4}$$

its characteristic function. If we define the delay operator

$$D = \exp(-j\, 2\, \pi f T) \tag{9.2.5}$$

we obtain from (9.2.4) the characteristic polynomial in $D$

$$G_p'(D) = \sum_0^N g_i D^i = \prod_{k=1}^N (D - D_k) \tag{9.2.6}$$

Since from (9.2.3) and (9.1.1)

$$G(f) = T G_p(f) u_R(f + f_N) \exp(-j\, 2\, \pi f t_0) \tag{9.2.7}$$

the spectral shaping is determined by the characteristic polynomial. We select $t_0 = -0.5\, NT$ so that $G(f)$ has a simplified analytic expression. In Table 9.1 are presented most common examples of PRS, of which duobinary and particularly the modified duobinary are the most useful. The duobinary is a special case of class 1 or polybinary PRS. In polybinary $g_i = 1$, $i = 1, 2, \ldots N$.

*Example* 9.2.1 Duobinary and modified duobinary PRS
For the duobinary signal ($N = 1$)

$$G_p'(D) = 1 + D \tag{9.2.8}$$

**Table 9.1 Examples of PRS the impulse response and transfer function**

| SIGNAL | $G_p'(D)$ | $g(t - t_0)$ | $g(t)$ | $G(f)$ | $G(f)$ $\quad f < f_N$ | $M_s$ |
|---|---|---|---|---|---|---|
| Class 1 Duobinary | $1 + D$ |  −2T −T 0 T 2T 3T t | $\frac{4}{\pi}\frac{\cos(\pi t/T)}{1 - (2t/T)^2}$ | 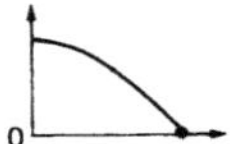 0 $f_N$ | $2T\cos(0.5\omega T)$, $\omega = 2\pi f$ | $2M - 1$ |
| Dicode | $1 - D$ | 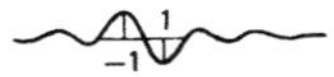 1 −1 | $\frac{8}{\pi}\frac{\cos(\pi t/T)(t/T)}{(2t/T)^2 - 1}$ | 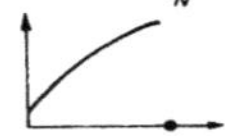 $f_N$ | $j2T\sin(0.5\omega T)$ | $2M - 1$ |
| Class 4 Modified Duobinary | $1 - D^2$ | 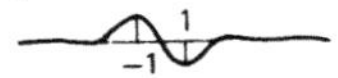 1 −1 | $\frac{2}{\pi}\frac{\sin(\pi t/T)}{(t/T)^2 - 1)}$ | 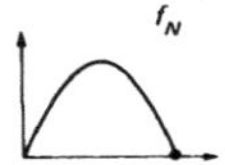 $f_N$ | $j2T\sin(\omega T)$ | $2M - 1$ |
| Class 2 | $1 + 2D + D^2$ | 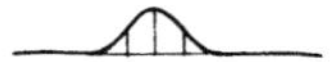 1 2 1 | $\frac{2}{\pi}\frac{\sin(\pi t/T)}{[1 - (t/T)^2](t/T)}$ | 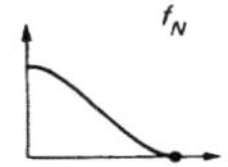 $f_N$ | $4T\cos^2(0.5\omega T)$ | $4M - 3$ |
| — | $1 + D - D^2 + D^3$ | 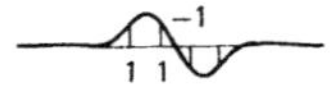 −1 1 1 | $-\frac{64}{\pi}\frac{\cos(\pi t/T)(t/T)}{[(2t/T)^2 - 1][(3t/T)^2 - 1]}$ | 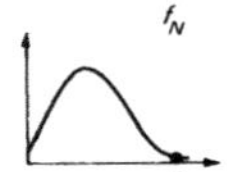 $f_N$ | $j4T\cos(0.5\omega T)\sin(\omega T)$ | $4M - 3$ |
| — | $1 - D - D^2 + D^3$ | 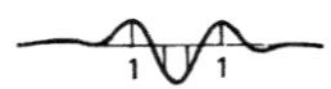 1 1 −1 −1 | $\frac{16}{\pi}\frac{\cos(\pi t/T)[(2t/T)^2 - 3]}{[(2t/T)^2 - 9][(2t/T)^2 - 1]}$ | 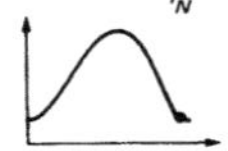 $f_N$ | $-4T\sin(0.5\omega T)\sin(\omega T)$ | $4M - 3$ |
| Class 5 | $1 - 2D^2 + D^4$ | 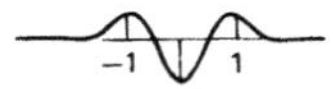 −1 1 −2 | $\frac{8}{\pi}\frac{\sin(\pi t/T)}{(t/T)^2 - 4}$ | 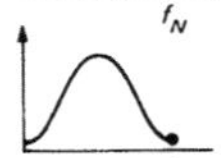 $f_N$ | $-4T\sin^2(\omega T)$ | $4M - 3$ |
| Class 3 | $2 + D - D^2$ | 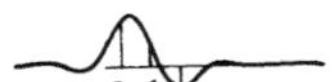 2 1 −1 | $\frac{1}{\pi}\frac{\sin(\pi t/T)(3t/T - 1)}{[(t/T)^2 - 1](t/T)}$ | 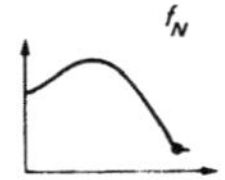 $f_N$ | $T(1 + \cos\omega T + j3\sin\omega T)$ | $4M - 3$ |
| — | $2 - D^2 - D^4$ | 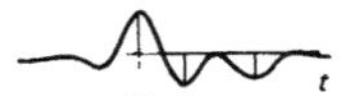 2 1 t | $\frac{2}{\pi}\frac{\sin(\pi t/T)(2 - 3t/T)}{[(t/T)^2 - 4](t/T)}$ | 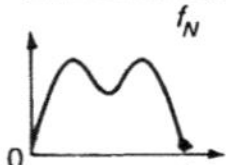 0 $f_N$ | $T(-1 + \cos(2\omega T) + j3\sin(2\omega T))$ | $4M - 3$ |

Hence

$$G_p(f) = 1 + \exp(-j\,2\,\pi f T) = 2\exp(-j\pi f T)\cos(\pi f T) \quad (9.2.9)$$

Selecting $t_0 = -0.5\,NT = -0.5\,T$, we obtain from (9.2.7)

$$G(f) = 2\,T\cos(\pi f T) u_R(f + f_N) \quad (9.2.10)$$

This function is zero for $f = \pm f_N$.

For the modified duobinary ($N = 2$)

$$G'_p(D) = (1 + D)(1 - D) = 1 - D^2 \quad (9.2.11)$$

Hence

$$G_p(f) = 2\,j\sin(2\,\pi f T)\exp(-j\,2\,\pi f T) \quad (9.2.12)$$

Selecting $t_0 = -\,0.5\,NT = -T$, we obtain from (9.2.7)

$$G(f) = 2\,Tj\sin(2\,\pi f T) u_R(f + f_N) \quad (9.2.13)$$

which is 0 for $f = 0, \pm f_N$. The 0 value at $f = 0$ is caused by the factor $1 - D$ of (9.2.11). Such a spectral shaping is very desirable in systems whose channel is unable to handle DC signals, as, for example, the telephone channel. Because (9.2.13) is continuous at the end points, $\pm f_N$, it can be well approximated.

All examples in Table 9.1 have the factors $1 + D$ or $1 - D$ (or both) in their characteristic polynomial. The value $t_0 = -0.5\,NT$ was selected to simplify the equation for $g(t)$, because this puts the time origin to the center of nonzero $g_i$ values. In Table 9.1 we also show the PRS both in the time and frequency domain.

The output of the detector filter in a system with PRS is

$$r_k = a_k g_0 + \sum_{i=1}^{N} a_{k-i} g_i + n_k \quad (9.2.14)$$

where the second term

$$I = \sum_{1}^{N} a_{k-i} g_i \quad (9.2.15)$$

is the controlled ISI, and $n_k$ is zero-mean Gaussian noise with variance

$$\sigma_n^2 = 0.5\, N_0 \int_{-\infty}^{\infty} |H_{RD}(f)|^2\, df \tag{9.2.16}$$

We assume that $a_i \in \{\pm 1, \pm 3, \ldots, \pm(M - 1)\}$. Thus in the noiseless case

$$r_k = s_k = \sum_0^N a_{k-i} g_i \tag{9.2.17}$$

which is a multilevel signal even when $a_i = \pm 1$ is only binary. The number of levels of $s_k$, $M_s$, depends on $M$ and the numerical values of $\{g_k\}$. $M_s$ is shown in the last column of Table 9.1.

*Example* 9.2.2 Duobinary PRS
In this case

$$s_k = a_k + a_{k-1}$$

Hence when $a_k = \pm 1$, $s_k$ has three values 0, $\pm 2$, while when $a_k = \pm 1, \pm 3$, $s_k$ has seven values 0, $\pm 2$, $\pm 4$, $\pm 6$.

Because $I$ is invariant to a replacement of $g_i$ by $|g_i|$ and to reordering of the terms (this was explained in detail in Section 4.4), the systems with the same set $\{|g_k|, k \neq 0\}$ and the same value of $g_0$, have the same error probability; hence only one system of the equivalent family must be considered.

*Example* 9.2.3 Equivalence of PRS
The duobinary, dicode, and modified duobinary are equivalent because in them $g_0 = 1$ and $\{|g_k|, k \neq 0\} = \{1\}$. Similarly $1 + 2D + D^2$ and $1 - 2D^2 + D^4$ are equivalent because $g_0 = 1$ and $\{|g_k|, k \neq 0\} = \{2, 1\}$.

## 9.3 ELIMINATION OF ISI BY DECISION FEEDBACK

At time $t_k$, when the decision is made about the value of $a_k$, we have the decisions about $a_{k-1}, a_{k-2}, \ldots, a_{k-N}$. Let these decisions be $\hat{a}_{k-i}$, $i = 1, 2, \ldots, N$, so that

$$\hat{I} = \sum_1^N \hat{a}_{k-i} g_i \tag{9.3.1}$$

is available at the detector prior to the current decision. If we feed back these decisions to the receiver by subtracting $\hat{I}$ from $r_k$, the result is

$$\hat{r}_k = r_k - \hat{I} = a_k g_0 + I_F + n_k \tag{9.3.2}$$

where

$$I_F = \sum_{1}^{N} (a_{k-i} - \hat{a}_{k-i}) g_i \tag{9.3.3}$$

Such a receiver, called obviously a *decision feedback receiver*, is shown in Fig. 9.1. Equation (9.3.2) is the same as eq. (4.2.1) with $r_k$ replaced by $\hat{r}_k$ and $I$ by $I_F$; hence, applying the methods of Chapter 4, the symbol error probability in the presence of (decision) feedback is

$$P_F(e) = 2(1 - M^{-1})\overline{Q((g_0 - I_F)/\sigma_n)} \tag{9.3.4}$$

where the average is over $I_F$. If we assume that the last $N$ decisions are correct, i.e., $\hat{a}_{k-i} = a_{k-i}$, $i = 1, 2, \ldots, N$, then $I_F = 0$, and we obtain a lower bound on $P_F(e)$

$$P_{FL}(e) = 2(1 - 1/M)Q(g_0/\sigma_n) \tag{9.3.5}$$

If one symbol is incorrect this error tends to propagate; hence $P_F(e) \geqq P_{FL}(e)$, but the difference will be small for practically small values of $P_F(e)$. If the noise samples $\{n_k\}$ are independent, upper bounds to $P_F(e)$ have been found in Ref. 9.22 for binary symbols and in Ref. 9.23 for $M$-ary symbols

$$P_{FU} = M^{N_1} P_{FL}(e) \tag{9.3.6}$$

where $N_1$ is the number of terms $\{g_i\}$ with nonzero values.

*Example* 9.3.1 Bounds to duobinary PRS
For duobinary PRS with binary symbols, $M = N_1 = 2$; hence

$$Q(g_0/\sigma_n) \leqq P_F(e) \leqq 4\, Q(g_0/\sigma_n) \tag{9.3.7}$$

The same result is obtained for dicode and modified duobinary PRS.

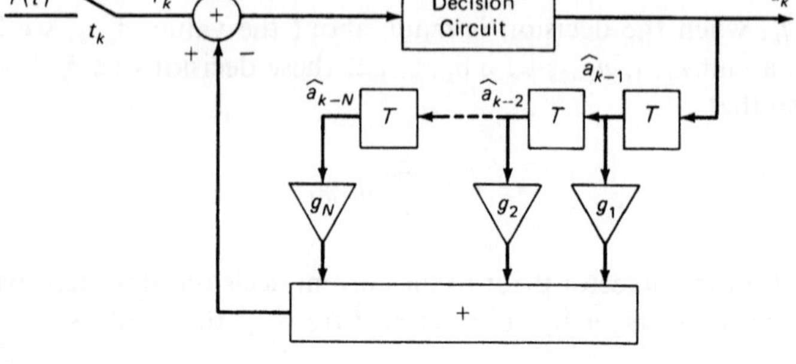


Fig. 9.1. PRS system with decision feedback.

In Ref. 9.23, the PRS system is modeled as a Markov chain, and the exact value $P_F(e)$ is obtained. The ratio $P_F(e)/P_{FL}(e)$ is given in Table 9.2 for various PRS systems and two values of $P_{FL}(e)$. This table is reproduced from Ref. 9.23.

**Table 9.2 The ratio of error probability and lower bound $P_F(e)/P_{FL}(e)$ in PRS systems**

| System | $P_{FL}(e) = 10^{-2}$ | | | $P_{FL}(e) = 10^{-3}$ | | |
|---|---|---|---|---|---|---|
| | $M = 2$ | 4 | 8 | 2 | 4 | 8 |
| $1 + D$, $1 - D$, $1 - D^2$ | 1.9 | 3.8 | 7.1 | 2.0 | 4.0 | 8.0 |
| $1 + 2D + D^2$, $1 - 2D + D^4$ | 3.7 | 11 | 28 | 4.0 | 13 | 43 |
| $2 + D - D^2$, $2 - D^2 - D^4$ | 1.9 | 3.7 | 7.1 | 2.0 | 4.0 | 8.0 |
| $1 + D - D^2 - D^3$<br>$1 - D - D^2 + D^3$ | 4.5 | 16 | 41 | 5.0 | 21 | 96 |



The ratio $g_0/\sigma_n$ is related to the signal-to-noise ratio per bit by

$$g_0/\sigma_n = \left[\eta \frac{3 \log_2 M}{M^2 - 1}(2 E_b/N)\right]^{1/2} \tag{9.3.8}$$

where

$$\eta = \frac{g_0^2}{E_C E_{RD}} \tag{9.3.9}$$

and $E_C$, $E_{RD}$ are defined in Section 4.2. We shall consider two cases

1. Model 1—Matched filter In this case

$$E_C = E_{RD} = \int_{-\infty}^{\infty} |G(f)| df = 2 \int_0^{f_N} |G(f)| df \tag{9.3.10}$$

Therefore

$$\eta = \eta_1 = \left(0.5 g_0 \Big/ \int_0^{f_N} |G(f)| df\right)^2 \tag{9.3.11}$$

In this method the noise samples $\{n_k\}$ are not independent.

2. Model 2—Transmitter shaping In this case

$$H_{RD}(f) = u_R(f + f_N), G_C(f) = G(f) \tag{9.3.12}$$

Hence

$$E_{RD} = 1/T, E_C = \int_{-\infty}^{\infty} |G(f)|^2 \, df = T \sum_0^N g_i^2 \tag{9.3.13}$$

Therefore

$$\eta = \eta_2 = \left[ \sum_0^N (g_i/g_0)^2 \right]^{-1} \tag{9.3.14}$$

In this model the samples are independent.

*Example* 9.3.2 Duobinary and modified duobinary PRS
From column 6 of Table 9.1 we obtain in both cases the same numerical result for the integral

$$\int_0^{f_N} |G(f)| df = \int_0^{f_N} 2\,T \cos(\pi f T)\, df = \int_0^{f_N} 2\,T \sin(2\,\pi f T)\, df = 2/\pi$$

Therefore

$$\eta_1 = (\pi/4)^2 = -2.1 \text{ dB}$$

and since in both cases the set $\{|g_i|\}$ is identical $\{1, 1\}$

$$\eta_2 = 0.5 = -3 \text{ dB}$$

The signal-to-noise ratio degradation relative to the ideal binary case $(g_0/\sigma_n = (2\,E_b/N_0)^{1/2})$ for various PRS with binary symbols and a bit error probability of $10^{-5}$ is shown in Table 9.3. In model 1 we have the degradation only for the lower bound (the true value and upper bound are unknown because the noise samples are dependent). For model 2 there are three entries that correspond to: the lower bound, the true value, and the upper bound. This table is reproduced from Ref. 9.23. The case of ISI elimination by precoding is discussed in the next section.
We note from this table that there is a penalty of at least 2.3 or 3.2 dB in signal-to-noise ratio per bit in using the PRS. This is the penalty for the

**Table 9.3 Signal-to-noise penalty (in dB) for PRS system with binary symbols and error probability of $P_b(e) = 10^{-5}$**

| system | MODEL 1 | | MODEL 2 | |
|---|---|---|---|---|
| | Dec. feed | Prec. | Dec. feed | Prec. |
| $1 \pm D$, $1 - D^2$ | 2.1 | 2.3 | 3–3.3–3.3 | 3.2 |
| $1 + 2D + D^2$<br>$1 - 2D + D^4$ | 6.0 | 6.3 | 7.8–8.4–8.4 | 3.0 |
| $2 + D - D^2$<br>$2 - D - D^4$ | 1.2 | 7.5 | 1.3–2.1–2.4 | 8.0 |
| $1 + D - D^2 - D^3$<br>$1 - D - D^2 + D^3$ | 4.6 | 4.9 | 6.0–6.7–6.9 | 6.3 |



greater spectral efficiency. Additional discussions of decision feedback can be found in Refs. 9.10, 9.11, 9.16, 9.24, and 9.25.

## 9.4 Elimination of ISI by precoding

In this method we assume that the original symbols $\{a_k\}$ belong to the set $\mathring{A}_0 = \{0, 1, \ldots, M - 1\}$ (this is no restriction because by a linear equation $a'_k = 2a_k - M + 1$ we may obtain the set $\mathring{A}_{\pm}$) and prior to transmission we *precode* them into symbols $b_k$, using the rule

$$b_k = a_k - \sum_{i=1}^{N} b_{k-i} g_k / g_0 \tag{9.4.1}$$

so that at the detector output we obtain

$$r_k = \sum_{i=0}^{N} b_{k-i} g_i + n_k = g_0 a_k + n_k \tag{9.4.2}$$

which is normally obtained in a system with no ISI. The only problem with (9.4.1) is that although $a_k$ is an $M$-ary symbol, $b_k$ is not.

*Example* 9.4.1 Duobinary PRS
Here $g_0 = g_1 = 1$. Hence from (9.4.1)

$$b_k = a_k - b_{k-1} \tag{9.4.3}$$

Let $b_0 = 1$, and let $a_1, a_2, a_3, a_4, a_5 = 0, 0, 1, 1, 0$ (we assume binary symbols). Then $b_1, b_2, b_3, b_4, b_5 = -1, 1, 0, 1, -1$, which are ternary.

This defficiency can be easily resolved by taking the modulo $M$ value of (9.4.1), i.e.

$$b_k = a_k - \sum_{1}^{N} b_{k-i}g_i/g_0 \qquad \text{(modulo } M)$$
$$= a_k - \sum_{1}^{N} b_{k-i}g_i/g_0 + cM \tag{9.4.4}$$

where $c$ is an integer so that $b_k$ is confined to $\mathring{A}_0$. thus at the receiver we obtain

$$r_k = \sum_{0}^{N} b_{k-i}g_i/g_0 + n_k = g_0\{a_k + cM\} + n_k \tag{9.4.5}$$

If there is no noise we can recover $a_k$ from $r_k$ by the decision rule

$$a_k = r_k/g_0 - cM = r_k/g_0 \qquad \text{(modulo } M) \tag{9.4.6}$$

In the presence of noise we shall obtain only the estimate of $a_k$

$$\hat{a}_k = r_k/g_0 \qquad \text{(modulo } M) \tag{9.4.7}$$

which may not be equal to $a_k$ because of noise. The system with precoding is shown in Fig. 9.2.

*Example* 9.4.2 Duobinary PRS with binary symbols
We assume binary symbols; hence from (9.4.4)

$$b_k = a_k - b_{k-1} \text{ (modulo 2)}$$
$$= a_k \oplus b_{k-1} = \begin{cases} 0 & a_k = b_{k-1} \\ 1 & a_k \neq b_{k-1} \end{cases} \tag{9.4.8}$$

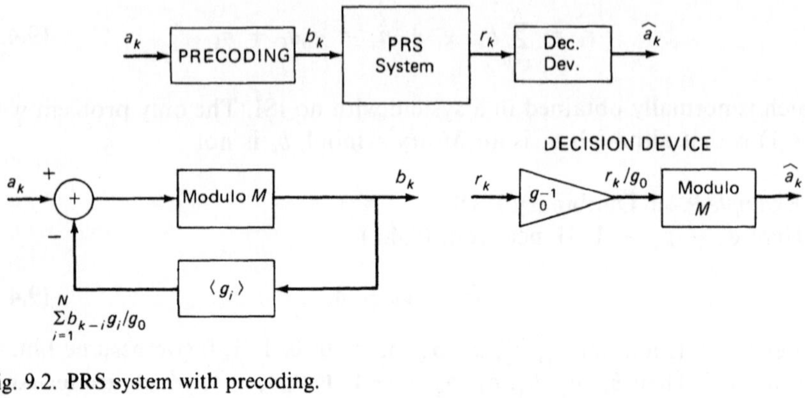


Fig. 9.2. PRS system with precoding.

Thus from (9.4.5)

$$r_k = b_k + b_{k-1} + n_k = s_k + n_k \tag{9.4.9}$$

We see from (9.4.8) that

$$a_k = b_k + b_{k-1} \text{ (modulo 2)} \tag{9.4.10}$$

Therefore the decision rule is

$$\hat{a}_k = r_k \text{ (modulo 2)} = s_k + n_k \text{ (modulo 2)} \tag{9.4.11}$$

which is the same as (9.4.10) in the absence of noise. For binary $b_k = 0, 1$, $s_k$ has three values $s_k = 0, 1, 2$, and in the absence of noise the rule is

$$\begin{aligned} s_k &= 0 \qquad \hat{a}_k = 0 \\ s_k &= 1 \qquad \hat{a}_k = 1 \\ s_k &= 2 \qquad \hat{a}_k = 0 \end{aligned}$$

as illustrated in Fig. 9.3. For Gaussian noise the decision borders are at points $r_k = 0.5, 1.5$. There will be an error if the noise, centered at these points crosses the boundaries. Thus

$$P_b(e|s_k = 0) = P(n_k > 0.5) = Q(0.5/\sigma_n) \tag{9.4.12}$$

$$P_b(e|s_k = 1) = P(|n_k| > 0.5) = 2\,Q(0.5/\sigma_n) \tag{9.4.13}$$

$$P_b(e|s_k = 2) = P(n_k \leqq -0.5) = Q(0.5/\sigma_n) \tag{9.4.14}$$

To compute the bit error probabilities, we need the probabilities $P(s_k = m)$, $m = 0, 1, 2$. Now

$$P(s_k = 0) = P(b_k = 0, b_{k-1} = 0) = 1/4 \tag{9.4.15}$$

$$P(s_k = 1) = P(b_k = 0, b_{k-1} = 1) + P(b_k = 1, b_{k-1} = 0) = 1/2 \tag{9.4.16}$$

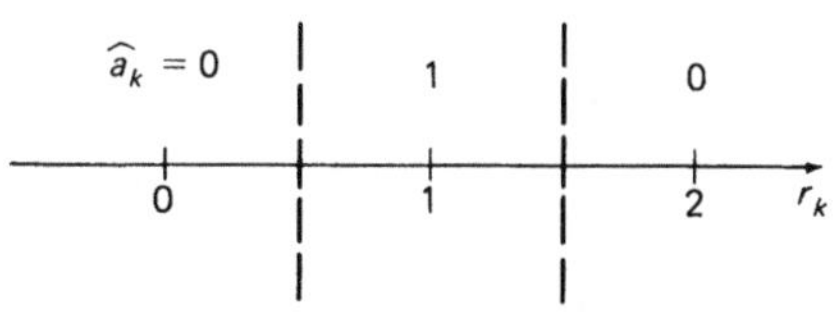


Fig. 9.3. Decision rule for duobinary PRS with binary symbols.

$$P(s_k = 2) = P(b_k = 1, b_{k-1} = 1) = 1/4 \tag{9.4.17}$$

When we combine (9.4.12)–(9.4.17), we obtain

$$P_b(e) = \sum_{m=0}^{2} P_b(e|s_k = m)P(s_k = m) = 1.5\, Q(0.5\, g_0/\sigma_n) \tag{9.4.18}$$

with $g_0 = 1$.

*Example* 9.4.3 Duobinary PRS with $M$-ary symbols
In this case in the absence of noise we have from (9.4.4)

$$a_k = b_k + b_{k-1} \text{ (modulo } M) = s_k \text{ (modulo } M) \tag{9.4.19}$$

which is also the decision rule when noise is present, i.e.

$$\hat{a}_k = s_k + n_k \text{ (modulo } M) \tag{9.4.20}$$

Because the values of $s_k$ are $0, 1, \ldots, 2(M-1)$, both $s_k = m$ and $s_k = M - 1 + m$ are interpreted as $\hat{a}_k = m$. The decision rule is shown in Fig. 9.4. The error probability is

$$P(e) = \sum_{m=0}^{2(M-1)} P(e|s_k = m)P(s_k = m) \tag{9.4.21}$$

Note from Fig. 9.4 that

$$P(e|s_k = m) = \begin{cases} P(n_k \geq 0.5) = Q(0.5/\sigma_n) & m = 0 \\ P(|n_k| \geq 0.5) = 2\, Q(0.5/\sigma_n) & 0 \leq m \leq 2(M-1) \\ P(n_k \leq -0.5) = Q(0.5/\sigma_n) & m = 2(M-1) \end{cases} \tag{9.4.22}$$

Therefore

$$P(e) = 2\, Q(0.5/\sigma_n) - Q(0.5/\sigma_n)\{P(s_k = 0) + P(s_k = 2(M-1))\} \tag{9.4.23}$$

Because

$$P(s_k = 0) = P(b_k = 0, b_{k-1} = 0) = M^{-2} \tag{9.4.24}$$

$$P(s_k = 2(M-1)) = P(b_k = M-1, b_{k-1} = M-1) = M^{-2} \tag{9.4.25}$$

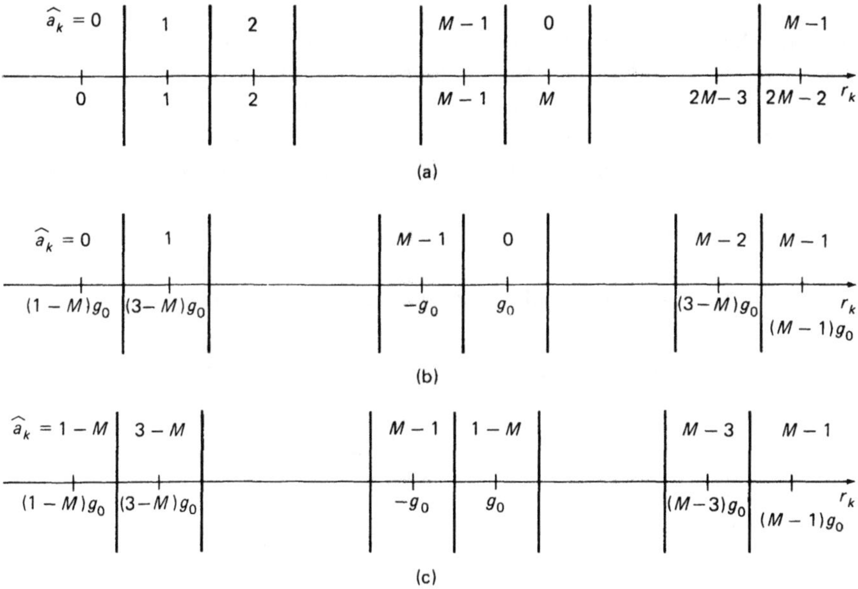


Fig. 9.4. Decision rule for duobinary PRS with $M$-ary symbols. (a) Original $\{a_k\}$ and precoded $\{b_k\}$ symbols from set $\mathring{A}_0$. (b) $\{a_k\} \in \mathring{A}_0$, $\{b_k\} \in \mathring{A}_\pm$. (c) $\{a_k\}$, $\{b_k\} \in \mathring{A}_\pm$.

after substitution into (9.4.23) leads to

$$P(e) = 2(1 - M^{-2})Q(0.5\, g_0/\sigma_n) \tag{9.4.26}$$

with $g_0 = 1$.

When we compare (9.4.26) with (9.3.5) there are apparently two differences

1. The multiplying factor is changed from $2(1 - M^{-1})$ to $2(1 - M^{-2})$.
2. The argument is changed from $g_0/\sigma_n$ to $0.5\, g_0/\sigma_n$.

The second difference is a result of using two different symbols sets, i.e., $\mathring{A}_\pm = \{\pm 1, \pm 3, \ldots, \pm(M - 1)\}$ when neighboring symbols are separated by a distance of 2 and $\mathring{A}_0 = \{0, 1, 2, M - 1\}$ where neighboring symbols are separated by a distance of 1. When we relate $0.5\, g_0/\sigma_n$ to the signal-to-noise ratio per bit, the result is

$$0.5\, g_0/\sigma_n = \left[\eta \frac{3 \log_2 M}{M^2 - 1}(2\, E_b/N_0)\right]^{1/2} \tag{9.4.27}$$

the same as in (9.3.8). The probability of error with precoding is thus

$$P_{PC}(e) = 2(1 - M^{-2})Q\left[\left(\eta \frac{3 \log_2 M}{M^2 - 1} 2\, E_b/N_0\right)^{1/2}\right] \tag{9.4.28}$$

which differs from the lower bound $P_{FL}(e)$ for decision feedback in (9.3.5) only by the multiplying factor. In Table 9.3 we also show the additional energy required when precoding is used with binary symbols.

Actually, we do not use symbols $b_i \in \mathring{A}_0$ for transmission, because, since $\overline{b_i} \neq 0$, this would mean a waste of energy in a DC component, as explained in Chapter 2. To circumvent this problem, we replace in transmission $b_k$ by

$$b'_k = 2\, b_k - M + 1 \in \mathring{A}_\pm \tag{9.4.29}$$

so that now $\overline{b'_k} = 0$. This will have an effect on $r_k$, and now

$$\begin{aligned} r_k &= \sum_0^M b'_{k-i} g_i + n_k = 2 \sum_0^M b_{k-i} g_i - (M-1) \sum_0^M g_i + n_k \\ &= 2\, g_0 \{a_k + cM\} - (M-1) \sum_0^M g_i + n_k \end{aligned} \tag{9.4.30}$$

Thus in order to recover $a_k$, the decision rule is

$$\hat{a}_k = \left( r_k + (M-1) \sum_0^M g_i \right) \Big/ (2\, g_0) \qquad (\text{modulo } M) \tag{9.4.31}$$

In fact, after the decision rule is established, we do not need the shifting and scaling operation in (9.4.31). The decision rule for the duobinary case would be as shown in Fig. 9.4(b).

Finally, if the original symbols $a_k$ are not from the set $\mathring{A}_0$ but rather from $\mathring{A}_\pm$, that simply means a relabeling of the symbols as shown for the duobinary case in Fig. 9.4(c).

We have assumed that $\{g_i\}$ are integers, the main reason for this being the requirement that $b_k$ are $M$-ary symbols. The precoding technique was generalized to arbitrary $\{g_i\}$ in Ref. 9.20.

## 9.5 ERROR MONITORING

It is important in a digital communications system to monitor the performance of the system from the receiver terminal. Excessive noise, a reduction in signal energy, or even an interrupted channel may not be detected by the receiver, which would continue to generate unreliable symbols. If the number of noiseless signal values at the detector output, $s_k$, is identical to the number of symbols and the transition from $s_k$ to $s_{k+1}$ is arbitrary, the detector is unable to recognize unreliable performance. With PRS there are certain rules whose frequent violation, which can be detected, is an indication of deterioration of the system. This point will be illustrated for duobinary PRS with binary symbols, but the same principles apply to other PRS and nonbinary symbols.

For duobinary PRS

$$s_k = b_k + b_{k-1},\ s_{k+1} = b_{k+1} + b_k \tag{9.5.1}$$

Thus the term $b_k$ is common to $s_k$ and $s_{k+1}$. Let $(b_k, b_{k-1})$ be the state of the system with output $s_k$. From state $(b_k, b_{k-1})$ we move to state $(b_{k+1}, b_k)$ the output of which is $s_{k+1}$. The system can be only in four states (0, 0), (0, 1) (1, 0), (1, 1). The state diagram and the transitions from state to state with the corresponding outputs are shown in Fig. 9.5. From the diagram we see the following rules:

a. There is no transition from (0, 0) to (1, 1), i.e., if $s_k = 0$, $s_{k+1} \neq 2$.
b. There is no transition from (1, 1) to (0, 0), i.e., if $s_k = 2$, $s_{k+1} \neq 0$.
c. If $s_k = s_{k+m} = 0$ and $s_{k+1} = s_{k+2} = \dots = s_{k+m-1} = 1$, then $m$ must be odd. Similarly if $s_k = s_{k+m} = 2$.
d. If $s_k = 0$, $s_{k+m} = 2$ (and vice versa), and $s_{k+1} = s_{k+2} = \dots = s_{k+m-1} = 1$, then $m$ is even.

In the presence of noise, it is quite possible that these rules are violated; for example $r_k$ may be in the region for which $s_k = 2$. In Fig. 9.6 we show a sequence of $\{s_k\}$ that is obtained from $\{r_k\}$ by quantizing

$$\begin{aligned} r_k &< 0.5 \rightarrow s_k = 0 \\ 0.5 \leq r_k &< 1.5 \rightarrow s_k = 1 \\ 1.5 < r_k & \quad\ \ \rightarrow s_k = 2 \end{aligned} \tag{9.5.2}$$

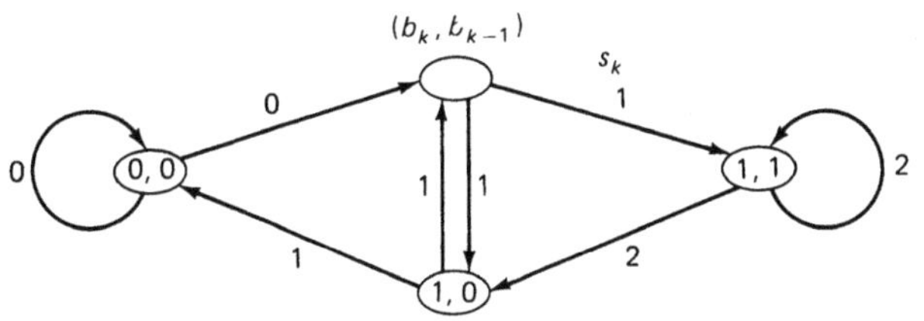


Fig. 9.5. State diagram of duobinary PRS with binary symbols.

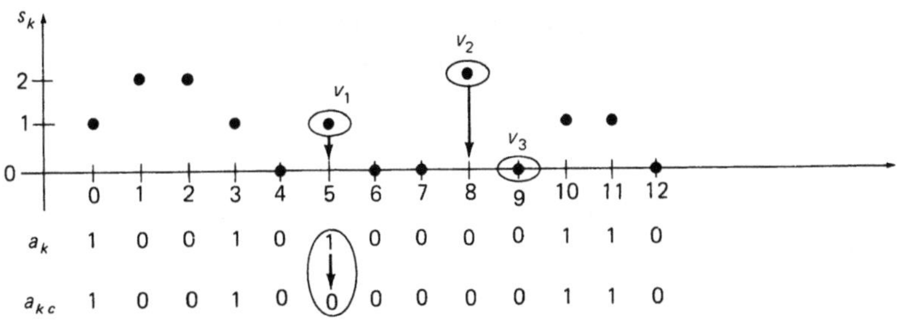


Fig. 9.6. Error monitoring in duobinary PRS with binary symbols.

The violations are indicated by circles. Since $a_k = s_k$ (modulo 2), we also show the sequence of symbols. When we recognize a rule violation the corresponding symbol is in error. By eliminating the violation we can correct that error. A corrected symbol sequence $a_{kc}$ is also shown in Fig. 9.6. Thus $V_1$ violates rule (c), $V_2$ violates rule (a), and $V_3$ violates rule (b). By eliminating violation $V_1$, the symbol is corrected from 1 to 0.

When the number of violations exceeds a critical value the system may be declared as faulty. When the number of violations is small, errors may be detected and even corrected. Error detection and correction techniques with and without null zones (a null zone is a set of $r_k$ values close to the decision boundaries where the decision is unreliable and a temporary "do not know" decision can be made) are presented in Refs. 9.10, 9.11, 9.16, and 9.25. In Fig. 9.7 we show the improvement that results in using a null zone of length $d$ = 0.125. The bit error falls in between curves $A$ and $B$. The penalty in signal-to-noise ratio is reduced to about 1.6 dB only. This curve is from Ref. 9.10. Other curves can be found in Refs. 9.16 and 9.25.

## 9.6 SUMMARY

In this chapter we have defined a PRS system in which the spectral efficiency is

$$\eta_B = \log_2 MR/f_N = 2 \log_2 M$$

rather than

$$\eta_B = 2 \log_2 M/(1 + \beta)$$

The resulting ISI may cause error propagation that can be eliminated by decision feedback or by precoding. In both cases the improvement in spectral efficiency is achieved by a penalty of about 2–3 dB in signal-to-noise ratio per bit for PRS system from class $1 \pm D^N$. The intrinsic rules of PRS may be used to monitor the system performance and for error detection and correction. Many references are given for further reading. Particularly for applications of PRS to digital radio systems, the reader is referred to Ref. 9.28. For error monitoring, the reader should also consult Ref. 9.27.

## 9.7 PROBLEMS

9.2.1 Derive the transfer functions $G(f)$ and the impulse response $g(t)$ for PRS with characteristic polynomial.

a. $1 - D^2$
b. $1 + 2D + D^2$
c. $1 - 2D^2 + D^4$

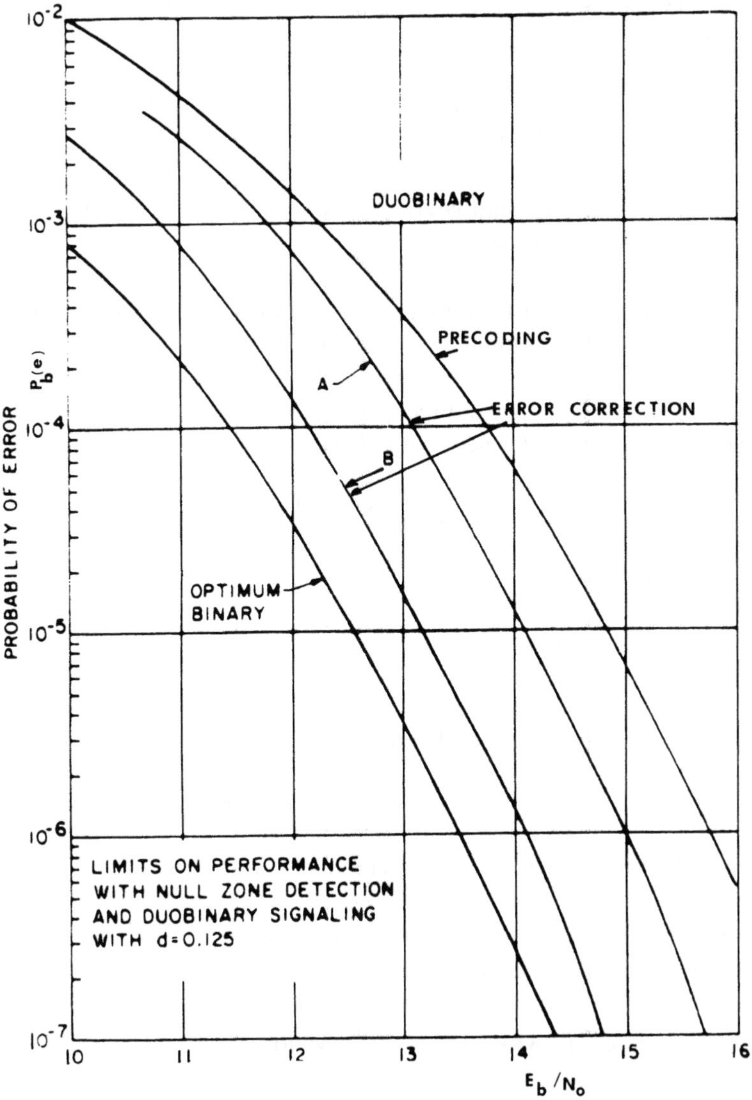


Fig. 9.7. Bit error probability as a function of signal-to-noise ratio per bit of duobinary PRS with binary symbols with and without error correction (J. W. Smith, "Error Control in Duobinary Data Systems by Means of Null Zone Detection," *IEEE Tr. Comm. Tech.*, Vol. COM-16, December 1968, pp. 825–830. Copyright © 1968 IEEE.

9.2.2 Specify the characteristic polynomial of PRS such that $G(f) = 0$ for $f = 0, \pm 0.5 f_N, \pm f_N$.

9.3.1 Compute the error probability of duobinary PRS with decision feedback and $M = 2$, 4 and 8 symbols.

9.3.2 Show that the noise samples of a PRS system in model 1 are dependent and in model 2 independent.

9.3.3 Compute the signal-to-noise ratio penalties $\eta_1$ and $\eta_2$ (in dB) for PRS with characteristic polynomial $1 - 2D^2 + D^4$.

9.4.1 Compute the sequence of precoded symbols $\{b_k\}$ $k = 1, 2, \ldots, 10$ if the sequence of original quaternary symbols is

$$a_1, a_2, a_3, \ldots a_{10} = 0, 3, 1, 2, 0, 0, 2, 1, 3, 1$$

and the systems are
a. duobinary
b. modified duobinary
and $b_0 = 0$.

9.4.2 The same as Problem 9.4.1, but the symbols are binary

$$a_1, a_2, \ldots, a_{10} = 1, 0, 0, 1, 1, 1, 0, 0, 1, 1$$

and the system has characteristic polynomial $1 + 2D + D^2$.

9.4.3 Derive an expression for the error probability as a function of $g_0/\sigma_n$ for the system with characteristic polynomial $1 + 2D + D^2$.

9.4.4 Explain in detail why eq. (9.4.27) is valid.

9.5.1 The following sequence of samples has been obtained at the detector output in duobinary PRS with binary symbols. Identify the violations

$$r_1, r_2, r_3, r_4, \ldots, r_{10} = -1.1, 1.1, 1, 0.9, 0.3\ 0.4, 1.7, 2.1, 1.6, 0.9, 0.1$$

9.5.2 In modified duobinary PRS with binary symbols
a. Specify the state diagram and the value of $s_k$ in each state.
b. Specify the transition rules for $s_k, s_{k+1}$.

## 9.8 REFERENCES


9.1 A. Lender, "The Duobinary Technique for High Speed Data Transmission," *AIEE Tr. Comm. Electron.*, Vol. 82, May 1963, pp. 214–218.

9.2 A. Lender, "Correlative Digital Communication Techniques," *IEEE Tr. Comm. Tech.*, Vol. COM-12, December 1964, pp. 128–135.

9.3 A. Lender, "A Synchronous Signal with Dual Properties for Digital Communication," *IEEE Tr. Comm. Tech.*, vol. COM-13, June 1965, pp. 202–208.

9.4 R. D. Howson, "An Analysis of the Capabilities of Polybinary Data Transmission," *IEEE Tr. Comm. Tech.*, Vol. COM-13, June 1965, pp. 312–319.

9.5 A. Lender, "Correlative Level Coding for Binary Data Transmission," *IEEE Spectrum*, Vol. 3, February 1966, pp. 104–115.

9.6 E. R. Kretzmer, "Generalisation of a Technique for Binary Data Transmission," *IEEE Tr. Comm. Tech.*, Vol. COM-14, February 1966, pp. 67–68.

9.7 F. K. Beker, E. R. Kretzmer, and J. R. Sheehan, "A New Signal Format for Efficient Data Transmission," *BSTJ*, Vol. 45, May–June 1966, pp. 755–758.

9.8 P. J. van Gerwen, "Efficient Use of Pseudo-Ternary Codes for Data Transmission," *IEEE Tr. Comm. Tech.*, Vol. COM-15, August 1967, pp. 558–660.

9.9 A. Lender, "Correlative Data Transmission with Coherent Recovery using Absolute Reference," *IEEE Tr. Comm. Tech.*, Vol. COM-16, February 1968, pp. 108–115.

9.10 J. W. Smith, "Error Control in Duobinary Data Systems by Means of Null Zone Detection," *IEEE Tr. Comm. Tech.*, Vol. COM-16, December 1968, pp. 825–830.

9.11 J. F. Gun and J. A. Lombardi, "Error Detection for Partial Response Systems," *IEEE Tr. Comm. Tech.*, Vol. COM-17, December 1979, pp. 734–737.

9.12 H. Kobayashi, "Coding Schemes for Reduction of Interference in Data Transmission Systems," *IBM J. Res. Develop.*, Vol. 14, July 1970, pp. 343–353.

9.13 H. Kobayashi and D. T. Tang, "Application of Partial Response Channel Coding to Magnetic Recording Systems," *IBM J. Res. Develop.*, Vol. 14, July 1970, pp. 368–375.

9.14 H. Kobayashi, "Application of Probabilistic Decoding to Digital Magnetic Recording Systems," *IBM J. Res. Develop.*, Vol. 15, June 1971, pp. 64–74.

9.15 M. Tomlison, "New Automatic Equalizer Employing Modulo Arithmetic," *Electron. Lett.*, Vol. 7, March 1971, pp. 138–139.

9.16 H. Kobayashi and D. T. Tang, "On Decoding of Correlative Level Coding Systems with Ambiguity Zone Detection," *IEEE Tr. Comm. Tech.*, Vol. COM-19, August 1971, pp. 467–477.

9.17 H. Kobayashi, "Correlative Level Coding and Maximum Likelihood Decoding," *IEEE Tr. Inf. Theory*, Vol. IT-17, September 1971, pp. 586–594.

9.18 H. Kobayshi, "A Survey of Coding Schemes for Transmission of Recoding of Digital Data," *IEEE Tr. Comm. Tech.*, Vol. COM-19, December 1971, pp. 1087–1100.

9.19 G. D. Forney, "Maximum Likelihood Sequence Elimination of Digital Sequences in the Presence of Intersymbol Interference," *IEEE Tr. Inf. Theory*, Vol. IT-18, May 1972, pp. 363–378.

9.20 H. Harashima and H. Miyakawa, "Matched Transmission Technique for Channels with Intersymbol Interference," *IEEE Tr. Comm.*, Vol. COM-20, August 1972, pp. 774–780.

9.21 B. M. Smith, "Some Results for the Eye Patterns of Class 4 Partial Response Data Signals," *IEEE Tr. Comm.*, Vol. COM-22, May 1974, pp. 696–698.

9.22 D. C. Duttweiler, J. E. Mazo, and D. G. Messershmitt, "An Upper Bound on the Error Probability of Decision-Feedback Equalization," *IEEE Tr. Inf. Theory*, Vol. IT-20, July 1974, pp. 490–497.

9.23 P. Kabal and S. Pasupathy, "Partial response signalling," *IEEE Tr. Comm.*, Vol. COM-23, September 1975, pp. 921–934.

9.24 R. D. Gitlin and E. Y. Ho, "A Null Zone Decision Feedback Equalizer Incorporating Maximum Likelihood Bit Detection," *IEEE Tr. Comm.*, Vol. COM-23, November 1975, pp. 1243–1250.

9.25 I. Korn, "A Partial Response Binary Communication System with Erasure," *IEEE Tr. Comm.*, Vol. COM-27, February 1979, pp. 493–498.

9.26 E. A. Newcombe and S. Pasupathy, "Error Rate Monitoring in a Partial Response System," *IEEE Tr. Comm.*, Vol. COM-28, July 1980, pp. 1052–1061.

9.27 E. A. Newcombe and S. Pasupathy, "Error Rate Monitoring for Digital Communications," *Proc. IEEE*, Vol. 70, August 1982, pp. 805–828.

9.28 K. Feher, *Digital Communication: Microwave Applications*, Prentice-Hall Inc., Englewood Cliffs, N.J. 1981, Chapter 7.

# 10 SYSTEM OPTIMIZATION

## 10.1 INTRODUCTION

A model of an ASK communication system is shown in Fig. 10.1. In this figure $G_T(f)$ represents all filtering in transmitter (i.e., the shaping and transmitter filters) and $H'_R(f)$ all filtering in the receiver (i.e., the receiver and detector filters). The symbols $\{a_i\}$ are from the set $\mathring{A}_{\pm} = \{\pm 1, \pm 2, \ldots, \pm(M - 1)\}$, are independent, and appear at the rate of $R = 1/T$ symbols/sec. The noise $n_C(t)$ is zero-mean, Gaussian with power spectral density $S_{nc}(f)$, which is not necessarily white.

In this chapter we pose and solve the following problem: given $H'_C(f)$, find $H'_R(f)$ and $G_T(f)$ so that the system is optimized in some sense. The optimization criteria and the exact formulation are presented in Section 10.2. We define a reasonable criterion that includes the mean square criterion and find the optimal receiver, given transmitter and vice versa, in Section 10.3.

In Section 10.4 we specify the optimal receiver and transmitter or receiver only with or without a constraint on the total system response. A summary is presented in Section 10.5 followed by problems in Section 10.6 and References in section 10.7.

## 10.2 FORMULATION OF OPTIMIZATION PROBLEM

The detector output is

$$r(t) = \sum a_i g(t - iT) + n(t) \tag{10.2.1}$$

where, from Figs. 10.1 and 10.2

$$G(f) = G'_C(f)H'_R(f) = G_C(f)H_R(f) \tag{10.2.2}$$

$$G'_C(f) = G_T(f)H'_C(f) = G_C(f)N^{-0.5}(f) \tag{10.2.3}$$

and $n(t)$ is zero-mean, Gaussian noise with variance

$$\sigma_n^2 = \int_{-\infty}^{\infty} S_n(f)\, df \tag{10.2.4}$$

$$S_n(f) = S_{nc}(f)|H'_R(f)|^2 = 0.5\, N_0|H_R(f)|^2 \tag{10.2.5}$$

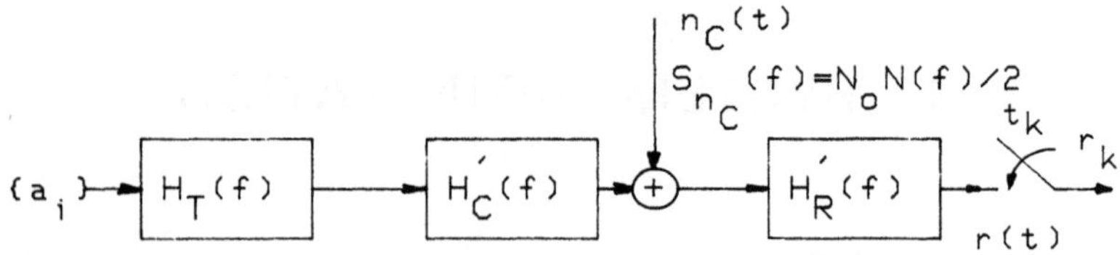


Fig. 10.1. ASK communication system with nonwhite noise.

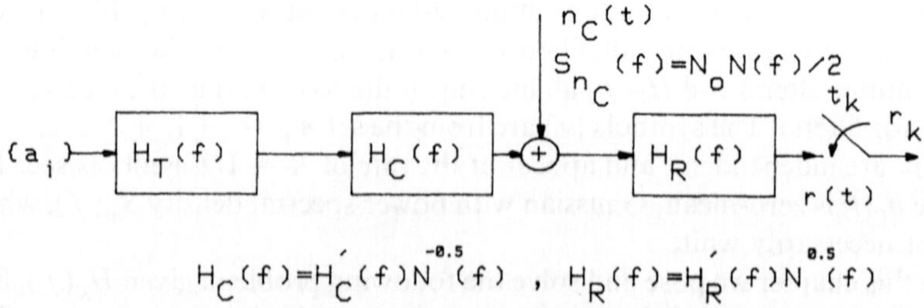


Fig. 10.2. Equivalent ASK communication system with white noise.

Since the systems in Figs. 10.1 and 10.2 are equivalent so long as

$$H_C(f) = H'_C(f)N^{-0.5}(f) \tag{10.2.6}$$

$$H_R(f) = H'_R(f)N^{0.5}(f) \tag{10.2.7}$$

we may assume in the future that the channel noise is white. We obtain the necessary results for the colored noise case by substituting (10.2.6) and (10.2.7) in the final formulas. After sampling at time $t_k = t_0 + kT$, we obtain

$$r_k = \sum_i a_i g_{k-i} + n_k \tag{10.2.8}$$

We may assume here, without loss in generality, that $t_0 = 0$, because if this is not true we may simply replace the signal $g(t)$ by $g(t - t_0)$. The average transmitted energy per symbol is

$$E_s = \sigma_a^2 E_T \tag{10.2.9}$$

where

$$\sigma_a^2 = \overline{a_i^2} = (M^2 - 1)/3 \tag{10.2.10}$$

and

$$E_T = \int_{-\infty}^{\infty} |G_T(f)|^2 \, df \tag{10.2.11}$$

We assume that the channel transfer function, $H_C(f)$, is given. The problem is to select $G_T(f)$ and $H_R(f)$ so that under certain constraints (as for example (10.2.11) with a fixed value of $E_T$) the system is optimized in some sense. There are several criteria of optimization that can be used.

a. *Minimum error probability*[10.1] It was shown in Chapter 4 that the error probability is

$$P(e) = 2(1 - M^{-1})\overline{Q((g_0 - I)/\sigma_n)} \tag{10.2.12}$$

where $Q(\ )$ is the integral of a Gaussian function, and

$$I = \sum_{i \neq 0} a_{k-i} g_i \tag{10.2.13}$$

is intersymbol interference (ISI). The problem is to find $G_T(f)$ and $H_R(f)$ that will give a set of $\{g_i\}$ that minimizes $P(e)$. This is the most meaningful criterion in digital communications. However, due to the nonlinear relation between $P(e)$ and $\{g_i\}$, very few analytical results can be obtained.[10.1]

b. *Minimization of maximal intersymbol interference* Here we minimize

$$I_{\max} = (M - 1) \sum_{i=0} |g_i| \tag{10.2.14}$$

which is equivalent to maximizing the eye opening in the absence of noise. This criterion is too conservative, because the probability that $I = I_{\max}$ is very small. It also ignores the noise.

c. *Minimum mean square error*[10.2–10.9] We assume that the desired output at time $t_k$ is

$$\hat{r}_k = \sum_i a_i d_{k-i} \tag{10.2.15}$$

while the actual output is as in (10.2.8). For example, in a system with no ISI, only $d_0 \neq 0$, but in the duobinary system, $d_0 = d_1 \neq 0$. The error between the desired and actual output is

$$e_k = r_k - \hat{r}_k = \sum_i a_i(g_{k-i} - d_{k-i}) + n_k \tag{10.2.16}$$

and the mean square error is

$$\varepsilon = \overline{e_k^2} = \sigma_a^2 \sum_i (g_i - d_i)^2 + \sigma_n^2 \tag{10.2.17}$$

It was shown in Section 4.3 that

$$g_i = \int_{-\infty}^{\infty} G(f) \exp(j\,2\,\pi f iT)\,df = \int_{f\in F} G_\Sigma(f) \exp(j\,2\,\pi f iT)\,df \quad (10.2.18)$$

where

$$G_\Sigma(f) = \sum_k G(f + kR),\ R = 1/T \quad (10.2.19)$$

and

$$F = \{f\colon |f| \leqq f_N\},\ f_N = R/2 \quad (10.2.20)$$

is a (simple) Nyquist interval. A similar expression can be written for $d_i$. On the other hand

$$G_\Sigma(f) = T \sum_i g_i \exp(-j\,2\,\pi f iT) \quad (10.2.21)$$

and

$$D_\Sigma(f) = T \sum_i d_i \exp(-j\,2\,f\pi iT) \quad (10.2.22)$$

which are periodic functions in $f$ with period $R = 1/T$.

Using these equations we can write

$$\sum_i (g_i - \mathrm{d_i})^2 = \sum_i (g_i - d_i) \int_{f\in F} \{G_\Sigma(f) - D_\Sigma(f)\} \exp(j\,2\,\pi f iT)\,df$$

$$= R \int_{f\in F} |G_\Sigma(f) - D_\Sigma(f)|^2\,df \quad (10.2.23)$$

Similarly, since $S_n(f) \geqq 0$, we can write

$$\sigma_n^2 = \int_{f\in F} S_{n\Sigma}(f)\,df \quad (10.2.24)$$

where

$$S_{n\Sigma}(f) = \sum_k S_n(f + kR) \quad (10.2.25)$$

Equations (10.2.18), (10.2.23), and (10.2.24) are also valid if $F$ in (10.2.20) is replaced by a generalized Nyquist interval (GNI) defined as follows

$$F = \left\{ f: f \in F \rightarrow -f \in F, f + kR \notin F \text{ all integer } k \neq 0, \int_F df = R \} \right\} \tag{10.2.26}$$

Note that if $G(f) \neq 0$ only in $f \in F$, then

$$G_\Sigma(f) = G(f) \qquad f \in F \tag{10.2.27}$$

i.e., the summation is reduced to a single term. This is the function with the minimum bandwidth. The same is true for $D_\Sigma(f)$, and we shall indeed assume that

$$D_\Sigma(f) = D(f) \qquad f \in F \tag{10.2.28}$$

There are many GNIs. For our purposes we shall select the one with the maximum channel transfer capability, i.e.

$$F = \{f: |H_C(f)| \geqq |H_C(f + kR)|, \text{ all integer } k \neq 0\} \tag{10.2.29}$$

and if there is equality for several frequencies we shall select the one with the smallest absolute value. Such a set is illustrated in Fig. 10.3. Note that $3\,R/4 \leqq |f| \leqq 5\,R/4$ is not in $F$, while $5\,R/4 \leqq |f| \leqq 3\,R/2$ is in $F$.

When we substitute (10.2.23), (10.2.24), and (10.2.28) into (10.2.17), we obtain the mean square error in the frequency domain

$$\varepsilon = \sigma_a^2 \mathrm{R} \int_{f \in F} |G_\Sigma(f) - D(f)|^2 \, df + \int_{f \in F} S_{n\Sigma}(f) \, df \tag{10.2.30}$$

## 10.3 OPTIMAL RECEIVER AND TRANSMITTER

We shall say that a criterion is reasonable if under this criterion an increase in noise power, $\sigma_n^2$, does not improve system performance. The minimum probability of error is a reasonable criterion so long as $g_0 \geqq I_{\max}$ and may be so even without this condition. The mean square error is certainly a reasonable criterion. We shall prove two theorems pertaining to the optimal receiver and optimal transmitter under a reasonable criterion, which have been originally proved (in a different form) in Refs. 10.10 and 10.11. The main difference is that in these references the desired system has no ISI.

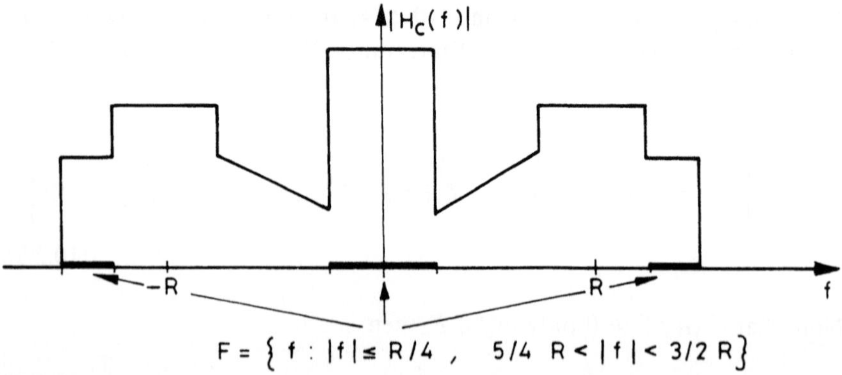


Fig. 10.3. Generalized Nyquist interval.

### 10.3.1 Optimal receiver

*Theorem 1* Let $G_C(f)$ be given (i.e., the transmitter and channel are given). The optimal receiver has the form

$$H_{Rop}(f) = G_C^*(f)C(f) \tag{10.3.1}$$

where $C(f)$ is a periodic function of $f$ with period $R$, i.e.

$$C(f) = C(f + kR). \tag{10.3.2}$$

*Proof*
Using the notation

$$X_k(f) = X(f + kR) \tag{10.3.3}$$

for all functions, we can write (10.2.19) using (10.2.2)

$$G_\Sigma(f) = \sum_k G_{ck}(f)H_{Rk}(f) \tag{10.3.4}$$

If we use the proposed optimal receiver we obtain from (10.3.4) and (10.3.2)

$$G_{op\Sigma}(f) = \sum_k |G_{ck}(f)|^2 C_k(f) = C(f) \sum_k |G_{ck}(f)|^2 \tag{10.3.5}$$

If we select

$$C(f) = G_\Sigma(f) \Big/ \sum_k |G_{ck}(f)|^2 \tag{10.3.6}$$

then

$$G_{op\Sigma}(f) = G_{\Sigma}(f) \tag{10.3.7}$$

and so far as the signal, $\{g_i\}$, is concerned, the optimal and the arbitrary receiver lead to identical results. However, for the noise we obtain with the optimal receiver

$$\begin{aligned} S_{nop\Sigma}(f) &= 0.5\, N_0 \sum_k |H_{Ropk}(f)|^2 \\ &= 0.5\, N_0 |C(f)|^2 \sum_k |G_{ck}(f)|^2 \end{aligned} \tag{10.3.8}$$

and after substitution of (10.3.6) and (10.3.4)

$$\begin{aligned} S_{nop\Sigma}(f) &= 0.5\, N_0 |G_{\Sigma}(f)|^2 \Big/ \sum_k |G_{ck}(f)|^2 \\ &\leqq 0.5\, N_0 \sum_k |H_{Rk}(f)|^2 = S_{n\Sigma}(f) \end{aligned} \tag{10.3.9}$$

where we have used Schwartz inequality

$$\left| \sum_k G_{ck}(f) H_{Rk}(f) \right|^2 \leqq \sum_k |G_{ck}(f)|^2 \sum_k |H_{Rk}(f)|^2 \tag{10.3.10}$$

Equality holds only if

$$H_{Rk}(f) = C(f) G_{ck}^{*}(f) \tag{10.3.11}$$

where $C(f)$ is independent of $k$, i.e., a periodic function in $f$ with period $R$. It follows from (10.3.9) and (10.2.24) that

$$\sigma_{nop}^2 \leqq \sigma_n^2 \tag{10.3.12}$$

with equality only if $H_{Rk}(f)$ is as in (10.3.11) i.e., $H_R(f)$ is as in (10.3.1).

Because $C(f)$ is periodic, it can be expressed as a Fourier series in the frequency domain

$$C(f) = \sum_i C_i \exp\,(-j\, 2\, \pi i f/R) \tag{10.3.13}$$

$$C_i = T \int_{f \in F} C(f) \exp\,(j\, 2\, \pi i f/R)\, df \tag{10.3.14}$$

Thus in the time domain

$$c(t) = \sum_i C_i \delta(t - iT) \tag{10.3.15}$$

The last expression can be realized by a circuit called a *transversal filter* (TF), or *tapped delay line* (TDL), shown in Fig. 10.4. It follows from Theorem 1 that the optimal receiver is composed of a matched filter in tandem with a TF. Referring to Fig. 10.4, we see that if $y(t)$ is the response of the matched filter, then

$$r(t) = \sum_i C_i y(t - iT) \tag{10.3.16}$$

$$r_k = \sum_i C_i y_{k-i} \tag{10.3.17}$$

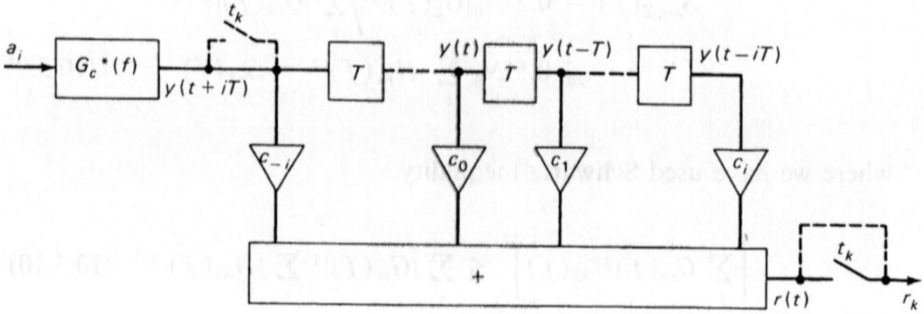


Fig. 10.4. Transversal filter.

In Fig. 10.4 the sampler is shown after the TF, but eq. (10.3.17) remains valid if the sampler is moved to the input of the TF, as shown in broken lines in the figure.

Because the matched filter compensates for any phase in $G_C(f)$, we may assume in the future for convenience that $G_C(f)$ is real. Finally if the noise is not white, using (10.2.6) and (10.2.7), the optimal receiver is

$$H'_{\text{Rop}}(f) = G_C^*(f)C(f)/N(f) \tag{10.3.18}$$

### 10.3.2 Optimal transmitter

*Theorem 2* Let $\{g_i\}$ (i.e., $G_\Sigma(f)$) be given. A transmitter, $G_T(f)$ with a constraint on its energy

$$\int_{f\in F} \sum_k |G_{Tk}(f)|^2 \, df = \int_{-\infty}^{\infty} |G_T(f)|^2 \, df = E_T \tag{10.3.19}$$

is optimal if $G_T(f) = 0$ for all $f \notin F$.

*Proof*

For an arbitrary $G_T(f)$ but with an optimal receiver

$$G_\Sigma(f) = C(f) \sum_k |G_{Tk}(f)|^2 |H_{ck}(f)|^2 \tag{10.3.20}$$

If we select now

$$|G_{Top}(f)|^2 = \frac{G_\Sigma(f)}{C(f)|H_C(f)|^2} I_F(f) \tag{10.3.21}$$

where here

$$I_F(f) = \begin{cases} 1 & f \in F \\ 0 & f \notin F \end{cases} \tag{10.3.22}$$

and substitute into (10.3.20), we obtain, using (10.2.27)

$$\begin{aligned} G_{op\Sigma}(f) &= C(f) \sum_k |G_{Topk}(f)|^2 |H_{ck}(f)|^2 \\ &= C(f)|G_{Top}(f)|^2 |H_C(f)|^2 = G_\Sigma(f) \end{aligned} \tag{10.3.23}$$

Thus the signal remains unchanged. In deriving (10.3.23) we have used the property that if

$$X(f) = X(f) I_F(f) \tag{10.3.24}$$

then

$$\left\{ \sum_k X_k(f) \right\} I_F(f) = X(f) I_F(f) \tag{10.3.25}$$

The signal energy with the optimal transmitter is

$$\begin{aligned} E_{Top} &= \int_{f \in F} |G_{Top}(f)|^2 \, df = \int_{f \in F} \frac{G_\Sigma(f)}{C(f)|H_C(f)|^2} \, df \\ &= \int_{f \in F} \sum_k |G_{Tk}(f)|^2 |H_{ck}(f)|^2 / |H_C(f)|^2 \, df \end{aligned} \tag{10.3.26}$$

Using the definition of $F$ in (10.2.29)

$$E_{Top} \leqq \int_{f \in F} \sum_k |G_{Tk}(f)|^2 \, df = E_T \tag{10.3.27}$$

with equality only if the arbitrary $G_T(f)$ satisfied already $G_T(f) = 0, f \notin F$.

To keep the energy fixed at value $E_T$, we can multiply $G_{Top}(f)$ by $K \geqq 1$, so that

$$K^2 E_{Top} = E_T \tag{10.3.28}$$

and simultaneously divide $H_R(f)$ by $K$, so that $G(f)$ remains unchanged. Doing so, the noise variance is

$$\sigma_{nop}^2 = 0.5\, N_0 \int_{-\infty}^{\infty} |H_R(f)|^2 df / K^2 = \sigma_n^2 / K^2 \leqq \sigma_n^2 \tag{10.3.29}$$

which is less than in the unoptimized system.

We thus conclude that the optimal transmitter filter is such that all its energy is allocated to the frequency band in which the channel transfer function has its maximum values in the sense of (10.2.29).

## 10.4 MINIMIZATION OF THE MEAN SQUARE ERROR

The results in Section 10.3 are valid for any reasonable criterion; the exact form of $C(f)$ will depend on the specific criterion. In this section we confine our discussion to the minimum mean square error criterion, which is stated again here in a convenient form

$$\varepsilon = \sigma_a^2 R \int_{f \in F} |G_\Sigma(f) - D(f)|^2\, df + 0.5\, N_0 \int_{-\infty}^{\infty} |H_R(f)|^2\, df \tag{10.4.1}$$

where $G(f)$ is given in (10.2.2) and (10.2.3). The optimal receiver is

$$H_{Rop}(f) = C(f) G_C^*(f) \tag{10.4.2}$$

and the optimal transmitter is

$$G_{Top}(f) = G_T(f) I_F(f) \tag{10.4.3}$$

We may minimize (10.4.1) with or without the constraint

$$G_\Sigma(f) = D(f) \tag{10.4.4}$$

With this constraint the mean square error is simplified to

$$\varepsilon = 0.5\, N_0 \int_{-\infty}^{\infty} |H_R(f)|^2\, df \tag{10.4.5}$$

The minimization of $\varepsilon$ with assumption

$$D(f) = d_0 T \tag{10.4.6}$$

was the subject of Refs. 10.4–10.9. The general result was first presented in Ref. 10.12.

### 10.4.1 Optimization of receiver

*With constraint (10.4.4)* With the optimal receiver

$$G(f) = |G_C(f)|^2 C(f) \tag{10.4.7}$$

Hence using the constraint (10.4.4)

$$C_{\text{op}}(f) = D(f)/G_{C2}(f) \tag{10.4.8}$$

where

$$G_{C2}(f) = \sum_k |G_C(f + kR)|^2 \tag{10.4.9}$$

Therefore

$$H_{R\text{op}}(f) = G_C^*(f) D(f)/G_{C2}(f) \tag{10.4.10}$$

and

$$\varepsilon = \varepsilon_1 = 0.5\, N_0 \int_{-\infty}^{\infty} |H_{R\text{op}}(f)|^2\, df = 0.5\, N_0 \int_{f \in F} |D(f)|^2/G_{C2}(f)\, df \tag{10.4.11}$$

*Example* 10.4.1
In this example we assume a modified duobinary signal

$$D(f) = jT \sin(2\, \pi f T)$$

and that

$$H_C(f) = 1$$

$$S_{nc}(f) = N_0/2$$

$$G_T(f) = (TE_T)^{0.5} I_F(f)$$

$$F = \{f: |f| \leqq R/2\}$$

In this case

$$G_C(f) = (TE_T)^{0.5} I_F(f)$$

Hence

$$C_{\text{op}}(f) = jT \sin(2\pi fT)/(TE_T)$$

$$H_{R\text{op}}(f) = (TE_T)^{-1/2} jT \sin(2\pi fT) I_F(f)$$

$$\varepsilon_1 = \frac{0.5\, N_0}{TE_T} \int_{-R/2}^{R/2} \{T \sin(2\pi fT)\}^2\, df = 0.25\, N_0/E_T \qquad (10.4.12)$$

*Without constraint (10.4.4)* When we use the optimal receiver in (10.4.1), we obtain

$$\varepsilon = \int_{f\in F} \{\sigma_a^2 R|G_{C2}(f)C(f) - D(f)|^2 + 0.5\, N_0 G_{C2}(f)|C(f)|^2\}\, df \qquad (10.4.13)$$

Letting

$$C(f) = C_I(f) + jC_Q(f),\; D(f) = D_I(f) + jD_Q(f) \qquad (10.4.14)$$

and denoting

$$A(f) = G_{C2}(f) + N_0/(2\,\sigma_a^2 R) \qquad (10.4.15)$$

we can rewrite (10.4.13) in a quadratic form

$$\varepsilon = \int_{f\in F} \{\sigma_a^2 RA(f) G_{C2}(f) \{(C_I(f) - D_I(f)/A(f))^2 + (C_Q(f) - D_Q(f)/A(f))^2\} + 0.5\, N_0 |D(f)|^2/A(f)\}\, df \qquad (10.4.16)$$

This is minimized when

$$C(f) = C_{\mathrm{op}}(f) = D(f)/A(f) \qquad (10.4.17)$$

The optimal receiver and minimal mean square error are

$$H_{R\mathrm{op}}(f) = G_C^*(f)D(f)/A(f) \qquad (10.4.18)$$

$$\varepsilon = \varepsilon_2 = 0.5\, N_0 \int_{f\in F} |D(f)|^2/A(f)\, df \qquad (10.4.19)$$

Note that when the signal-to-noise ratio is large, i.e.

$$G_{C2}(f) \gg N_0/(2\, \sigma_a^2 R) \qquad (10.4.20)$$

then

$$A(f) \simeq G_{C2}(f) \qquad (10.4.21)$$

and eqs. (10.4.18) and (10.4.19) are identical to (10.4.10) and (10.4.11)

*Example* 10.4.2
We use the data of Example 10.4.1 with the assumption that the symbols are binary; hence $\sigma_a^2 = 1$, and

$$A(f) = 0.5\, N_0 T + TE_T$$

The mean square error is

$$\varepsilon_2 = \frac{0.25\, N_0}{0.5\, N_0 + E_T} = (0.25\, N_0/E_T)(1 + 0.5\, N_0/E_T)^{-1} \qquad (10.4.22)$$

Both $1/\varepsilon_1$ and $1/\varepsilon_2$ are shown in Fig. 10.5 as a function of the signal-to-noise ratio.

## 10.4.2 Optimization of receiver and transmitter

When we optimize the transmitter we have to set a limit to transmitter energy. Hence we minimize (10.4.13) with constraint (10.2.11). This is equivalent to minimizing

$$V = \varepsilon + \lambda \int_{-\infty}^{\infty} |G_T(f)|^2\, df = \varepsilon + \lambda \int_{f\in F} G_{T2}(f)\, df \qquad (10.4.23)$$

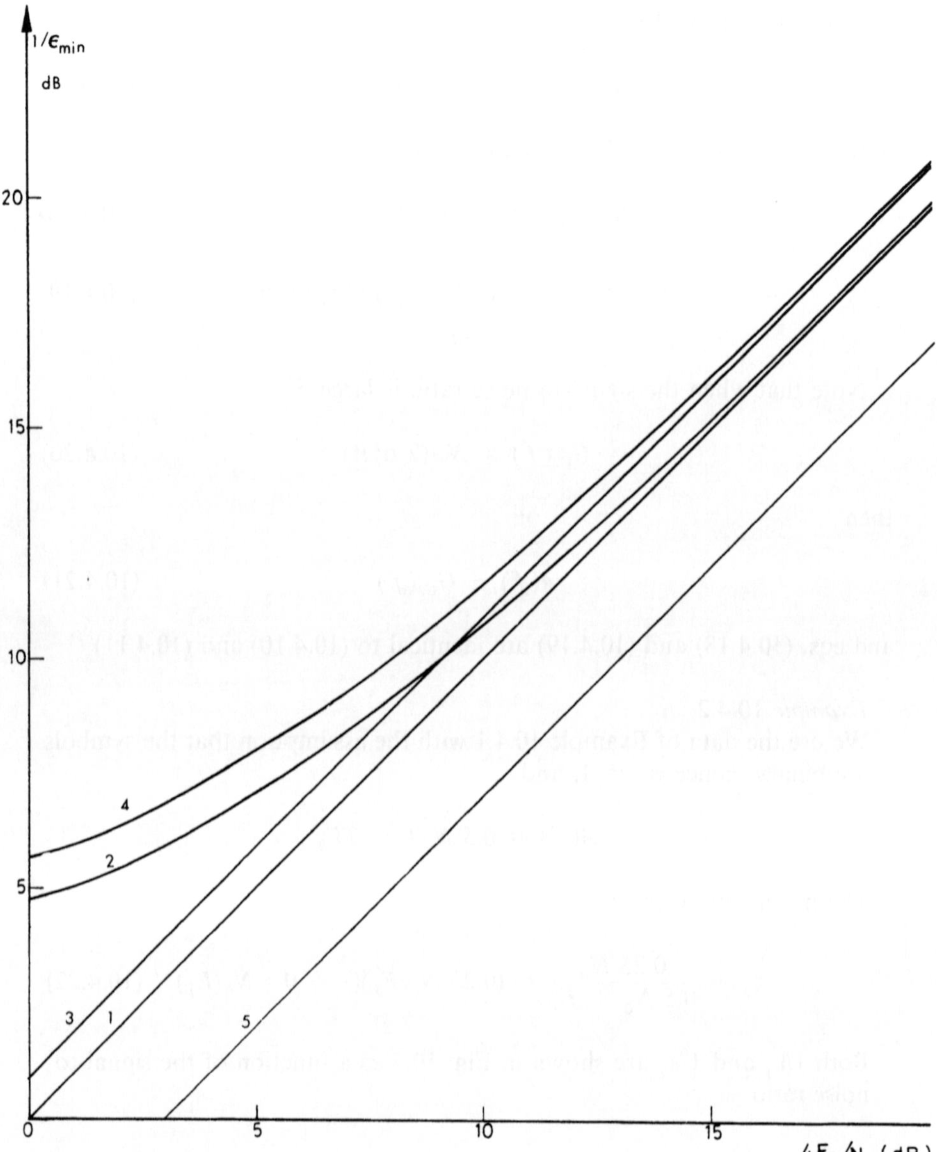


Fig. 10.5. The inverse of mean square error as a function of signal-to-noise ratio for a system with duobinary signal. (1) Optimal receiver with constraint on total system response. (2) Optimal receiver without constraint on total system response. (3) Optimal receiver and transmitter with constraint on total system response. (4) Optimal receiver and transmitter without constraint on total system response. (5) Optimal receiver and transmitter for a 100% excess bandwidth raised cosine signal with no intersymbol interference (I. Korn, "Optimisation of Receiver and Transmitter for Partial Response Signals," *IEEE Proc.*, Vol. 129, pt. F. October 1982, pp. 347–351.)

where

$$G_{T2}(f) = \sum_k |G_T(f + kR)|^2 \tag{10.4.24}$$

and $\lambda$ is a constant (called Lagrange multiplier), chosen so that constraint (10.2.11) is satisfied. We already know that the optimal transmitter is confined to $F$; hence

$$V = \int_{f \in F} \{\sigma_a^2 R||G_C(f)|^2 C(f) - D(f)|^2 + 0.5\, N_0 |C(f) G_C(f)|^2 + \lambda |G_T(f)|^2\}\, df \tag{10.4.25}$$

Again we can optimize the system with or without constraint (10.4.4).

*With constraint (10.4.4)* In this case

$$C_{\text{op}}(f) = D(f)/|G_C(f)|^2 \tag{10.4.26}$$

Hence

$$V = \int_{f \in F} \left\{0.5\, N_0 \left| \frac{D(f)}{G_T(f) H_C(f)} \right|^2 + \lambda |G_T(f)|^2 \right\} df \tag{10.4.27}$$

Substitute

$$|G_T(f)|^2 = |G_{T\text{op}}(f)|^2 + \delta O^2(f) \tag{10.4.28}$$

where $O(f)$ is an arbitrary, but nonzero, function in $f$, and $\delta$ is a constant. Because $G_{T\text{op}}(f)$ is optimal, $V$ is minimal with respect to $\delta$ if $\delta = 0$. Thus taking the derivative we obtain from

$$\left. \frac{dV}{d\delta} \right|_{\delta=0} = 0 \tag{10.4.29}$$

$$|G_{T\text{op}}(f)|^2 = \lambda^{-1/2} |D(f)/H_C(f)| I_F(f) \tag{10.4.30}$$

After substitution into (10.2.11), the result is

$$\lambda = (B_1/E_T)^2 \tag{10.4.31}$$

where

$$B_1 = \int_{f \in F} |D(f)/H_C(f)|\, df \tag{10.4.32}$$

When we substitute (10.4.31) into (10.4.30), the optimal transmitter filter is

$$|G_{T\text{op}}(f)|^2 = (E_T/B_1)|D(f)/H_C(f)|I_F(f) \qquad (10.4.33)$$

When we substitute (10.4.33) into (10.4.26), (10.4.2), and (10.4.5), we obtain

$$C_{\text{op}}(f) = (B_1/E_T)/|H_C(f)| \qquad (10.4.34)$$

$$|H_{R\text{op}}(f)|^2 = (B_1/E_T)|D(f)/|H_C(f)|I_F(f)| \qquad (10.4.35)$$

$$\varepsilon = \varepsilon_3 = 0.5\, N_0 B_1^2/E_T \qquad (10.4.36)$$

*Example* 10.4.3
We continue here Example 10.4.2, except that $G_T(f)$ is not as in Example 10.4.1, but will be optimized. In this case

$$D(f)/H_C(f) = jT \sin(2\,\pi f T)$$

Hence from (10.4.32)

$$B_1 = T \int_{-R/2}^{R/2} |\sin(2\,\pi f T)|\, df = 2/\pi$$

The optimal transmitter, receiver, and mean square errors are from (10.4.33), (10.4.35), and (10.4.36)

$$|G_{T\text{op}}(f)|^2 = (E_T/B_1) T \sin(2\,\pi f T) I_F(f)$$

$$|H_{R\text{op}}(f)|^2 = 2(\pi E_T)^{-1}\, T \sin(2\,\pi f T) I_F(f) \qquad (10.4.37)$$

$$\varepsilon_3 = (0.25\, N_0/E_T)(8/\pi^2)$$

A plot of $\varepsilon_3^{-1}$ is also shown in Fig. 10.5.

<u>*Without constraint (10.4.4)*</u> Using (10.4.14) and (10.2.3), we can rewrite (10.4.25) in the form

$$V = \int_{f\in F} \{\sigma_a^2 R|H_C(f)|^4|C(f)|^2|G_T(f)|^4 + \{0.5\, N_0|H_C(f)|^2|C(f)|^2 + \lambda - 2\,\sigma_a^2 R|H_C(f)|^4(C_I(f)D_I(f) + C_Q(f)D_Q(f))\}|G_T(f)|^2 + \sigma_a^2 R|D(f)|^2\}\, df \qquad (10.4.38)$$

or in a form similar to (10.4.16)

$$V = \int_{f \in F} \{\sigma_a^2 R A(f) |G_T(f)|^2 |H_C(f)|^2 \{(C_I(f) - D_I(f)/A(f))^2 + (C_Q(f) - D_Q(f)/A(f))^2\} + 0.5\, N_0 |D(f)|^2/A(f) + \lambda |G_T(f)|^2\}\, df \tag{10.4.39}$$

where $A(f)$ is as in (10.4.15)

$$A(f) = |G_T(f)|^2 |H_C(f)|^2 + N_0/(2\, \sigma_a^2 R) \tag{10.4.40}$$

When we substitute (10.4.28) into (10.4.38), we obtain from

$$\left. \frac{\partial V}{\partial \delta} \right|_{\delta = 0} = 0 \tag{10.4.41}$$

and the fact that $O^2(f)$ is arbitrary, the equation for the optimal transmitter

$$2\, \sigma_a^2 R |H_C(f)|^4 |C(f)|^2 |G_{Top}(f)|^2 + 0.5\, N_0 |H_C(f)|^2 |C(f)|^2 + \lambda - 2\sigma_a^2 R |H_C(f)|^4 (C_I(f) D_I(f) + C_Q(f) D_Q(f)) = 0 \tag{10.4.42}$$

We obtain simultaneously from (10.4.39) that the optimal $C(f)$ is as in (10.4.17)

$$C_{op}(f) = D(f)/A(f) \tag{10.4.43}$$

or using (10.4.40)

$$(2\, \sigma_a^2 R |H_C(f)|^2 |G_T(f)|^2 + N_0) C_{op}(f) = 2\, \sigma_a^2 R D(f) \tag{10.4.44}$$

It thus follows from (10.4.44) that for optimality

$$C_I(f) D_I(f) + C_Q(f) D_Q(f) = \frac{2\, \sigma_a^2 R |H_C(f)|^2 |G_{Top}(f)|^2 + N_0}{2\, \sigma_a^2 R} |C_{op}(f)|^2 \tag{10.4.45}$$

Hence (10.4.42) can be simplified to

$$0.5\, N_0 |H_C(f)|^2 |C_{op}(f)|^2 = \lambda \tag{10.4.46}$$

Thus

$$C_{op}(f) = (2\, \lambda / N_0)^{0.5} / H_C(f) \tag{10.4.47}$$

Taking the absolute value of (10.4.44) and substituting (10.4.47), we obtain the optimal transmitter

$$|G_{T\text{op}}(f)|^2 = \frac{|D(f)|}{|C_{\text{op}}(f)||H_C(f)|^2} - \frac{N_0}{2\,\sigma_a^2 R|H_C(f)|^2}$$

$$= (2\,\lambda/N_0)^{-0.5}|D(f)/H_C(f)| - N_0/(2\,\sigma_a^2 R|H_C(f)|^2) \tag{10.4.48}$$

Applying now the constraint (10.2.11), we obtain from (10.4.48)

$$E_T = (2\,\lambda/N_0)^{-0.5}B_1 - N_0 B_2 \tag{10.4.49}$$

where $B_1$ was defined in (10.4.32) and

$$B_2 = \int_{f\in F} (2\,\sigma_a^2 R|H_C(f)|^2)^{-1}\,df \tag{10.4.50}$$

Thus

$$(2\,\lambda/N_0)^{0.5} = B_1/(E_T + N_0 B_2) \tag{10.4.51}$$

and

$$C_{\text{op}}(f) = B_1(E_T + N_0 B_2)^{-1}/H_C(f) \tag{10.4.52}$$

The optimal receiver and transmitter are finally

$$\begin{aligned}|H_{R\text{op}}(f)|^2 &= |G_{T\text{op}}(f)H_C(f)C_{\text{op}}(f)|^2\\ &= |G_{T\text{op}}(f)|^2 B_1^2/(E_T + N_0 B_2)^2\end{aligned} \tag{10.4.53}$$

$$|G_{T\text{op}}(f)|^2 = \{(E_T + N_0 B_2)|D(f)/H_C(f)|/B_1 - N_0/(2\,\sigma_a^2 R|H_C(f)|^2)\}I_F \tag{10.4.54}$$

The minimal mean square error is

$$\begin{aligned}\varepsilon = \varepsilon_4 &= \int_{f\in F} 0.5\,N_0|D(f)|^2/A(f)\,df\\ &= 0.5\,N_0 B_1^2/(E_T + N_0 B_2)\end{aligned} \tag{10.4.55}$$

If the signal-to-noise ratio is large, i.e., if

$$2\,\sigma_a^2 R|H_C(f)|^2|G_T(f)|^2 \gg N_0$$

then eqs. (10.4.52)–(10.4.55) are reduced to (10.4.33)–(10.4.36).

*Example* 10.4.4
We continue here with Example 10.4.3. Because in this example $H_C(f) = 1$ and $\sigma_a^2 = 1$, we obtain from (10.4.50)

$$B_2 = (2\ \sigma_a^2)^{-1}$$

and $B_1$ is as in example 10.4.3, namely

$$B_1 = 2/\pi$$

Thus

$$|G_{Top}(f)|^2 = \{(E_T + N_0/(2\ \sigma_a^2))T \sin(2\ \pi f T)\pi/2 - 0.5\ N_0 T\} I_F$$

$$|H_{Rop}(f)|^2 = 4|G_{Top}(f)|^2/(\pi(E_T + 0.5\ N_0))^2$$

$$\varepsilon_4 = 0.25\ (N_0/E_T)(1 + 0.5\ N_0/E_T)^{-1}(8/\pi^2) \qquad (10.4.56)$$

A plot of $\varepsilon_4{}^{-1}$ is also shown in Fig. 10.5.

One can see from fig. 10.5 that when the signal-to-noise ratio is large (large $E_T/N_0$), the minimum mean square error is the same whether there is or is not a constraint on the system response.

*Example* 10.4.5
If in the system of example 10.4.1 a raised cosine signal with 100% excess bandwidth

$$G(f) = \begin{cases} T(1 + \cos(2\ \pi f/R)) & |f| \leqq R/2 \\ 0 & \text{otherwise} \end{cases} \qquad (10.4.57)$$

is required, the optimal receiver, transmitter, and minimum mean square error, under condition of no intersymbol interference, are

$$|G_{Top}(f)|^2 = E_T G(f) \qquad (10.4.58)$$

$$|H_{Rop}(f)|^2 = G(f)/E_T \qquad (10.4.59)$$

$$\varepsilon = \varepsilon_5 = 0.5\ N_0/E_T \qquad (10.4.60)$$

This is also shown in Fig. 10.5.

## 10.5 SUMMARY

In this chapter we have derived the optimal receiver or receiver and transmitter with or without a constraint on the overall system response under a reasonable criterion. The desired system response may be of the partial response type. Specific formulas have been given for the mean square error criterion. The noise in the system may be colored, because it was shown that such a system is equivalent to another system with white noise. The minimal mean square error for the system with white noise is given in (10.4.11), (10.4.19), (10.4.36), and (10.4.55), respectively. If we account for the colored noise

$$S_{nc}(f) = 0.5\, N_0 N(f) \tag{10.5.1}$$

we have to replace $H_C(f)$ by $H_C(f)N^{-0.5}(f)$ and $H_R(f)$ by $H_R(f)N^{0.5}(f)$. The results are

$$\varepsilon_1 = 0.5\, N_0 \int_{f\in F} |D(f)|^2 \Big/ \sum_k |G_T(f + kR)H_C(f + kR)N^{-0.5}(f + kR)|^2\, df \tag{10.5.2}$$

$$\varepsilon_2 = 0.5\, N_0 \int_{f\in F} |D(f)|^2 \Big/ \Big( \sum_k |G_T(f + kR)H_C(f + kR)N^{-0.5}(f + kR)|^2 + N_0/(2\,\sigma_a^2 R) \Big)\, df \tag{10.5.3}$$

$$\varepsilon_3 = 0.5\, N_0 \left( \int_{f\in F} |D(f)N^{0.5}(f)/H_C(f)|df \right)^2 \Big/ E_T \tag{10.5.4}$$

$$\varepsilon_4 = 0.5\, N_0 \left( \int_{f\in F} |D(f)N^{0.5}(f)/H_C(f)|df \right)^2 \Big/ \left\{ E_T + N_0 \int_{f\in F} (N(f)/(2\,\sigma_a^2 R|H_C(f)|^2))\, df \right\} \tag{10.5.5}$$

## 10.6 PROBLEMS

10.2.1 Show that the systems in Fig. 10.1 and Fig. 10.2 are identical so far as the overall signal response and noise variance are concerned.

10.2.2 Assume that $G(f)$ is the raised cosine function ($R = 1/T$)

$$G(f) = T \cos^2 (0.5\, \pi f/R) u_{2R}(f + R)$$

Compute

$$G_\Sigma(f) = \sum_k G(f + kR)$$

10.2.3 Compute $D_\Sigma(f)$ for the duobinary and modified duobinary signals.

10.2.4 Show that (10.2.29) defines a generalized Nyquist interval.

10.2.5 Compute the generalised Nyquist interval in the sense of (10.2.29) if the channels are as in Fig. P10.2.5.

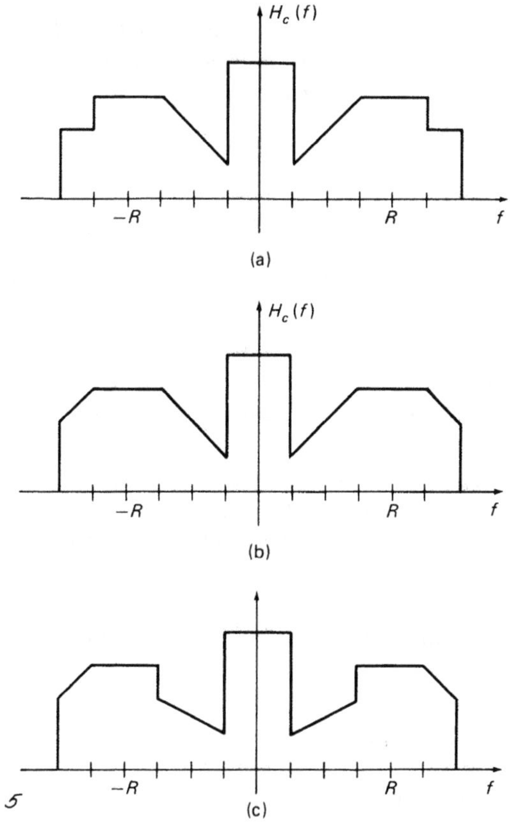


Fig. P10.2.5

10.3.1 Assume that

$$C(f)u_R(f + 0.5\ R) = jT \sin(2\ \pi f T)u_R(f + 0.5\ R)$$

Specify the tap values $\{C_i\}$ of a transversal filter that realizes this function.

10.3.2 Given the channels in Problem 10.2.5, in which frequency band will the signal energy be allocated if optimal transmitter filters are used?

10.3.3 Prove eq. (10.3.25).

10.4.1 Assume a system with binary symbols. The desired system has no intersymbol interference, i.e., $d_0 \neq 0$, $d_i = 0$, $i \neq 0$. Assume that the channel transfer function is

$$H_C(f) = \cos(0.5\,\pi f/R)u_{2R}(f + R)$$

and that the noise is white with power spectral density $0.5\,N_0$. Compute the mean square error, $\varepsilon$, and the ratio $\rho = d_0^2/\varepsilon$ for the following cases

a. The transmitter and receiver are

$$G_T(f) = (E_T T)^{0.5} H_C(f)$$

$$G_R(f) = u_{2R}(f + R)$$

b. The transmitter is as in (a), but the receiver is optimal with constraint (10.4.4).

c. The same as (b), but without constraint (10.4.4).

d. The transmitter and receiver are optimal with constraint (10.4.4).

e. The same as (d), but without constraint (10.4.4).

10.4.2 Write expressions for the optimal receiver, transmitter, and minimum mean square error if the noise is not white instead of eqs. (10.4.10), (10.4.11), (10.4.18), (10.4.19), (10.4.33), (10.4.35), (10.4.36), (10.4.53), (10.4.54), and (10.4.55).

10.4.3 Repeat problem 10.4.1 if the noise is nonwhite with power spectral density

$$S_{nC}(f) = 0.5\,N_0 H_C(f)$$

10.4.4 Prove eq. (10.4.30).

10.4.5 Prove eq. (10.4.42).

## 10.7 REFERENCES


10.1 M. R. Aaron and D. W. Tufts, "Intersymbol Interference and Error Probability," *IEEE Tr. Inf. Theory*, Vol. IT-12, January 1966, pp. 26–34.

10.2 D. W. Tufts, "Summary of Certain Intersymbol Interference Results," *IEEE Tr. Inf. Theory*, Vol. IT-10, October 1964, pp. 308–000.

10.3 D. A. George, "Matched Filters for Interfering Signals," *IEEE Tr. Inf. Theory*, Vol. IT-11, January 1965, pp. 153–154.

10.4 D. W. Tufts, "Nyquist's Problem—The Joint Optimisation of Transmitter and Receiver in Pulse Amplitude Modulation," *Proc. IEEE*, Vol. 51, March 1965, pp. 248–259.

10.5 J. W. Smith, "The Joint Optimisation of Transmitted Signal and Receiver Filter for Data Transmission Systems," *BSTJ*, Vol. 44, December 1965, pp. 2363–2392.

10.6 S. T. Berger and D. W. Tufts, "Optimum Pulse Amplitude Modulation. Part 1: Transmitter-Receiver Design and Bounds from Information Theory," *IEEE Tr. Inf. Theory*, Vol. IT-13, April 1967, pp. 196–208.

10.7 R. W. Chang and S. L. Feeny, "Hybrid Digital Transmission Systems—Part 1: Joint Optimization of Analog and Digital Repeaters," *BSTJ*, Vol. 47, October 1968, pp. 1663–1686.

10.8 D. Chan and R. W. Donaldson, "Optimum Pre- and Post-filtering of Sampled Signals with Application to Pulse Modulation and Data Compression Systems," *IEEE Tr. Comm. Tech.*, Vol. COM-19, April 1971, pp. 141–157.

10.9 B. Dejon and E. Hansler, "Optimal Multiplexing of Sampled Signals in Noisy Channels," *IEEE Tr. Inf. Theory*, Vol. IT-17, May 1971, pp. 257–262.

10.10 T. Ericson, "Structure of Optimum Receiving Filters in Data Transmission Systems," *IEEE Tr. Inf. Theory*, Vol. IT-17, May 1971, pp. 352–353.

10.11 T. Ericson, "Optimum Band Filters are Always Band Limited," *IEEE Tr. Inf. Theory*, Vol. IT-19, July 1973, pp. 570–572.

10.12 I. Korn, "Optimisation of Receiver and Transmitter for Partial Response Signals," *IEEE Proc.*, Vol. 129, pt. F, October 1982, pp. 347–351.

# 11 EQUALIZATION

## 11.1 INTRODUCTION

We showed in Chapter 10 that the optimal receiver is composed of a matched filter and a transversal filter (TF) with an infinite number of taps. A model of such a system is shown in Fig. 11.1. In this figure $\{a_i\}$ are independent symbols from the set $\mathring{A}_{\pm} = \{\pm 1, \pm 3, \ldots, \pm(M-1)\}$, and $g_T(t)$, $h_C(t)$, $h_F(t)$, and $h_E(t)$ are the impulse responses of transmitter, channel, fixed (matched), and equalizer (transversal) filters, respectively. If the transmitter and channel filters are known and the overall system response is given, we can compute the optimal receiver as suggested in Chapter 10. The results of Chapter 10 are, however, deficient and incomplete for two practical reasons. The first problem is the unrealizibility of a transversal filter with an infinite number of taps. When the number of taps is made finite, the separation of the receiver filter into a matched filter and TF is not any more optimal. We may instead decompose the receiver filter into a fixed filter (not necessarily a matched filter) and a TF and then optimize the finite number of tap gains.

The second reason is more fundamental. In Chapter 10 it was assumed that the channel characteristics are known. In practice the channel may not be known precisely or if known initially may change with time. For example, in a switched telephone system the link between any two subscribers is established via various lines; hence the channel varies from call to call. In a radio channel the signal may be subjected to frequency selective fading. This implies that the optimal receiver cannot be fixed, but must be allowed to vary according to the changing conditions in the channel. Because the signal at receiver output must remain as desired, independent of the channel variation, the receiver must incorporate a component that will undo these variations, namely, an *equalizer*. The TF with a finite number of taps with variable gains can serve as an equalizer. The equalizer is called *adaptive* if the tape gains adapt to the changes in the channel. The equalizer is called *automatic* if the adaptation does not require a manual intervention, but is rather performed by electronic means. The modern equalizer is both adaptive and automatic.

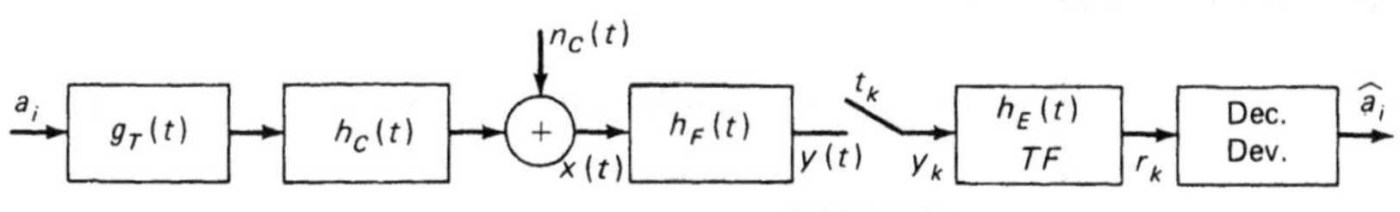


Fig. 11.1. Model of baseband system.

In Section 11.2 we define precisely the problem of optimization of the adaptive, automatic equalizer. In Section 11.3 we discuss various configurations of equalizers. In Section 11.4 we derive the optimal tap gains under a mean square error criterion. In Section 11.5 we derive the optimal tap gains under a zero-forcing criterion. In Section 11.6 we discuss nonlinear equalization. In Section 11.7 we present a summary, followed by problems in 11.8 and references in 11.9.

## 11.2 DEFINITION OF THE PROBLEM

Referring to Fig. 11.1, the output of the fixed receiver filter is

$$y(t) = \sum_i a_i g_F(t - iT) + n_F(t) \tag{11.2.1}$$

where

$$g_F(t) = g_C(t) * h_F(t) = g_T(t) * h_C(t) * h_F(t) \tag{11.2.2}$$

and $n_F(t)$ is zero-mean, Gaussian noise with power spectral density

$$S_{nF}(f) = S_{nC}(f)|H_F(f)|^2 \tag{11.2.3}$$

where $H_F(f)$ is the Fourier transform of $h_F(t)$. Samples are taken every $T$ seconds at times, $t_k = t_0 + kT$, so that the input to the equalizer is

$$y_k = \sum_k a_i g_{F,k-i} + n_{F,k} \tag{11.2.4}$$

where

$$y_k = y(t_k),\ g_{F,k} = g_F(t_k),\ n_{F,k} = n_F(t_k) \tag{11.2.5}$$

The equalizer has an impulse response

$$h_E(t) = \sum_n c_n \delta(t - nT) \tag{11.2.6}$$

where $\{c_n\}$ are the tap gains and $\delta(t)$ is the impulse function, so that the output of the equalizer is

$$r_k = \sum_n c_n y_{k-n} = \sum_i a_i g_{k-i} + n_k \tag{11.2.7}$$

where

$$g_k = \sum_n c_n g_{F,k-n},\ n_k = \sum_n c_n n_{F,k-n} \tag{11.2.8}$$

Identical equations can be obtained if the sampler in Fig. 11.1 is moved from the input to the output of the TF. If this is done, then $\{g_k\}$ and $\{n_k\}$ are samples of

$$g(t) = g_F(t) * h_E(t) = \sum_n c_n g_F(t - nT) \tag{11.2.9}$$

$$n(t) = n_F(t) * h_E(t) = \sum_n c_n n_F(t - nT) \tag{11.2.10}$$

$n(t)$ is zero-mean, Gaussian noise with variance

$$\sigma_n^2 = \int_{-\infty}^{\infty} S_{nC}(f)|H_F(f)H_E(f)|^2 \, df \tag{11.2.11}$$

where $H_E(f)$ is the Fourier transform of $h_E(t)$.

$$H_E(f) = \sum_n c_n \exp(-j\,2\,\pi f n T) \tag{11.2.12}$$

It was shown in Chapters 4 and 10 that

$$g_k = \int_{-0.5R}^{0.5R} G_\Sigma(f) \exp(j\,2\,\pi f t_k) \, df \tag{11.2.13}$$

where $R = 1/T$ and

$$G_\Sigma(f) = \sum_k G(f + kR) = \sum_k G_F(f + kR) H_E(f + kR) \tag{11.2.14}$$

In (11.2.14) $G(f)$ and $G_F(f)$ are the Fourier transforms of $g(t)$ and $g_F(t)$, respectively. Since $H_E(f)$ is a periodic function of $f$ with period $R$, we obtain

$$G_\Sigma(f) = H_E(f) G_{F\Sigma}(f) \tag{11.2.15}$$

where

$$G_{F\Sigma}(f) = \sum_k G_F(f + kR) \tag{11.2.16}$$

Let the desired response at time $t_k$ be

$$\hat{r}_k = \sum_i a_i d_{k-i} \tag{11.2.17}$$

(for example in a system with no intersymbol interference the desired response is $d_0 = 1$ and $d_i = 0, i \neq 0$, while in a duobinary system $d_0 = d_1 = 1$ and all other $d_i$ are 0), which can be realized by a system with transfer function

$$D(f) = \sum_i d_i \exp(-j2\pi fiT) \tag{11.2.18}$$

If there is no restriction on the number of taps in the equalizer, the desired response can be obtained by selecting

$$H_E(f) = G_\Sigma(f)/G_{F\Sigma}(f) = D(f)/G_{F\Sigma}(f) \tag{11.2.19}$$

i.e., by selecting the tap values

$$c_i = T \int_{-0.5R}^{0.5R} D(f)/G_{F\Sigma}(f) \exp(j2\pi fiT)\, df \tag{11.2.20}$$

If the number of taps is finite, (11.2.19) cannot be satisfied. The difference between the actual and desired response is

$$e_k = r_k - \hat{r}_k = \sum_i a_i(g_{k-i} - d_{k-i}) + n_k \tag{11.2.21}$$

The problem is to select $\{c_n\}$ so that the system is optimized in some sense. There are several criteria of optimization that can be used.

*Zero forcing* In this criterion, we ignore the noise term in (11.2.21) (this is usually justified in the telephone channel, where the signal-to-noise ratio is large and the intersymbol interference is the dominant factor), and we select the tap gains to minimize

$$D = \sum_i |g_i - d_i|/d_0 \tag{11.2.22}$$

This is proportional to the maximal error

$$|e_k|_{\max} = (M-1)\sum_i |g_i - d_i| \tag{11.2.23}$$

For example if we assume that $g_0 = d_0 = 1$ and $d_i \neq 0, i \neq 0$, then $D$ is proportional to the maximal value of intersymbol interference, and the eye opening, as shown in Fig. 11.2, is

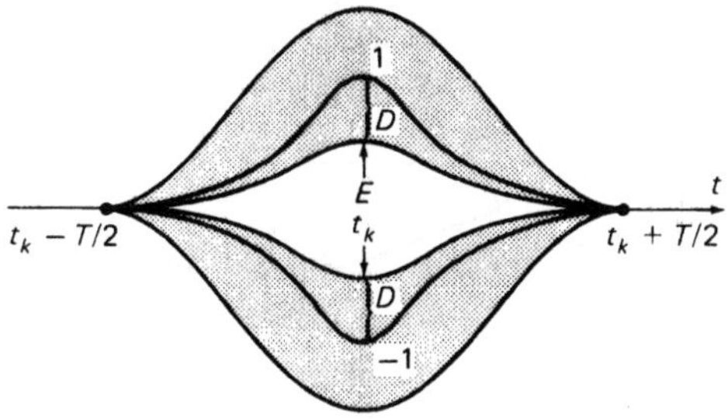


Fig. 11.2. Eye opening and zero-forcing criterion.

$$E = 2(1 - D) \tag{11.2.24}$$

Thus with this criterion we maximize the eye opening.

Mean square error The tap gains, $\{c_n\}$ are selected so that the mean square error

$$\varepsilon_k = \overline{e_k^2} = \sigma_a^2 \sum_i (g_i - d_i)^2 + \sigma_n^2 \tag{11.2.25}$$

is minimized. In (11.2.25) the bar denotes statistical expectation and

$$\sigma_a^2 = \overline{a_i^2} = (M^2 - 1)/3 \tag{11.2.26}$$

Note that in (11.2.25) $\varepsilon_k$ does not depend on $k$; therefore whenever it will be convenient we shall drop the index.

Probability of error The tap gains are selected to minimize the error probability. This criterion leads to nonlinear equations for the tap gains that are at present not very useful.

The zero-forcing criterion was analyzed first,[11.1–11.6] but most analytic results are avaliable for the mean square error criterion.[11.7–11.42] Although the mean square error and minimum error probability criteria are not identical, in many practical situations, they lead to similar performance.[11.38]

## 11.3 STRUCTURE OF EQUALIZERS

In 11.1 and 11.2 we identified the equalizer with the transversal filter. The equalizer may be improved by a more elaborate circuit in which the TF is put into a feedback configuration before or after the decision device. In this section we consider several structures for the equalizer.

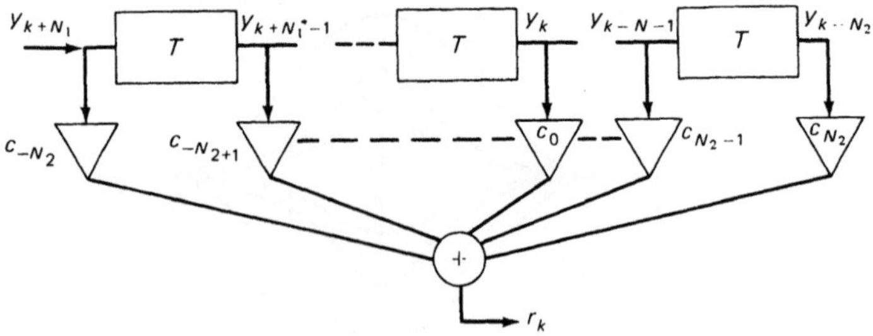


Fig. 11.3. Forward equalizer.

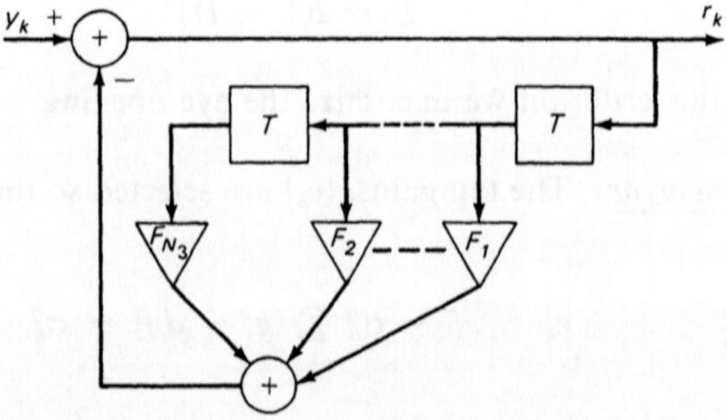


Fig. 11.4. Recursive equalizer.

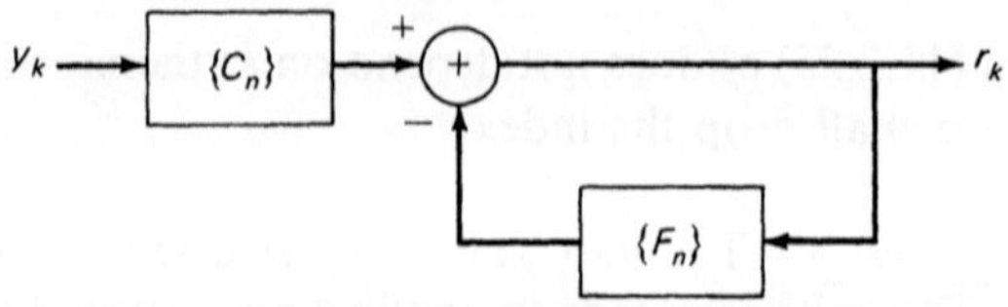


Fig. 11.5. Composite forward and recursive equalizer.

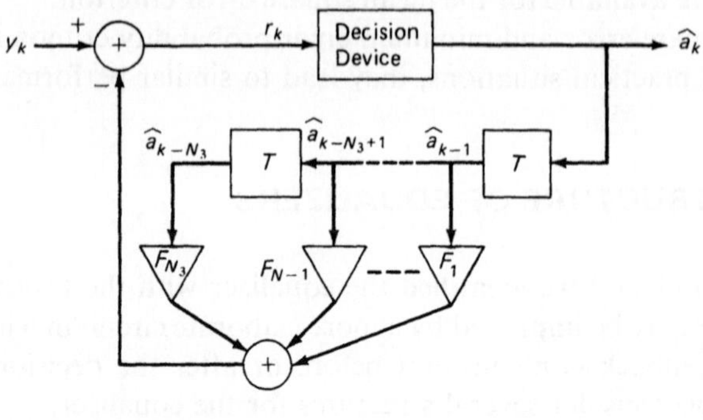


Fig. 11.6. Decision feedback equalizer.

### 11.3.1 Forward (nonrecursive) equalizer

This is the simplest equalizer, formed by the TF only. The equalizer is shown in Fig. 11.3. The relation between input and output is

$$r_k = \sum_{n=-N_1}^{N_2} c_n y_{k-n} \tag{11.3.1}$$

### 11.3.2 Feedback (recursive) equalizer

This equalizer is shown in Fig. 11.4. The tap gains are denoted here by $\{F_i\}$, $i = 1, \ldots, N_3$. The relation between input and output is

$$r_k = y_k - \sum_{i=1}^{N_3} F_i r_{k-i} \tag{11.3.2}$$

or

$$\sum_{i=0}^{N_3} F_i r_{k-i} = y_k \tag{11.3.3}$$

with $F_0 = 1$.

### 11.3.3 Composite forward and feedback equalizer

The equalizer is shown in Fig. 11.5. The relation between input and output is

$$\sum_{i=1}^{N_3} F_i r_{k-i} = \sum_{n=-N_1}^{N_2} c_n y_{k-n} \tag{11.3.4}$$

where the number of taps in the forward TF is $N_1 + N_2 + 1$ and in the feedback TF $N_3$.

### 11.3.4 Decision feedback equalizer

This equalizer is shown in Fig. 11.6. Note that the feedback is taken after the decision device. The relation between input and output is

$$r_k = y_k - \sum_{i=1}^{N_3} F_i \hat{a}_{k-i} \tag{11.3.5}$$

When we substitute (11.2.4) we obtain

$$
\begin{aligned}
r_k &= \sum_i a_{k-i} g_{F,i} + n_{F,k} - \sum_{i=1}^{N_3} \hat{a}_{k-i} F_i \\
&= a_k g_{F,0} + \sum_{i=1}^{N_3} (a_{k-i} - \hat{a}_{k-i}) g_{F,1} + \sum_{i=1}^{N_3} (g_{F,i} - F_i) \hat{a}_{k-i} \\
&\quad + \sum_{\substack{i<0 \\ i>N_3}} a_{k-i} g_{F,i} + n_{F,k}
\end{aligned}
\tag{11.3.6}
$$

If the system is such that $g_{F,i} = 0$ for $i < 0$ and $i > N_3$, and we select

$$F_i = g_{F,i},\ i = 1, \ldots, N_3 \tag{11.3.7}$$

then

$$r_k = a_k g_{F,0} + \sum_{i=1}^{N_3} (a_{k-i} - \hat{a}_{k-i}) g_{F,i} + n_{F,k} \tag{11.3.8}$$

If the probability of error is very small, we may assume that the last $N_3$ symbols have been received correctly, i.e.

$$\hat{a}_{k-i} = a_{k-i},\ i = 1, 2, \ldots, N_3 \tag{11.3.9}$$

Hence

$$r_k = a_k g_{F,0} + n_{F,k} \tag{11.3.10}$$

which means that all intersymbol interference from past symbols is eliminated. To eliminate intersymbol interference from future symbols we need a forward TF.

### 11.3.5 Composite forward and decision feedback equalizer

This equalizer is shown in Fig. 11.7. The relation between $r_k$ and $y_k$ is, using (11.2.7)

$$
\begin{aligned}
r_k &= \sum_{n=-N_1}^{N_2} c_n y_{k-n} - \sum_{i=1}^{N_3} F_i \hat{a}_{k-i} \\
&= \sum_i a_{k-i} g_i + n_k - \sum_{i=1}^{N_3} F_i \hat{a}_{k-i}
\end{aligned}
\tag{11.3.11}
$$

This equation can be reordered as in (11.3.6)

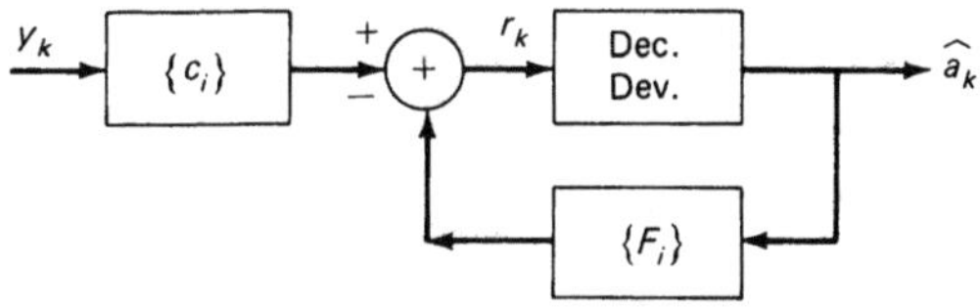


Fig. 11.7. Composite forward and decision feedback equalizer.

$$r_k = a_k g_0 + \sum_{i=1}^{N_3} (a_{k-i} - \hat{a}_{k-i}) g_i + \sum_{i=1}^{N_3} (g_i - F_i)\hat{a}_{k-i}$$

$$+ \sum_{\substack{i<0 \\ i>N_3}} a_{k-i} g_i + n_k \tag{11.3.12}$$

If we select

$$F_i = g_i,\ i = 1, 2, \ldots, N_3 \tag{11.3.13}$$

and the error probability is small, we obtain

$$r_k = a_k g_0 + \sum_{\substack{i<0 \\ i>N_3}} a_{k-i} g_i + n_k \tag{11.3.14}$$

The forward TF reduces the effect of the second term.

In analyzing this equalizer it is always assumed in the literature that the past $N_3$ decisions are correct; otherwise the problem is nonlinear. The nonlinearity is caused by the dependence of $\hat{a}_i$ on the error probability, which is a nonlinear function of tap gains.

Other equalizers, which will not be discussed here, are Kalman filter equalizers and their modification. The most popular equalizers in practice are the forward with or without the decision feedback TF.

## 11.4 MINIMUM MEAN SQUARE ERROR

In this section we optimize the equalizer composed of a forward and decision feedback TFs as in Fig. 11.7. The total number of tap gains in $N$, where

$$N = N_1 + N_2 + N_3 + 1 \tag{11.4.1}$$

$N_1 + N_2 + 1$ is the number of taps in the forward TF, and $N_3$ is the number in the feedback TF. First we present a formal solution to the optimal tap values and the minimal mean square error. Next we present an iterative algorithm and show that indeed this solution converges to the optimal solution. Finally, we present a practical solution.

### 11.4.1 Formal solution

Assuming that the last $N_3$ decisions are correct, the difference between the desired and actual response is

$$e_k = r_k - \hat{r}_k = \sum_{i=-N_1}^{N_2} c_i y_{k-i} - \sum_{i=1}^{N_3} F_i a_{k-i} - \sum_i d_i a_{k-i}$$
$$= \sum_i (g_i - d_i - F_i) a_{k-i} + n_k \tag{11.4.2}$$

The mean square error is independent of $k$ (for a fixed set of $\{c_i\}$, $\{F_i\}$), namely

$$\varepsilon = \overline{e_k^2} = \sigma_a^2 \sum_i (g_i - d_i - F_i)^2 + \sigma_n^2 \tag{11.4.3}$$

where $\sigma_n^2$ is given in (11.2.11) or, using (11.2.8)

$$\sigma_n^2 = \overline{n_k^2} = \sum_i \sum_j c_i c_j R_{nF}((i - j)T) \tag{11.4.4}$$

and

$$R_{nF}(\tau) = \int_{-\infty}^{\infty} S_{nC}(f) |H_F(f)|^2 \exp(j\, 2 f \pi \tau)\, df \tag{11.4.5}$$

It would be more convenient if we express (11.4.2) in the form of products of vectors. Thus, let

$$\mathbf{v}_c = (c_{-N_1}, \ldots c_0, \ldots, c_{N_2}) \tag{11.4.6}$$

$$\mathbf{v}_{a,k} = (a_{k-1}, a_{k-2}, \ldots, a_{k-N_3}) \tag{11.4.7}$$

$$\mathbf{v}_{y,k} = (y_{k+N_1}, \ldots y_k, \ldots, y_{k-N_2}) \tag{11.4.8}$$

$$\mathbf{v}_F = (F_1, F_2, \ldots, F_{N_3}) \tag{11.4.9}$$

and we rewrite (11.4.2)

$$e_k = \mathbf{v}_c \mathbf{v}^T{}_{y,k} - \mathbf{v}_F \mathbf{v}^T{}_{a,k} - \hat{r}_k \tag{11.4.10}$$

where $\mathbf{x}^T$ is the transpose of vector $\mathbf{x}$. We can further simplify if we combine the two tap vectors into a single one and the same for the inputs, namely, let

$$\mathbf{C} = (C_1, C_2, \ldots, C_N) = (\mathbf{v}_C, \mathbf{v}_F) \tag{11.4.11}$$

$$Y_k = (Y_1, Y_2, \ldots, Y_N) = (\mathbf{v}_{y,k}, -\mathbf{v}_{a,k}) \tag{11.4.12}$$

Thus

$$e_k = \mathbf{C}\mathbf{Y}_k^T - \hat{r}_k = \mathbf{Y}_k\mathbf{C}^T - \hat{r}_k \tag{11.4.13}$$

the mean square error is using the last equation

$$\varepsilon = \overline{e_k^2} = \overline{(\mathbf{C}\mathbf{Y}_k^T - \hat{r}_k)(\mathbf{Y}_k\mathbf{C}^T - \hat{r}_k)} \tag{11.4.14}$$

To minimize $\varepsilon$ we take the derivative of (11.4.14) with respect to the tap gains. Thus from (11.4.14) and (11.4.13)

$$\frac{\partial \varepsilon}{\partial C_j} = 2\, \overline{e_k \frac{\partial e_k}{\partial C_j}} = 2\, \overline{e_k Y_j} = 0 \tag{11.4.15}$$

This will indeed give the minimum value because

$$\frac{\partial^2 \varepsilon}{\partial C_j^2} = \overline{\frac{2\, \partial e_k}{\partial C_j} Y_j} = 2\, \overline{Y_j^2} > 0 \tag{11.4.16}$$

Let

$$\mathbf{V} = (\partial\varepsilon/C_1, \partial\varepsilon/\partial C_1, \ldots, \partial\varepsilon/\partial C_N) \tag{11.4.17}$$

be the gradient of $\varepsilon$. When we substitute (11.4.15) into (11.4.17), we obtain

$$\mathbf{V} = 2\, \overline{e_k Y_k} = 2\, \overline{(\mathbf{C}\mathbf{Y}_k^T - \hat{r}_k) Y_k} = 2(\mathbf{C}M_Y - \mathbf{v}_{rY}) \tag{11.4.18}$$

where $M_Y$ is the matrix

$$M_Y = \overline{\mathbf{Y}_k^T \mathbf{Y}_k} \tag{11.4.19}$$

and $\mathbf{v}_{rY}$ is the vector

$$\mathbf{v}_{rY} = \overline{\hat{r}_k \mathbf{Y}_k} \tag{11.4.20}$$

It can be shown (see Problem 11.4.1) that $M_Y$ is a symmetric matrix with real terms, i.e.

$$M_Y = M_Y^T \tag{11.4.21}$$

When we equate (11.4.18) to zero, we obtain the vector of optimal gains

$$\mathbf{C}_{\text{op}} M_Y - \mathbf{v}_{rY} = 0 \tag{11.4.22}$$

$$\mathbf{C}_{\text{op}} = \mathbf{v}_{rY} M_Y^{-1} \tag{11.4.23}$$

where $M_Y^{-1}$ is the inverse matrix of $M_Y$. When we substitute (11.4.23) into (11.4.14), we obtain the minimal mean square error

$$\varepsilon_{\min} = \overline{(\mathbf{C}_{\text{op}} \mathbf{Y}_k^T - \hat{r}_k)(\mathbf{Y}_k \mathbf{C}_{\text{op}}^T - \hat{r}_k)} = \overline{\hat{r}_k^2} - \mathbf{v}_{rY} M_Y^{-1} \mathbf{v}_{rY}^T \tag{11.4.24}$$

We define the vector of tap gain errors by

$$\mathbf{C}_e = \mathbf{C} - \mathbf{C}_{\text{op}} \tag{11.4.25}$$

Thus the gradient is, from (11.4.22) and (11.4.18)

$$\mathbf{V} = 2\,\mathbf{C}_e M_Y \tag{11.4.26}$$

and the mean square error is, from (11.4.14)

$$\begin{aligned}\varepsilon &= \overline{((\mathbf{C}_e + \mathbf{C}_{\text{op}})\mathbf{Y}_k^T - \hat{r}_k)(\mathbf{Y}_k(\mathbf{C}_e + \mathbf{C}_{\text{op}})^T - \hat{r}_k)} \\ &= \varepsilon_{\min} + \mathbf{C}_e M_Y \mathbf{C}_e^T\end{aligned} \tag{11.4.27}$$

### 11.4.2 Iterative solution

The optimal tap gains are given by eq. (11.4.23). This equation cannot be implemented in practice because of the large dimensions of the matrix and the complexity in the computation of its inverse. An alternative algorithm is the iterative solution

$$\mathbf{C}^{(i+1)} = \mathbf{C}^{(i)} - \delta \mathbf{V}(\mathbf{C}^{(i)}) \tag{11.4.28}$$

where $\mathbf{C}^{(i)}$ is the vector of tap gains at the $i$th iteration, $\mathbf{V}(\mathbf{C}^{(i)})$ is the gradient when the tap gain vector is $\mathbf{C}^{(i)}$, and $\delta$ is a constant ($\delta$ may in fact vary with iteration, but the analysis is simpler if we have it constant). The algorithm in (11.4.28) is not the only one available. This particular one in which the tap gains are proportional only to the gradient of the error is called the steepest descent method. This algorithm is illustrated in one dimension (for the $k$th component of $\mathbf{C}^{(i)}$) in Fig. 11.8. When we substitute

$$\mathbf{V}(\mathbf{C}^{(i)}) = 2(\mathbf{C}^{(i)} - \mathbf{C}_{\text{op}}) M_Y \tag{11.4.29}$$

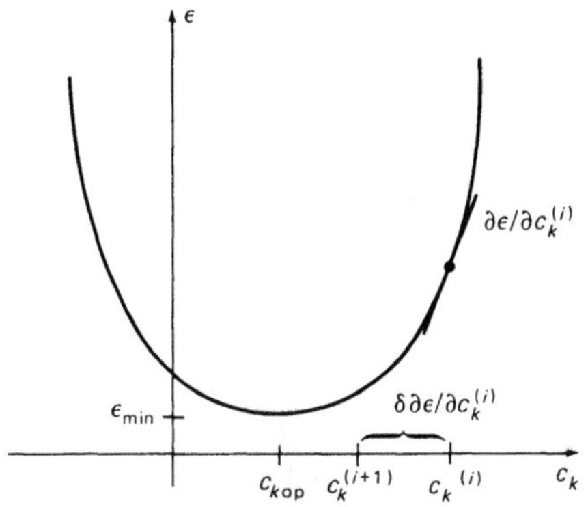


Fig. 11.8. Steepest descent algorithm.

into (11.4.28), we obtain

$$\mathbf{C}^{(i+1)} = \mathbf{C}^{(i)} - 2\,\delta(\mathbf{C}^{(i)} - \mathbf{C}_{\text{op}})M_Y \tag{11.4.30}$$

We subtract from both sides of (11.4.30) the vector $\mathbf{C}_{\text{op}}$, and using the notation

$$\mathbf{C}_i = \mathbf{C}^{(i)} - \mathbf{C}_{\text{op}} \tag{11.4.31}$$

we obtain

$$\mathbf{C}_{i+1} = \mathbf{C}_i(I - 2\,\delta M_Y) \tag{11.4.32}$$

where $I$ is the identity matrix of dimension $N \times N$. The mean square error at the $i$th iteration is from (11.4.27), adjusting for the notation in (11.4.31)

$$\varepsilon_i = \varepsilon_{\min} + \mathbf{C}_i M_Y \mathbf{C}_i^T \tag{11.4.33}$$

*Eigenvalues and eigenvectors*

Our intention is to prove that $\mathbf{C}_i \to 0$ and $\varepsilon_i \to \varepsilon_{\min}$. In doing that we shall investigate the *eigenvalues* and *eigenvectors* of $M_y$. $\lambda_k$ is an eigenvalue, and $\mathbf{v}_k$ is an eigenvector of $M_Y$ if

$$\mathbf{v}_k M_Y = \lambda_k \mathbf{v}_k \qquad k = 1, \ldots, N \tag{11.4.34}$$

The set of equations (11.4.34) can be combined into a single equation

$$M_v M_Y = \Lambda M_v \tag{11.4.35}$$

where $\Lambda$ is a diagonal matrix

$$\Lambda = \begin{pmatrix} \lambda_0 & 0 \, . \, 0 \, \ldots & 0 \\ 0 & \lambda_1 \, . & 0 \\ \vdots & & . \\ 0 \, . & . & 0 \; \lambda_{N-1} \end{pmatrix} \tag{11.4.36}$$

and $M_v$ is the matrix, whose rows are the eigenvectors

$$M_v = \begin{pmatrix} \mathbf{v}_1 \\ \mathbf{v}_2 \\ \vdots \\ \mathbf{v}_N \end{pmatrix} \tag{11.4.37}$$

Since the eigenvectors are orthogonal, i.e.

$$\mathbf{v}_i \mathbf{v}_j^T = \begin{cases} 1 & i = j \\ 0 & i \neq j \end{cases} \tag{11.4.38}$$

the product of $M_v$ and its transpose is

$$M_v M_v^T = I \tag{11.4.39}$$

Hence

$$M_v^T = M_v^{-1} \tag{11.4.40}$$

Applying (11.4.40) to (11.4.35), we obtain

$$M_v M_Y M_v^T = \Lambda \tag{11.4.41}$$

$$M_Y = M_v^T \, \Lambda \, M_v \tag{11.4.42}$$

Because $M_Y$ is a *positive definite matrix* (i.e., for any nonzero vector $\mathbf{x}$

$$\mathbf{x} M_Y \mathbf{x}^T = \overline{\mathbf{x}\mathbf{Y}_k^T \mathbf{Y}_k \mathbf{x}^T} = z^2 > 0$$

where $z = \mathbf{x} Y_k^T$) all eigenvalues are positive.

Let

$$M'_Y = I - 2\,\delta M_Y \tag{11.4.43}$$

We can see from (11.4.34) that $\{\mathbf{v}_k\}$ are also the eigenvectors of $M'_Y$; however the eigenvalues are

$$\lambda'_k = 1 - 2\,\delta\lambda_k \tag{11.4.44}$$

Let $\Lambda'$ be the diagonal matrix, similar to (11.4.36), but with entries $\lambda'_k$; then as in (11.4.41) and (11.4.42)

$$M_v M'_Y M_v^T = \Lambda' \tag{11.4.45}$$

$$M'_Y = M_v^T \Lambda' M_v \tag{11.4.46}$$

Convergence We substitute (11.4.43) and (11.4.46) into (11.4.32) and obtain

$$\mathbf{C}_{i+1} = \mathbf{C}_i M_v^T \Lambda' M_v \tag{11.4.47}$$

Similarly we substitute (11.4.42) into (11.4.33) and obtain

$$\varepsilon_i = \varepsilon_{\min} + \mathbf{C}_i M_v^T \Lambda M_v \mathbf{C}_i^T \tag{11.4.48}$$

At this stage it is convenient to define a modified vector of tap gain errors at the $i$th iteration

$$\mathbf{C}'_i = \mathbf{C}_i M_v^T \tag{11.4.49}$$

so that (11.4.47) after postmultiplying by $M_v^T$ is

$$\mathbf{C}'_{i+1} = \mathbf{C}'_i \Lambda' = \mathbf{C}'_0 (\Lambda')^i \tag{11.4.50}$$

where $\mathbf{C}'_0$ is the initial value of the modified tap gain error vector. $(\Lambda')^i$ is a diagonal matrix, the $k$th entry of which is

$$(\lambda'_k)^i = (1 - 2\,\delta\lambda_k)^i \tag{11.4.51}$$

Thus if

$$|\lambda'_k| < 1, \; k = 1, \ldots, N \tag{11.4.52}$$

$$\lim_{i\to\infty} \mathbf{C}'_{i+1} = \mathbf{C}'_0 \lim_{i\to\infty} (\Lambda')^i = 0 \tag{11.4.53}$$

which implies, from (11.4.49), that

$$\lim_{i\to\infty} \mathbf{C}_i = 0 \tag{11.4.54}$$

When we substitute (11.4.49) into (11.4.48), we obtain

$$\varepsilon_i = \varepsilon_{\min} + \mathbf{C}'_i \Lambda \mathbf{C}'^T_i = \varepsilon_{\min} + \mathbf{C}'_0 (\Lambda')^i \Lambda (\Lambda')^i \mathbf{C}'^T_0 \tag{11.4.55}$$

$(\Lambda')^i\Lambda(\Lambda')^i$ is also a diagonal matrix, the $k$th element of which is

$$(\lambda_k')^{2i}\lambda_k = (1 - 2\,\delta\lambda_k)^{2i}\lambda_k \qquad (11.4.56)$$

which also converges to zero for large $i$. Thus

$$\lim_{i\to\infty} \varepsilon_i = \varepsilon_{\min} \qquad (11.4.57)$$

*Settling time* Condition (11.4.52) implies that

$$|1 - 2\,\delta\lambda_k| < 1 \rightarrow 0 < \delta < 1/\lambda_k \qquad (11.4.58)$$

Let $\lambda_m$ and $\lambda_M$ be the minimal and maximal eigenvalues; then (11.4.58) is certainly satisfied if the constant $\delta$ is selected so that

$$0 \leqq \delta \leqq 1/\lambda_M \qquad (11.4.59)$$

However a more uniform convergence for all tap gains occurs if

$$\delta = 1/(\lambda_m + \lambda_M) \qquad (11.4.60)$$

The speed of convergence depends on the spread of the eigenvalues. If all eigenvalues are identical, with value $\lambda$, then by selecting

$$\delta = 0.5/\lambda \qquad (11.4.61)$$

convergence occurs in a single iteration. Because the eigenvalues are not identical, the tap gains will converge to their optimal values at different rates. Let $C'_{i,k}$ be the $k$th component of $\mathbf{C}'_i$. We obtain from (11.4.50)

$$C'_{i+1,k} = C'_{0,k}(1 - 2\,\delta\lambda_k)^i = C'_{0,k}\exp(-iT_I/\tau_k) \qquad (11.4.62)$$

where $T_I$ is the time interval between two successive iterations, and $\tau_k$ is a time constant

$$\tau_k = -T_I/\ln(1 - 2\,\delta\lambda_k) \qquad (11.4.63)$$

If we assume that $\delta\lambda_k \ll 1$, which is often satisfied in practice, (11.4.63) is simplified to

$$\tau_k = T_I/(2\,\delta\lambda_k) \qquad (11.4.64)$$

We may assume that after four time constants, the tap gains have been settled close to their optimal value; hence the settling time for the tap gain is

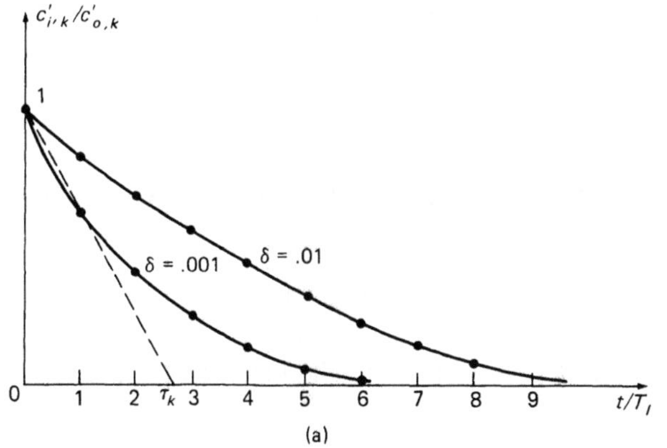


Fig. 11.9. Settling time.

$$T_k = 4\,\tau_k = 2\,T_l/(\delta\lambda_k) \qquad (11.4.65)$$

The average settling time is

$$T_{av} = \sum_{k=1}^{N} T_k/N = 2\,T_l/(\delta\lambda_{eq}) \qquad (11.4.66)$$

where

$$N/\lambda_{eq} = \sum_{k=1}^{N} 1/\lambda_k \qquad (11.4.67)$$

The settling time for the mean square error is, from (11.4.55) and (11.4.56), half the settling time for the tap gains. The settling time is illustrated in Fig. 11.9.

### 11.4.3 Practical solution

The solutions presented in Sections 11.4.1 and 11.4.2 are valid provided the gradient

$$\mathbf{V} = 2\,\overline{e_k Y_k} = 2\,\mathbf{C}_e M_Y \qquad (11.4.68)$$

or the gradient at the $i$th iteration

$$\mathbf{V}_i = 2\,\mathbf{C}_i M_Y \qquad (11.4.69)$$

are known precisely. In practice it is impossible to compute the statistical average in (11.4.68). Thus, instead of a true gradient, an estimate of the gradient $\hat{\mathbf{V}}_i$ is used. A convenient estimate of the gradient is, from (11.4.68), simply

$$\hat{\mathbf{V}}_i = 2\, e_i \mathbf{Y}_i \tag{11.4.70}$$

In this case the tap gains are updated every $T$ seconds, i.e., at the symbol rate, so that the iteration time is

$$T_I = T \tag{11.4.71}$$

A better estimate, which is closer to the true gradient, is

$$\hat{\mathbf{V}}_i = 2 \sum_{k=(i-1)K}^{iK} e_k \mathbf{Y}_k / K \tag{11.4.72}$$

The tap gains are updated here every $KT$ seconds, so that

$$T_I = KT \tag{11.4.73}$$

Fractional updating, in which the input to the equalizer is sampled at a rate greater than the symbol rate, so that $K$ samples are available during a $T_I = T$ interval, has also been considered in the literature; however we shall not discuss this method further.

Gradient noise Note that the estimate of the gradient is a random variable, the average of which is the true gradient. Thus the estimate is an *unbiased estimate.* Let

$$\boldsymbol{\eta}_i = \mathbf{V}_i - \hat{\mathbf{V}}_i \tag{11.4.74}$$

be the error in the gradient, or in other words the *gradient noise*. It is zero mean with covariance matrix

$$M_\eta = \overline{\boldsymbol{\eta}_i^T \boldsymbol{\eta}_i} \tag{11.4.75}$$

The tap upgrading algorithm is, instead of (11.4.28)

$$\mathbf{C}^{(i+1)} = \mathbf{C}^{(i)} - \delta \hat{\mathbf{V}}_i = \mathbf{C}^{(i)} - \delta \mathbf{V}_i + \delta \boldsymbol{\eta}_i \tag{11.4.76}$$

This is illustrated in the form of a block diagram in Fig. 11.10. We subtract from both sides of (11.4.76) the optimal vector, $\mathbf{C}_{\text{op}}$ and obtain, as in (11.4.32)

$$\mathbf{C}_{i+1} = \mathbf{C}_i M'_Y + \delta \boldsymbol{\eta}_i \tag{11.4.77}$$

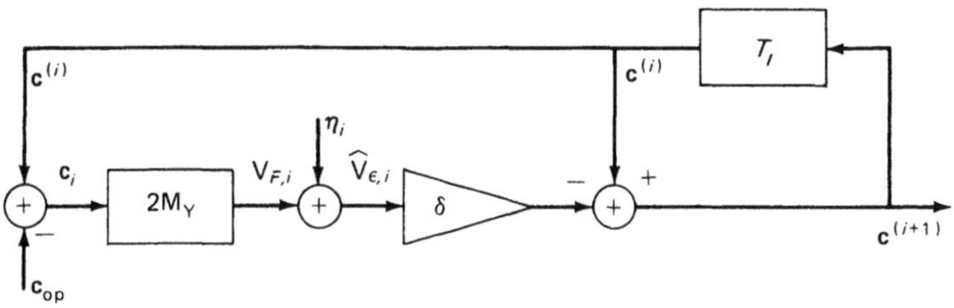


Fig. 11.10. Block diagram for algorithm with noisy gradient.

where we have also used (11.4.43). Because $\boldsymbol{\eta}_i$ is a random vector, the tap gains $\mathbf{C}^{(i)}$ and $\mathbf{C}_i$ are random, but their average value is the same as in the last section.

In the initial stages the deterministic component in (11.4.77) (the average value) is dominant; hence $\mathbf{C}_i$ will decrease exponentially with $i$. In the steady state, the random component is dominant, because even if $\mathbf{C}_i = 0$, at the next iteration

$$\mathbf{C}_{i+1} = \delta\boldsymbol{\eta}_i \tag{11.4.78}$$

will not be zero, but rather fluctuate around zero. In the steady state, the tap values are close to their optimal values

$$\mathbf{C}^{(i)} \simeq \mathbf{C}_{\text{op}} \tag{11.4.79}$$

hence the true gradient is close to zero, which means that the error $e_i$ and the input $\mathbf{Y}_i$ are approximately uncorrelated. Thus

$$\boldsymbol{\eta}_i \simeq -\hat{\mathbf{V}}_i = -2\, e_i\mathbf{Y}_i \tag{11.4.80}$$

where we have used (11.4.70). A theoretical justification for this assumption can be found in Ref. 11.39. We shall make the additional assumptions (which are justified by simulations) that $e_i^2$ is uncorrelated with the inputs $\{Y_1^2, Y_2^2, \ldots, Y_N^2\}$. Thus the covariance matrix of $\boldsymbol{\eta}_i$ is

$$M_\eta = \overline{\boldsymbol{\eta}_i^T\boldsymbol{\eta}_i} = 4\,\overline{e_i^2 Y_i^T Y_i} = 4\,\overline{e_i^2 M_Y} = 4\,\varepsilon_{\min} M_Y \tag{11.4.81}$$

where $\varepsilon_{\min}$ is the minimal mean square error when the true gradient is used. If we use in (11.4.80) the better gradient estimate of (11.4.72), the covariance matrix is

$$M_\eta = 4\,\varepsilon_{\min} M_Y/K \tag{11.4.82}$$

If we postmultiply (11.4.77) by $M_r^T$, we obtain, as in (11.4.50)

$$\mathbf{C}'_{i+1} = \mathbf{C}'_i\Lambda' + \delta\boldsymbol{\eta}'_i \tag{11.4.83}$$

where we have denoted

$$\boldsymbol{\eta}_i' = \boldsymbol{\eta}_i M_r^T \tag{11.4.84}$$

The covariance matrix of $\boldsymbol{\eta}_i'$ is, using (11.4.82) and (11.4.41)

$$M_\eta' = \overline{\boldsymbol{\eta}_i'^T \boldsymbol{\eta}_i'} = M_r \overline{\boldsymbol{\eta}_i^T \boldsymbol{\eta}_i} M_r^T = 4\,\varepsilon_{\min} M_r M_Y M_r^T / K = (4\,\varepsilon_{\min}/K)\Lambda \tag{11.4.85}$$

Thus the variance of $\eta_{i,k}'$, the $k$th component of $\boldsymbol{\eta}_i'$ is

$$\overline{(\eta_{i,k}')^2} = 4\,\varepsilon_{\min}\lambda_k/K \tag{11.4.86}$$

<u>*Tap gain variance*</u> The variance of $C_{i,k}'$, the $k$th component of $\mathbf{C}_i'$ is from (11.4.83)

$$\overline{(C_{i+1,k}')^2} = (\lambda_k')^2\overline{(C_{i,k}')^2} + \delta^2\overline{(\eta_{i,k}')^2} \tag{11.4.87}$$

which in steady state is not dependent on the iteration number. Thus (11.4.87) is simplified to

$$\overline{(C_k')^2} = \frac{4\,\delta^2\varepsilon_{\min}\lambda_k}{K(1-(\lambda_k')^2)} \tag{11.4.88}$$

where $C_k'$ is the $k$th component of $\mathbf{C}_i'$ in steady state. Applying (11.4.44), we obtain

$$\overline{(C_k')^2} = \delta\varepsilon_{\min}/\{K(1 - \delta\lambda_k)\} \tag{11.4.89}$$

If we assume that $\delta$ is such that

$$\delta\lambda_k \ll 1 \tag{11.4.90}$$

eq. (11.4.90) is further simplified to

$$\overline{(C_k')^2} = \delta\varepsilon_{\min}/K \tag{11.4.91}$$

<u>*Excess mean square error*</u> The mean square error is from (11.4.55)

$$\varepsilon_i = \varepsilon_{\min} + \mathbf{C}_i'\Lambda\mathbf{C}_i'^T = \varepsilon_{\min} + \sum_{k=1}^{N} \lambda_k (C_k')^2 \tag{11.4.92}$$

which is also a random variable, because $\{C_k'\}$ are random variables. The average value of $\varepsilon_i$ is in steady state not $\varepsilon_{\min}$, but contains an extra term

$$\varepsilon = \overline{\varepsilon_i} = \varepsilon_{\min} + \sum_{k=1}^{N} \overline{\lambda_k (C_k')^2} = \varepsilon_{\min} + (\delta\varepsilon_{\min}/K) \sum_{k=1}^{N} \lambda_k/(1 - \lambda_k)$$

$$= \varepsilon_{\min} + (\delta\varepsilon_{\min}/K) \sum_{k=1}^{N} \lambda_k \tag{11.4.93}$$

where we have used (11.4.89) and (11.4.91). The excess mean square error, caused by the gradient noise, is from (11.4.93)

$$\varepsilon_{\text{exc}} = \delta\varepsilon_{\min} N\lambda_{\text{av}}/K \tag{11.4.94}$$

where

$$\lambda_{\text{av}} = \sum_{k=1}^{N} \lambda_k/N \tag{11.4.95}$$

is the average eigenvalue. We thus see that the excess mean square error is proportional to the iteration step size, $\delta$, and to the number of taps $N$. However, $\varepsilon_{\min}$ is a decreasing (at least nonincreasing) function of $N$, as can be deduced from (11.4.29); thus the optimal $N$, which minimizes $\varepsilon_{\text{exc}}$, cannot be specified without the knowledge of $M_Y$ and $\mathbf{v}_{rY}$.

We can also relate the excess mean square error to the average settling time. When we substitute (11.4.64) into (11.4.95), we obtain

$$\lambda_{\text{av}} = T_I/(2\,\delta\tau_{\text{eq}}) \tag{11.4.96}$$

where

$$N/\tau_{\text{eq}} = \sum_{k=1}^{N} 1/\tau_k \tag{11.4.97}$$

It was stated in the previous section that the settling time for the mean square error is half the settling time for the tap gains. Thus

$$T_{\text{eq}} = 2\,\tau_{\text{eq}} \tag{11.4.98}$$

$$\delta\lambda_{\text{av}} = T_I/T_{\text{eq}} = KT/T_{\text{eq}} \tag{11.4.99}$$

Combining (11.4.99) and (11.4.94), the result is

$$\varepsilon_{\text{exc}} = \varepsilon_{\min}(T/T_{\text{eq}})N \tag{11.4.100}$$

Because $T_{\text{eq}}$ is an equivalent settling time, we see that the excess bandwidth is inversely proportional to the settling time.

In practice $\delta$ and $N$ are chosen so that

$$\delta N \lambda_{av}/K \leqq 0.1 \tag{11.4.101}$$

Hence

$$\varepsilon_{exc} \leqq \varepsilon_{min}/10 \tag{11.4.102}$$

Typical curves for the random nature of the mean square error are shown in Fig. 11.11.

*Relation to system response* We can relate $\varepsilon_{exc}$ to the system transfer function and to the power at the output of the fixed filter in the receiver. The trace of the matrix $M_Y$ is from (11.4.42)

$$\text{tr}(M_Y) = \sum_{k=1}^{N} (M_Y)_{kk} = \sum_{k=1}^{N} \lambda_k \sum_{j=1}^{N} v_{jk}^2 = \sum_{k=1}^{N} \lambda_k = N\lambda_{av} \tag{11.4.103}$$

where $(M_Y)_{kk}$ is the $k$th diagonal element of $M_Y$, and we have used the orthogonality condition of (11.4.39). On the other hand, from (11.4.19), (11.4.12), (11.4.8), and (11.4.7)

$$\text{tr}(M_Y) = \sum_{i=1}^{N} \overline{Y_i^2} = \sum_{j=-N_1}^{N_2} \overline{y_{kj}^2} + \sum_{j=1}^{N_3} \overline{a_{k-j}^2} = (N_1 + N_2 + 1)\overline{y_k^2} + N_3\sigma_a^2 \tag{11.4.104}$$

where, from (11.2.4)

$$\overline{y_k^2} = \sigma_a^2 \sum_i g_{F,i}^2 + \sigma_{nF}^2 \tag{11.4.105}$$

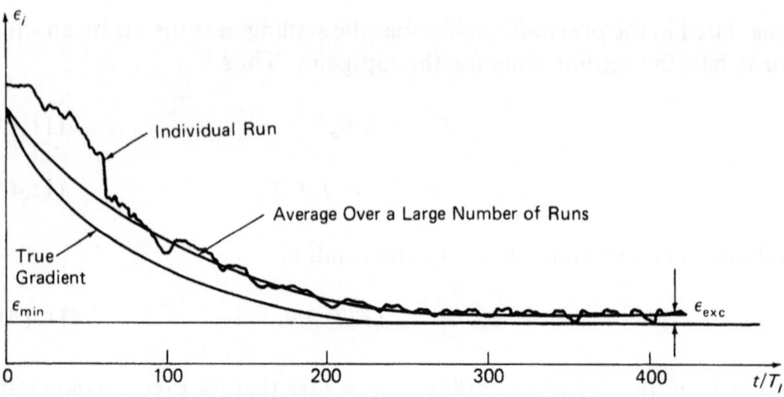


Fig. 11.11. Convergence of mean square error.

When we combine (11.4.103)–(11.4.105), the result is

$$\lambda_{av} = (\sigma_a^2/N)\left\{N_1 + N_2 + 1)\left(\sum_i g_{F,i}^2 + \sigma_{nF}^2/\sigma_a^2\right) + N_3\right\} \quad (11.4.106)$$

Since

$$y_k^2 = \int_{-\infty}^{\infty} S_y(f)\, df$$

$$= \int_{-\infty}^{\infty} (\sigma_a^2 R|G_F(f)|^2 + S_{nC}(f)|H_F|^2)\, df = P_Y \quad (11.4.107)$$

we also obtain

$$\lambda_{av} = (P_Y/N)(N_1 + N_2 + 1 + N_3\sigma_a^2/P_Y) \quad (11.4.108)$$

### 11.4.4 Automatic and adaptive equalization

According to (11.4.76) and (11.4.70), the tap values are upgraded according to

$$\mathbf{C}^{(i+1)} = \mathbf{C}^{(i)} - 2\,\delta e_i \mathbf{Y}_i \quad (11.4.109)$$

which from (11.4.12), (11.4.8), and (11.4.7) is tapwise

$$C_j^{(i-1)} = C_j^{(i)} - 2\,\delta e_i y_{i-j} \qquad j = -N_1, \ldots, 0, \ldots, N_2 \quad (11.4.110)$$

$$F_j^{(i+1)} = F_j^{(i)} + 2\delta e_i \hat{a}_{i-j} \qquad j = 1, \ldots, N_3 \quad (11.4.111)$$

Since

$$e_i = r_i - \hat{r}_i = r_i - \sum_k \hat{a}_{i-k} d_k \quad (11.4.112)$$

eqs. (11.4.110)–(11.4.112) can be mechanized as in Fig. 11.12.

In automatic equalization, a learning or training period may be established during which a known sequence of symbols is transmitted from transmitter to receiver. In the training mode the switches in Fig. 11.12 are connected to terminals $T$. During that period, which is longer than the settling time, the tap gains converge to their optimal position. When the switches are connected to terminal $A$, the equalizer is in the adaptive mode during which

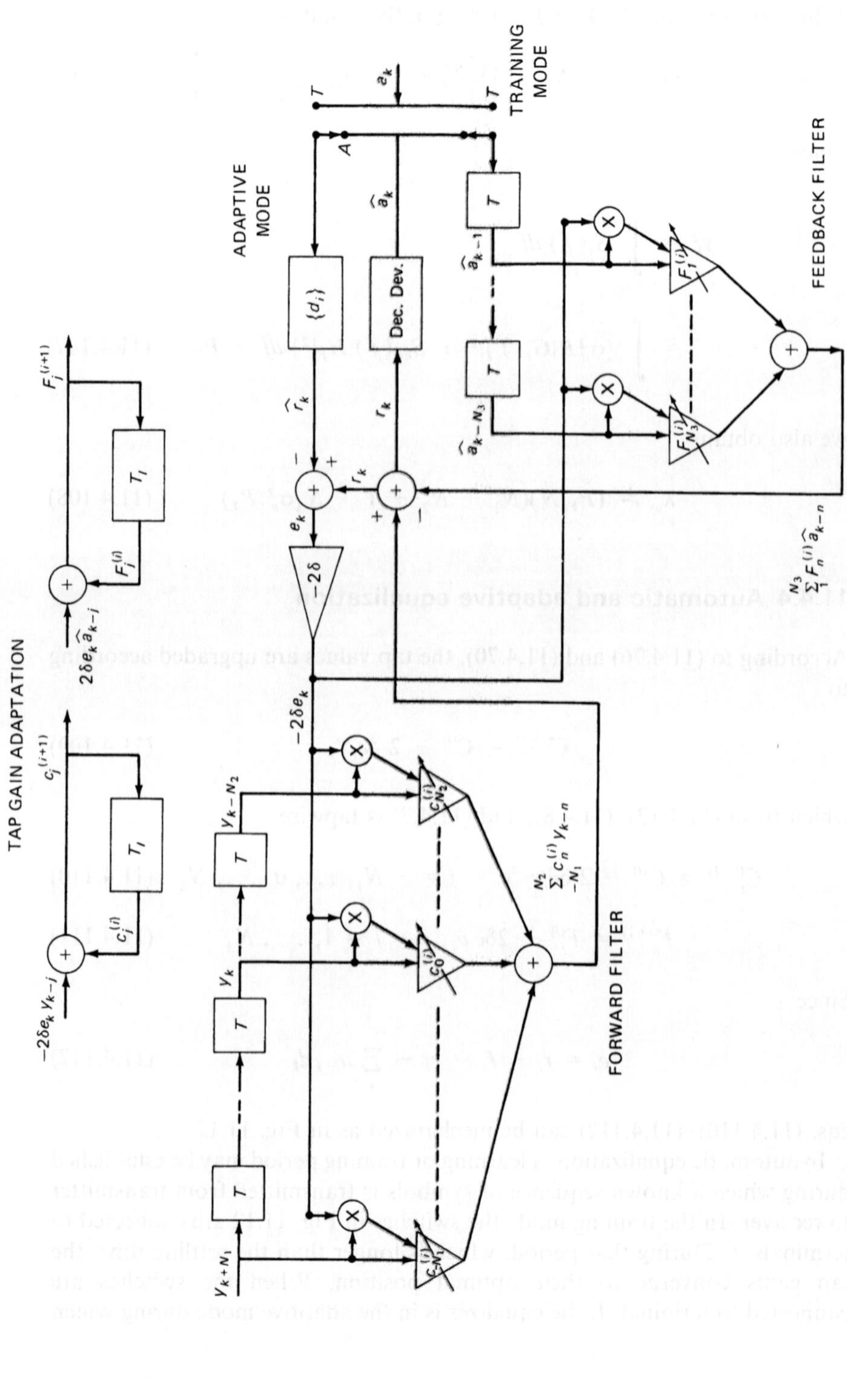


Fig. 11.12. Automatic, adaptive equalizer.

the decision symbols are used for continuing tap upgrading. In some practical systems the taps are upgraded only if $2\, e_i Y_{i-j}$ or more generally

$$\left| 2 \sum_{k=K_i}^{K_{i+1}} e_k Y_{k-j} \right| \tag{11.4.113}$$

exceeds a certain threshold. In (11.4.113) $K_i$ is a random integer, the instant when the $i$th upgrading was required. The realization is simplified if $e_i$, $y_i$, or both are quantized to their sign, because this eliminates multipliers. Various systems of this type have been studied in Refs. 11.26 and 11.27. They are presented in Table 11.1

**Table 11.1 Systems with practical tap upgrading**

| SYSTEM | TAP UPGRADING | NUMBER OF TAPS | | |
|---|---|---|---|---|
| | | $N_1$ | $N_2$ | $N_3$ |
| 1 | $e_i Y_{i-j}$ | 3 | 0 | $N-4$ |
| 2 | $Y_{i-j}$ sign $e_i$ | 3 | 0 | $N-4$ |
| 3 | $e_i Y_{i-j}$ | 3 | $N-4$ | 0 |
| 4 | $e_i$ sign $Y_{i-j}$ | 3 | $N-4$ | 0 |
| 5 | $Y_{i-j}$ sign $e_i$ | 3 | $N-4$ | 0 |
| 6 | sign $e_i$ sign $Y_{i-j}$ | 3 | $N-4$ | 0 |

The first two systems contain a composite forward and decision feedback equalizer. The last four contain only a forward equalizer. The settling time and mean square error as a function of number of tap gains, $N$, are shown in Fig. 11.13. In all these systems it was assumed that the system response, up to the equalizer, has samples

$$g_{F,0} = 1,\ g_{F,-1} = 0.3,\ g_{F,2} = 0.25$$

$$g_{F,-2} = g_{F,1} = g_{F,3} = 0.2,\ g_{F,-3} = 0.15$$

and the desired response is $\hat{r}_i = a_i$ (i.e., $d_0 = 1, d_i = 0, i \neq 0$). It was assumed that the step size is $\delta = 0.02$. It can be seen from this figure that if the error, $e_i$, is quantized, both the settling time and mean square error increase significantly. The signals $\{Y_i\}$ may be quantized (curve 4) without a great penalty in performance. We can also see that with unquantized values there is an optimal number of taps that minimize the mean square error, as predicted in the previous subsection.

Other simulations have been reported in Ref. 11.19 and are presented in Fig. 11.14. $g_F(t)$, which contains a telephone channel, is shown in Fig. 11.14(a). Here also the symbols are binary, with a bit rate of 7200 bps, and

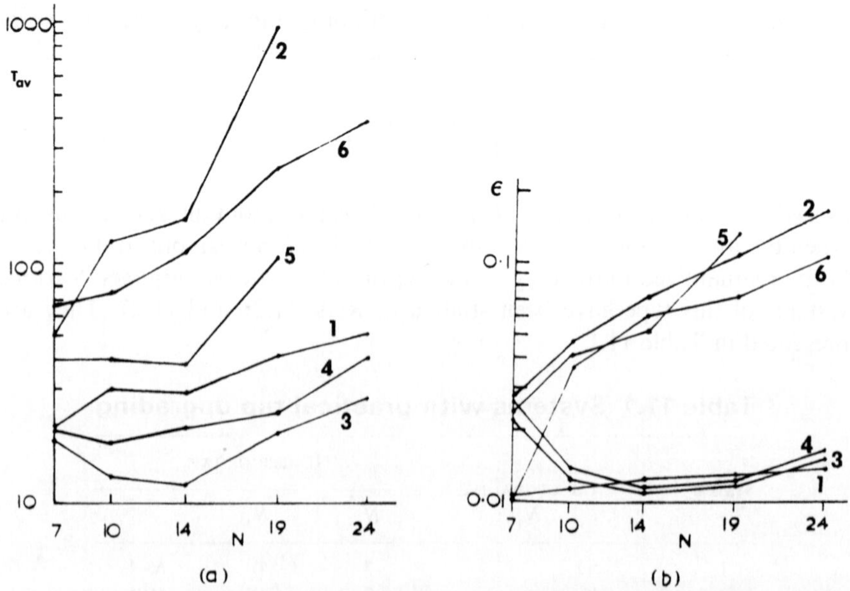


Fig. 11.13. (a) Settling time and (b) mean square error for systems defined in Table 11.1 as a function of number of tap gains (C. J. Macleod, E. Ciapala, and Z. J. Jelonek, "Study of Recursive Equalizers for Data Transmission with a Comparison of the Performance of Six Systems," *Proc. IEE*, Vol. 122, October 1975, pp. 1097–1104).

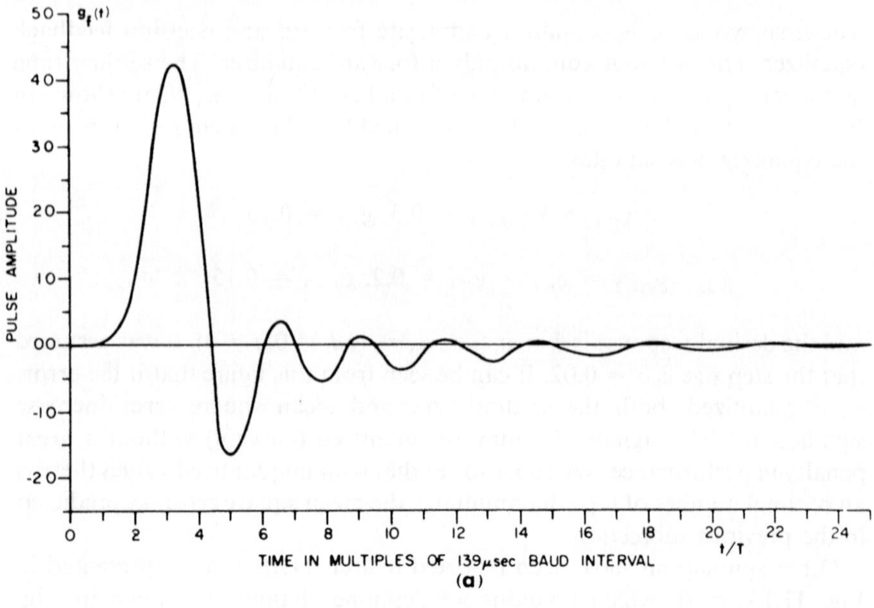


Fig. 11.14(a)

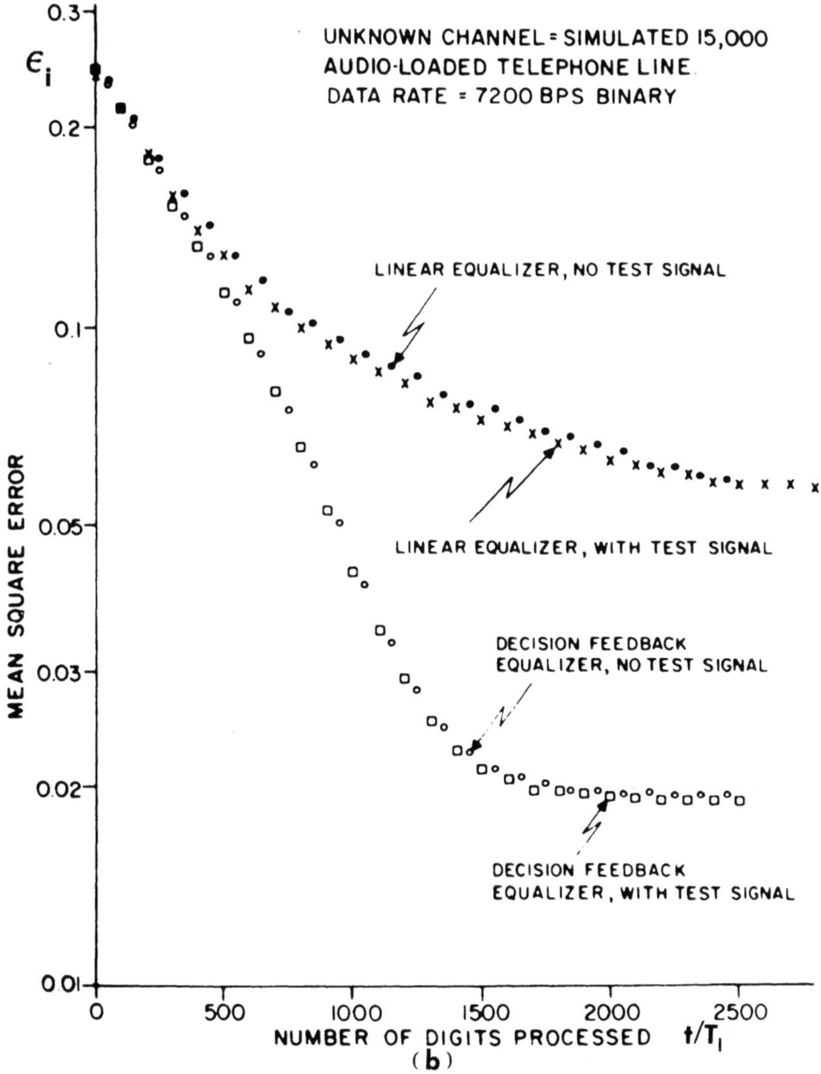


Fig. 11.14. (a) System impulse response and (b) mean square error for forward only or composite equalizer as a function of time D. A. George, R. R. Bowen, and J. R. Storey, "An Adaptive Decision Feedback Equalizer," *IEEE Tr. Comm. Tech.*, Vol. COM-19, June 1971, pp. 281–293. Copyright © 1971 IEEE).

the desired response is $r_i = a_i$. A forward equalizer with $N = 11$ taps was compared to a composite equalizer with various distributions of taps. The best selection was 4 forward taps and 7 feedback taps. It can be seen that the mean square error is almost the same whether a training sequence is used or not. The mean square error for the system with the composite equalizer is by an order of magnitude smaller then for the system with forward equalizer only.

### 11.4.5 Fast adaptive algorithm

We have already noted in Section 11.4.2 that if all eigenvalues are equal we can achieve convergence in a single step by selecting

$$\delta = 0.5/\lambda \tag{11.4.114}$$

The settling time depends on the difference between the largest and smallest eigenvalues $\lambda_M - \lambda_m$, and the settling time is achieved in a single step if the difference is zero. The idea of reducing the settling time is related to a reduction of the spread of eigenvalues. Thus, let us use instead of (11.4.28) the algorithm

$$\mathbf{C}^{(i+1)} = \mathbf{C}^{(i)} - \delta M_Q \mathbf{V}_i \tag{11.4.115}$$

Hence

$$\mathbf{C}_{i+1} = \mathbf{C}_i(I - 2\,\delta M_Q M_Y) \tag{11.4.116}$$

where $M_Q$ is a matrix. Let

$$M'_Q = I - 2\,\delta M_Q M_Y \tag{11.4.117}$$

If $M_Y$ is known we can select

$$M_Q = M_Y^{-1} \tag{11.4.118}$$

and all eigenvalues of $M'_Q$ are identical. If $M_Y$ is not known exactly, an estimated $\hat{M}_Y$ can be obtained from $L$ measurements of the system response, $\{M_{Yj}\}$ (for example, the telephone channels have a typical characteristic)

$$\hat{M}_Y = \sum_{j=1}^{L} M_{Yj}/L \tag{11.4.119}$$

If we take

$$M_Q = \hat{M}_Y^{-1} \tag{11.4.120}$$

we obtain

$$M'_Q = I - 2\,\delta \hat{M}_Y^{-1} M_Y \tag{11.4.121}$$

the eigenvalues of which are less spread than the eigenvalues of $M'_Y = 1 - 2\,\delta M_Y$. This particular method was suggested in Ref. 11.25. Another suggestion was to take

$$M_Q = M_d^{-1} \tag{11.4.122}$$

where $M_d$ is similar to $M_Y$, but with $\{g_{F,i}\}$ replaced by the desired response $\{d_i\}$, i.e., it is assumed that

$$y_k = \sum_i a_i d_{k-i} \tag{11.4.123}$$

instead of eq. (11.2.4).

Another fast training algorithm was proposed in Ref. 11.22. There the input to the equalizer is not $v_{y,k}$, but rather

$$\mathbf{v}'_{y,k} = M_p \mathbf{v}_{y,k} \tag{11.4.124}$$

so that

$$r_k = \mathbf{v}_C M_P^T \mathbf{v}'^T_{y,k} \tag{11.4.125}$$

where $M_P$ is a proper matrix. Instead of the matrix $M'_Y$, we have the matrix

$$M'_P = I - \delta M_P^T M_Y M_P \tag{11.4.126}$$

and $M'_P$ is selected so that

$$M_P^T M_Y M_P = I \tag{11.4.127}$$

Here again if $M_Y$ is unknown, an estimate of $M_Y$, $\hat{M}_Y$ is substituted into (11.4.127). An example is given in Ref. 11.22, in which the settling time was reduced dramatically.

Two other methods are proposed in Ref. 11.28: the conjugate gradient method, and the Fletcher-Powell method, which is identical to the method of Ref. 11.25. The general algorithm is

$$\mathbf{C}^{(i+1)} = \mathbf{C}^{(i)} + \delta \mathbf{S}^{(i)} \tag{11.4.128}$$

If

$$\mathbf{S}^{(i)} = -V_i \tag{11.4.129}$$

we have the steepest descent method, which was discussed at length up to this point. In the conjugate gradient method

$$\mathbf{S}^{(i)} = -\mathbf{V}_i + \beta \mathbf{S}^{(i-1)},\ \mathbf{S}^{(0)} = -\mathbf{V}_0 \tag{11.4.130}$$

where $\beta$ is a constant. With this method the settling time does not exceed $N$ iteration times. A generalization of (11.4.130) is

$$\mathbf{S}^{(i)} = -\mathbf{V}_i + \beta_1 \mathbf{S}^{(i-1)} + \beta_2 \mathbf{S}^{(i-2)} \tag{11.4.131}$$

where $\beta_1$, $\beta_2$ are constants. An equalizer with a short settling time and cyclic tap updating is described in Ref. 11.29. Additional algorithms (for example, with automatically adjustable steps, $\delta$) can be found in Refs. 11.31 and 11.32.

### 11.4.6 Equalization of passband systems

Up til now we have considered the equalization of a baseband (ASK) system. Because of the equivalence of baseband and bandpass systems, all results are applicable without change to ASK passband systems. Equalization of a QASK passband system, which is equivalent to a complex baseband system, requires complex tap gain values, or in fact two equalizers, one in the inphase path and the second in the quadrature phase path. Passband equalization is discussed in depth in Refs. 11.28 and 11.33–11.37.

## 11.5 ZERO-FORCING EQUALIZATION

In zero-forcing equalization the tap gains are selected to minimize the distortion

$$D = D(\mathbf{v}_C) = \sum_k |g_k - d_k|/d_0 \tag{11.5.1}$$

where from (11.2.8) and (11.4.6)

$$g_k = \mathbf{v}_C \mathbf{g}_{F,k}^T \tag{11.5.2}$$

$$\mathbf{g}_{F,k} = (g_{F,k+N_1}, \ldots, g_{F,k}, \ldots, g_{F,k-N_2}) \tag{11.5.3}$$

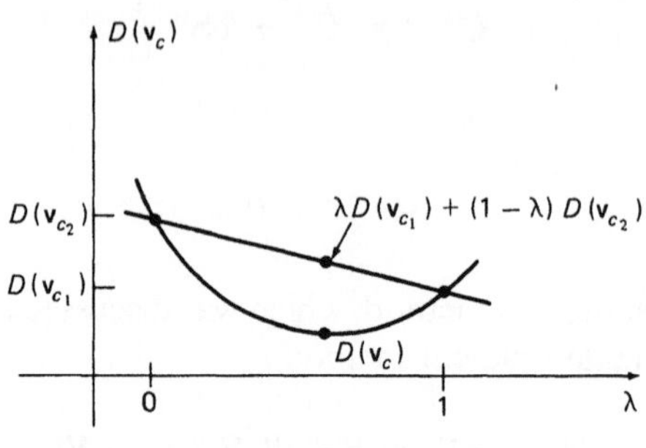


Fig. 11.15. Convex function.

Note that here we assume that the equalizer is composed of a forward transversal filter only. We shall show that $D(\mathbf{v}_C)$ has a unique minimum so long as $\sum_i |g_{F,i}| \leqq 2g_{F,0}$, i.e., the eye is opened before equalization. The optimal tap gains are such that $g_k = d_k$ for $k = -N_1, \ldots, -1, 0, 1, \ldots N_2$. If the desired response is $d_0 \neq 0$, $d_k = 0$, $k \neq 0$, the optimal tap gains force zero values for $g_k$, $k = -N_1, \ldots, -1, 1, \ldots, N_2$. For this reason the criterion is called *zero-forcing equalization.* To prove this statement we need three theorems.

*Theorem 1* $D(\mathbf{v}_C)$ is a convex function of $\mathbf{v}_C$.

*Proof*
We have to prove that if

$$\mathbf{v}_C = \lambda \mathbf{v}_{C1} + (1 - \lambda)\mathbf{v}_{C2},\ 0 \leqq \lambda \leqq 1 \tag{11.5.4}$$

then

$$D(\mathbf{v}_C) \leqq \lambda D(\mathbf{v}_{C1}) + (1 - \lambda) D(\mathbf{v}_{C2}) \tag{11.5.5}$$

where $\mathbf{v}_{C1}$, $\mathbf{v}_{C2}$ are two arbitrary vectors of tap gains. A convex function in one dimension is illustrated in Fig. 11.15.

We substitute (11.5.4) into (11.5.1) and obtain

$$\begin{aligned} D(\mathbf{v}_C) &= \sum_k |(\lambda \mathbf{v}_{C1} + (1 - \lambda)\mathbf{v}_{C2})\mathbf{g}_{F,k}^T - d_k|/d_0 \\ &= \sum_k |\lambda(\mathbf{v}_{C1}\mathbf{g}_{F,k}^T - d_k) + (1 - \lambda)(\mathbf{v}_{C2}\mathbf{g}_{F,k}^T - d_k)|/d_0 \\ &\leqq \lambda \sum_k (\mathbf{v}_{C1}\mathbf{g}_{F,k}^T - d_k)/d_0 + (1 - \lambda) \sum_k (\mathbf{v}_{C2}\mathbf{g}_{F,k}^T - d_k)/d_0 \\ &= \lambda D(\mathbf{v}_{C1}) + (1 - \lambda) D(\mathbf{v}_{C2}) \end{aligned}$$

*Conclusions*: If there is a minimum, the minimum is unique.

*Theorem 2* $D(\mathbf{v}_C)$ is minimum if $g_{k_j} = d_{k_j}$ for a set of $N = N_1 + N_2 + 1$ indices $\{k_1, k_2, \ldots, k_N\}$.

*Proof*
Since $|x| = x \text{ sign } x$, we can rewrite (11.5.1)

$$\begin{aligned} D(\mathbf{v}_C) &= \sum_k (\mathbf{v}_C \mathbf{g}_{F,k}^T - d_k) \text{ sign } (g_k - d_k)/d_0 \\ &= \mathbf{v}_C \sum_k \mathbf{g}_{F,k}^T \text{ sign } (g_k - d_k)/d_0 - \sum_k d_k \text{ sign } (g_k - d_k)/d_0 \\ &= \sum_{n=-N_1}^{N_2} c_n b_n - w \end{aligned}$$

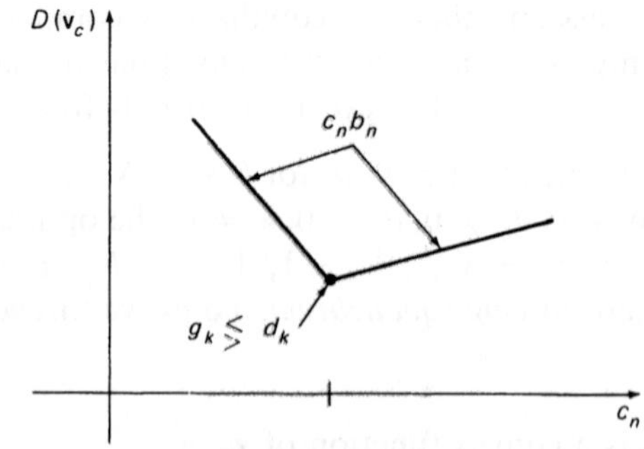


Fig. 11.16. Piecewise linear function with break point.

where

$$b_n = \sum_k g_{F,k-n} \text{ sign } (g_k - d_k)/d_0$$

$$w = \sum_k d_k \text{ sign } (g_k - d_k)/d_0$$

The coefficient $b_n$ does not depend on $\{c_n\}$ so long as $\{g_k - d_k\}$ do not change their signs. Whenever this happens there may be a jump in the value of $b_n$. Therefore $D(\mathbf{v}_C)$ is a piecewise linear function of $\{c_n\}$ with break points whenever one of the terms $\{g_k - d_k\}$ changes sign. This is illustrated in one dimension in Fig. 11.16. The minimum can occur only at a break point. With $N$ tap gains there can only be $N$ break points $\{k_1, k_2, \ldots, k_N\}$.

*Theorem 3* If

$$\sum_{k \neq 0} |g_{F,k}| < g_{F,0} \tag{11.5.6}$$

then $D(\mathbf{v}_C)$ is minimum for

$$g_k = d_k \qquad k = -N_1, \ldots, 0, 1, \ldots, N_2 \tag{11.5.7}$$

*Proof*
Assume that $\mathbf{v}_C$ is such that $D(\mathbf{v}_C)$ is minimum and for some $n_j \in \{-N_1, \ldots, 0, 1, \ldots, N_2\}$, $g_{nj} \neq d_{nj}$. We shall show that this is impossible. In fact, instead of $\mathbf{v}_C$, we propose $\mathbf{v}_C^*$ such that

$$c_n^* = \begin{cases} c_n & n \neq n_j \\ c_{nj} - \delta \text{ sign}(g_{nj} - d_{nj}) & n = n_j \end{cases}$$

Thus

$$g_k^* - d_k = v_c^* \mathbf{g}_{F,k}^T - d_k = \mathbf{v}_C g_{F,k}^T - d_k - \delta g_{F,k-nj} \operatorname{sign}(g_{nj} - d_{nj})$$
$$= g_k - d_k - \delta g_{F,k-nj} \operatorname{sign}(g_{nj} - d_{nj}) \quad (11.5.8)$$

If $k \neq n_j$, we obtain

$$|g_k^* - d_k| \leqq |g_k - d_k| + \delta |g_{F,k-nj}|$$

while if $k = n_j$, we obtain

$$|g_{nj}^* - d_{nj}| \leqq (|g_{nj} - d_{nj}| - \delta g_{F,0}) \operatorname{sign}(g_{nj} - d_{nj})$$

If we select $\delta$ so that

$$0 < \delta < |g_{nj} - d_{nj}|/g_{F,0}$$

we obtain

$$|g_{nj}^* - d_{nj}| \leqq |g_{nj} - d_{nj}| - \delta g_{F,0} \quad (11.5.9)$$

We substitute (11.5.8) and (11.5.9) into (11.5.1) and obtain

$$D(\mathbf{v}_C^*) = \sum_k |g_k^* - d_k|/d_0 \leqq \sum_k |g_k - d_k|/d_0$$
$$+ \delta\left(\sum_{k \neq nj} |g_{F,k-nj}| - g_{F,0}\right) \Big/ d_0$$
$$= D(\mathbf{v}_C) + \delta\left(\sum_{k \neq 0} |g_{F,k}| - g_{F,0}\right) \Big/ d_0$$

Thus so long as

$$\sum_k |g_{F,k}| < 2\, g_{F,0}$$

$$D(\mathbf{v}_C^*) < D(\mathbf{v}_C)$$

and the assumption that $D(\mathbf{v}_C)$ was minimum is contradicted.

*Optimal tap values* We thus conclude that the optimal $\mathbf{v}_C$ satisfies the set of equations

$$\mathbf{v}_{Cop} \mathbf{g}_{F,k}^T = d_k, \; k = -N_1, \ldots, 0, 1, \ldots, -N_2 \quad (11.5.10)$$

and the minimum distortion is

$$D_{\min} = D(\mathbf{v}_{Cop}) = \sum_{\substack{k<-N_1 \\ k>N_2}} |\mathbf{v}_{Cop}\mathbf{g}_{F,k}^T - d_k|/d_0 \tag{11.5.11}$$

Let $M_F$ be the matrix whose columns are the vectors $\mathbf{g}_{F,-N1}, \ldots, \mathbf{g}_{F,N2}$, i.e.

$$M_F = (\mathbf{g}_{F,-\mathrm{N1}}^T, \ldots, \mathbf{g}_{F,0}^T, \ldots, \mathbf{g}_{F,N2}^T) \tag{11.5.12}$$

and let $\mathbf{d}$ be the vector

$$\mathbf{d} = (d_{-N1}, \ldots, d_0, \ldots, d_{N2}) \tag{11.5.13}$$

When we substitute (11.5.12) and (11.5.13) into (11.5.10), the result is

$$\mathbf{v}_{Cop} M_F = \mathbf{d} \tag{11.5.14}$$

Hence

$$\mathbf{v}_{Cop} = \mathbf{d} M_F^{-1} \tag{11.5.15}$$

<u>*Iterative solution*</u> Equation (11.5.14) can be solved using iteration

$$\mathbf{v}_C^{(i+1)} = \mathbf{v}_C^{(i)} - \delta \mathbf{V}_i \tag{11.5.16}$$

where $\delta$ is the step size, and $\mathbf{V}_i$ is the gradient

$$\mathbf{V}_i = (\partial D_i/\partial c_{-N1}^{(i)}, \ldots, \partial D_i/\partial c_0^{(i)}, \ldots, \partial D_i/\partial c_{N2}^{(i)}) \tag{11.5.17}$$

and

$$D_i = D(\mathbf{v}_C^{(i)}) \tag{11.5.18}$$

The $n$th component of the gradient is

$$\begin{aligned} \partial D_i/\partial c_n^{(i)} &= d_0^{-1} \sum_k \partial\{(g_k^{(i)} - d_k) \operatorname{sign}(g_k^{(i)} - d_k)\}/\partial c_n^{(i)} \\ &= d_0^{-1} \sum_k \operatorname{sign}(g_k^{(i)} - d_k)\partial g_k^{(i)}/\partial c_n^{(i)} \\ &= \sum_k g_{F,k-n} \operatorname{sign}(g_k^{(i)} - d_k)/d_0 \end{aligned} \tag{11.5.19}$$

The terms

$$(g_k^{(i)} - d_k)\partial \operatorname{sign}(g_k^{(i)} - d_k)/\partial c_n^{(i)}$$

are missing in (11.5.19) because

$$x \frac{d \operatorname{sign} x}{dx} = 0 \tag{11.5.20}$$

If we assume that (11.5.6) is satisfied, we can approximate (11.5.19) by its dominant term, namely

$$\partial \hat{D}_i / \partial c_n^{(i)} = g_{F,0} \operatorname{sign} (g_n^{(i)} - d_n)/d_0 \tag{11.5.21}$$

The iterative solution (11.5.16) will converge to the optimal value because, from (11.5.16) and (11.5.21)

$$\begin{aligned} g_k^{(i+1)} - d_k &= \sum_{n=-N_1}^{N_2} c_n^{(i+1)} g_{F,k-n} - d_k = \sum_{n=-N_1}^{N_2} c_n^{(i)} g_{F,k-n} - d_k \\ &\quad - (\delta g_{F,0}/d_0) \sum_{n=-N_1}^{N_2} g_{F,k-n} \operatorname{sign} (g_n^{(i)} - d_n) \\ &= g_k^{(i)} - d_k - (\delta g_{F,0}^2/d_0) \operatorname{sign} (g_k^{(i)} - d_k) \\ &\quad - (\delta g_{F,0}/d_0) \sum_{\substack{n=-N_1 \\ n \neq k}}^{N_2} g_{F,k-n} \operatorname{sign} (g_n^{(i)} - d_n) \\ &= (|g_k^{(i)} - d_k| - \delta g_{F,0}^2/d_0) \operatorname{sign} (g_k^{(i)} - d_k) \\ &\quad - (\delta g_{F,0}/d_0) \sum_{\substack{n=-N_1 \\ n \neq k}}^{N_2} g_{F,k-n} \operatorname{sign} (g_n^{(i)} - d_n) \end{aligned} \tag{11.5.22}$$

Taking the absolute value

$$\begin{aligned} |g_k^{(i+1)} - d_k| &\leqq \big| |g_k^{(i)} - d_k| - \delta g_{F,0}^2/d_0 \big| + (\delta g_{F,0}/d_0) \sum_{\substack{n=-N_1 \\ n \neq 0}}^{N_2} |g_{F,n}| \\ &\leqq \big| |g_k^{(i)} - d_k| - \delta g_{F,0}^2/d_0 \big| + \delta g_{F,0}^2/d_0 \end{aligned} \tag{11.5.23}$$

If we select

$$\delta \leqq |g_k^{(i)} - d_k| d_0 / g_{F,0}^2 \tag{11.5.24}$$

we obtain

$$|g_k^{(i+1)} - d_k| \leqq |g_k^{(i)} - d_k| \tag{11.5.25}$$

Hence

$$D_{i+1} \leqq D_i \tag{11.5.26}$$

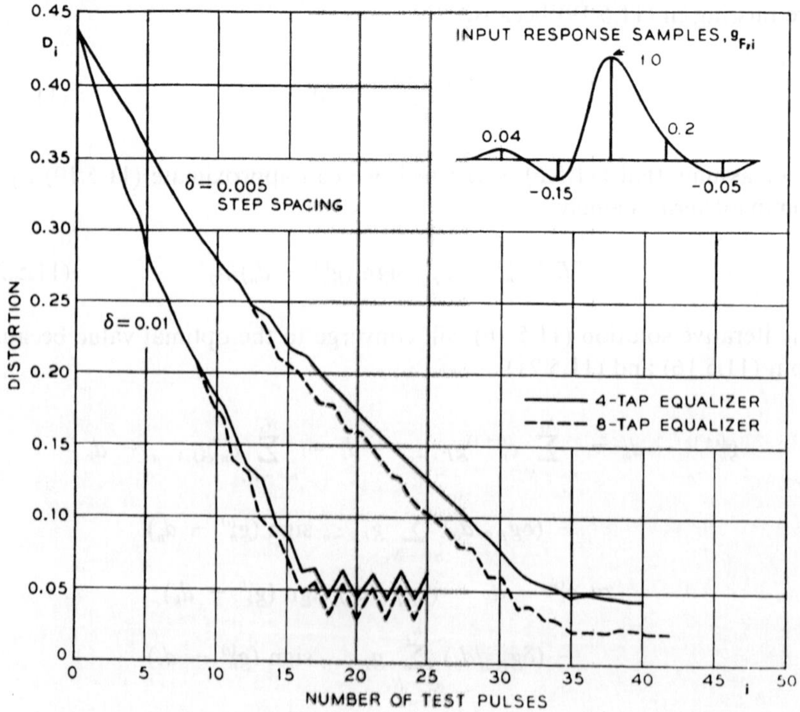


Fig. 11.17. Distortion of zero-forcing equalizer as a function of iteration number (reprinted with permission from *The Bell System Technical Journal.* Copyright 1975, AT&T).

With any fixed $\delta$, there will be an iteration $i$ so that (11.5.24) is not satisfied any more. In that case we obtain from (11.5.23)

$$|g_k^{(i+1)} - d_k| \leqq 2\,\delta g_{F,0}^2/d_0 \tag{11.5.27}$$

Thus

$$D_{i+1} \leqq 2\,\delta N g_{F,0}^2/d_0 + \sum_{\substack{k<-N_1 \\ k>N_2}} |\mathbf{v}_C \mathbf{g}_{F,k}^T - d_k|/d_0 \tag{11.5.28}$$

When the first term in (11.5.28) is sufficiently small (by a proper selection of $\delta$), that means that (11.5.10) is approximately satisfied; hence the second term is very close to the optimal value in (11.5.11). However, even when $i \to \infty$, there will be an excess distortion, $D_{\text{exc}}$, caused by the usage of the estimate of the gradient, which from (11.5.28) is proportional to the step size $\delta$. The settling time, however, is inversely related to $\delta$.

A detailed analysis of automatic and adaptive zero-forcing equalizers is

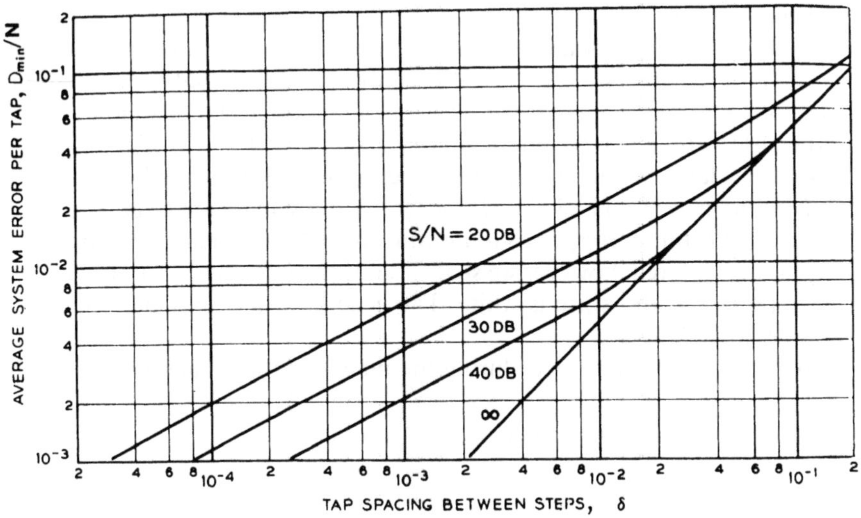


Fig. 11.18. Distortion of zero-forcing equalizer as a function of iteration step size with signal-to-noise ratio as parameter (reprinted with permission from *The Bell System Technical Journal*. Copyright 1975, AT&T).

presented in Refs. 11.4 and 11.6. They show that if the system response is: $g_{F,0} = 1$, $g_{F,1} = 0.2$, $g_{F,-1} = -0.15$, $g_{F,2} = -0.05$, $g_{F,-2} = 0.04$, the desired response is: $d_0 = 1$, $d_i = 0$, $i \neq 0$, and the symbols are binary, the value of $D_i$ as a function of $i$ and two values of δ is shown in Fig. 11.17. In Fig. 11.18 is shown for the same case the minimum distortion as a function of δ with signal-to-noise ratio as a parameter.

## 11.6 NONLINEAR EQUALIZATION

As we can see from Fig. 11.1, the input to the receiver filter is

$$x(t) = \sum_i a_i g_c(t - iT) + n_c(t) = s(t) + n_c(t) \tag{11.6.1}$$

where

$$g_C(t) = g_T(t) * h_C(t) \tag{11.6.2}$$

and $n(t)$ is white, Gaussian noise with power spectral density (PSD) 0.5 $N_0$ and bandwidth, $B$, which is much greater than the bandwidth of $G_C(f)$. We assume that $g_C(t)$ has a duration longer than $T$, so that

$$x(t_0) = \sum_i a_i g_C(t_0 - iT) + n_C(t_0)$$

is affected by $N_2$ past symbols and $N_1$ future symbols (if $N_1T < t_0 < (N_1 + 1)T$). We shall assume for convenience that $t_0 = 0$ (this simply means that $g_C(t)$ is replaced by $g_C(t - t_0)$) because this will simplify the notation. Therefore, it makes sense that our decision on the value of $a_0$ should be based on the observation of $x(t)$ over an interval $I = \{t: -NT < t < NT\}$, where $N > N_1, N_2$ is large enough so that the effect of the tails is negligible. This was indeed done in Refs. 11.43–11.53. Generally the symbols may be $M$-ary or even complex (this corresponds to an equivalent LSK system), and the noise $n_C(t)$ may be colored; however we shall assume here that the symbols are real, binary ($\pm 1$) and the noise is white. The general results may be found, for example, in Ref. 11.53.

Given that $a_0 = m = \pm 1$, during the interval $I$ the sequence of symbols

$$\mathbf{a}(m) = \{a_{-N}, \ldots, a_{-1}, m, a_1, \ldots a_N\} \tag{11.6.3}$$

has been received. There are

$$L = 2^{2N} \tag{11.6.4}$$

such sequences, all of which are equiprobable. Let

$$\mathbf{a}_\iota(m) = \{a_{-N}(\iota), \ldots, a_{-1}(\iota), m, a_1(\iota), \ldots, a_N(\iota)\} \tag{11.6.5}$$

be the $\iota$th sequence $1 \leqq \iota \leqq L$, and let

$$s(t, \mathbf{a}_\iota(m)) = mg_C(t) + \sum_{i \neq 0} a_i(\iota) g_C(t - iT) \tag{11.6.6}$$

be the corresponding signal for $t \in I$. Given $\mathbf{a}_\iota(m)$, we can compute the pdf (probability density function) of $x(t)$, $t \in I$.

$$\begin{aligned} p_{x(t)|\mathbf{a}(m)}(x(t)|\mathbf{a}_\iota(m)) &= p_{nc(t)}(x(t) - s(t, \mathbf{a}_\iota(m))) \\ &= C \exp\left( -0.5 \int (x(t) - s(t, \mathbf{a}_\iota(m)))^2/\sigma_{nc}^2 \, dt \right) \end{aligned} \tag{11.6.7}$$

and the integration is over $I$. Equation (11.6.7) may be proved by replacing the continuous functions $x(t)$, $n_C(t)$, and $s(t, \mathbf{a}_\iota(m))$ by a vector $\mathbf{Z} = \{Z_0, Z_1, Z_2, \ldots, Z_K\}$, where $Z_0 = Z(-NT)$, $Z_i = Z(-NT + i\Delta T)$, $\Delta T = (2N + 1)T/K$ ($Z(t)$ stands for $x(t)$, $n_C(t)$, and $s(t, \mathbf{a}_\iota(m))$ and then taking the limit when $K \to \infty$. For any finite $K$, $\mathbf{n}_C$ is a Gaussian vector. Details of this derivation may be found, for example, in Ref. 11.54. To obtain the conditional pdf (probability density function) of $x(t)$, given $a_0 = m$ only, we have to take the average over all sequences $a(m)$

$$p_{x(t)\,a_0}(x(t)|m) = \int_{\mathbf{a}(m)} p_{x(t);\mathbf{a}(m)}(x(t)|\mathbf{a}_\iota(m))p_{\mathbf{a}(m)}(\mathbf{a}_\iota(m))\, d\mathbf{a}(m)$$

$$= (C/L)\sum_{\iota=1}^{L} \exp\left\{-0.5\int (x(t) - s(t, \mathbf{a}_\iota(m)))^2\, dt/\sigma_{nc}^2\right\} \tag{11.6.8}$$

The maximum likelihood decision rule, which minimizes the error probability is

$$\hat{a}_0 = 1 \text{ if } p_{x(t)|a_0}(x(t)|1) \geqq p_{x(t)|a_0}(x(t)|-1) \tag{11.6.9}$$

and vice versa if the inequality is reversed. Equivalently, $\hat{a}_0 = 1$ if the likelihood ratio

$$\Lambda = \lambda_1/\lambda_{-1} \geqq 1 \tag{11.6.10}$$

where

$$\lambda_m = \sum_{\iota=1}^{L} \exp\,(\lambda_\iota(m)/\sigma_{nc}^2) \tag{11.6.11}$$

$$\lambda_\iota(m) = \int x(t)s(t, \mathbf{a}_\iota(m))\, dt - 0.5\int s^2(t, \mathbf{a}_\iota(m))\, dt \tag{11.6.12}$$

We substitute (11.6.6) into (11.6.12) and obtain

$$\lambda_\iota(m) = \sum_i a_i(\iota)\int x(\tau)g_c(\tau - iT)\, d\tau - 0.5\sum_i\sum_j a_i(\iota)a_j(\iota)$$

$$\int g_C(t - iT)g_C(t - jT)\, dt \tag{11.6.13}$$

with $a_0(\iota) = m$.
Denote

$$y(t) = x(t) * g_C(-t) = \int g_C(-t + \tau)x(\tau)\, d\tau \tag{11.6.14}$$

$$g(t) = \int g_C(\tau - t)g_C(\tau)\, d\tau = \int_{-\infty}^{\infty} |G_C(f)|^2 \cos\,(2\,\pi f t)\, df \tag{11.6.15}$$

i.e., $y(t)$ is the response to $x(t)$ of a filter that is matched to $g_C(t)$, and $g(t)$ is the response of this filter to $g_C(t)$. Thus

$$\lambda_1(m) = my_0 + \sum' a_i(1)y_i - 0.5\left\{(2N+1)g_0 + 2m\sum_i' a_i(1)g_i + \sum_i'\sum_{j\neq i}' a_i(1)a_j(1)g_{i-j}\right\} \tag{11.6.16}$$

where

$$y_i = y(iT),\ g_i = g(iT) \tag{11.6.17}$$

and the prime in the summation means that the zero term is omitted. When we substitute (11.6.1) into (11.6.14) we obtain

$$y(t) = \sum_i a_i g(t - iT) + n(t) \tag{11.6.18}$$

and

$$y_k = \sum_i a_i g_{k-i} + n_k \tag{11.6.19}$$

where $n(t)$ is zero mean, Gaussian noise with PSD $0.5\ N_0|G_C(f)|^2$ and variance

$$\sigma_n^2 = 0.5\ N_0 g_0 \tag{11.6.20}$$

Instead of computing $\Lambda \gtreqless 1$, we can also compute $\ln \Lambda \gtreqless 0$, or equivalently

$$r = 0.5\ \sigma_{nc}^2 \ln \Lambda \gtreqless 0 \tag{11.6.21}$$

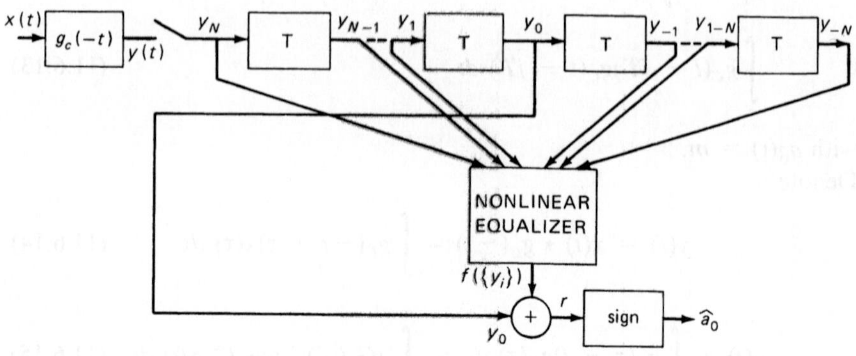


Fig. 11.19. Communication system with nonlinear equalizer.

When we substitute (11.6.10)–(11.6.16) into (11.6.21), we obtain

$$r = y_0 + f(\mathbf{y}) \tag{11.6.22}$$

where

$$\mathbf{y} = (y_{-N}, \ldots, y_{-1,}, y_1, \ldots, y_N) \tag{11.6.23}$$

and

$$\begin{aligned} f(\mathbf{y}) = 0.5\, \sigma_{nc}^2 \ln \Bigg[ \sum_{i=1}^{L} \exp \Bigg\{ \Bigg( \sum_i{}' a_i(\iota)(y_i - g_i) \\ - 0.5 \sum_i{}' \sum_{j \neq i}{}' a_i(\iota) a_j(\iota) g_{i-j} \Bigg) \Bigg/ \sigma_{nc}^2 \Bigg\} \Bigg/ \sum_{i=1}^{L} \\ \exp \Bigg\{ \Bigg( \sum{}' a_i(\iota)(y_i + g_i) \\ - 0.5 \sum_i{}' \sum_{j \neq i}{}' a_i(\iota) a_j(\iota) g_{i-j} \Bigg) \Bigg/ \sigma_{nc}^2 \Bigg\} \Bigg] \end{aligned} \tag{11.6.24}$$

The decision is

$$\hat{a}_0 = \text{sign } r \tag{11.6.25}$$

and can be computed as shown in Fig. 11.19. This figure is very similar to Fig. 11.3, the difference being in the replacement of the linear summation by the nonlinear operation $f(\mathbf{y})$. From eq. (11.6.22) or from Fig. 11.19, we draw the following conclusions:

1. The optimal, nonlinear receiver is composed of a filter matched to $g_C(t)$ and a transversal filter followed by a nonlinear operator. Thus, except for the nonlinear operator, the receiver is the same as in Chapter 10.
2. The decisions are based solely on $\mathbf{y}$, which means that all information about the symbols that originally was concealed in $x(t)$ is present in $\mathbf{y}$. This property of $\mathbf{y}$ makes it a *sufficient statistic.*
3. If $g_i = 0$ for $i \neq 0$, which means that there is no intersymbol interference (ISI), we obtain $f(\mathbf{y}) = 0$

$$r = y_0 = a_0 g_0 + n_0 \tag{11.6.26}$$

and there is no need for an equalizer.
4. If

$$f(\mathbf{y}) = \sum_i c_i' y_i \tag{11.6.27}$$

the equalizer is linear. This could have happened if the symbols $\{a_i\}$ were Gaussian rather than binary. This statement can be proved as follows. We write (11.6.19) in the form

$$y_k = a_0 g_k + u_k \tag{11.6.28}$$

where

$$u_k = \sum_i{}' a_i g_{k-i} + n_k \tag{11.6.29}$$

is a zero mean, Gaussian rv with correlation

$$R_u(k - \iota) = \overline{u_k u_\iota} = 0.5\, N_0 g_{k-\iota} + \sum_i g_{k-i} g_{\iota-i} \tag{11.6.30}$$

Given that $a_0 = m = \pm 1$, we can write

$$\mathbf{y} = m\mathbf{g} + \mathbf{u} \tag{11.6.31}$$

where $\mathbf{g}$ and $\mathbf{u}$ are vectors similar to (11.6.23). The conditional probabilities are thus

$$p_{\mathbf{y}|a_0}(\mathbf{y}|m) = p_{\mathbf{u}}(\mathbf{y} - m\mathbf{g}) = C \exp\{-0.5\,(\mathbf{y} - m\mathbf{g})R_u^{-1}(\mathbf{y} - m\mathbf{g})^T\} \tag{11.6.32}$$

where $R_u^{-1}$ is the inverse of the matrix $R_u$, the $k$, $\iota$th element of which is $R_u(k - \iota)$. Thus the likelihood ratio is

$$\Lambda = \exp\,(2\,\mathbf{y}R_u^{-1}\mathbf{g}^T) \tag{11.6.33}$$

and

$$\ln \Lambda = 2\,\mathbf{y}R_u^{-1}\mathbf{g}^T = \sum_i c_i y_i \tag{11.6.34}$$

with

$$c_i = 2 \sum_{j=-M}^{M} (R_u^{-1})_{ij} g_j \tag{11.6.35}$$

Here $(R_u^{-1})_{ij}$ is the element in the $i$th row and $j$th column of the matrix $R_u^{-1}$.

### 11.6.1 Small ISI

Here we ignore the double summation terms in (11.6.24). While the single summation term is the effect of ISI on $a_0$, the double summation term is the effect of ISI on the other symbols. When $|g_j|, j \neq 0$ is relatively small, we may ignore the latter terms. Thus $f(\mathbf{y})$ is simplified to

$$f(\mathbf{y}) = 0.5\,\sigma_{nc}^2 \ln\left[\sum_{\iota=1}^{L} \exp\left(\sum_i{}' a_i(\iota)(y_i - g_i)/\sigma_{nc}^2\right) \Big/ \sum_{i=1}^{L} \exp\left(\sum_i{}' a_i(\iota)(y_i + g_i)/\sigma_{nc}^2\right)\right] \quad (11.6.36)$$

It is not difficult to show that

$$f(y) = 0.5\,\sigma_{nc}^2 \sum_i{}' \ln \frac{\cosh\left((y_i - g_i)/\sigma_{nc}^2\right)}{\cosh\left((y_i + g_i)/\sigma_{nc}^2\right)} = \sum_i{}' c(y_i) \quad (11.6.37)$$

The function

$$c(y) = 0.5 \ln\left(\cosh(y - g)/\cosh(y + g)\right) \quad (11.6.38)$$

has the following properties

a. $c(0) = 0 \; c(-y) = -c(y)$

b. for $g = 0$, $c(y) = 0$. For $g > 0$, $c(y)$ is a decreasing function of $y$

c. $\lim_{y\to\infty} c(y) = -g$

This is illustrated in Fig. 11.20, from which we see that it has the form of a soft limiter. We can approximate this function by

$$c(y) \simeq L(y) = \begin{cases} -g \text{ sign } y & |y| > g \\ -y \text{ sign } g & |y| \leqq g \end{cases} \quad (11.6.39)$$

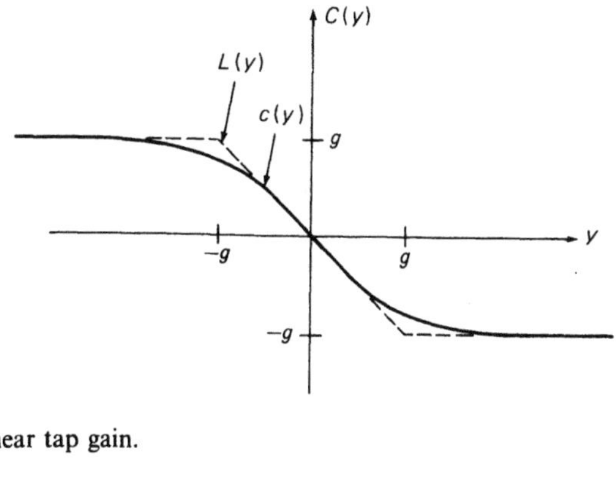


Fig. 11.20. Nonlinear tap gain.

which is also shown in Fig. 11.20 in a broken line. We can give an intuitive explanation to this result. We substitute (11.6.37) and obtain

$$r = y_0 + \sum_i{}' c(y_i) = a_0 g_0 + \sum_i{}' (a_i g_i + c(y_i)) + n_0 \quad (11.6.40)$$

Ideally if

$$c(y_i) = -a_i g_i \quad (11.6.41)$$

we would have eliminated the ISI. When $|y_i|$ is large we may estimate with great confidence that $a_i = \text{sign } y_i$. Indeed in (11.6.39) we have for large $|y_i|$

$$c(y_i) = -g_i \text{ sign } y_i = -\hat{a}_i g_i \quad (11.6.42)$$

and

$$r = a_0 g_0 + \sum_i{}' (a_i - \hat{a}_i) g_i + n_0 \quad (11.6.43)$$

When $|y_i|$ is small we do not have this confidence, and the result is

$$r = y_0 - \sum_i y_i \text{ sign } g_i \quad (11.6.44)$$

which is again a linear equalizer. This equalizer has the form of Fig. 11.3 with $c_0 = 1$ and all other linear amplifiers $c_i$, replaced by the nonlinear amplifier $c(y_i)$.

### 11.6.2 Large signal-to-noise ratio

When $\sigma_{nc}^2$ in (11.6.11) is small we can use the approximation

$$\lambda_m \simeq \exp (\Lambda(m)/\sigma_{nc}^2) \quad (11.6.45)$$

where

$$\Lambda(m) = \max_i \{\lambda_i(m)\} \quad (11.6.46)$$

Therefore

$$r = 0.5\, \sigma_{nc}^2 \ln \Lambda = 0.5\, \sigma_{nc}^2 (\Lambda(1) - \Lambda(-1)) = y_0 + f_1(\mathbf{y}) \quad (11.6.47)$$

where

$$f_1(\mathbf{y}) = 0.5\left\{\sum_i{}' a_i(1)(y_i - g_i) - 0.5 \sum_i{}' \sum_{j\neq i}{}' a_i(1)a_j(1)g_{i-j}\right.$$
$$\left. - \sum_i{}' a_i(-1)(y_i + g_i) + 0.5 \sum_i{}' \sum_{j\neq i}{}' a_i(-1)a_j(-1)g_{i-j}\right\} \qquad (11.6.48)$$

where $\{a_i(m)\}$, $i \neq 0$ is the sequence that maximizes $\lambda_\iota(m)$. If these sequences are identical for $m = \pm 1$, we obtain

$$f_1(\mathbf{y}) = -\sum_i{}' a_i(1)g_i \qquad (11.6.49)$$

If indeed this was the transmitted sequence, then $a_i(1) = a_i$ and

$$r = y_0 - \sum_i{}' a_i g_i = a_0 g_0 + \sum_i{}' a_i g_i - \sum_i{}' a_i g_i + n_0$$
$$= a_0 g_0 + n_0 \qquad (11.6.50)$$

and again the ISI is virtually eliminated.

We could have obtained immediately eq. (11.6.48) if, instead of the maximum likelihood criteria of (11.6.9), we used the rule

$$\hat{a}_0 = 1 \text{ if } \max_{\mathbf{a}(1)} p_{x(t)|\mathbf{a}(1),a_0}(x(t)|\mathbf{a}(1), 1) \geq \max_{\mathbf{a}(-1)} p_{x(t)|\mathbf{a}(-1),a_0}(x(t)|\mathbf{a}(-1), -1) \qquad (11.6.51)$$

which in fact selects the most likely sequence (MLS). If the MLS contains $a_0 = m = \pm 1$, our decision is $a_0 = m$.

When we have to our disposition the set $\{y_i\}$, the determination of the MLS is rather a complicated task, because we have to compute the 2 $L$ values $\{\lambda_\iota(m),\ \iota = 1, \ldots, L,\ m = \pm 1\}$. However, using the Viterbi decoding method,[11.49–11.56] which is in fact a version of dynamic programming,[11.57] this can be done sequentially, reducing the computational complexity.

*Example* 11.6.1

We assume that $g_C(t)$ is a raised cosine of duration $T_0 > T$

$$g_C(t) = \cos^2(\pi t/T_0)u_{T_0}(t + 0.5\,T_0)$$

Hence after the matched filter

$$g(t) = (T_0 - |t|)(1 + 0.5\cos(2\pi t/T_0)) + 0.75\sin(2\pi|t|/T_0)u_{2T_0}(t + T_0)$$

Because $g(t)/g(0) < 0.01$ for $|t| > 0.75\,T_0$, we may assume that there are $K = 0.75\,T_0/T$ significant interfering terms instead of $T_0/T$. The number of

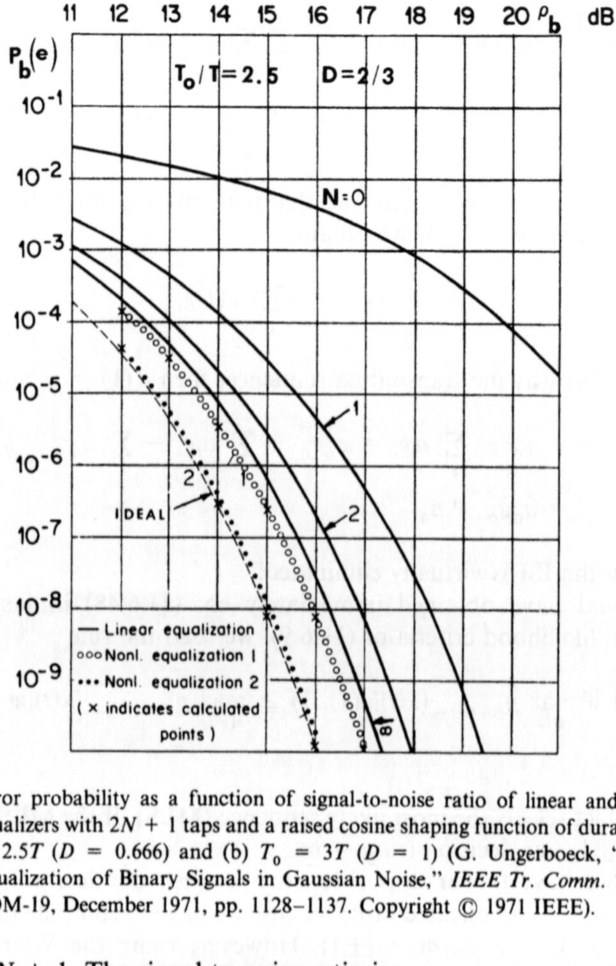


Fig. 11.21. Error probability as a function of signal-to-noise ratio of linear and nonlinear equalizers with $2N + 1$ taps and a raised cosine shaping function of duration (a) $T_0 = 2.5T$ ($D = 0.666$) and (b) $T_0 = 3T$ ($D = 1$) (G. Ungerboeck, "Nonlinear Equalization of Binary Signals in Gaussian Noise," *IEEE Tr. Comm. Tech.*, Vol. COM-19, December 1971, pp. 1128–1137. Copyright © 1971 IEEE).

taps is $2N + 1$. The signal-to-noise ratio is

$$\rho_b = g_0^2/\sigma_n^2 = 0.75\, T_0/N_0$$

and the peak, normalized ISI is

$$D = \sum_i{}' g_i/g_0$$

The results are shown in Fig. 11.21, reproduced from Ref. 11.49. Note that for $D = 1$ the eye is closed. The nonlinear equalizer for high signal-to-noise ratio (called in Fig. 11.21 equalizer 2) is more effective in reducing the effect of ISI then the nonlinear equalizer for small ISI (called here equalizer 1), and both are better than the linear equalizer. In fact, with only 5 taps

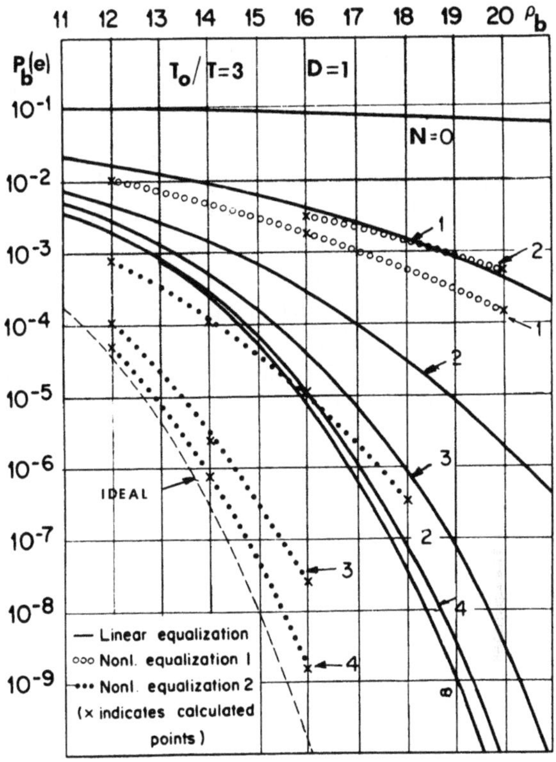


Fig. 11.21. *(con't.)*

for $D = 0.666$ and 9 taps for $D = 1$, the error probability is very close to the ideal, i.e.

$$P_b(e) = Q((2\ \rho_b)^{0.5})$$

## 11.7 SUMMARY

In this chapter we have discussed the optimal equalizer with a finite number of tap gains under a mean square error and maximal eye opening criteria. First we introduced various configurations of equalizers. For the mean square error criterion we analyzed the composite forward and decision feedback equalizers. We have presented a formal solution, an iterative algorithm, and a practical algorithm in which the true gradient is replaced by an unbiased estimate of the gradient. We have shown that with this algorithm the solution converges to the optimal one, with the settling time being a decreasing function of step size, $\delta$, used in the iterative algorithm. We have also shown that the estimated, noisy gradient causes an excess mean square error beyond the mathematical minimal value that is proportional to $\delta$. We have presented several methods for the reduction of the settling time.

A separate section was devoted to the zero-forcing equalizer, where it was shown that a simple, iterative algorithm converges to the optimal solution.

We have discussed briefly the problem of nonlinear equalization. We have shown in fact that a linear equalizer is optimal only if the symbols are Gaussian rvs instead of being discrete rvs. We have shown that for high signal-to-noise ratios the optimal nonlinear equalizer produces the most likely sequence of symbols, rather than the most likely single symbol. We have mentioned that the practical algorithm in finding the most likely sequence is the Viterbi algorithm, but we did not discuss this method at any length.

We have also not mentioned the family of equalizers based on Kalman filters.[11.58–11.63] To give the last two topics any fair treatment here would extend this chapter beyond the original intentions.

## 11.8 PROBLEMS

11.4.1 Show that

a. $M_Y$ is a real symmetric matrix.

b. $M_Y$ is a positive definite matrix.

11.4.2 Show that the mean square error can be expressed as in eq. (11.4.27).

11.4.3 Assume a system in which

$$g_{F,0} = 1, g_{F,-1} = 0.3, g_{F,2} = 0.25$$

$$g_{F,-2} = g_{F,1} = g_{F,2} = 0.2, g_{F,-2} = 0.15$$

the desired response is $d_0 = 1, d_i = 0\ i \neq 0$, the symbols are binary, and the noise can be ignored.

a. Compute $M_Y$, $\mathbf{v}_{rY}$, $\mathbf{c}_{op}$, and $\varepsilon_{min}$, assuming a forward equalizer with $N = N_1 + N_2 + 1$ $(N_1 = N_2)$ tap gains. Assume $N_1 = 1, 2, 3, 4$. Plot $\varepsilon_{min}$ as a function of $N$.

b. Repeat (a) assuming a decision feedback equalizer with $N = N_3$ tap gains. Assume $N_3 = 1, 2, \ldots, 9$ taps. Plot $\varepsilon_{min}$ as a function of $N$.

c. Repeat (a) assuming a composite forward and decision feedback equalizer with $N = N_1 + N_3 + 1$ tap gains $(N_2 = 0)$. Assume $N_1 = N_3 = 1$,

2, 3, 4. Plot $\varepsilon_{min}$ as a function of $N$.

d. Which is the best equalizer?

11.4.4 Assume the data of Problem 11.4.3 and a forward equalizer with $N = N_1 + N_2 + 1$ ($N_1 = N_2$) tap gains.

a. Compute the eigenvalues of the matrix $M_Y$ for $N_1 = 1, 2, 3, 4$.

b. Compute the average eigenvalue.

c. Compute the settling time for each tap gain and the average settling time if $\delta = 1/\lambda_M$ and $\lambda_M$ is the maximal eigenvalue.

d. Compute the excess mean square error.

11.4.5 Prove that the eigenvectors are orthogonal.

11.5.1 Assume a system in which

$$g_{F,0} = 1,\ g_{F,1} = 0.2,\ g_{F,-1} = -0.15,\ g_{F,2} = -0.05,\ g_{F,-2} = 0.04$$

the desired system response is $d_0 = 1$, $d_i = 0$ $i \neq 0$, binary symbols, and ignore the noise. A zero-forcing equalizer with $N = N_1 + N_2 + 1$ tap gains is used ($N_1 = N_2$).

a. Compute the matrix $M_F$ for $N_1 = 1, 2, 3, 4$.

b. Compute in each case the vector of optimal tap gains, $\mathbf{v}_{Cop}$.

c. Compute in each case the minimal distortion $D_{min}$.

d. Plot $D_{min}$ as a function of $N$.

e. Compute $\varepsilon_{min}$ (using a mean square error criterion) for $N_1 = 1, 2, 3, 4$. Plot $\varepsilon_{min}^{0.5}$ as a function of $N$, and compare with (d).

11.6.1 Show that for binary equiprobable symbols eq. (11.6.36) is simplified to (11.6.37).

11.6.2 Derive the optimal maximum likelihood equalizer for $M$-ary symbols.

a. Simplify the equalizer, assuming the ISI is small.

b. Simplify the equalizer, assuming the signal-to-noise ratio is large.

## 11.9 REFERENCES


11.1 M. A. Rappaport, "Automatic Equalization of Data Transmission Facility Distortion using Transversal Equalizers," *IEEE Tr. Comm. Tech.*, Vol. COM-12, September 1964, pp. 65–73.

11.2 F. K. Becker, L. N. Holzman, R. W. Lucky and E. Pof, "Automatic Equalization of Digital Communication," *Proc. IEEE*, Vol. 53, January 1965, pp. 96–97.

11.3 E. D. Gibson, "Automatic Equalization using Time Domain-Equalizers," *Proc. IEEE*, Vol. 53, August 1965, p. 1140.

11.4 R. W. Lucky, "Automatic Equalization for Digital Communication," *BSTJ*, Vol. 45, April 1965, pp. 547–588.

11.5 E. Gorog, "A New Approach to Time Domain Equalization," IBM Res. Develop., Vol. 9, July 1965, pp. 228–232.

11.6 R. W. Lucky, "Techniques for Adaptive Equalization of Digital Communication Systems," *BSTJ*, Vol. 45, February 1966, pp. 255–286.

11.7 R. W. Lucky and H. R. Rudin, "Generalised Automatic Equalization for Communication Channels," *Proc. IEEE*, Vol. 54, March 1966, pp. 439–440.

11.8 P. L. Zador, "Error Probabilities in Data System Pulse Regenerator with DC Restoration," *BSTJ*, Vol. 45, July 1966, pp. 479–984.

11.9 C. W. Niessen, "Automatic Channel Equalization Algorithm," *Proc. IEEE*, Vol. 55, May 1967, p. 689.

11.10 B. Widrow, *Adaptive Filters, I: Fundamentals*, Stanford Electron Lab., Stanford University, Stanford, Calif. Technical Report G764–6, December 1966.

11.11 H. Rudin, "Automatic Equalization using Transversal Filters," *IEEE Spectrum*, Vol. 4, January 1967, pp. 53–59.

11.12 R. W. Lucky and H. R. Rudin, "An Equalizer for General Purpose Communication Channels," *BSTJ*, Vol. 46, November 1967, pp. 2179–2208.

11.13 M. K. Simon, "Extensions to the Analysis of Regenerative Repeaters with Quantized Feedback," *BSTJ*, Vol. 46, October 1967, pp. 1831–1851.

11.14 M. J. DiToro, "Communication in Time Frequency Spread Media using Adaptive Equalization," *Proc. IEEE*, Vol. 56, October 1968, pp. 1653–1679.

11.15 D. W. Lytle, "Convergence Criteria for Transversal Equalizers," *BSTJ*, Vol. 47, October 1968, pp. 1775–1801.

11.16 A. Gersho, "Adaptive Equalization of Highly Dispersive Channels for Data Transmission," *BSTJ*, Vol. 48, January 1969, pp. 55–70.

11.17 J. G. Proakis and J. H. Miller, "An Adaptive Filter for Digital Signalling through Channels with Intersymbol Interference," *IEEE Tr. Inf. Theory*, Vol. IT-15, July 1969, pp. 484–497.

11.18 L. D. Davisson, "Steady State Error in Adaptive Mean Square Minimization," *IEEE Tr. Inf. Theory*, Vol. IT-16, July 1970, pp. 382–385.

11.19 D. A. George, R. R. Bowen, and J. R. Storey, "An Adaptive Decision Feedback Equalizer," *IEEE Tr. Comm. Tech.*, Vol. COM-19, June 1971, pp. 281–293.

11.20 D. Monsen, "Feedback Equalization for Fading Dispersive Channels," *IEEE Tr. Inf. Theory*, Vol. IT-17, January 1971, pp. 56–64.

11.21 T. J. Schonfield and M. Schwartz, "A Rapidly Converging First Order Training Algorithm for an Adaptive Equalizer," *IEEE Tr. Inf. Theory*, Vol. IT-17, July 1971, pp. 431–439.

11.22 R. W. Chang and E. Y. Ho, "A New Equalizer Structure for Fast Start Up Digital Communications," *BSTJ*, Vol. 50, July–August 1971, pp. 1969–2014.

11.23 R. D. Gitlin, J. F. Mazo, and M. G. Taylor, "On the Design of Gradient Algorithms for Digitally Implemented Adaptive Filters," *IEEE Tr. Cir. Theory*, Vol. CT-20, March 1973, pp. 125–136.

11.24 J. Salz, "Optimum Mean Square Decision Feedback Equalization," *BSTJ*, Vol. 52, October 1973, pp. 1341–1373.

11.25 K. H. Muller, "A New Fast Converging Mean Square Algorithm for Adaptive Equalizers with Partial Response Signalling," *BSTJ*, Vol. 54, January 1975, pp. 143–153.

11.26 C. J. Macleod, E. Ciapala, and *Z. J. Jelonek*, "Quantization of Non-recurrsive Equalization for Data Transmission," *Proc. IEE*, Vol. 122, October 1975, pp. 1105–1110.

11.27 C. J. Macleod, E. Ciapala, and Z. J. Jelonek, "Study of Recursive Equalizers for Data Transmission with a Comparison of the Performance of Six Systems," *Proc. IEEE*, Vol. 122, October 1975, pp. 1097–1104.

11.28 J. G. Proakis, "Advances in Equalization for Intersymbol Interference," *Advances in Communication Systems* (A. Balakrishnan, ed.) 1975, pp. 123–198.
11.29 R. W. Muellar and D. A. Spaulding, "Cyclic Equalization: A New Rapidly Converging Technique for Synchronous Data Communication," *BSTJ*, Vol. 54, February 1975, pp. 369–406.
11.30 B. Widrow, J. M. McCool, M. G. Larimore, and C. R. Johnson, "Stationary and Nonstationary Learning Characteristic of LMS Adaptive Filter," *Proc. IEEE*, Vol. 64, August 1976, pp. 1151–1162.
11.31 A. Cantoni and K. C. K. Kwong, "Application of Richardson's Non-stationary Iterative Procedure to the Design of Adaptive Equalizers," *IEEE Tr. Inf. Theory*, Vol. IT-22, September 1976, pp. 560–567.
11.32 E. Cecchi, G. Martinelli, G. Orlandi, and M. Salerno, "Possibility of Automatically Acquiring the Optimal Adjusting Step in Adaptive Equalizers," *Proc. IEE*, Vol. 125, July 1978, pp. 626–632.
11.33 R. D. Gitlin, E. Y. Ho, and J. E. Mazo, "Passband Equalization for Differentially Phase Modulated Data Signals," *BSTJ*, Vol. 52, February 1973, pp. 219–238.
11.34 D. D. Falconer and G. J. Foschini, "Theory of Minimum Mean Square Error QAM systems Employing Decision Feedback Equalization," *BSTJ*, Vol. 52, December 1973, pp. 1821–1849.
11.35 D. D. Falconer, "Jointly Adaptive Equalization and Carrier Recovery in Two-Dimensional Digital Communication Systems," *BSTJ*, Vol. 55, March 1976, pp. 317–334.
11.36 D. D. Falconer, "Application of Passband Decision Feedback Equalization in Two-Dimensional Data Communication Systems," *IEEE Tr. Comm.*, Vol. COM-24, October 1976, pp. 1159–1166.
11.37 D. D. Falconer, "Analysis of Gradient Algorithm for Simultaneous Passband Equalization and Carrier Phase Recovery," *BSTJ*, Vol. 55, April 1976, pp. 403–428.
11.38 R. W. Pulleyblank, "A Comparison of Receivers Designed on the Basis of Minimum Mean Square Error and Probability of Error for Channels with Intersymbol Interference and Noise," *IEEE Tr. Comm.*, Vol. COM-21, December 1973, pp. 1434–1438.
11.39 J. E. Mazo, "On the Independence Theory of Equalizer Convergence," *BSTJ*, Vol. 58, May–June 1979, pp. 963–982.
11.40 J. Krishnamurthy and H. M. Dante, "Bounds on Probability of Error in Decision Feedback Equalizers," *IEEE Tr. AES*, Vol. AES-12, January 1976, pp. 173–177.
11.41 E. Dalle Mese and D. Guili, "Generalised Decision Feedback Equalization of Digital Communication Channels," *Electronics Circuits and Systems*, Vol. 3, July 1979, pp. 145–151.
11.42 C. A. Belfiore and J. H. Park, "Decision Feedback Equalization," *Proc. IEEE*, Vol. 67, August 1979, pp. 1143–1156.
11.43 J. M. Aein, J. C. Hancock, "Reducing the Effects of Intersymbol Interference with Correlation Receivers," *IEEE Tr. Inf. Theory*, Vol. IT-9, July 1963, pp. 167–175.
11.44 R. W. Chang and J. C. Hancock, "On Receiver Structures for Channels Having Memory," *IEEE Tr. Inf. Theory*, Vol. IT-12, October 1966, pp. 463–468.
11.45 R. A. Gonsalves, "Maximum Likelihood Receiver for Digital Transmission," *IEEE Tr. Comm. Tech.*, Vol. COM-16, June 1968, pp. 392–398.
11.46 K. Abend, T. J. Harley, B. D. Fritchman and G. Gumacos, "On Optimum Receivers for Channels Having Memory," *IEEE Tr. Inf. Theory*, Vol. IT-14, November 1968, pp. 819–820.
11.47 R. R. Bowen, "Bayesian Decision Procedures for Interfering Digital Signals," *IEEE Tr. Inf. Theory*, Vol. IT-15, July 1969, pp. 506–507.
11.48 K. Abend, B. D. Fritchman, "Statistical Detection for Communication Channels with Intersymbol Interference," *Proc. IEEE*, Vol. 58, May 1970, pp. 779–785.

11.49 G. Ungerboeck, "Nonlinear Equalisation of Binary Signals in Gaussian Noise," *IEEE Tr. Comm. Tech.*, Vol. COM-19, December 1971, pp. 1128–1137.
11.50 G. D. Forney, "Maximum Likelihood Sequence Estimation of Digital Sequences in the Presence of Intersymbol Interference," *IEEE Tr. Inf. Theory*, Vol. IT-18, May 1972, pp. 363–378.
11.51 F. R. Magee and J. G. Proakis, "Adaptive Maximum Likelihood Sequence Estimation for Digital Signaling in the Presence of Intersymbol Interference," *IEEE Tr. Inf. Theory*, Vol. IT-19, January 1973, pp. 120–124.
11.52 S. U. H. Qureshi and E. E. Newhall, "An Adaptive Receiver for Data Transmission over Time Dispersive channels," *IEEE Tr. Inf. Theory*, Vol. IT-19, July 1973, pp. 448–457.
11.53 G. Ungerboeck, "Adaptive Maximum Likelihood Receiver for Carrier Modulated Data Transmission Systems," *IEEE Tr. Comm.*, Vol. COM-22, May 1974, pp. 624–636.
11.54 A. Viterbi, *Principles of Coherent Communications*, McGraw-Hill Book Co., New York, N.Y., 1966.
11.55 A. J. Viterbi, "Error Bounds for Convolutional Codes and an Asymptotical Optimum Decoding Algorithm," *IEEE Tr. Inf. Theory*, Vol. IT-13, April 1967, pp. 260–269.
11.56 J. K. Omura, "On the Viterbi Decoding Algorithm," *IEEE Tr. Inf. Theory*, Vol. IT-15, January 1969, pp. 177–179.
11.57 R. Bellman, *Dynamic Programming*, Princeton Univ. Press, Princeton, N.J., 1957.
11.58 R. E. Lawrence and H. Kaufman, "The Kalman Filter for the Equalization of a Digital Communication Channel," *IEEE Tr. Comm. Tech.*, Vol. COM-19, December 1971, pp. 1137–1141.
11.59 J. W. Mark, "A Note on the Modified Kalman Filter for Channel Equalization," *Proc. IEEE*, April 1973, pp. 481–482.
11.60 D. Goddard, "Channel Equalization using a Kalman Filter for fast Data Transmission," *IBM Res. Develop*, Vol. 18, May 1974, pp. 267–273.
11.61 S. Benedetto and E. Biglieri, "On Linear Receivers for Digital Transmission Systems," *IEEE Tr. Comm.*, Vol. COM-22, September 1973, pp. 1205–1215.
11.62 G. Nicholson and J. P. Norton, "Kalman Filter Equalization for a Time Varying Communication Channel," *ATR*, Vol. 13, 1979, pp. 3–11.
11.63 E. Dalle Mese and G. Corsini, "Adaptive Kalman Filter Equaliser," *Electronic Lett.*, Vol. 16, July 1980, pp. 547–549.

# 12 LINE CODING

## 12.1 INTRODUCTION

In the telephone system speech and other analogue signals (such as picturephone and television) may be transmitted as digital signals using pulse code modulation (PCM). In PCM, speech is sampled at a rate of 8000 samples per second, and each sample is represented by seven (mainly in North America and Japan) or eight (in rest of the world) bits. The result is a sequence of bits, called *Marks* (for "1") and *Spaces* (for "0" or "− 1") at the rate of 56 kbps or 64 kbps. For efficient usage of telephone cables, several PCM signals are multiplexed into higher bit rates. The first hierarchy of this multiplexing combines 24 (in North America and Japan) or 30 (in the rest of the world) basic PCM signals, generating binary sequences at the rate of 1.544 Mbps or 2.048 Mbps, the extra bits arising from signaling and other information. The PCM structures are shown in Tables 12.1 and 12.2.

**Table 12.1 PCM plan in North America**

| LEVEL | RATE (MBPS) | VOICE CHANNELS | MEDIUM | REPEATER SPACING (MILES) | ERROR RPOBABILITY |
|---|---|---|---|---|---|
| 1 | 1.544 | 24 | Wire | 1 | $10^{-6}$ |
| 2 | 6.312 | 96 | Coax | 2.5 | $10^{-7}$ |
| 3 | 44.736 | 672 | Coax | – | – |
| 4 | 274.176 | 4032 | Coax | 1 | $10^{-6}$ |
| 5 | 560.160 | 8064 | Coax | 1 | $4 \times 10^{-9}$ |
| 6 | 18,500 | 233,000 | Waveguide<br>Optical fiber | 25 | |

**Table 12.2 PCM plan in North America, Japan, and Europe**

| LEVEL | | 1 | 2 | 3 | 4 | 5 |
|---|---|---|---|---|---|---|
| Bit rate | North America | 1.544 | 6.312 | 44.736 | 274.176 | 560.160 |
| (Mbps) | Japan | 1.544 | 6.312 | 32.064 | 97.728 | 400.352 |
| | Europe | 2.048 | 8.446 | 32.368 | 139.264 | 560 |
| No. of | North America | 24 | 96 | 672 | 4032 | 8064 |
| channels | Japan | 24 | 96 | 480 | 1440 | 5760 |
| | Europe | 30 | 120 | 480 | 1920 | 7680 |

The channels in the telephone system consist of single pair and multipair cables for lower bit rates and coaxial cables for higher bit rates. Because of attenuations in the cable, the digital signal must be regenerated at regular points along the cable by repeaters, the output of which is ideally a noise-free, undistorted version of its input. The regenerators, as well as the telephone sets (with a PCM chip), operate on a power supply from the other end of the cable, hence the DC path cannot be used by the signal. The digital signal is AC-coupled to the cable. Hence to prevent excessive intersymbol interference (ISI) due to low-frequency distortion, the power spectral density (PSD) of the signal must be DC-free and must have low values at low frequencies. Because the PSD is a statistical average, a DC-free signal may still have temporary DC accumulation. This can be represented by a running digital sum (RDS)

$$\text{RDS} = \sum_{n}^{k} a_i \qquad k \geq n \tag{12.1.1}$$

where $n$ is arbitrary, and $a_i = 0, +1, -1$ are the symbols (here we anticipate that the binary symbols may be represented by ternary symbols and the shaping function is NRZ (nonreturn to zero)). The difference between the maximal value of RDS and the minimal value of RDS is called the *digital sum variation* (DSV)

$$\text{DSV} = (\text{RDS})_{\max} - (\text{RDS})_{\min} \tag{12.2.2}$$

and is an indication of the DC accumulation.

The cable also attenuates high-frequency signals, while crosstalk in multipair cables is increased at high frequencies. Thus the PSD of the signal must be low at high frequencies.

The repeaters need timing information to regenerate the signal at the correct rate. This information is obtained from transitions in the signal levels of the digital signal. Therefore we must ensure that for any binary sequence (including a sequence with a large number of consecutive spaces) there is a sufficient number of transitions. This makes the system transparent to the binary symbols.

Simplicity of generating the digital signal is a very important factor. With digital chips it is convenient to generate rectangular waveforms; thus in PCM the shaping functions that are best candidates are NRZ (nonreturn to zero), RZ (return to zero), and BP (biphase), already described in Chapter 3.

In any communications system we have to monitor the performance by estimating the error probability without actually knowing the transmitted sequence. In PCM the binary symbols are independent, all sequences are possible, and there is no redundancy. Hence monitoring is impossible unless coding is introduced. In the latter case ternary symbols represent the original binary symbols, without an increase in the transmission rate, and the resulting redundancy is used for monitoring.

Chapter 3 showed that the PSD of a baseband signal depends on two factors: the shaping function and the symbol correlation. In line coding we introduce correlation, so that a large family of PSDs is created with an NRZ shaping function only. In summary, when we transmit binary symbols in a cable we use a line code with the following desirable properties of the resulting signal

1. The PSD has no DC and has low values for both high and low frequencies.
2. The signal has sufficient number of transitions.
3. Error monitoring is possible.
4. A low value for the DSV.
5. The code should be simple.
6. The signal should have a minimum power consistent with the required error probability and crosstalk.
7. If possible the code should reduce the transmission rate on the line.

In this chapter we describe various line codes used in PCM systems. In Section 12.2 we discribe several binary encoding techniques. In 12.3 we shall describe linear ternary codes, the most significant of which is the bipolar. In 12.4 we discuss codes in which $N$ binary symbols are encoded into $K$ ternary symbols. Such codes are alphabetic. The PST, MS43, and 4B-3T are examples of such codes. In 12.5 we consider substitution codes, in which a sequence of $n$ consecutive zeroes in a bipolar code are replaced by a sequence of symbols that violate the normal bipolar code rule. HDBn, CHDBn, TIBn, and BnZS are examples of such codes. We compare the various properties of these line codes, particularly their PSDs.

Bipolar codes are introduced in Ref. 12.1 and other papers in the same issue of *Bell System Technical Journal.* A PST code is described in Ref. 12.2 The MS43 code is presented in Ref. 12.3. The B6ZS code is analyzed in Ref. 12.4. HDB, CHDB, and TIB codes are described in Refs. 12.5 and 12.6. Refs. 12.5 and 12.7–12.9 review the various line coding techniques. A new method of design of alphabetic codes with small low-frequency contents is presented in Ref. 12.10. The PSD of alphabetic codes is computed in Ref. 12.11 and that of nonalphabetic codes in Refs. 12.12 and 12.13.

In 12.6 we present a summary, which is followed by problems in 12.7 and a list of references in 12.8.

## 12.2 BINARY CODES

Chapter 3 showed that a baseband signal with a common shaping function, $h(t)$

$$s(t) = \sum_i a_i h(t - iT) \tag{12.2.1}$$

has a PSD (see eq. (3.4.8))

$$S_s(f) = |H(f)|^2 \, S_a(f)/T \tag{12.2.2}$$

where $S_a(f)$ depends on the correlation between the symbols

$$S_a(f) = \sum_k R_a(k) \exp(-j\, 2\, \pi f Tk) \tag{12.2.3}$$

$$R_a(k) = \overline{a_0 a_k} \tag{12.2.4}$$

and the bar denotes the statistical average. For independent symbols

$$S_a(f) = \overline{a_0^2} - (\overline{a_0})^2 + (\overline{a_0})^2 \sum_k \delta(f - k/T)/T \tag{12.2.5}$$

Hence the PSD depends only on the spectrum of the shaping function, $H(f)$ (except for discrete line frequencies, which may be useful in timing). Figure 12.1 shows several binary digital signals in which a mark is "1" and a space is "−1" or "0." In NRZ-L, the shaping function is NRZ. Hence for equiprobable symbols $a_i = \pm 1$, we obtain

$$S_s(f)/E = \mathrm{sinc}^2(fT) \tag{12.2.6}$$

where

$$\mathrm{sinc}\, x = \sin(\pi x)/(\pi x) \tag{12.2.7}$$

and $E$ is the energy in the NRZ pulse. The PSD is shown in Fig. 12.2.

In NRZ-M a mark is represented by a change in level, and a space by no change (the opposite is true for NRZ-S). This signal can be described by

$$s(t) = \sum_i b_i h(t - iT) \tag{12.2.8}$$

where

$$b_i = -b_{i-1} a_i \qquad (b_{-1} = 1) \tag{12.2.9}$$

Hence if $a_i = \pm 1$ are independent, $b_i = \pm 1$ are independent. Thus the PSD is the same as in (12.2.6). This is also true for NRZ-S. These three signals have two defficiencies:

1. $S_s(0) \neq 0$.
2. A long string of spaces (or marks) is a DC signal with no timing information.

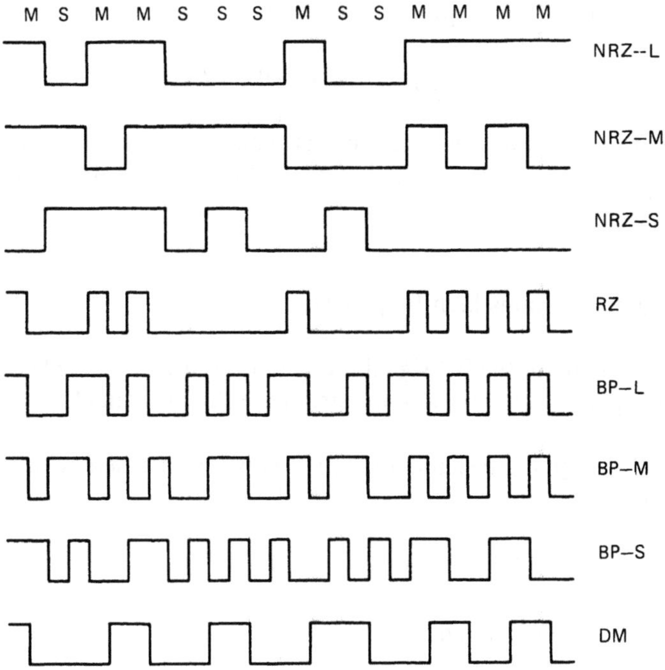


Fig. 12.1. Binary coded symbols.

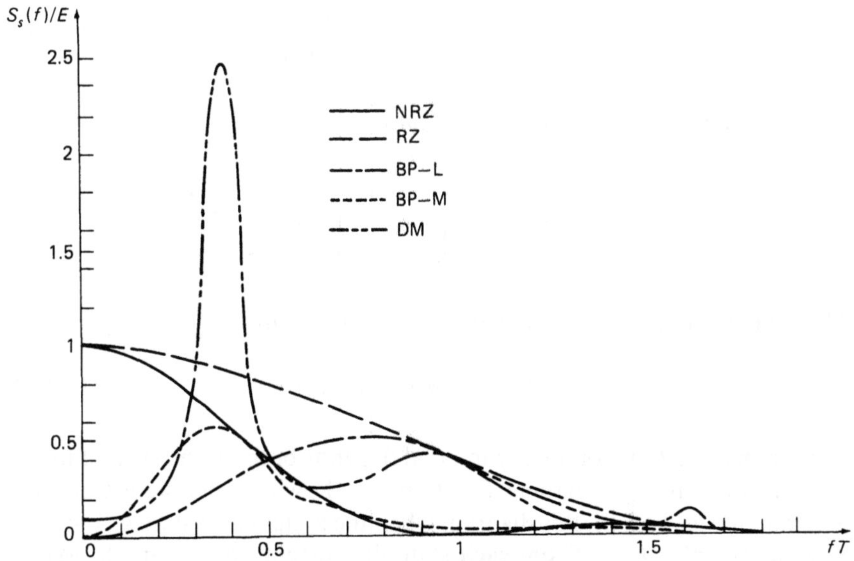


Fig. 12.2. The power spectral density of binary coded signals.

In the RZ signal with equiprobable symbols $a_i = \pm 1$ the PSD is

$$S_s(f)/E = \text{sinc}^2\,(0.5\,fT) \tag{12.2.10}$$

which is also shown in Fig. 12.2. In this signal, there is a transition at the beginning of each interval and in the middle of each interval, but the defficiencies are

1. $S_s(0) \neq 0$.
2. The PSD contains high frequencies.

In another version of the RZ signal the symbols are $a_i = 0, 1$. This version is shown in Fig. 12.1. The continuous part of the PSD is as in (12.2.10) divided by 4.

In the BP-L signal the shaping function is BP. Hence here with equiprobable symbols $a_i = \pm 1$

$$S_s(f)/E = \sin^2\,(0.5\,\pi fT)\,\text{sinc}^2\,(0.5\,fT) \tag{12.2.11}$$

There is no DC in this signal, and the only defficiency is the high-frequency content.

In the BP-M signal there is a transition at the beginning of each interval. A mark has an additional transition in the middle of the interval. Here a space is represented by either of the two NRZ pulses

$$h_1(t) = -h_2(t) = \begin{cases} 1 & 0 \leq t \leq T \\ 0 & \text{otherwise} \end{cases} \tag{12.2.12}$$

and a mark by either of the two BP pulses

$$h_3(t) = -h_4(t) = \begin{cases} 1 & 0 \leq t \leq 0.5T \\ -1 & 0.5T \leq t \leq T \\ 0 & \text{otherwise} \end{cases} \tag{12.2.13}$$

This signal cannot be represented by (12.2.1), but by

$$s(t) = \sum_i h(t - iT, a_i) \tag{12.2.14}$$

and the shaping function in any interval depends both on the symbol in this interval and previous shaping function, as shown in the state transition diagram in Fig. 12.3. In this diagram when the system is in state $k$, $k = 1, 2, 3, 4$, the signal is $h_k(t)$. From each state the current symbol, mark (M), or space (S) will lead to the next state, with probability $p$ for mark and $q = 1 -$

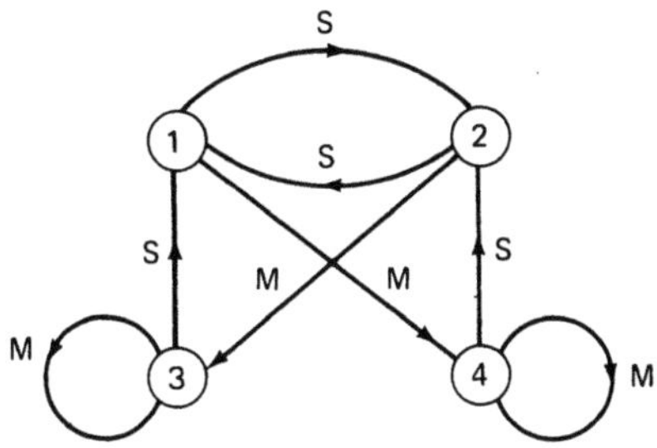


Fig. 12.3. The transition diagram of biphase mark.

$p$ for space. Let $P_k$ be the probability of being in state $s_k$ and $Q_{kj}$ be the conditional probability that the next state is $s_k$ if the present state is $s_j$. We have from the state diagram the matrix $Q$ with elements $Q_{kj}$.

$$Q = \begin{pmatrix} 0 & q & q & 0 \\ q & 0 & 0 & q \\ 0 & p & p & 0 \\ p & 0 & 0 & p \end{pmatrix} \tag{12.2.15}$$

and in steady state

$$P_k = \sum_{j=1}^{4} Q_{kj} P_j \tag{12.2.16}$$

The PSD can be computed from eq. (3.4.2)

$$S_s(f) = \sum_i S_{h,i}(f) \exp(-j\, 2\, \pi f T i)/T \tag{12.2.17}$$

where in the present case

$$S_{h,i}(f) = \overline{H(f, a_i) H^*(f, a_0)} = \sum_{k=1}^{4} \sum_{j=1}^{4} H_k(f) H_j^*(f) Q_{kj}^{(i)} P_j \tag{12.2.18}$$

where $Q_{kj}^{(i)}$ is the conditional probability of being in state $k$, $i$ intervals after occurrence of state $j$. $Q_{kj}^{(i)}$ is the $k, j$th element of the matrix $Q^i$; hence $Q_{kj}^{(1)} = Q_{kj}$, and

$$Q_{kj}^{(0)} = \begin{cases} 1 & k = j \\ 0 & k \neq j \end{cases} \tag{12.2.19}$$

We assume that

$$\lim_{i \to \infty} Q_{kj}^{(i)} = P_k \tag{12.2.20}$$

which means that after a long time the states are independent. We can thus write from (12.2.17)

$$S_s(f) = \left\{\sum_{k=1}^{4} |H_k(f)|^2 P_k + 2\,\mathrm{Re}\left\{\sum_{k=1}^{4}\sum_{j=1}^{4} H_k(f)H_j^*(f)Q_{kj}(f)P_j\right\}\right\}\Big/T \tag{12.2.21}$$

where

$$Q_{kj}(f) = \sum_{i}^{\infty} Q_{kj}^{(i)} \exp(-j\,2\,\pi f T i) \tag{12.2.22}$$

For $p = q = 0.5$, we obtain $P_k = 1/4$, $k = 1, \ldots 4$

$$Q = \begin{pmatrix} 0 & 0.5 & 0.5 & 0 \\ 0.5 & 0 & 0 & 0.5 \\ 0 & 0.5 & 0.5 & 0 \\ 0.5 & 0 & 0 & 0.5 \end{pmatrix} \tag{12.2.23}$$

and for all $i \geq 2$

$$Q^i = 0.25\begin{pmatrix} 1 & 1 & 1 & 1 \\ 1 & 1 & 1 & 1 \\ 1 & 1 & 1 & 1 \\ 1 & 1 & 1 & 1 \end{pmatrix} \tag{12.2.24}$$

Thus

$$S_s(f) = \left\{0.25\sum_{k=1}^{4} |H_k(f)|^2 + 2\,\mathrm{Re}\left\{\sum_{k=1}^{4}\sum_{j=1}^{4} H_k(f)H_j^*(f)\right.\right.$$

$$\left.\left.(Q_{kj} - 0.25)0.25\exp(-j\,2\,\pi f T)\right\}\right\}\Big/T \tag{12.2.25}$$

When we substitute (12.2.12), (12.2.13), (12.2.23), and (12.2.24) into (12.2.25), we obtain

$$S_s(f) = \{|H_1(f)|^2 \sin^2(\pi f T) + |H_3(f)|^2 \cos^2(\pi f T)\}/T \tag{12.2.26}$$

where $|H_1(f)|^2/T^2$ is given in eq. (12.2.6) and $|H_3(f)|^2/T^2$ in eq. (12.2.11). The PSD is shown in Fig. 12.2 The PSD of BP-S is the same as for BP-M for equiprobable symbols.

In DM (delay modulation) (this is also called *Miller coding*) a mark is represented by a transition in the middle of the interval, and a space by no transition, except when followed by another space, in which case there is a

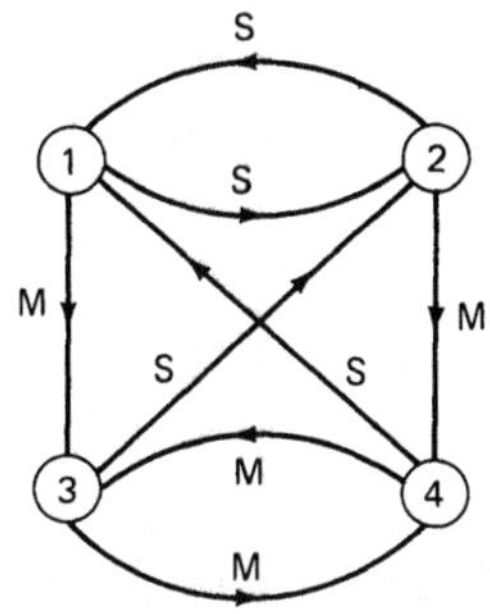


Fig. 12.4. The transition diagram of delay modulation.

transition at the end of the interval. Here a mark and a space are represented as in (12.2.12) and (12.2.13), but the state transition diagram is as in Fig. 12.4. The $Q$ matrix is here

$$Q = \begin{pmatrix} 0 & q & 0 & q \\ q & 0 & q & 0 \\ p & 0 & 0 & p \\ 0 & p & p & 0 \end{pmatrix} \tag{12.2.27}$$

For $p = q = 0.5$, we obtain $P_k = 1/4$, and the PSD was derived in Ref. 12.14. The result is

$$\begin{aligned} S_s(f)/E = \{&23 - 2\cos\delta - 22\cos(2\delta) - 12\cos(3\delta) + 5\cos(4\delta) \\ &+ 12\cos(5\delta) + 2\cos(6\delta) - 8\cos(7\delta) + 2\cos(8\delta)\}/ \\ &\{2\delta^2(17 + 8\cos(8\delta))\} \end{aligned} \tag{12.2.28}$$

where

$$\delta = \pi f T \tag{12.2.29}$$

The PSD of delay modulation is also shown in Fig. 12.2. With this code most of the energy lies in the vicinity of $fT = 0.35$; however, there is a DC component.

Because states (and signals) in the last two codes can appear only in specified order, the violation of this order can be used to monitor errors. For example, it follows from Fig. 12.4 that state 1 cannot follow state 3. Hence if this happens at the receiver, this indicates an error.

## 12.3 LINEAR TERNARY CODES

In these codes the shaping function is common and is an NRZ pulse. The binary symbols $a_i = \pm 1$ are encoded into ternary symbols $b_i = 0, \pm 1$ using the linear relation

$$b_i = \sum_{k=0}^{k} C_k a_{i-k} \tag{12.3.1}$$

where the coefficients $\{C_k\}$ define the code. These codes are pseudoternary, because the ternary symbols deliver the same amount of information as the binary symbols. The partial response signals (PRS) described in Chapter 9 can also be described equivalently by (12.3.1). Thus with $C_1 = C_0 = 0.5$ (all other $C_i = 0$), we obtain the duobinary code; with $C_0 = -C_2 = 0.5$, we obtain the modified duobinary code; with $C_1 = -C_0 = 0.5$, we obtain the twinned binary (TB) code; and with $C_0 = -C_1 = 0.5$, we obtain the dicode. The signal here is

$$s(t) = \sum_i b_i h(t - iT) = \sum_i a_i h_1(t - iT) \tag{12.3.2}$$

where

$$h_1(t) = \sum_{k=0}^{k} C_k h(t - kT) \tag{12.3.3}$$

Several codes are shown in Fig. 12.5. The dicode is not shown because it is the negative of TB. Note that in the TB code, a pulse is created only if there is a change in symbol, and the pulses are alternately positive and negative.

The PSD of these signals is given by (12.2.2) with

$$S_a(f) = \left| \sum_{k=0}^{K} C_k \exp(-j\, 2\, \pi f T k) \right|^2 \tag{12.3.4}$$

Thus

$$S_a(f) = \begin{cases} \cos^2 (\pi f T) & \text{duobinary} \\ \sin^2 (2\pi f T) & \text{modified duobinary} \\ \sin^2 (\pi f T) & \text{twinned binary} \end{cases} \tag{12.3.5}$$

The PSD is shown in Fig. 12.6. The problem with these signals is error propagation, i.e., a single error may affect the error probability of the next $K$ symbols. To prevent error propagation, the symbols $\{a_i\}$ may be precoded, prior to application of (12.3.1). This was discussed for PRS in Chapter 9. For the TB code the result of precoding is the Bipolar or AMI (alternative mark inversion) code. In this code a mark is encoded into alternating positive and negative pulses and a space into a zero pulse. In the receiver a nonzero pulse is recognized as a mark. Hence there is no error propagation. Precoding does not change the PSD. Hence the PSD of the bipolar signal is the same as for the TB signal. This can also be shown directly from (12.2.2) with $R_a(k)$ replaced by

$$R_b(k) = \overline{b_0 b_k} = \begin{cases} 0.5 & k = 0 \\ 0.25 & k = \pm 1 \\ 0 & |k| > 1 \end{cases} \tag{12.3.6}$$

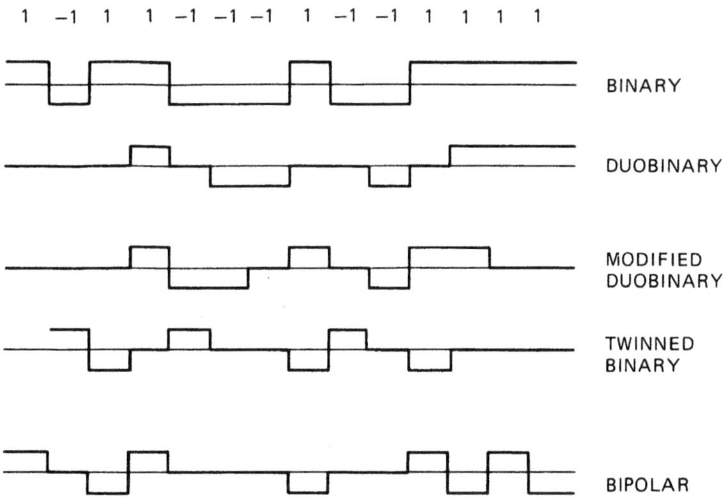


Fig. 12.5. Signals generated with linear ternary codes.

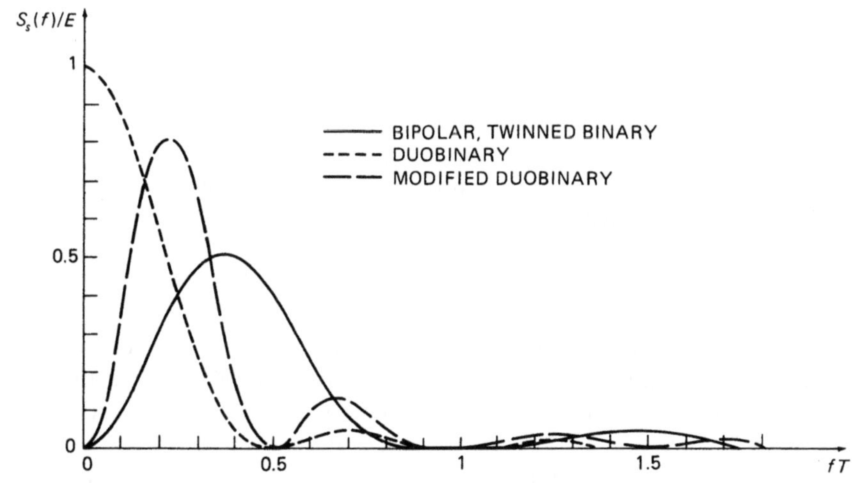


Fig. 12.6. The power spectral density of linear ternary codes.

The digital sum variation (DSV) of the bipolar code is the minimum possible, namely 1. There is no DC component. The only disadvantage of the code is that a long sequence of spaces generates a zero signal with no energy and no timing information.

We obtain interleaved pseudoternary codes if we apply the codes to the even and odd bits separately and combine the resulting sequences. In this process the DSV is doubled, but each frequency in the PSD is reduced to half. In fact, the modified duobinary is an interleaved Dicode.

*Example* 12.3.1 Bipolar code
Denoting the binary symbols by 0, 1 and the ternary symbols by 0, +, −, we show a binary sequence and the encoded bipolar sequence

| | |
|---|---|
| Binary sequence | 1 1 00 1 1 0000 1 1 1 1 1 00 |
| Bipolar sequence | + − 00 + − 0000 + − + − + 00 |

Note that the VDS is 1.

*Example* 12.3.2 Interleaved bipolar code

| | |
|---|---|
| Binary sequence | 1 1 0000 1 1 1 0 1 1 00 1 0 |
| Odd bipolar code | + 0 0 − + − 0 + |
| Even bipolar code | + 0 0 − 0 + 0 0 |
| Interleaved bipolar code | + + 0000 − − + 0 − + 00 + 0 |

Note that the VDS is 2.

## 12.4 ALPHABETIC CODES

Nonlinear codes are divided into alphabetic and zero-substitution codes. In alphabetic codes the sequence of binary numbers is grouped into words (or blocks) of $N$ symbols, and each word is encoded into a word of $K$ ternary symbols. $N$ and $K$ satisfy the condition

$$N \leq K \log_2 3 \tag{12.4.1}$$

Let us call the rate of the ternary symbols the *line rate*, because these symbols are transmitted through the line (channel). We assume that the pulses that represent both the binary and ternary symbols have the same duration $T$. Therefore if $K = N$, the line rate is the same as the bit rate, though if $K < N$, the line rate is less than the bit rate. Hence either the bandwidth of the channel may be reduced, or the bit rate may be increased.

A code without rate change is the PST (pair selected ternary) code in which $K = N = 2$. Hence pairs of binary symbols are encoded into pairs of ternary symbols, as shown in Table 12.3.

**Table 12.3 PST code**

| BINARY WORD | TERNARY WORD | |
|---|---|---|
| | MODE A (RDS = 0) | MODE B (RDS = 1) |
| 00 | − + | − + |
| 01 | 0 + | 0 − |
| 10 | + 0 | − 0 |
| 11 | + − | + − |

In this table + (−) means a ternary +1 (−1). Mode A is used when the RDS is zero, and mode B when the RDS is one. Note that the mode changes every time the sequence 01 or 10 is transmitted so that a DC balance is achieved.

*Example* 12.4.1
The binary and ternary sequences are

| | | | | | | | | | |
|---|---|---|---|---|---|---|---|---|---|
| | 10 | 11 | 00 | 01 | 11 | 10 | 00 | 11 | 01 |
| | +0 | +− | −+ | 0− | +− | +0 | −+ | +− | 0− |
| Mode | A | B | B | B | A | A | B | B | B |

The 4B-3T (four binary-three ternary) and MS43 are examples of codes with a rate change of 3/4. In both codes, words of four binary symbols are encoded into words of three ternary symbols, as shown in Tables 12.4 and 12.5, respectively.

In 4B-3T there are two modes of operation depending on the value of the RDS. Six words that have all three symbols (hence a digital sum of zero) are common to both modes. They do not change the RDS. The remaining 10 words have a nonzero digital sum; hence to achieve a DC-free signal the mode changes. When the RDS = −1, −1, −3, we use mode A, but when RDS = 0, 1, 2, we use mode B. The VDS is here 7. The VDS is reduced to 5 in the MS43 code, which has three modes: in mode A, RDS = 1; in mode B, RDS = 2, 3, and in mode C, RDS = 4.

With all alphabetic codes there is a problem of framing, because there is no extra symbol for word separation. Because not all ternary sequences are used (for example 00 is not used in PST, and 000 is not used in 4B-3T and MS43) the occurrence of such a sequence indicates frame violation. After framing is established, the same sequences can be used for error monitoring.

**Table 12.4 4B-3T code**

| BINARY WORD | TERNARY WORD MODE A RDS = −1, −2, −3 | TERNARY WORD MODE B RDS = 0, 1, 2 |
|---|---|---|
| 0000 | + 0 − | + 0 − |
| 0001 | − + 0 | − + 0 |
| 0010 | 0 − + | 0 − + |
| 0011 | + − 0 | + − 0 |
| 0100 | + + 0 | − − 0 |
| 0101 | 0 + + | 0 − − |
| 0110 | + 0 + | − 0 − |
| 0111 | + + + | − − − |
| 1000 | + + − | − − + |
| 1001 | − + + | + − − |
| 1010 | + − + | − + − |
| 1011 | + 0 0 | − 0 0 |
| 1100 | 0 + 0 | 0 − 0 |
| 1101 | 0 0 + | 0 0 − |
| 1110 | 0 + − | 0 + − |
| 1111 | − 0 + | − 0 + |

**Table 12.5 MS43 code**

| BINARY WORD | TERNARY WORD MODE A RDS = 1 | TERNARY WORD MODE B RDS = 2, 3 | TERNARY WORD MODE C RDS = 4 |
|---|---|---|---|
| 0000 | + + + | − + − | − + − |
| 0001 | + + 0 | 0 0 − | 0 0 − |
| 0010 | + 0 + | 0 − 0 | 0 − 0 |
| 0100 | 0 + + | − 0 0 | − 0 0 |
| 1000 | + − + | + − + | + − − |
| 0011 | 0 − + | 0 − + | 0 − + |
| 0101 | − 0 + | − + 0 | − 0 + |
| 1001 | 0 0 + | 0 0 + | − − 0 |
| 1010 | 0 + 0 | 0 + 0 | − 0 − |
| 1100 | + 0 0 | + 0 0 | 0 − − |
| 0110 | − + 0 | − + 0 | − + 0 |
| 1110 | + − 0 | + − 0 | + − 0 |
| 1101 | + 0 − | + 0 − | + 0 − |
| 1011 | 0 + − | 0 + − | 0 + − |
| 0111 | − + + | − + + | − − + |
| 1111 | + + − | + − − | + − − |

**Table 12.6 FOMOT code**

| BINARY WORD | TERNARY WORD MODE A RDS = −2 | MODE B RDS = −1, 0 | MODE C RDS = 1, 2 | MODE D RDS = 3 |
|---|---|---|---|---|
| 0000 | + − + | + − + | + − + | − − − |
| 0001 | 0 + − | 0 + − | 0 + − | 0 + − |
| 0010 | 0 − + | 0 − + | 0 − + | 0 − + |
| 0011 | 0 + + | 0 + + | 0 − − | 0 − − |
| 0100 | − + 0 | − + 0 | − + 0 | − + 0 |
| 0101 | 0 + 0 | + − − | 0 + 0 | + − − |
| 0110 | − + + | 0 − 0 | − + + | 0 − 0 |
| 0111 | + − 0 | + − 0 | + − 0 | + − 0 |
| 1000 | − 0 + | − 0 + | − 0 + | − 0 + |
| 1001 | + + − | 0 0 − | + + − | 0 0 − |
| 1010 | 0 0 + | − − + | 0 0 + | − − + |
| 1011 | + 0 − | + 0 − | + 0 − | + 0 − |
| 1100 | + 0 0 | − 0 0 | + 0 0 | − 0 0 |
| 1101 | + + 0 | + + 0 | − 0 − | − 0 − |
| 1110 | + 0 + | + 0 + | − − 0 | − − 0 |
| 1111 | + + + | − + − | − + − | − + − |

FOMOT (four-mode ternary) is a code with four modes, shown in Table 12.6, has better framing and the same DSV as MS43. Ternary codes with constraints on the PSD have been developed in Ref. 12.15.
There are also variable length (VL) codes. For example in VL43 code four or eight binary symbols are encoded into ternary code words of length three and six, respectively, so that the line rate is constant.[12.3] The DSV in this code is only 4, and there is more timing information.

The signal generated by the alphabetic codes can be written as

$$s(t) = \sum_i \left( \sum_{k=1}^{K} b_i^{(k)} h(t - (k - 1)T - iT_K) \right) \tag{12.4.2}$$

where

$$T_K = KT \tag{12.4.3}$$

and $b_i^{(k)}$ is the $k$th symbol in the $i$th word

$$\mathbf{b}_i = (b_i^{(1)}, b_i^{(2)}, \ldots, b_i^{(K)}), \; b_i^{(k)} = 0, \pm 1 \tag{12.4.4}$$

The PSD of the codes can be computed using a signal flow graph method[12.4] or an algebraic method.[12.11] The result is

$$S_s(f) = T_K^{-1} |H(f)|^2 \sum_i \mathbf{V} R_i \mathbf{V}^{*T} \exp(-j\, 2\, \pi f T_K i) \tag{12.4.5}$$

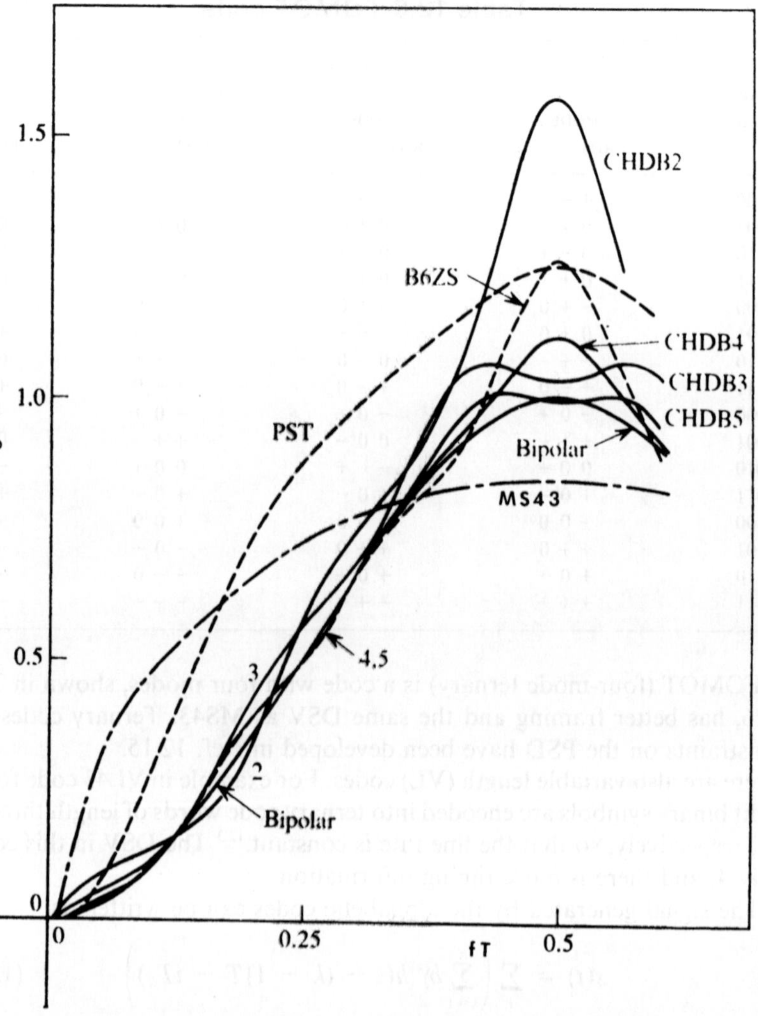


Fig. 12.7. The power spectral density of nonlinear ternary codes (from A. Croisier, "Introduction to Pseudoternary Transmission Codes," IBM J. Res. Develop, Vol. 14, July 1970, pp. 354–364. Copyright © 1970 by International Business Machines Corporation; reprinted with permission).

where **V** is the vector

$$\mathbf{V} = (v, v^2, \ldots, v^k), \; v = \exp(j\,2\,\pi f T) \tag{12.4.6}$$

$\mathbf{V}^{*T}$ is the transpose of the conjugate of **V**, and $R_i$ is the correlation matrix.

$$R_i = \overline{\mathbf{b}_0{}^T\mathbf{b}_i} \tag{12.4.7}$$

For the PST code with equiprobable binary symbols the PSD is

$$S_s(f) = |H(f)|^2(1 + \cos\beta)(7 + 4\cos\beta + 2\cos^2\beta)/(8T) \tag{12.4.8}$$

where

$$\beta = 2\pi fT \tag{12.4.9}$$

A formula for the MS43 code can be found in Ref. 12.11. The results are shown in Fig. 12.7, which is reproduced from Ref. 12.5.

## 12.5 NONALPHABETIC CODES

The only deficiency of the bipolar code was the lack of timing information in a long string of zeroes. In the zero substitution codes, which are nonlinear and nonalphabetic, such a string is replaced by a ternary sequence, some symbols of which violate the bipolar rule (the rule is that two successive nonzero pulses have opposite polarity). This violation is recognized by the decoder. Hence the zero string will be reinserted into the sequence.

We shall use the following notation: B represents a normal, nonzero, bipolar pulse; and V represents a nonzero pulse that violates the bipolar rule. In BnZS (bipolar $n$ zero substitution) codes a string of $n = 4$ zeroes is replaced by VBVB, $n = 6$ zeros by 0VB0VB and for $n > 6$ by 000 ... 0VB0VB (other potential substitution words are V0BV0B or B0VB0V). For $n < 4$, we must have more than one substitution word. They are 0V and BV for $n = 2$ and 00V and B0V for $n = 3$. They are used according to Table 12.7.

**Table 12.7 B2ZS and B3ZS codes**

| | B2ZS | | B3ZS | |
|---|---|---|---|---|
| LAST SUBSTITUTION or LAST PULSE | 0 + or + + | 0 − or − − | 0 0 + or + 0 + | 0 0 − or − 0 − |
| + | − − | 0 + | − 0 − | 0 0 + |
| − | 0 + | + + | 0 0 − | + 0 + |

The DSV of this code is 3.

In HDB$n$ (high-density bipolar $n$) code $n + 1$ zeroes are replaced by one of two sequences os length $n + 1$

$$\text{B00} \ldots \text{0V} \quad \text{or} \quad \text{000} \ldots \text{0V} \tag{12.5.1}$$

and they are selected so that the number of B pulses between two consecutive V pulses is odd (this makes the consecutive V pulses of opposite polarity). The DSV here is only 2, and the power is less than in BnZS (because in the substitution sequence there are more zeroes).

*Example* 12.5.1 HDB 3
The binary and ternary sequences are

```
1 1 000 1 00 1 1 1 0 0 0 0 1 1 0 0 0 1
+ − 00 − + 00 − + − + 0 + 0 − + − 0 − +
B B 00 V B 00 B B B B 0 V 0 B B B 0 V B
```

In CHDB$n$ (compatible HDB$n$) the substitution sequences are

$$000 \ldots \mathrm{B0V} \quad \text{or} \quad 000 \ldots \mathrm{0V} \tag{12.5.2}$$

the advantage being that the decoder is independent of $n$.

We have already noted that when we interleave two sequences the resulting PSD is compressed by a factor of 2 in frequency, but the DSV is increased by the same factor. In TIB$n$ (transparent interleaved bipolar $n$) code we interleave two bipolar sequences (i.e., the even and the odd bits are encoded separately as bipolar subsequences), but $n + 1$ zeroes in the interleaved sequence are replaced by

$$00 \ldots 00\mathrm{XXVV}$$

where V is a bipolar violation in its subsequence, and X is other 0 or B, selected so that the number of B pulses, between two successive V pulses in each subsequence, is odd. The V pulses in the substitution sequence have opposite polarity. This code has a DSV of 2, the PSD is 0 at $f = 0$ and $fT = 0.5$, and the number of consecutive 0s is $n$.

*Example* 12.5.2. TIB5
The binary sequence, the odd bipolar subsequence, the even bipolar subsequence, and the ternary sequence before and after TIB5 coding is given by

```
1 1 1 1 0000 1 00 0 0 0 0 00 0 0 0 0 1 00 0 0 0 0 00 1 1
 −   +   0 0 −  0 0  0  0   0   0  00  0   0 +
   +   −  0 0  0 0  0   0 0   0   + 0  0  0 0   −
− + + − 0000 − 00 0 0 0 0 00 0 0 0 0 + 00 0 0 0 0 00 + −
− + + − 0000 − 00 + 0 + − 00 − + − + + 00 − 0 − + 00 + −
```

A nonalphabetic code that is not derived from the bipolar code is the TPC (time polarity control) code in which during the odd time intervals the nonzero pulses are positive and during the even time intervals the pulses are negative.

The zero-substitution codes may be viewed as variable-length alphabetic codes. Such a representation of an HDB2 code is given in Table 12.8. The HDB2 and B3ZS codes are identical.

**Table 12.8 HDB2 code**

| BINARY WORDS | LAST VIOLATION + | | LAST VIOLATION − | |
|---|---|---|---|---|
| | RDS 1 | RDS 0 | RDS 0 | RDS −1 |
| 1 | − | + | − | + |
| 01 | 0 − | 0+ | 0− | 0 + |
| 001 | 0 0 − | 0 0 + | 0 0 − | 0 0 + |
| 000 | − 0 − | 0 0 − | 0 0 + | + 0 + |

In view of this the PSD of the nonalphabetic codes can be computed using signal-flow graphs[12.12] or algebraic methods.[12.13] The second method leads to more general results. Thus for BnZs codes the PSD is with

$$P(a_i = 1) = p,\ P(a_i = 0) = q \tag{12.5.3}$$

$$\begin{aligned} S_s(f) = |H(f)|^2 \Bigg\{ p\mathrm{Re}\left\{\frac{1 - v}{1 + v(p - q)}\right\} + \frac{pq^n}{1 - q^n} \Bigg\{ |\alpha(v)|^2 \\ - 2\mathrm{Re}\{\{(1 - q^n)(1 - qv)\alpha(v) - v^{n+1}p(1 - q^n v^n)\alpha^*(v) \\ - q^n v^n (1 - qv)|\alpha(v)|^2\}/\{(1 - q^n v^*)(1 + z(p - q))\}\}\Bigg\} \end{aligned} \tag{12.5.4}$$

where

$$\alpha(v) = \sum_{i=1}^{n} b_i v^i \tag{12.5.5}$$

and

$$\mathbf{b} = (b_i, \ldots, b_n) \tag{12.5.6}$$

## Table 12.9 Properties of codes without rate change

| PARAMETER \ CODE | BIPOLAR | PST | HDB2 | HDB3 | B6ZS | HDB5 |
|---|---|---|---|---|---|---|
| DSV | 1 | 3 | 2 | 2 | 3 | 2 |
| Timing content | 1 | 1.25 | 1.57 | 1.02 | 1.28 | 0.98 |
| Average power | 1 | 1.50 | 1.21 | 1.10 | 1.06 | 1.02 |
| Number of consecutive zeroes | ∞ | 2 | 2 | 3 | 5 | 5 |

## Table 12.10 Properties of alphabetic codes

| PARAMETER \ CODE | PST | 4B-3T | MS43 | FOMOT |
|---|---|---|---|---|
| Bits per word $N$ | 2 | 4 | 4 | 4 |
| Symbols per word $K$ | 2 | 3 | 3 | 3 |
| Bit rate/line rate | 1 | 1.33 | 1.33 | 1.33 |
| Redundancy % | 58.5 | 18.8 | 18.8 | 18.8 |
| DSV | 3 | 7 | 5 | 5 |
| Timing content | 1.25 | 0.76 | 0.84 | 0.84 |
| Average power | 1.50 | 1.36 | 1.26 | 1.34 |
| Number of modes | 2 | 2 | 3 | 4 |
| Number of zeroes | 2 | 4 | 4 | 4 |

is the substitution sequence. For HDB$n$ and CHDB$n$ codes, the PSD is

$$S_s(f) = \frac{2p}{(1 - q^{n+1})(2 - q^{n+1})} \operatorname{Re}\left\{\frac{\{1 + q^{n+1}v + (1 - q^{n+1})\gamma(v)\}\{1 - q^{n+1}v + \beta(v)\}}{(1 + \gamma(v))(1 - \beta(v))}\right\} \tag{12.5.7}$$

where

$$\beta(v) = -pv\frac{1 - q^{n+1}v^{n+1}}{1 - qv} \tag{12.5.8}$$

and

$$\gamma(v) = \beta(v) + q^{n+1}v^{n+1} \tag{12.5.9}$$

Assuming $p = q = 0.5$, the PSD is shown in Fig. 12.7. Various properties of ternary codes are presented in Tables 12.9 and 12.10. The redundancy is given by

$$\text{Redundancy} = (K/N)\log_2 3 - 1 \qquad (12.5.10)$$

In the codes without rate change ($K = N$), the redundancy is 58.5%. The timing content and average power are normalized with respect to the bipolar code. The ternary codes do not exhaust all possible line codes. In the systems with low noise, multilevel line codes should also be considered for efficient utilization of the channel bandwidth.

## 12.6 SUMMARY

In this section we reviewed line codes: linear, nonlinear, alphabetic, and nonalphabetic. We described various properties of many codes and presented particularly their power spectral density. A selection of a particular code depends on the requirements: freedom of DC, ease of filtering, simple encoding and decoding, error monitoring, crosstalk, etc. In general nonlinear codes offer more versatility: simultaneously we can control the position of spectral zeroes, increase timing content, and reduce line rate.

## 12.7 PROBLEMS

12.2.1 Compute the PSD of the bipolar-M signal

a. assuming that $p = q = 0.5$
b. assuming that $p \neq q$.

12.2.2 Compute the PSD of the bipolar-S signal.

12.2.3 Compute the PSD of the delay modulation signal assuming that $p = q = 0.5$.

12.2.4 Compute the RDS and DVS of NRZ-L, NRZ-M, NRZ-S, and DM.

12.3.1 The binary sequence is

011011111001101111

a. Compute and sketch the duobinary signal.
b. Compute and sketch the modified duobinary signal.
c. Compute and sketch the twinned binary signal.
d. Compute and sketch the bipolar signal.

12.3.2 Compute and sketch the PSD of the following interleaved signals.
   a. duobinary and duobinary
   b. twinned binary and twinned binary
   c. bipolar and bipolar
   d. Compute in each case the RDS before and after interleaving.
   e. Compute in each case the DSV before and after interleaving.

12.4.1 Compute the PSD of the PST signal assuming that $p = q = 0.5$.

12.4.2 Compute the PSD of a 4B-3T signal assuming that $p = q = 0.5$.

12.4.3 Compute the PSD of a MS43 signal assuming that $p = q = 0.5$.

12.4.4 Compute the PSD of a FOMOT signal assuming that $p = q = 0.5$.

12.4.5 Given the binary sequence

110001100111100101001110011

compute
   a. The PST sequence.
   b. The 4B-3T sequence.
   c. The MS43 sequence.
   d. The FOMOT sequence.
   e. Compute in each case the RDS.
   f. Compute in each case the DSV.

12.5.1 Compute the PSD of B2ZS and B3ZS signal assuming that $p = q = 0.5$.

12.5.2 Compute the PSD of HDB3 signal assuming that $p = q = 0.5$.

12.5.3 Compute the PSD of TIB3 signal assuming that $p = q = 0.5$.

12.5.4 Given the binary sequence

1100000100010000111000001000

compute
   a. The B2ZS sequence.
   b. The B3ZS sequence.
   c. The HDB3 sequence.
   d. The TIB3 sequence.
   e. Compute in each case the RDS.
   f. Compute in each case the DSV.

12.5.5 Compute the properties of the codes in Table 12.9.

12.5.6 Compute the properties of the codes in Table 12.10.

## 12.8 REFERENCES


12.1 M. R. Aaron, "PCM Transmission in the Exchange Plant," *BSTJ*, Vol. 41, January 1962, pp. 99–142.

12.2 J. M. Sipress, "A New Class of Selected Ternary Pulse Transmission Plans for Digital Transmission Lines," *IEEE Tr. Comm. Tech.*, Vol. COM-13, September 1965, pp. 366–372.

12.3 P. A. Franaszek, "Sequence State Coding for Digital Transmission," *BSTJ*, Vol. 47, Janaury 1968, pp. 143–157.

12.4 V. I. Johannes, A.G. Kaim, and T. Walzman, "Bipolar Pulse Transmission with Zero Extraction," *IEEE Tr. Comm. Tech.*, Vol. COM-17, April 1969, pp. 303–310.

12.5 A. Croisier, "Introduction to Pseudoternary Transmission Codes," *IBM J. Res. Develop*, Vol. 14, July 1970, pp. 354–366.

12.6 A. Croisier, "Compatible High Density Bipolar Codes: An Unrestricted Transmission Plan for PCM Carriers," *IEEE Tr. Comm. Tech.*, Vol. COM-18, June 1970, pp. 265–268.

12.7 H. Kobayashi, "A Survey of Coding Schemes for Transmission or Recording of Digital Data," *IEEE Tr. Comm. Tech.*, Vol. COM-19, December 1971, pp. 1087–1100.

12.8 R. C. Houts and T. A. Green, "Comparing Bandwidth Requirements for Binary Baseband Signals," *IEEE Tr. Comm.*, Vol. COM-21, June 1973, pp. 776–781.

12.9 N. Q. Duc, "Line Coding Techniques for Baseband Digital Transmission," *Aust. Telecom. Res.* (ATR), Vol. 9, 1975, pp. 3–17.

12.10 V. A. Dieulus, "Spectrum Shaping with Alphabetic Codes with Finite Autocorrelation Sequence," *IEEE Tr. Comm. Tech.*, Vol. COM-26, April 1978, pp. 474–478.

12.11 G. L. Cariolaro and G. P. Tronca, "Spectra of Block Coded Digital Signals," *IEEE Tr. Comm.*, Vol. COM-22, October 1974, pp. 1555–1563.

12.12 W. Debus, "General Method for Calculating the Spectrum of a Zero Substitution Coded Signal," *IEEE Tr. Comm.*, Vol. COM-27, November 1979, pp. 1637–1643.

12.13 G. L. Cariolaro, G. L. Pierobon, and S. G. Popolin, "Spectral Analysis of Variable Length Coded Digital Signals," *IEEE Tr. Inf. Theory*, Vol. IT-28, May 1982, pp. 473–481.

12.14 M. Hecht and A. Guida, "Delay Modulation," *Proc. IEEE*, Vol. 57, July 1969, pp. 1314–1316.

12.15 E. Gorog, "Redundant Alphabets with Desirable Frequency Spectrum properties," *IBM J. Res. Develop*, Vol. 12, 1968, pp. 234–241.

# COMMONLY USED FUNCTIONS AND SYMBOLS

$\mathring{A}_0 = \{0, 1, \ldots, M - 1\}$

$\mathring{A}_1 = \{1, 2, \ldots, M\}$

$\mathring{A}_\pm = \{\pm 1, \pm 3, \ldots, \pm(M - 1)\}$

$$H_{id}(f) = \begin{cases} 1 & |f| \leqq W \\ 0 & |f| > W \end{cases}$$

$M$—number of symbols
$P(e)$ = symbol error probability
$P_b(e)$ = bit error probability

$$Q(x) = \int_x^\infty (2\pi)^{-0.5} \exp(-0.5t^2)\, dt$$

$R = 1/T$ symbol rate
$R_b = 1/T_b$ bit rate

$$\text{sign } t = \begin{cases} 1 & 0 < t \\ -1 & t < 0 \end{cases}$$

$\text{sinc } x = \sin(\pi x)/(\pi x)$

$\hat{\sin}\, x = \sin(xM)/(M \sin x)$

$T$—symbol duration
$T_b$—bit duration

$$u(t) = \begin{cases} 1 & 0 \leqq t \\ 0 & t < 0 \end{cases}$$

$$u_T(t) = \begin{cases} 1 & 0 \leqq t \leqq T \\ 0 & t < 0, t \geqq T \end{cases}$$

$X(f)$ = Fourier transform of $x(t)$
$X'(s)$ = Laplace transform of $x(t)$
$x_I$ = Re($x$) = real part of complex $x$
$x_Q$ = Im($x$) = imaginery part of complex $x$

# LIST OF ABBREVIATIONS

AC —alternating current
ACI —adjacent channel interference
AM —amplitude modulation
AMI —alternate mark inversion
ASK —amplitude shift keying
APSK —amplitude phase shift keying
AWGN —additive, white, Gaussian noise
bps —bits per second
B*n*ZS —bipolar *n* zero substitution
BP —biphase
BP-L —biphase level
BP-M —biphase mark
BP-S —biphase space
crv —continuous random variable
CHDB*n* —compatible high density bipolar *n*
CPDF —complementary probability distribution function
CPFSK —continuous phase FSK
drv —discrete random variable
DC —direct current
DM —delay modulation
DPSK —differential phase shift keying
DSB —double side band
DSV —digital sum variation
FFSK —fast frequency shift keying
FM —frequency modulation
FOMOT—four-mode ternary
FSK —frequency shift keying
FT —Fourier transform
GNI —general Nyquist interval
HDB*n* —high-density bipolar *n*
HS —half-cycle of sinusoid
HT —Hilbert transform
IFT —inverse Fourier transform
ISI —intersymbol interference
LSK —linear shift keying
LT —Laplace transform
ML —maximum likelihood

MLS —most likely sequence
MSK —minimum shift keying
NRZ —nonreturn to zero
NRZ-L —NRZ level
NRZ-M —NRZ mark
NRZ-S —NRZ space
OOK —on-off keying
OQASK —offset quadrature amplitude shift keying
OQPSK —offset quaternary phase shift keying
PCM —pulse code modulation
pdf —probability density function
PDF —probability distribution function
PM —phase modulation
PPM —pulse position modulation
PRS —partial response signal
PSD —power spectral density
PSK —phase shift keying
PST —pair selected ternary
QAM —quadrature amplitude modulation
QASK —quadrature amplitude shift keying
QCI —quadrature channel interference
QPSK —quadrature phase shift keying
rv —random variable
rp —random process
RC —raised cosine
RDS —running digital sum
RZ —return to zero
SFSK —sinusoidal frequency shift keying
SSB —single side band
SP —split phase
SQASK —staggered quadrature amplitude shift keying
TB —twinned binary
TDL —tapped delay line
TF —transversal filter
TIB*n* —transparent interleaved binary *n*
TPC —time polarity control
TR —triangular
TWT —traveling wave tube
VL43 —variable length 43
VSB —vestigial side band
wssp —wide sense stationary process

# INDEX


Aaron, M. R., 339, 578, 655
Abend, K., 631
Abramowitz, M., 339
Adjacent channel interference (ACI), ix, 159, 345, 357, 359, 363, 364, 383, 384, 390, 398, 403–405, 407, 408, 413, 416, 418, 430, 432, 434
Aein, J. M., 631
Amoroso, F., 156, 256
Amplifier, 236, 624
  linear,249
  nonlinear, 119, 144, 152, 249, 381, 624
  power, 119
Amplitude, viii, 2–4, 27, 103, 109, 115, 239, 471
  modulation, 236, 475
Amplitude Phase Shift Keying (APSK). *See* QASK
Amplitude Shift Keying (ASK), viii, 454, 502
  bandpass system, 109, 113, 142, 148, 324–331, 343, 369
    antipodal, 482
    coherent, 517
    DSB, 109, 110, 112, 113, 142, 343, 344, 348, 349, 350, 355
    equivalent baseband system 343, 345
    SSB, x, 111–114, 142, 343, 344, 355,
    VSB, x, 112, 113, 142, 343, 344, 355
    with Butterworth filter, 348
    with matched filter, 348
    with nonsymmetric filter, 349
    with Nyquist filter, 348
  baseband system, 142, 148, 151, 152, 259, 261, 306, 308, 309, 324–331, 412, 413
    condition for no ISI, 275
    decision function, 263, 264
    decision regions, 262, 265
    effect of ISI, 285
    error probability. *See* Error probability of ASK
    maximum likelihood decision rule, 261
    relation to LSK, OQASK, QASK, 260
    with Butterworth filter, 315–319, 322, 325–333
    with causal filter, 311, 321
    with finite number of poles, 312, 321
    with HS shaping function, 309, 311
    with matched filter, 269, 370
    with NRZ shaping function, 309, 311
    with Nyquist function system response, 306
    with raised cosine system response, 307, 308
    with SP shaping function, 309, 312
Anderson, J. B., 536
Anderson, R. R., 156, 257
Arthurs, E., 436, 469, 534
Aulin, T., 156, 157, 223, 224, 228, 256, 257, 536
Austin, M. C., 157, 175, 256, 491, 493, 534
Autocorrelation, 7, 76, 88, 100, 165, 166, 320–322
  of noise, 456
Average, 52–54, 60, 66, 72, 88, 218, 496
  conditional, 61, 62, 72
  energy per bit, 273, 324, 351
  energy per symbol, 272, 273, 347, 366
  error probability, 385
  of complex conjugate, 165
  of sum, 73
  of product, 160, 166, 218
  operation, 159
  power, 77, 79, 272, 347
  statistical, 160, 285

Bandwith, vii, viii, 18, 26, 36, 84, 105, 106, 132, 159, 249, 281, 282, 479, 531, 537, 617
  3-dB, 248, 314, 323, 349, 398, 406, 434
  99%, 170, 176, 199, 215, 222, 233, 251
  authorized channel, 246
  effective, 176
  efficiency, 176, 283
  excess, 261, 280, 283, 306, 537
  in which x% of power is contained, 162, 170, 174
  mask of, 159
  minimum, 249, 275, 279, 503, 537, 561
  narrow, 249
  noise equivalent filter, 475

normalised, 517
Nyquist, 279, 333
of baseband, 159, 170, 174, 175, 251
of Butterworth filter, 445
of channel, 101, 159, 247, 250, 644
of complex envelope, 161
of DPSK, 251
of filter, 28, 324
for digital radio, 246, 250
of FSK, 209, 214–216, 222
of LSK (ASK, OQASK, QASK), 170, 175, 180, 246, 251
of modulated signal, 160
of modulating signal, 109
of MSK, 251
of noise, 339
optimal, 403, 531
of PSK, 174, 178–180, 251
of raised cosine function, 280
of signal, 26
Barnett, W. T., 437
Baud, 102, 104, 259
Bayes rule
for probabilities, 42, 43
for probability densities, 58
for random vector, 69
Bayless, J. W., 341
Benedetto, S., 340, 436, 444, 445, 447, 468, 469, 632
Bennet, W. R., ix, 256, 437, 535
Berger, S. T., 579
Bessel function, 97, 344, 424, 456, 488
Biglieri, E. M., 340, 436, 444, 445, 447, 468, 469, 632
Biphase (BP). *See* Shaping function, biphase or split phase
BP–L, 637, 638
BP–M, 637, 638, 640
BP–S, 640
Bipolar code rule, 635, 649
violation of, 649
Bit Error Rate (BER), 273. *See* Error probability
Blanco, M. A., 339
Bobilin, R. T., 535
Borjesson, P. O., 339
Bowen, R. R., 607, 630, 631
Busgang, J. J., 469
Butterworth filter, 23, 92, 248, 250, 261, 315, 319, 322–324, 326, 330, 333, 335, 339, 348, 352, 360, 398–400, 403, 412, 432, 434, 445, 446, 456, 457, 462, 466–468, 491, 492, 497, 498, 514, 532, 533
3-dB bandwith of, 315
autocorrelation of output of, 332
residue of, 316
system with, 324, 326, 330, 348, 352, 387, 389, 390, 398, 399

Cable
coaxial, 101, 422, 634
telephone, 101, 634
multipair, 634
Cahn, C. R., 156, 468
Calandrino, L., 469
Carlson, A. B., 99
Carrier, 126
frequency, 126
local, 124
locally generated, 357
orthogonal, vii, 113
transmitted, 124
Castellani, V., 436, 447, 469
Cattermolle, K. W., 535
Cecchi, E., 631
Celebiler, M. I., 156, 339, 436, 468, 469
Chadwick, H. D., 534
Chan, D., 579
Chang, M. V., 157, 175, 256
Chang, R. W., 579, 630, 631
Channel, 101–103, 106, 259, 471
bandpass, 102, 103, 108
bandwith, 159
baseband, 101, 103
broadband, 108
coaxial cable, 422
copper wire, 422
quadrature, 117
radio, 422–424, 581
telephone, 106, 284, 584, 605, 608
transfer function, 424, 559
waveguide, 422
with flat fading, 422
with frequency selective fading, 360, 422
Chebyshev filter, 248, 250
Cherney, N. I., 535
Chernoff bound, 300, 301, 412
Ciapala, E., 606, 630
Click, 507, 520
noise, 514
Code, 104
Gray, 107
line. *See* line coding
Manchester, 106

Miller, 640
Coherent demodulation, 344
Cohn, J., 535
Collins, A. A., 341
Communication
analog, 249
digital, vii, 119, 559
satellite, vii, 119, 236
Communication system, vii, 1, 102–104, 249, 620, 634
ASK, 306, 557, 558
binary, 59, 95, 532
digital, vii, 1, 43, 89, 101, 104, 113, 159, 282, 550
Constellation
circular, ix, 115, 120, 357, 360, 365, 372, 382, 432, 439
general, 360, 375, 376
hexagonal, 381
of symbols, 114, 378, 380
optimal, 377
rectangular, 115, 357, 360, 365, 366, 368–382, 412, 432
symbol, 152
symmetrical, 173
triangular, 380–382
two dimensional, 356
Continuous Phase FSK (CPFSK). *See* FSK
Conversion
AM-to-AM, 236, 237, 255
AM-to-PM, 236, 237
Convolution, 6, 13, 18
Correlation, 1, 60, 76, 170, 496, 522, 622
cross, 7
of noise, 7, 11
Corsini, G., 632
Covariance, 60, 61, 66
matrix, 68, 73
Crippa, G., 469
Criterion
maximal eye opening, 627
mean square error, 429, 557, 582, 585, 589, 627
minimum error probability, 558, 561, 585
reasonable, 557, 576
zero forcing, 582, 584, 589
Croisier, A., 648, 655
Crosstalk, 634, 635, 653

Dalle Mese, G., 631, 632
Dante, H. M., 631
Davenport, W. B., 99
Davey, J. R., ix, 535
Davies, R. C., 536
Davisson, L. D., 630
De Buda, R., 156, 536
Debus, W., 655
Decibell (dB), 272, 478
Decision
device, 260, 473, 474, 585
feedback, 517, 537, 542, 545, 550, 552, 554
function, 264
interval, 43
regions, 259, 260, 262, 263, 265, 364, 365, 369, 372, 376, 410, 433, 482
rule, 261, 263, 264, 285, 334, 455, 475, 477, 480, 484, 494, 510, 521, 522, 533, 546, 547, 548–551, 619
De Jagger, F., 156
Dejon, B., 579
Dekker, C. B., 156
Demodulator, 103
Detection
coherent, 473
envelope, 473
noncoherent, 473
symbol by symbol, 260
Detector
coherent, 357
envelope, 483, 490
filter, 473, 484, 490–492, 505, 508, 531, 540
frequency, 473
integrate and dump, 311
matched filter, 398
sampling, 309–311, 316, 320–324, 333, 387, 412, 432
square law, 483, 490
De Vincentis, G., 340
Dieulus, V. A., 655
Differential Phase Shift Keying (DPSK), ix, 124–126, 138, 152, 439, 452
baseband equivalent model, 453
error probability in, 451, 461–466
ideal, 455
Digital Sum Variation (DSV), 634, 635, 644, 647, 649, 650, 653, 654
Discriminator, 474, 475, 494, 499, 511, 531
receiver, 474
Distortion, 617
excess, 615
minimum, 615
DiToro, B., 579
Diversity
frequency, 426

space, 426
time, 426
with maximal ratio combining, 426
with selection combining, 426, 427
Divsalar, D., 243, 256
Donaldson, R. W., 579
Doppler effect, 487
Duc, N. Q., 655
Durrani, S. H., 114, 156, 378, 382, 436
Duttweiler, D. C., 555
Dym, H., 469, 534

Efficiency, vii
factor of filter, 367
spectral, 281, 282, 396, 403, 433, 434, 441, 545, 552
Eigenvalue, 300, 593, 594, 596, 600, 608, 609, 629
Eigenvector, 300, 593, 629
Energy, 1, 6, 9, 10, 16, 19, 90, 91
average per bit, 324, 475
in shaping function, 324
of function, 267
of signal, viii, 424, 475, 565
Envelope, 26, 27, 37, 105, 116, 120, 152, 236
complex, 27, 30, 32, 34, 37, 93, 99, 105, 115–117, 119, 120, 141, 151, 234, 236, 238, 239, 354, 358, 439
constant, 249
Equalization, 260, 284, 285, 581
adaptive, 603
automatic, 603
conjugate gradient method, 609
fast adaptive algorithm of, 608
Fletcher-Powell method of, 609
nonlinear, ix, 582, 617, 628
of passband system, 610
steepest descent method of, 592, 593, 609
zero forcing, 610, 611
Equalizer, 284, 582, 584, 589, 610, 611, 627
adaptive, ix, 285, 581, 582, 604, 616
adaptive mode of, 603
automatic, ix, 285, 581, 582, 604, 616
composite, 586–589, 605, 607, 608, 627, 628
decision feedback, 586–589, 605, 627, 628
filter, 581
forward, 586, 588, 589, 605, 607, 608, 627–629
impulse response of, 582
Kalman filter, 589
linear, 622, 623, 626
nonlinear, 620, 626, 627
optimal, 627
recursive, 586, 587
training period of, 603
zero forcing, 616, 617, 628, 629
Ericson, T., 579
Error correction, 537, 552, 553
Error detection, 537, 552
Error monitoring, 550–552, 635, 645
Error probability, vii, viii, 102, 132, 138, 249, 261, 262, 269, 270, 272, 282, 286, 287, 290, 429, 537, 542, 543, 545, 547–549, 553, 554, 559, 561, 586, 587, 619, 626, 634, 635
bounds to, viii, 261, 415–418, 542, 543, 550
nominal, 429
of bit, 307
of symbol, 102, 260, 263
Error probability of ASK, 273–275, 366
bound by finite number of terms, 293
bounds and approximation of Jenq, 302
bounds on dependent symbols, Chernoff bounds, 300, 301
for system with Nyquist filter, 306–308
in system with Butterwoth filters, 324–332
Legendre series expansion, 295
lower bound to, 294
of finite number of terms, 291
Taylor series expansion, 295
upper bound, 293, 294
using bounds to probability density, 300
using quadrature formula, 297, 298
with ISI, 286, 290, 351
with nonsymmetric bandpass filter, 349
worst case bound, 292, 293
without ISI, 272–275
Error probability of DPSK
bounds to, 461, 464, 465
in ideal system, 451
with ISI, 464–466
without ISI, 463, 465
Error probability of FSK, 480–482, 485, 488, 495, 499, 505, 517, 518, 531, 532
binary, 483, 500, 501
upper bound to, 480, 481
wideband, 488–494
with coherent detector, 478, 479
with discriminator detector, 511–516
with envelope detector, 485, 486, 490
with noncoherent detector, 486
with square law detector, 488–494
Error probability of MSK, 399–408
effect of ACI and ISI, 408

with Butterworth filters, 389, 400
with nonnegative impulse response, 403–408
Error probability of OQASK, 360, 365, 378, 399
bounds to, 377
effect of interference, 382, 384–386, 390, 391, 396, 398–402, 404, 406–408
effect of phase offset, 389, 390
in system with Butterworth filters, 307, 389, 390, 399–403
in system with Nyquist filters, 386–388
with circular constellation, 360, 365, 370, 373, 374
with general constellation, 360, 365, 375–380
with quaternary symbols, 370, 374
with rectangular constellation, 360, 366, 368
Error probability of PSK, 122, 371, 395, 442–447, 451, 483
bounds to, 373, 442
extension of bounds of Jenq, 413
in ideal system, 451
with Nyquist filter, 395, 418, 420, 422
Error probability of QASK, 360, 365, 378, 394, 395, 470, 476
bounds to, 373
effect of ACI and ISI, 390, 391, 396
effect of interference, 382, 384–386
effect of phase offset, 388, 390
effect of QCI and ISI, 384
in system with Butterworth filterrs, 387, 390
in system with circular constellation, 360, 370, 373, 374, 394
in system with general constellation, 360, 375–380
in system with Nyquist filer, 386–388, 394, 395
in system with Rayleigh fading, 425, 426
in system with rectangular constellation, 360, 366–368
with quaternary symbols, 370, 374, 376
Error propagation, 537, 552, 642
Estimate
of gradient, 598
unbiased, 615
Euclidian distance, 262, 522
Event, 40, 44, 50, 62, 66
joint, 56
Eye diagram, 288–290, 293, 308
opening, 288, 559, 584, 585
Fading, 424, 425, 492
diversity for, 426
flat, 422, 424, 433
frequency selective, 360, 422, 427, 581
radio channel, 423
Rayleigh, 425
Fang, J. R., 156, 436, 437, 468, 469
Fast FSK (FFSK). *See* MSK and FSK
Feeny, S. L., 579
Feher, K., 157, 437, 469, 555
Filter, viii, 1, 2, 24, 491, 492, 503, 604. *See also* systems
bandlimiting, 22, 93
bandpass, viii, 1, 2, 23, 26–29, 32, 33, 37, 84, 85, 89, 93, 103, 112, 233–235, 344, 345, 349, 357, 473
baseband, 1, 2, 26–29, 89, 93, 94, 103, 259
baseband equivalent, viii, 30–33, 37, 38, 345, 358, 473
brick wall, 487, 517
Butterworth, 23, 314, 316, 387, 491, 492. *See also* Butterworth filter
causal, 20, 23, 310, 311, 321, 503
channel, 259, 311, 357
Chebyshev, 248, 250
demodulator, 103
detector, 259–261, 309, 320, 345, 357, 475, 476, 484, 487, 488, 492, 540
efficiency factor of, 367
equalizing, 259
fixed, 284
Gaussian, 406
ideal, 23, 28, 79, 84, 85, 500
linear, 1, 19, 20, 89, 233, 246, 422
lowpass, 23, 28, 79, 112, 113, 349
matched, 260, 261, 269, 309–311, 316, 324, 332, 334, 350, 387, 403, 473, 475, 477, 487, 505, 543, 564, 581
memoryless, 235
narrowband, 1, 37, 398
nonlinear, 235
bandpass, 233
receiver, 103, 259, 261, 271, 284, 309, 311, 312, 357, 398, 403, 422, 487, 499, 500, 517
response to sinusoid, 21
shaping, 259
SSB, 30, 31, 37, 38, 109
symmetric, 30, 38
time invariant, 19, 20, 422
time variant, 24
transfer function of, 20, 28
transmitter, 103, 259, 261, 309, 311, 312,

349, 357, 398, 403, 422, 475, 514
transversal, ix, 564, 577, 581, 583, 585, 588, 589, 611, 621
variable, 284
VSB, 30, 31, 37, 38, 109, 112
with finite number of poles, 312, 321
Fletcher-Powell method, 629
Forney, G. D., 536, 555, 632
Foschini, G. J., 156, 436, 631
Fourier series, 1, 10, 89–91, 165, 235, 456, 515
cooficients, 10, 517, 563
Fourier Transform (FT), viii, 11–17, 20, 28, 35, 37, 78, 81, 89, 91, 95, 106, 109–111, 159, 161, 163, 164, 166, 169, 170, 177, 186, 199, 224, 240, 259, 260, 312, 391, 502, 582, 583
Double (DFT), 167
Inverse (IFT), 11–13, 28, 35, 36, 111, 267, 283, 427
of signals, 12
pair, 11–13
properties of, 12
Single (SFT), 167, 177, 187, 193, 195, 209, 211, 219, 220
Franaszek, P. A., 655
Frederick, D. K., 99
Frequency, viii, 2, 22, 124
3–dB, 23
band, 101, 108
carrier, 30, 33, 103, 108, 126, 160, 235, 471
center, 101, 103, 473, 483
deviation, 126, 127, 132, 198, 472
average, 129
maximum, 473
normalised, 129, 171, 198, 199, 202, 482, 500, 517, 531
optimal, 531
instantanous, 126, 127
modulation, 507
microwave, 429
notch, 427, 429
Nyquist, 405
separation, 430, 511
Frequency Shift Keying (FSK), viii, ix, 109, 119, 126, 127, 128, 130, 141, 142, 144, 151, 152, 154, 155, 166, 403, 471–473, 478, 479, 507, 511, 517
as MSK, 133
binary, 130
coherent, ix, 473, 477, 476, 479, 481, 524, 532
optimal, 531, 532
orthogonal, 479, 532
error probability. *See* error probability of FSK
Fast (FFSK), 133
multi-h, 132, 133
narrowband, ix, 473, 474, 476, 531
noncoherent, ix, 473, 476, 483, 524, 531, 532
with envelope detector, 483, 487
orthogonal, 476, 479, 481, 524, 532
quaternary, 127
sinusoidal (SFSK), 119, 226
wide band, ix, 473, 474, 531
with continuous phase (CPFSK), 126, 127, 129
with discriminator, ix, 473, 474, 476, 494, 498, 503, 520, 531, 533
and detector filter, ix, 505, 507, 510, 511, 514–518
with noncontinous phase, 130, 131, 472
with observation interval larger than T, 520, 524–530
with PRS, 145
Fritchman, B. D., 631
Function, 2, 43
bandpass, 29, 30, 36
baseband equivalent, 35
brick wall, 537
causal, 271, 288
characteristic, 53, 538
concave, 338
continuous, 50, 220
convex, 611
decreasing, 50, 52
delta, 15
even, 11, 78, 84, 87, 173, 279
exponential, 2, 48
hypergeometric, 488
impulse, 2, 20, 45, 47, 111, 475, 582
increasing, 50, 52
inverse, 50
linear, 51, 126
nonlinear, 235, 413
odd, 11, 38, 47, 53, 54, 83, 84
orthogonal, 8, 90, 296
orthonormal, 9
periodic, 11, 90, 165, 277, 560, 562, 582
piecewise linear, 611
raised cosine, 280, 281, 576, 625, 626
ramp, 272
real, 11, 35, 279
sign, 2
sinusoid, 2, 21, 22
unit step, 2, 103, 111, 173, 235, 471

Garrison, C. Y., 214, 215, 222, 256
Gatkin, N. G., 535
Gauss, R. C., 257
Gaussian
curve, 443
filter, 360, 406, 434, 435, 517, 518, 532
system with, 408, 432
function, 295, 559
probability density, 266
Gaussian noise, 88, 260–262, 267, 290, 292, 294, 295, 300, 301, 345, 366, 375, 404, 432, 435, 477, 494, 540, 547, 557, 582, 583, 617, 620
nonwhite, 286, 292
white, 99, 260, 358, 473
Gaussian random process, 75, 77, 80, 82, 98, 360, 505
autocorrelation of, 77, 88
average of, 77
independent, 87, 360
uncorrelated, 87
Gaussian random variable, 48, 51, 54, 96, 97, 265, 267, 439, 441, 448, 462, 474, 478, 480, 483, 488, 494, 519, 622, 628
average value of, 54
characteristic function of, 54
complex, 447
independent, 61, 69
jointly, 57, 61
linear function of, 51
pdf, 75, 266
transformation of, 64
uncorrelated, 61, 69
variance of, 54
Gaussian random vector, 68, 74, 97, 618
characteristic function of, 74
covariance matrix of, 68
linear transformation of, 70, 71
George, D. A., 578, 607, 630
Geranim, V. A., 535
Gersho, A., 630
Gibson, E. D., 629
Giger, A. J., 437
Gitlin, R. D., 156, 436, 556, 630, 631
Glave, F. E., 340
Glenn, A. B., 489, 490, 534
Goddard, D., 632
Golub, G. H., 340
Gonsalves, R. A., 631
Gorog, E., 630, 655
Gradient
estimate, 594
noise, 598–600
noisy, 628
Gray code, 104, 273, 274
two-dimensional, 368
Greenstein, L. J., 179, 190, 247, 256, 257, 437
Green, T. A., 655
Gronemeyer, S. A., 156
Guida, A., 655
Guili, D., 631
Gulko, P., 157
Gumacos, G., 631
Gun, J. F., 555

Hancock, J. C., 631
Hansler, G., 579
Harada, V., 157
Harashima, H., 555
Harley, T. J., 631
Hermite plynomial, 295
Hilbert Transform (HT), viii, 1, 24, 25, 89, 92
of bandpass signal, 25
of signals, 25
of sinusoid, 24
Hill, F. S., 339
Hirade, K., 436
Ho, E. Y., 339, 436, 556, 630, 631
Hoffman, E., 535
Holzman, E., 629
Houts, R. C., 655
Howson, R. D., 555
Hubbard, W. M., 469

Immovili, G., 469
Impulse response, 19, 20, 35, 94, 98, 99, 429, 582
of bandpass filter, 30
of baseband filter, 30
of channel filter, 311, 357, 581
of receiver filter, 311, 357, 581
of transmitter filter, 311, 357, 581
Integrate and dump circuit, 475, 505
Interference, vii, 122, 382, 383. *See also* ACI, ISI, QCI
cochannel, 466
effect of, 382, 408
from adjacent channel, 159, 345, 357, 359
intersymbol, 359
quadrature channel, 359
Intersymbol Interference (ISI), viii, ix, 249, 260, 271, 279, 282, 285–289, 292, 306, 316, 332, 333, 335, 359, 362, 364, 383, 390, 403, 413, 416, 432, 439, 443, 450, 463, 491, 494,

502, 511, 513, 518, 531–533, 537, 544, 552, 559, 570, 575, 578, 584, 586, 623, 624, 626, 634
as random variable, 285, 286
controlled, 540
degradation by, 407, 408
effect on eye diagram, 288, 289, 290
elimination of, 541, 544, 545
maximal, 559
Nyquist condition for no, 275
probability density of, 285, 291
properties of, 286
ranking of terms of, 287
Ishizuka, M., 436

Jacobian, 63, 64, 70, 299
Jacobs, I. M., ix, 536
Jain, P. C., 535
Jelonek, Z. J., 606, 630
Jensen's inequality, 338
Jenq, Y. C., 302, 340, 413, 436
Jenq's
bounds, 302
extension of, 411
method, 411
Jitter, 288, 290
in sampling time, 281, 335
Johannes, V. I., 655
Johnson, C. R., 631

Kabal, P., 157, 555
Kabaswa, S., 468
Kaim, A. G., 655
Kalet, I., 156
Kalman filter, 589, 628
Karnovsky, M. I., 535
Kaufman, H., 632
Klapper, J., 535
Kobayashi, H., 555, 655
Korn, I., 140, 157, 230, 232, 256, 257, 319, 323, 325–327, 329–331, 339–341, 352, 354, 389, 390, 399, 408, 436, 437, 535, 536, 556, 570, 579
Krasnyy, L. G., 535
Kretzmer, E. R., 555
Krishnamurthy, J., 631
Kuo, F. K., 341, 354
Kwon, S. Y., 534
Kwong, K. C. K., 631

Lagrange multiplier, 571
Laplace
pdf, 48
random variable, 48
Laplace Transform (LT), viii, 1, 16–18, 89, 92, 312, 315
Inverse (ILT), 17, 19, 314
properties of, 17, 18
Larimore, M. G., 631
Lawrence, R. E., 632
Legendre series, 296–298
coeficients, 297
expansion, 412
polynomials, 10, 297
Leiter, M., 469
Lender, A., 555
Le-Ngoc, T., 157
L'Hopital's rule, 188
Likelihood ratio, 619, 622
Limiter
bandpass, 490, 497
hard, 152, 236, 237, 244, 246, 255
soft, 152, 255
Lind, L. F., 341
Lindsey, W. C., x, 354, 534
Linear Shift Keying (LSK), 108, 109, 142, 144, 148, 151, 152, 233, 249, 355, 441, 618
bandpass system, 260
with PRS, 148
Line code, 106, 635, 653
4B–3T, 635, 645, 646, 654
alphabetic, 635, 644, 645, 647, 653
Alternative Mark Inversion (AMI), 642
binary, 635, 643
bipolar, 635, 642–644, 648, 653, 654
BnZS, 635, 648, 649, 651, 654
CHDBn, 635, 648, 650, 652
Delay Modulation (DM), 640, 641, 653
duobinary, 642, 643, 653, 654
FOMOT, 647, 654
HDBn, 635, 649, 651, 652, 654
linear ternary, 635
modified duobinary, 642–644, 653
MS43, 635, 645, 646, 648, 649, 654
multilevel, 653
nonalphabetic, 635, 649, 653
nonlinear, 644, 649
properties of, 652
PSD of, 634–640, 642–644, 647–649, 652–654
pseudoternary, 642, 644
PST, 635, 645, 648, 649, 654
ternary, 641, 643, 653
TIBn, 635, 650, 654

TPC, 651
transition diagram of, 641
twinned binary, 642, 644, 653, 654
variable length, 647, 651
zero substitution, 635, 644, 649
Line coding, 106, 633, 635
Liu, B., 340, 436
Lombardi, J. A., 555
Lucky, R. W., x, 534, 629, 630
Lugannani, R., 340
Lundgren, C. W., 437
Luntz, M. B., 536
Luvison, A., 340
Lytle, D. W., 630

Macleod, C. J., 606, 630
Magee, F. R., 632
Manchester code, 104
Mark, J. W., 632
Markov chain, 543
Marcum, Y. I., 469
Marcum function, 462, 497
Martinelli, G., 631
Mask
emission, 246–249
Matched filter, 260, 261, 269, 283, 284, 334, 348, 620, 621, 625
as correlator, 271
as integrate and dump circuit, 271
bank of, 473, 477
detection, 445
detector, 398
for HS, 334
for NRZ, 270, 334, 487
for SP, 270, 334
realization, 271
Matrix, 63, 614
correlation, 648
covariance, 68, 73, 598, 599
diagonal, 594–596
inverse, 591
positive definite, 594
symmetric, 590
Matthews, J. W., 340
Maximum Apoteriori (MAP) decision rule, 332
Maximum Likelihood (ML)
decision region, 365
decision rule, 261, 263, 264, 333, 364, 521, 533, 619
decoder, 537
Mazo, J. E., 535, 555, 630, 631
McBride, A. C., 156
McCool, J. M., 631
McLane, P. J., 340
Mean square error, 429, 557, 561, 567, 570, 572, 576, 590, 591, 593, 597, 601, 605–607
excess, 600, 601, 628, 629
minimum, 559, 566, 569, 574–576, 578, 592, 599, 602
Messershmitt, D. G., 555
Miller, J. H., 630
Miller coding, 640
Milstein, L. B., 493, 534
Minimum Shift Keying (MSK), ix, 119, 133, 134, 137, 139, 141–143, 149–151, 154, 155, 224, 387, 403
as a form of DPSK, 138
as a special case of FSK, 133
binary, 138, 224
effect of ISI and ACI, 408
error probability, 399–402
equivalence to modified OQASK, 138
equivalence to quaternary OQASK, 134, 137
general, 229
M-ary, 134, 138
quaternary, 140, 231, 232
with Butterworth filters, 389, 399–402
with duobinary shaping function, 150
Miyakawa, H., 555
Modulation, 26, 104, 105, 108, 141, 144, 471
amplitude, 104
delay, 640, 641, 653
digital, viii, 271
frequency, 104
methods, viii, 119, 148
nonlinear, 144
phase, 236
Modulator, 103
quadrature, 344
Monsen, D., 630
Montgomery, G. F., 534
Mori, S., 157
Morinaga, N., 468
Muellar, R. W., 631
Muilwijk, D., 256
Muller, K. H., 630
Murphy, J, V., 340

Nader, S. E., 341
Namekawa, T., 468
Namet, M., 352, 354
Nelson, E. A., 535

Newcombe, E. A., 339
Newhall, E. E., 632
Nicholson, G., 632
Niessen, C. W., 630
Noise, 75, 88, 89, 122
autocorrelation of, 370
bandwith, 339
bandpass, 84, 85, 87–89
baseband, 79, 84, 85, 87, 88
baseband equivalent, 85, 88, 98
circularly symmetric, 481
complex envelope of, 89
Gaussian, 88, 99, 262, 358, 404, 540, 547
gradient, 598, 600
impulse, 466
margin, 288
variance of, 320, 566
vector, 365, 480
white, 88, 99, 358, 442
Nonlinearity, 236
bandpass, 233, 235, 237–239
complex, 236
memoryless, 233, 237, 238
No-Return to Zero (NRZ), 634, 636, 637. *See also* Shaping function NRZ
NRZ-L, 636, 637, 653
NRZ-M, 636, 637, 653
NRZ-S, 636, 637, 653
Norton, J. P., 632
Nuttal, D. H., 256
Nyquist
bandwith, 278–280, 333
condition of no ISI, 261, 275, 276
filter, 284, 348, 403, 476
frequency, 276, 405, 537
function, 276, 277, 280, 282, 283, 306, 332, 334, 406, 434, 454, 462, 537, 538
function approximation, 332
interval, 560–562, 577
square root of, 456
system response, 306
system with, 386, 388, 391, 418, 420, 422, 432
transfer function, 353

Oberst, T. F., 156
Oetting, T. D., 156
Offset Quadrature Amplitude Shift Keying (OQASK), ix, 117–120, 134, 137–139, 142, 143, 148, 151–155, 249, 355, 369, 384, 387, 432, 433, 502
bandpass system, 355
baseband equivalent system, 358, 359
bounds to error probability, 373
condition of no interference, 360
constellation for, 366, 367, 370, 373, 375, 377
decision regions, 364, 376, 410
effect of interference, 382, 384, 390, 391, 396, 398–402, 404, 406, 408
effect of phase offset, 389
equivalence to ASK, 369
equivalence to MSK, 119, 387
error probability of, 365, 378, 399
maximum likelihood decision rule, 364
modified, 138–141
symbol constellation, 356
system with Butterworth filter, 387, 390, 399
system with no interference, 364
system with Nyquist filter, 386
with coherent detector, 357
with constant envelope, 119
with PRS, 148
Offset Quadrature PSK (OQPSK), 122, 226. *See also* OQASK
O'Mahony, M. J., 535
Omura, J. K., 632
On-Of Keying (OOK), 333
Optical fiber, 101
Optimization
criteria, 557, 559
of receiver, 567, 569
of transmitter, 569
system, 557
Orlandi, G., 631
Osborne, W. P., 536
Oscillator, 132
Oshita, S., 469

Papantoni-Kazakos, P., 535
Papoulis, A., 99
Park, J. H., 631
Partial Response Signal (PRS), ix, 104, 144, 146, 147, 174, 520, 537-540, 543, 546, 550, 552, 576. *See also* Shaping function PRS
characteristic polynomial of, 538, 539, 552, 554
dicode, 538, 541, 542
duobinary, 538, 539, 541, 542, 544–546, 548–552, 554, 577
impulse response of, 539
modified duobinary, 538–542, 544, 555, 567, 577
polybinary, 538

precoding of, 537, 552
transfer function of, 539
Parseval's formula, 16
Pasupathy, S., 156, 157, 339, 555, 556
Pawula, R. F., 459, 460, 469, 535
Paz, I. M., 535
Pederson, R. D., 341
Pelchat, M. G., 536
Phan Van, H., 157
Phase, viii, 2–4, 22, 26, 33, 103, 115, 120, 123, 124, 236, 239, 471, 475
absolute, 138
coherence, 124
continuous, 249, 472
deviation, 156
difference, 125, 138, 150
instantanous, 126
Locked Loop (PLL), 345
modulation, 236
noise, 505, 506
offset, 410
path, 130
random, 160, 357
split, 505
trajectory, 130, 521, 524
transition, 132, 133
tree, 130–134, 155, 156
trellis, 133, 134, 151, 155
Phase Shift Keying (PSK), ix, 109, 115, 121, 124, 130, 141, 142, 144, 149, 151, 154–156, 166, 373, 374, 394, 412, 428, 432, 434, 439, 441, 478, 479, 482, 517. *See also* QASK with circular constellation
baseband model of, 439, 440
effect of interference, 408
error probability of, 420, 442–447, 451
equivalence to LSK, 441
equivalence to QASK, 122, 441
Quaternary (QPSK), 122, 123, 531
signatures of, 430, 431
with frequency selective fading, 428
with Nyquist function response, 388, 420
with PRS, 149
with various shaping functions, 443–447
Pierobon, G. L., 257, 655
Pof, E., 629
Poisson random variable, 48
probability, 532
process, 507
Pollak, H. O., 256
Popolin, S. G., 655
Power, 1, 6, 602
average, 77, 79, 87, 272
contained in bandwith, 161
efficient, 119
inband, 162, 199, 204
in line components, 181, 191, 192
normalized, 162, 247, 248
out-of-band, 171, 175, 180, 185, 186, 225–227, 229–232, 234
outside bandwidth, 162, 170
total, 162
transmitted, 247
Power spectral Density (PSD), 1, 78–81, 85, 88, 89, 98, 99, 105, 106, 159, 160, 165, 166, 321, 359, 473, 557, 578, 582, 617, 620
of ASK, 169–173, 175, 184, 190–193, 345
of baseband signal, 152, 168–171, 174, 253
of complex envelope, 159, 161, 162
of FSK, 170, 171, 175, 194, 198–208, 213–216, 222–224
of line codes, 634–640, 642–644, 647–649, 652–654
of LSK, 172
of modulated signal, 152, 161, 162
of MSK, 224–230, 234
of optimal signal, 175
of OQASK, 173
with hard limiter, 243, 244, 246
with nonlinear bandpass filter, 233, 238
of PSK, 174, 177, 178–186, 188–194, 273
of QASK, 173
with hard limiter, 240, 242
with nonlinear bandpass filter, 233, 238
of white noise, 273, 443
Prabhu, V. K., 156, 256, 339, 340, 436, 437, 446, 468, 469
Precoding, 532, 552
Proakis, J. G., 630–632
Probability, 40–44, 47, 57, 59, 66, 68, 70, 75, 91
a posteriori, 43
a priori, 43
joint, 108
marginal, 108
of erasure, 95
of error, 95
of event, 56
of joint event, 56
of symbol, 196
Probability density function (pdf), 45–48, 50, 52–54, 64, 72, 75, 88, 95, 97, 357, 447, 487, 508, 618
binary, 48

binomial, 48
conditional, 58, 69, 95
exponential, 48
Gaussian, 48, 266, 447
joint, 56, 68, 76, 96, 97, 439, 509
Laplace, 48
marginal, 68
normal, 48, 49, 54, 266
of frequency, 495
of phase, 505
of phase difference, 344, 459, 509
of product, 65
of sum, 64, 71
of vector, 67, 71
Poisson, 48
Rayleigh, 48, 449
Rician, 449, 484
uniform, 48, 96
Probability Distribution Function (PDF), 44–46, 50, 56, 57, 95, 495, 496, 508
Complementary (CPDF), 45, 49, 50
conditioned on event, 58
joint, 56, 62
marginal, 56
of vector, 57
Prolate spheroidal wave function, 175, 229
Pseudorandom sequence, 515, 517
Pulleyblank, R. W., 631
Pulse, 487
BP, 638
Code Modulation (PCM), 633, 634
NRZ, 122, 472, 475, 505, 638, 641
Position Modulation (PPM), 141
rectangular, 2, 103
Pupolin, S. G., 257

Quadrature Amplitude Modulation (QAM), viii, 114. *See* QASK
Quadrature Amplitude Shift Keying (QASK), viii, x, 113, 115, 116, 119, 122, 142, 148, 151, 152, 249, 307, 355, 369, 384, 387, 394, 430–434, 438
bandpass system, 355
baseband equivalent system, 358, 359, 363
bounds to error probability, 373
condition of no interference, 360
decision regions, 364, 376, 410
effect of ACI and ISI, 390, 391, 396
effect of interference, 382, 408
effect of phase offset, 388, 390
effect of QCI and ISI, 384
equivalence to ASK, 369
equivalence to PSK, 357, 373
error probability of 365, 378, 394, 395, 420, 426
with circular constellation, 370, 373, 394
with general constellation, 375
with rectangular constellation, 366, 367
in digital radio, 430
maximum likelihood decision rule, 364
optimal constellation, 377
outage area of, 431
signatures of 430, 431
symbol constellation of, 356, 357
system with Butterworth filter, 387, 390
system with no interference, 364
system with Nyquist filter, 386, 388, 422
with coherent detection, 357
with flat fading, 422
with frequency selective fading, 422, 427, 428
with Rayleigh fading, 423, 425, 426
Quadrature Channel Interference (QCI), ix, 359, 363, 364, 390, 403, 430, 432
Qureshi, S. U. H., 632

Rabsel, N., 156
Radio
digital, vii, 246, 247, 249, 429
Raised cosine family, 261, 280, 281, 306, 332, 430. *See also* Nyquist function, Shaping function
excess bandwith of 280, 307, 308
spectral efficiency of, 281, 282
Random process (rp), 1, 2, 74, 75, 79, 82, 108
autocorrelation of, 76–80, 83, 88–90, 98
average of, 76, 77, 88, 98
bandpass, 1, 2, 84, 99
baseband, 1, 2, 80, 84
coloured, 79
complex, 160
cross-correlation of, 77, 81, 83, 89
cyclostationary, 160, 162
Gaussian, 75, 77, 82, 87, 88, 98, 360
independent, 87, 160, 360
narrowband, 84
stationary, 75–77, 108
variance of 98
white, 79, 80
wide sense stationary (wss), 76–79, 83, 108, 160, 251
Random variable (rv), 1, 2, 38, 43–45, 50, 52, 55, 59, 62, 66, 73, 75, 80, 98, 357, 600
average of, 52–54, 60, 66, 72, 98

binary, 137, 241, 301, 414
characteristic function of 53–55
complex, 2, 65, 165, 439, 447, 448, 461
conditional average of, 61, 62
continuous (crv), 1, 47, 51, 53, 57
covariance of, 66
discrete (drv), 1, 47, 51–53, 57, 59, 68, 75, 96
discrete transformation of, 52
dispersion of, 53
equiprobable, 137, 241, 287, 290, 404
even, 266
exponential, 301
function of, 50
Gaussian, 51, 61, 64, 68, 69, 75, 80, 95–97, 363, 423, 439, 441, 447, 448
independent, 60, 61, 65, 68, 69, 72–75, 82, 96–98, 137, 241, 286, 287, 290, 405, 412, 423, 441, 448, 488, 497, 533
joint characteristic function of, 62
jointly Gaussian, 57
mixed, 47, 68
moment of, 53, 54, 60, 62, 487
normal, 50, 55
standard deviation of, 53
symmetric, 266, 285, 409
transformation of, 62, 63, 69
uncorrelated, 61, 66, 69, 80, 82, 98
variance of, 53–55, 64, 66, 98
Random vector, 2, 66, 67, 69, 70–75, 97
average of 69, 72
characteristic function of, 74
Gaussian, 70, 71, 74, 75, 97
orthogonal, 74
transformation of, 69, 70
uncorrelated, 74
Rappaport, M. A., 629
Rate
bit, 104, 174, 276, 281, 282
bit error, 104, 273. *See also* error probability
symbol, 104, 174. *See also* baud
symbol error, 104. *See also* error probability
Rayleigh
fading, 425
pdf, 48, 63, 435, 449
random variable, 48, 63, 449
Razin, B., 157
Receiver, ix, 101, 103, 106, 126, 474, 519
coherent, ix, 521
decision feedback, 542
filter, 473, 487, 499, 500, 517, 582, 617
noncoherent, 473, 474
nonlinear, 621
optimal, ix, 477, 557, 561, 562, 564, 565, 567–570, 572, 574, 575, 578, 581, 582, 603, 621
Repeater, 634
Rice "click" theory, 507
Rice, S. O., 469, 535
Rician random variable, 449
Roberts, J. H., 469, 535
Rosenbaum, A. S., 156, 469
Rowe, H. E., 256
Rudin, H. R., 630
Rummler, W. D., 437
Running Digital Sum (RDS), 634, 645, 653, 654
Rydbeck, N., 223, 224, 228, 256, 536

Saleh, A. A. M., 256
Salermo, M., 631
Saltzberg, B. S., 340
Salz, J., x, 156, 256, 468, 534, 535, 630
Sample space, 38, 43
Sampling time, 405, 494
offset, 331
optimal, 316
Sasase, I., 157
Schilling, D. L., 156, 535
Schonfield, T. J., 630
Schonhoff, T. A., 156, 527, 536
Schwartz, M., ix, 437, 535, 630
Schwartz inequality, 7, 8, 269, 337, 563
Series, 8
Fourier, 8
orthogonal, 8
Set, 38, 121
complementary, 38, 39
disjoint, 39
empty, 38
intersection of, 38, 39
M-ary, 471
subset, 38, 40, 43
symbol, 263
symmetric, 290
union of, 38, 39
Seth, B., 389, 399, 436
Settling time, 597, 605, 606, 608–610, 628, 629
average, 597, 600
Shaping function, viii, 103–105, 113, 122, 129, 137, 140, 141, 143, 147, 148, 150, 154, 155, 170, 171, 471, 638
Biphase (BP), 106

common, 104, 105, 169, 172, 175, 177, 187, 194, 197, 213, 221, 224, 231, 344, 635
complex, 111
constant envelope, 119
duobinary, 144, 146, 148, 150, 188, 213–215, 254
equivalent, 105, 138, 141, 144, 146, 152
full response, 103, 105, 106
Half Sinusoidal (HS), 106, 115, 116, 119, 120, 139, 144, 146, 152, 154, 155, 170–172, 183, 185, 190, 313, 334, 396
modified duobinary, 144, 272, 254
noncommon, 231
Non Return to Zero (NRZ), 106, 115, 123, 125, 127–129, 132–134, 137–140, 151, 155, 170–175, 178, 180, 183, 185, 313, 334, 350, 357, 396, 412, 443, 445, 471, 515, 524, 532, 635
nonoverlapping, 103, 104, 106, 139, 173, 466
of duration 2T, 177, 194
of duration KT, 216
of duration T, 177, 194
optimal, 175–177, 186
optimization of, 175
overlapping, 104, 144, 145, 147, 173, 177, 249, 439
Partial Response (PRS), 104, 144, 146, 147, 174, 520
PPM, 232
Raised Cosine (RC), 106, 144, 155, 170, 171, 183, 184, 190–192, 215, 216, 222–228, 443, 446, 447, 467, 625, 626
Return to Zero (RZ), 106, 107, 155, 170, 334
rectangular, 183, 185, 439, 446, 447, 466
Split Phase (SP), 106, 121, 130, 154, 313, 533
symbol dependent, 139, 141
trapezoidal, 182, 184
Triangular (TR), 106, 107, 130, 131, 145, 170, 171, 182, 184, 189, 190, 443, 446
Sheehan, J. R., 555
Shehadeh, N. M., 534
Shimbo, O., 156, 339, 436, 437, 468, 469
Signal, 1, 2, 12, 18, 35
analog, 633
analytic, 25, 37, 89, 93
bandpass, viii, 1, 2, 26, 27, 32, 33, 36, 89, 101, 103, 111, 124, 236, 347
baseband, viii, 1, 2, 26, 36, 89, 101–103, 105–108, 110, 113, 121, 124, 126–108, 139, 144, 145, 148, 150, 152–156, 168, 170, 234, 471, 635
baseband equivalent, viii, 33, 37
carrier, viii, 103, 104, 471
causal, 4, 6
complex, 2, 3, 13
constant envelope, 249, 432
correlative level, 146, 537
demodulated, 357
deterministic, 1–3, 89
digital, 75, 631, 634
duobinary. *See* Partial Response Signal
electromagnetic, 101
flow graph, 647
full response, 537
imaginary, 4, 13
impulse, 20
inphase, 4, 172
interfering, 357
lowpass, 101
modified duobinary. *See* Partial Response Signal
modulated, viii, 14, 101–105, 108–113, 119, 120, 123, 124, 128, 130, 141, 148, 150, 152, 154, 155, 249, 452, 471
modulating, 109, 515
multilevel, 541
narrowband, 1
nonoverlapping, 105
orthogonal, 476, 479, 480, 531
path, 506
periodic, 1, 5, 6, 14, 90, 515
PRS. *See* Partial Response Signal
quadrature, 4, 172
raised cosine, 570, 575
random, viii, 81, 89, 515
real, 2, 4, 13, 16, 20, 25, 26, 109
spectrally efficient, ix, 537
SSB, 110, 111
transmitted, 475
VSB, 110, 112
Signature of
PSK, 430, 431
QASK, 430, 431
Signal-to-noise ratio, vii, viii, 272, 307, 324, 344, 367, 442, 459, 460, 475, 476, 478, 482, 488, 508, 511, 518, 522, 523, 537, 543, 549, 552, 553, 569, 570, 575, 584, 617, 624, 626
degradation, 407, 543
penalty in, 545
Simon, M. K., x, 156, 225–227, 230, 243, 256, 354, 534, 630

Singh, H., 535
Single Side Band (SSB), 161. *See* ASK-SSB
Sipress, J. M., 655
Slepian, P., 256
Smith, B. M., 555
Smith, E. F., 534
Smith, J. G., 156
Smith, J. W., 340, 553, 555, 579
Source, 101–103
  binary, 104, 115, 117
Spilker, J. J., 354
Spaulding, D. A., 631
Springett, J. C., 534
Staggered QASK (SQASK), 115. *See* OQASK
State
  diagram, 551
  steady, 600
  transition, 551
Stegun, I. A., 339
Stein, S., ix, 437, 463, 469, 534, 535
Stiffler, J. J., x
Stochastic process, 89. *See* random process
Storey, J. R., 607, 630
Sundberg, C. E. W., 156, 157, 223, 224, 228, 256, 257, 339, 536
Svenson, A., 157
Symbols, viii, 43, 95, 101, 121, 137
  average value of, 108
  binary, 104, 107, 115, 127, 133, 137, 138, 141, 146, 148, 150, 383, 471, 481, 503, 551
  complex, 113, 114, 122
  constellation, 113, 172
  dependent, 306
  equiprobable, 108, 168, 169, 172, 173, 194, 197, 221
  independent, 108, 168, 169, 187, 194, 210, 213, 218, 259, 383, 471, 581
  M-ary, 101, 104, 113, 135, 259, 618
  mean square value of, 108
  multilevel, 306
  precoded, 554
  quaternary, 107, 115, 122, 126, 127, 139, 152, 154, 155, 215, 365
  random, 108
  rate, 102, 127
  source, 125
  stationarity of, 166, 167
  stationary, 163, 165, 166
  symmetric set of, 172
  transmitted, 124
  two dimensional, 113
  uncorrelated, 169, 170
  vector of, 146
Synchronization, vii, viii, ix, 106
  carrier, 344
  circuit, 345
  non linear timing circuit, 282
  phase, ix, 344
  timing, viii, 282
System, 1, 9, 20. *See also* filter
  bandpass, 88, 108, 349
  baseband, 88, 108
  baseband equivalent, 35, 94, 349
  digital radio, 552
  linear, 1, 19, 20, 22, 77, 81, 98, 144
  linear time invariant, 1, 19, 20, 22, 77
  nonlinear, 144
  real, 22
  response, 311, 607
  telephone, 581, 633, 634

Tan, C. H., 535
Tang, D. T., 555
Tap gain, ix, 587, 589, 605, 627, 629
  complex, 610
  nonlinear, 623
  optimal, 611, 613, 629
Tapped Delay Line (TDL), 564
Taylor, M. G., 630
Taylor series, 295, 298, 337, 412
Television, 633
Thomas, C. M., 114, 156, 378, 382, 436
Thomas, J. B., 340, 436
Tjeng, T., 216, 256
Tjhung, T., 204, 216, 256, 534
Tobin, E. M., 340
Tomlinson, M., 535, 555
Transfer function, 19, 20, 233, 584
  baseband equivalent, 88, 427
  lowpass equivalent, 234
  Nyquist, 353
  of bandpass filter, 28, 32
  of frequency selective fading channel, 427 428
  of system, 602
Transmitter, ix, 101, 102, 113, 259, 557, 561, 564–66, 569, 570, 572–575, 577, 578, 603
Transversal filter, ix, 564, 577, 581, 583, 585, 588, 589, 611, 621
taps of, 581, 607
Travelling Wave Tube (TWT), 236, 237, 382
Tronca, G. P., 257, 655
Tsang, Y., 326, 330, 341, 390, 436
Tufts, D. W., 339, 578, 579

Ungerboeck, G., 626, 632

Van Gerven P. J., 555
Venn diagram 39
Vestigial Side Band (VSB), 161. *See* ASK-VSB
Vitello, D., 247, 257
Viterbi, A. J., ix, 632
Viterbi
  algorithm, 628
  decoder, 537
  decoding, 625
Von Bayer, H. J., 256

Walzman, T., 655
Waveguide, 101, 422
Weidener, M. Y., 114, 156, 378, 382, 436
Weinstein, S. B., 156, 436, 469
Weldon, E. J., x, 534
Welsh, J. H., 340
Widrow, B., 630, 631
Wilson, S. G., 256
Wittke, P. H., 535
Wozencraft, J. M., ix, 536

Yao, K., 340
Yeh, Y. W., 339

Zador, P. L., 530

MIX
Papier aus verantwortungsvollen Quellen
Paper from responsible sources
FSC® C105338

If you have any concerns about our products,
you can contact us on
**ProductSafety@springernature.com**

In case Publisher is established outside the EU,
the EU authorized representative is:
**Springer Nature Customer Service Center GmbH**
**Europaplatz 3, 69115 Heidelberg, Germany**

Printed by Libri Plureos GmbH
in Hamburg, Germany